# The management of labour

**THIRD EDITION**

# The management of labour

**THIRD EDITION**

**Sir Sabaratnam Arulkumaran** PhD, FRCOG, FRCS
Professor and Head of Obstetrics and Gynecology
St George's University of London
London, United Kingdom

**Gita Arjun** FACOG
Director and Consultant Obstetrician and Gynecologist
EV Kalyani Medical Centre
Chennai, India

**Leonie K Penna** FRCOG
Consultant Obstetrician and Gynecologist
King's College Hospital
London, United Kingdom

Universities Press

**Universities Press (India) Private Limited**

*Registered Office*
3-6-747/1/A & 3-6-754/1, Himayatnagar, Hyderabad 500 029 (A.P.), India
email: info@universitiespress.com, www.universitiespress.com

*Distributed by*
Orient Blackswan Private Limited

*Registered Office*
3-6-752 Himayatnagar, Hyderabad 500 029 (A.P.), India

*Other Offices*
Bengaluru / Bhopal / Bhubaneshwar / Chandigarh / Chennai / Ernakulam / Guwahati
Hyderabad / Jaipur / Kolkata / Lucknow / Mumbai / New Delhi / Noida / Patna

© Universities Press (India) Private Limited 2011

First published by Orient Longman Private Limited 1996
Reprinted 1997 (twice), 2001 (twice), 2003
Second Edition 2005
Reprinted 2006
First Universities Press Impression 2008
Third edition 2011

*Cover and book design:*
© Universities Press (India) Private Limited 2011

ISBN 978 81 7371 746 8

All rights reserved. No part of the material may be reproduced or utilised in any form, or by any means, electronic or mechanical, including photocopying, recording, or by any information storage and retrieval system, without written permission from the publisher.

*Cover design*
OSDATA, Hyderabad 500 049

*Typeset in* Sabon LT Std 10.5/12.8 *by*
OSDATA, Hyderabad 500 049

*Printed in India by*   SS Colour Impression Pvt. Ltd., Chennai 600 106.

*Published by*
Universities Press (India) Private Limited
3-6-747/1/A & 3-6-754/1, Himayatnagar, Hyderabad 500 029 (A.P.), India

Care has been taken to confirm the accuracy of information presented in this book. The editors and the publisher, however, cannot accept any responsibility for errors or omissions or for consequences from application of the information in this book and make no warranty, express or implied, with respect to its contents.

# PREFACE TO THE THIRD EDITION

The woman in labour is the focus of every dedicated obstetrician. Being able to provide optimum care for the mother and the unborn child is the goal for which we all strive. The Third Edition of *The Management of Labour* arms the practising obstetrician with clear, evidence-based guidelines to provide such care.

The Millennium Development Goal 5 is to achieve 75 per cent reduction in maternal mortality by the year 2015. Recent reports suggest a decline in maternal deaths from 550,000 to 350,000 per year – a 1.5 per cent decline that is slower than the expected 6 per cent decline. To achieve this global goal, more reduction is needed in Sub-Saharan Africa and South Asia. This is particularly important in India, which has the largest number of births per year (27 million) in the world. With its high maternal mortality of about 300 to 500 per 100,000 births, about 75,000 to 150,000 maternal deaths occur every year in India.

Nearly 75 per cent of maternal deaths are during the intrapartum period or within the first 48 hours after delivery. For every woman who dies, there are 20 who have severe morbidity; mortality is merely the tip of the iceberg. Confidential enquiries into maternal deaths and morbidity reveal that 60 per cent to 80 per cent are avoidable, even in developed countries. Hence, it is imperative to provide the best care in labour.

Three to four million infant deaths are recorded each year during the antenatal period, during labour and immediately afterwards. A third are due to infection and another third due to birth asphyxia; many of these deaths could be avoided with good management of labour.

The authors of various chapters, and the editors, have produced the third edition of *The Management of Labour* to provide practitioners unambiguous practice guidelines to help them achieve the above goals.

Evidence-based knowledge, along with clear interpretation of current scientific evidence, is provided in this book to improve care for the woman in labour. The contributors and the editors, have scanned the literature and consulted evidence-based reviews, such as the Cochrane Database, and utilised guidelines from the National Institute of Clinical Excellence, the Royal College of Obstetricians and Gynaecologists from the UK, The American College of Obstetricians and Gynecologists and that of other National Societies in constructing these chapters. Evidence changes from time to time and the new edition of this book is brought out in a timely manner by the publishers to make the literature current and relevant.

Professionalism in a physician demands an implicit commitment and devotion to compassionate care. Care of the pregnant woman, especially when she is in labour, requires empathy, technical and communication skills. These must be learnt by apprenticeship under a learned and skilled mentor.

The publisher and editors are most grateful to the authors who have generously contributed to this book and thank the readers for using this book and applying the knowledge in practice. There are many more topics that could be included in such a text, but for the sake of brevity and practical considerations, we have distilled the essentials. There may be errors or controversies in management described in this book. We ask your help by writing to the publishers or editors with your comments, so that we can correct and enhance the chapters in the next reprint or edition.

Sir Sabaratnam Arulkumaran<br>
Gita Arjun<br>
Leonie Penna

# PREFACE TO THE FIRST EDITION

Passage through the birth canal is the shortest but possibly the most hazardous journey made by an individual in his or her life. Hypoxia, trauma and infection are inherent risks. The risks are increased if they are associated with preterm and postterm birth, prelabour rupture of the membranes or antepartum hemorrhage and when labour is induced as a consequence of medical or obstetric disorders in pregnancy. The mother faces problems of anxiety, pain, infection and if labour is prolonged, the possibility of operative delivery, trauma, postpartum hemorrhage and long-term morbidity. At times, she runs the risk of losing her life because of complications during childbirth. The women and babies who face these risks every day deserve care to the best of our ability. The art of intrapartum care has evolved and is evidence based. The knowledge of scientific principles should be available to everyone who provides care to the pregnant mother, a healthy baby and emotional satisfaction to those involved, including members of the family. These can be achieved by acquiring knowledge, skill and through compassionate team care with attention to details of the needs of the mother, the fetus and the process of labour.

This multi-author volume tries to achieve the goal of providing the knowledge of intrapartum management to the caregiver. It also covers closely related topics which may be of importance just prior to or just after the process of labour. Where possible, the book is adequately illustrated. The references cited in each chapter should prove especially useful as they provide recent knowledge in key areas of the field. As editors we have used our vast experience in the subject to fine tune each chapter. We hope that this book will serve the needs of many obstetricians, midwives and trainees who offer valuable care to the pregnant mother in labour.

S Arulkumaran
S S Ratnam
K Bhasker Rao

# LIST OF CONTRIBUTORS

**K Ambujam**
Additional Professor,
Government Medical College
Thrissur, India

**Amarnath Bhide**
Consultant, Department of
Obstetrics and Gynecology
Fetal Medicine Unit
St. George's Hospital,
London, United Kingdom

**Anita Dutta**
Guy's and St Thomas' NHS
Foundation Trust
London, United Kingdom

**T P Baskaran**
Maternal Fetal Medicine Unit
Department of Obstetrics and
Gynecology,
Hospital Kuala Lumpur
Malaysia

**Cleave Gass**
Consultant Anaesthetist
and Postgraduate Education
Director, St George's Hospital
London, United Kingdom

**Cruz Winston Justin**
Consultant in Obstetrics and
Gynecology,
Southend University Hospital,
Westcliff-on-Sea, United
Kingdom

**Daisy Nirmal**
Consultant Obstetrician and
Gynecologist
Norfolk & Norwich University
Hospital, NHS Trust, Norwich,
United Kingdom

**David I Fraser**
Consultant Obstetrician and
Gynecologist
Norfolk & Norwich University
Hospital
NHS Trust
Norwich, United Kingdom

**Dhiraj Uchil**
Specialist Registrar
Department of Obstetrics
and Gynecology
University Hospital
London, United Kingdom

**Duru Shah**
Chairman, Gynaecworld
Consultant Obstetrician and
Gynecologist
Breach Candy Hospital/
Jaslok Hospital/Sir H N
Hospital, Mumbai, India

**Edwin Chandraharan**
Consultant Obstetrician and
Gynecologist,
Lead Clinician-Labour Ward,
St. George's Healthcare
NHS Trust
London, United Kingdom

**Evita Fernandez**
Managing Director and
Consultant Obstetrician
Fernandez Hospital for
Women and the Newborn
Hyderabad, India

**Gita Arjun**
Director and Consultant
Obstetrician and Gynecologist
EV Kalyani Medical Centre
Chennai, India

**Humera Bukhari**
Honorary Clinical Fellow
St. George's Healthcare
NHS Trust,
London, United Kingdom

**Lakshmi Seshadri**
Professor, Department of
Obstetrics and Gynecology
Christian Medical College
Hospital, Vellore, India

**Leonie K Penna**
Clinical Director,
Womens' Services and
Consultant Obstetrician/Lead
for the Labour Ward,
King's College Hospital
London, United Kingdom

**W C Maina**
Staff Grade, Obstetrics and
Gynecology
Consultant Obstetrician and
Gynecologist
Norfolk and Norwich
University Hospital NHS Trust,
Norwich, United Kingdom

**Melina Georgiou**
Specialist Registrar/Clinical
Fellow in Obstetrics and
Gynecology
Kings College Hospital
London, United Kingdom

**Michael Stephen Robson**
Consultant Obstetrician and
Gynecologist and
Master of the Department of
Obstetrics and Gynecology,
The National Maternity Hospital
Dublin, Republic of Ireland

**Mirudhubashini Govindarajan**
Director, Women's Center and Hospital, Coimbatore, India

**Muralidhar V Pai**
Professor and Unit Head,
Department of Obstetrics and Gynecology
Kasturba Medical College,
Manipal, India

**Nigel Kennea**
Consultant Neonatologist
St George's Healthcare Trust
London, United Kingdom

**Nuzhat Aziz**
Consultant Obstetrician,
Head of the Department,
Obstetrics
Fernandez Hospital for Women and the Newborn
Hyderabad, India

**V P Paily**
Professsor Jubilee Mission Medical College,
Consultant, Mother Hospital and Raji Nursing Home,
Thrissur, India

**Pankaj Desai**
Chief of Unit in Ob-gyn (VRS)
Medical College and SSG Hospital
Baroda, India

**Purvi Patel**
Assistant Professor
Department of Obstetrics and Gynecology, Medical College and S.S.G. Hospital
Baroda, India

**Pranathi Reddy**
Consultant Obstetrician and Urogynecologist
Clinical Director
Maternal–Fetal Medicine
Rainbow Hospital for Women and Children
Hyderabad, India

**S Rajasri**
Consultant Obstetrician and Gynecologist, EV Kalyani Medical Centre Chennai, India

**Rehana Iqbal**
Consultant Anesthetist
St George's Hospital
London, United Kingdom

**Rohan D'Souza**
Clinical Fellow
Fetal Medicine Unit
St. George's Hospital
London, United Kingdom

**Sabaratnam Arulkumaran**
Professor and Head of Obstetrics and Gynecology
St George's University of London
London, United Kingdom

**Sambit Mukhopadhyay**
Consultant Obstetrician and Gynecologist
Norfolk and Norwich
University Hospital NHS Trust
Norwich, United Kingdom

**K N Sreelakshmi**
Assistant Professor, Department of Obstetrics and Gynecology
Kasturba Medical College
Manipal, India

**Shobhana Mahadevan**
Consultant Obstetrician and Gynecologist
Seethapathy Clinic and Hospital
Chennai, India

**Soumya Balakrishnan**
Consultant Obstetrician and Gynecologist
E V Kalyani Medical Centre
Chennai, India

**Sudeshna Ray**
Diploma (Gynec Endoscopy)
Consultant Obstetrician and Gynecologist

Jaslok Hospital and Research Centre, Mumbai, India

**Sunil T Pandya**
Director, Prerna Anaesthesia and Critical Care Services
Head, Department of Anesthesia, Pain and Critical Care, Fernandez Hospital
Hyderabad, India

**Surabhi Nanda**
Research Fellow in Fetal Medicine
Harris Birthright Research Centre for Fetal Medicine,
King's College Hospital,
London, United Kingdom

**Ted Gasiorowski**
Specialist Registrar and Clinical Fellow in Neonatal Pediatrics
St George's Hospital
London, United Kingdom

**Terence Lao**
Associate Professor
Chinese University of Hong Kong, The New Territory
Hong Kong

**Tulika Singh**
Consultant in Obstetrics and Gynecology
Newham University Hospital,
London, United Kingdom

**Uma Ram**
Consultant Obstetrician and Gynecologist, Seethapathy Clinic and Hospital, Chennai, India

**Vinotha Thomas**
Registrar in Obstetrics and Gynecology, EV Kalyani Medical Centre, Chennai, India

**Vivek Nama**
Specialist Registrar, Obstetrics and Gynecology, St. George's Hospital, London, United Kingdom

# CONTENTS

1. Physiopharmacology of labour
   *Humera Bukhari and Edwin Chandraharan* — 1
2. The Management of the first stage of labour
   *Daisy Nirmal, David I Fraser and Sambit Mukhopadhyay* — 30
3. Pain relief in labour
   *Sunil T Pandya* — 56
4. Consent in labour
   *Cleave Gass and Rehana Iqbal* — 77
5. Intrapartum fetal monitoring
   *Rohan D'Souza and Sabaratnam Arulkumaran* — 85
6. Uterine contractions
   *Rohan D'Souza, Vivek Nama and Sabaratnam Arulkumaran* — 112
7. The management of intrapartum fetal distress
   *Rohan D'Souza and Sabaratnam Arulkumaran* — 126
8. Fluid management in labour
   *W C Maina, David I Fraser and Sambit Mukhopadhyay* — 138
9. Management of second stage of labour
   *Pankaj Desai and Purvi Patel* — 152
10. Operative vaginal delivery
    *Cruz Winston Justin and Tulika Singh* — 170
11. Shoulder dystocia
    *VP Paily and K Ambujam* — 188
12. Episiotomy
    *Terence Lao* — 205
13. Breech delivery
    *Lakshmi Seshadri* — 215
14. Strategies to reduce the rate of cesarean section
    *Michael Stephen Robson* — 237
15. Cesarean section: procedure and technique
    *Gita Arjun, S Rajasri, Soumya Balakrishnan and Vinotha Thomas* — 248
16. Vaginal birth after cesarean delivery
    *Pranathi Reddy* — 266

| | | |
|---|---|---|
| 17. | Antepartum hemorrhage<br>*Amarnath Bhide* | 277 |
| 18. | The third stage of labour<br>*Melina Georgiou and Leonie K Penna* | 289 |
| 19. | Management of postpartum hemorrhage<br>*Gita Arjun, S Rajasri, Soumya Balakrishnan and Vinotha Thomas* | 303 |
| 20. | Postpartum collapse<br>*Surabhi Nanda and Leonie K Penna* | 319 |
| 21. | The management of obstetric perineal trauma<br>*Terence Lao* | 348 |
| 22. | Prostaglandins in labour<br>*Uma Ram and Shobana Mahadevan* | 355 |
| 23. | Induction of labour<br>*Duru Shah and Sudeshna Ray* | 368 |
| 24. | Prelabour rupture of membranes<br>*Mirudhubashini Govindarajan* | 387 |
| 25. | Preterm labour and delivery– management issues<br>*T P Baskaran* | 402 |
| 26. | Prolonged pregnancy<br>*Amarnath Bhide* | 420 |
| 27. | Prolonged and obstructed labour<br>*Pankaj Desai and Purvi Patel* | 429 |
| 28. | Peripartum hysterectomy<br>*Anita Dutta and Edwin Chandraharan* | 444 |
| 29. | Rupture uterus<br>*Muralidhar V Pai and K N Sreelakshmi* | 453 |
| 30. | Management of severe preeclampsia and eclampsia<br>*Evita Fernandez and Nuzhat Aziz* | 463 |
| 31. | Neonatal resuscitation and the management of immediate neonatal problems<br>*Ted Gasiorowski and Nigel Kennea* | 486 |
| 32. | Complications of the puerperium<br>*Dhiraj Uchil* | 495 |
| | *Index* | 515 |

# CHAPTER 1

# PHYSIOPHARMACOLOGY OF LABOUR

*Humera Bukhari and Edwin Chandraharan*

Human labour is a complex process and is characterised by the onset of effective uterine contractions leading to progressive effacement and dilatation of the cervix, resulting in the expulsion of the fetus, placenta and the membranes. The complexity of human parturition is exemplified by the term 'labour', which has been coined in recognition of the hard work that the parturient as well as the uterine myometrium have to perform in order to deliver the fetus.

Understanding the physiopharmacology of labour may help clinicians to manage this process more efficiently and thereby potentially modify this process when required, by the use of pharmacological agents to stimulate or inhibit labour. Unlike parturition in animals, most notably sheep, the exact physiology of labour in humans has not been fully understood. It appears that human parturition is not preceded by sudden and dramatic changes in the maternal concentrations of estradiol and progesterone, as seen in sheep. Moreover, fetal cortisol, which plays a major role in ovine parturition, neither peaks before labour nor affects the placental endocrine function in humans. Hence, it is unlikely to play a predominant role in human labour.

At the molecular level, the formation of gap junctions between the myometrial cells, to make them function as an efficient 'functional syncytium' increase prior to established uterine contractions. There is also an increase in the concentration of oxytocin receptors in the myometrium, making the latter more sensitive to oxytocin. In addition, increased prostaglandin synthesis by the membranes and the decidua is considered to play a vital role. The period during which these molecular events are initiated is often termed 'prelabour'. It is characterised by both cervical ripening and myometrial excitement, which finally culminate in labour. Estrogen, progesterone, oxytocin, prostaglandins, relaxin, second messengers, corticosteroids, calcium and sympathetic amines (Roy et al 1984; Roy and Arulkumaran 1991) are all thought to play a role in human labour (Table 1.1).

> 'Prelabour' is characterised by both cervical ripening and myometrial excitement, which finally culminate in labour.

## The Myometrium and the Cervix

It is important to appreciate that although the uterine myometrium and the cervix are part of the same uterus, they are different in terms of histology and function. The myometrium is mainly composed of bundles of interlacing smooth muscle fibres with sparse connective tissue, whereas the cervix is predominantly composed of fibrous tissue. This distinct histologic framework helps them to perform two opposing functions during pregnancy and labour. During pregnancy, the myometrium has to remain relaxed and progressively distend to allow the growth and functional maturity of the fetus in utero. The cervix on the other hand has to act as a firm 'door' to guard and to protect the uterine contents, until the time is ripe for their expulsion.

> The distinct histological difference between the myometrium and the cervix helps them to perform two opposing functions during pregnancy and labour.

During prelabour, the excitability of the myometrium increases, as it prepares to expel the uterine contents (fetus, placenta and membranes). The cervix ripens (becomes soft and stretchable), so that it may loosen and yield to pressure from above, allowing the products to pass through without difficulty. Finally, during labour, there are efficient, strong and progressive myometrial contractions associated with progressive dilatation and effacement of the cervix, resulting in the descent of the presenting part. Hence, there is considerable synergy between the myometrium and the cervix. Any deviation in the above process could result in preterm labour, uterine inertia and cervical dystocia, which may contribute to increased maternal and fetal morbidity and mortality.

## The myometrium and its gap junctions

The myometrium is essentially composed of smooth muscle cells arranged in longitudinal, transverse and oblique directions as well as in a criss-cross manner with intervening blood vessels. This arrangement is often referred to as 'living ligatures' and is the main mechanism in the control of postpartum hemorrhage. Under the influence of the placental sex steroids, the myometrium undergoes remarkable growth, both by hyperplasia and hypertrophy during pregnancy. Its weight increases by about 15-fold and intrauterine volume increases about 1000-fold. The smooth

> The arrangement of the myometrial cells around the blood vessels is often referred to as 'living ligatures' and is the main mechanism in the control of postpartum hemorrhage.

**Table 1.1** Factors associated with the onset of labour

| |
|---|
| **Mother** |
| Sex steroids (estrogens and progesterone) |
| Prostaglandins |
| Peptides |
| Oxytocin |
| Relaxin |
| VIP/Prolactin/CRH |
| ? Autonomic nervous system |
| Cervical ripening (effacement and dilatation) |
| Inflammatory mediators and cytokines/interleukins |
| Myometrial contractility |
| **Fetus** |
| VIP: Vasoactive intestinal polypeptides |
| CRH: Corticotropin releasing hormone |

muscle cells are embedded in an extracellular matrix composed mainly of collagen fibres (Huszar and Walsh 1989).

Electron microscopy has shown that plasma membranes from the two opposing cells have intermembranous protein particles (called 'connexins'), protruding through each membrane and spanning the gap between the membranes (Fig 1.1). These are called 'gap junctions' and are believed to represent low resistance pathways to the flow of excitation. They allow communication between adjacent cells, which may be electrical or metabolic or both, and also allow the passage of inorganic ions and small molecules (Cole and Garfield 1986). Electrical signals (e.g. action potentials) can be rapidly transmitted to all neighbouring myometrial cells, leading to efficient contraction as a functional syncytium. It has been recognised that the development of these gap junctions is one of the earliest changes occurring during the process of prelabour. Several animal studies have shown that myometrial gap junctions begin to increase before term and their number becomes significantly higher during labour and falls rapidly in the postpartum period (Garfield and Hayashi 1980; Saito et al 1985). This implies that during the 'preparatory phase', the excitability of the myometrium as well as its capacity to contract in a coordinated manner, increase.

> 'Gap junctions' allow rapid transmission of electrical signals to all neighbouring myometrial cells, leading to efficient contraction. Development of these gap junctions is one of the earliest changes occurring during the process of prelabour.

It has also been shown that estrogen and prostaglandins induce the formation of gap junctions, while progesterone inhibits it (Garfield and Hayashi 1980). The permeability of gap junctions to various substances appears to be regulated by both calcium ions and cyclic adenosine monophosphate (cAMP) (Cole and Garfield 1986, 1988; Garfield et al 1987). Research has revealed that in humans, the number of gap junctions present was found to be higher in both term and preterm labour in the presence of good uterine contractions. They were few in number in women with infrequent uterine contractions and were absent in non-pregnant women (Garfield and Hayashi 1980, 1981; Balducci et al 1992). Also, the levels of mRNA (messenger RNA) coding for the gap junction protein 'connexin-43', were elevated in the human myometrium towards term and with the onset of labour (Chow and Lye 1994). It is believed that oxytocin does not have the ability to induce the formation of gap junctions and cannot stimulate the myometrium in the absence of gap junctions.

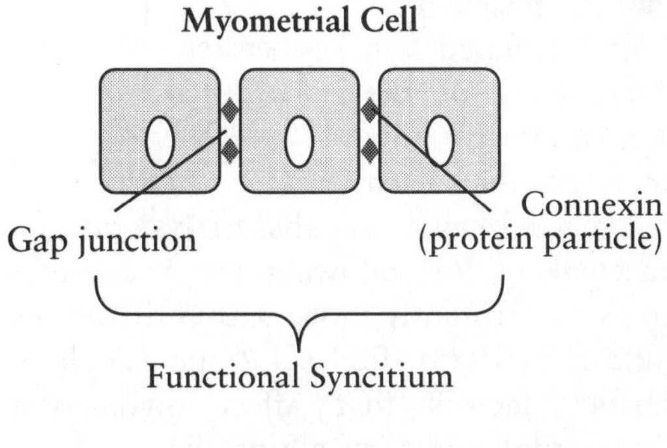

**Figure 1.1** Myometrial cells and gap junctions

## Regulation of Uterine Contractility

The uterine musculature has the property of retraction, which refers to the partial shortening of muscle fibres which have been in a state of contraction. This property keeps the individual myometrial cell from going back to its original muscle fibre length at the end of each contraction and hence, helps in the expulsion of the fetus.

The myometrium is rich in smooth muscle cells arranged in bundles in all directions and is embedded in a connective tissue stroma, which predominantly consists of collagen. This arrangement aids in the transmission of the tension generated during contractions uniformly throughout the tissue. The fundamental process involved in the myometrial contractions is actin–myosin interaction, which is similar to that seen in other smooth muscles (Huszar and Walsh 1989). Myosin is the principal protein of muscle contraction and the process is dependent on calcium. Entry of calcium ions into the myometrial cells initiates a cascade of events, culminating in myometrial contraction. Initially, the intracellular calcium interacts with calmodulin to activate myosin light chain kinase, which in turn phosphorylates the light chains of myosin. This leads to the exposure of the actin–myosin binding sites and the phosphorylated myosin interacts with actin to bring about a contraction (Fig 1.2). Hence, myometrial contraction is an active process requiring energy in the form of adenosine triphosphate (ATP).

During relaxation, calcium ions are pumped back into the sarcoplasmic reticulum, which again is an energy requiring process. A fall in calcium ions leads to dephosphorylation of myosin chains and a return to the resting state. However, unlike the other smooth muscles, the myometrium is not richly innervated (Garfield et al 1987). Therefore, neural activity does not appear to be a prerequisite for myometrial contractions. Endocrinological and biochemical signals play a vital role in initiating and maintaining uterine contractions. It is indeed noteworthy that despite the lack of significant neural activity, myometrial contractions are usually well coordinated during labour. Gap junctions play a vital role in this process of coordination by allowing both metabolic and electrophysiologic communications between the cells.

To initiate spontaneous electrical activity, it is necessary for some cells to have a lower resting membrane potential than others. These are called pacemaker cells. In the human uterus, there appears to be no constant pacemaker area (Wolfs and Van Leewan 1979), which is contrary to the previous belief that pacemakers were situated in the cornua of the uterus. It is now accepted that each myometrial cell is capable of becoming a pacemaker, thus allowing the pacemaker areas to constantly move within the uterus (Osa et al 1983). Tables 1.2 and 1.3 show various factors that affect myometrial contractility and cervical ripening.

> There appears to be no constant pacemaker area in the human uterus. Each myometrial cell is capable of becoming a pacemaker, thus allowing the pacemaker areas to constantly move within the uterus.

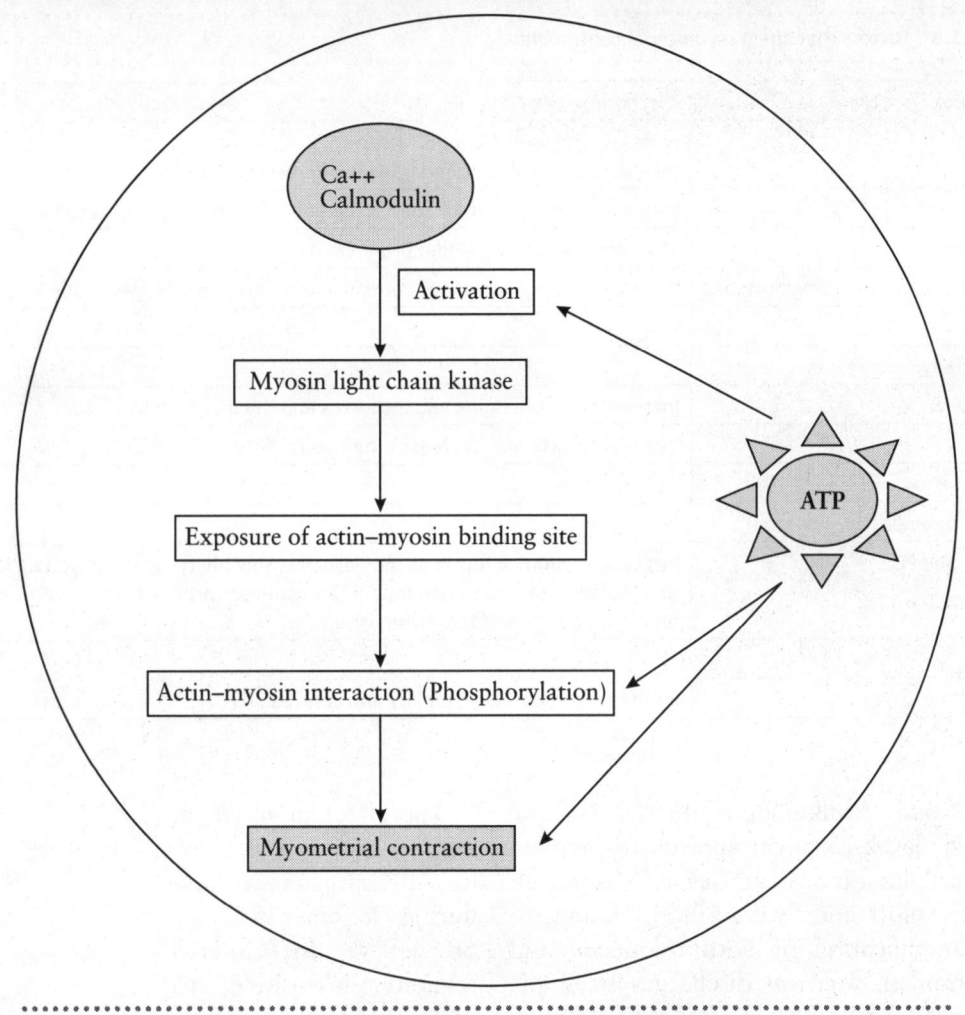

## Figure 1.2 Basic physiology of muscle contraction

Ca++ Calmodulin → Activation → Myosin light chain kinase → Exposure of actin–myosin binding site → Actin–myosin interaction (Phosphorylation) → Myometrial contraction

ATP

**Table 1.2** Changes occurring in the cervix and the myometrium

|  | Cervix | Myometrium |
|---|---|---|
| Pre-pregnancy/ early pregnancy | Firm | Quiescent |
| Pre-labour | Ripening | Excitable |
| Labour | Effacement and dilatation | Contraction and retraction |

# Role of Peptide Hormones
## Oxytocin

Oxytocin was found to induce contractions in a previously sensitised uterus. It also increases the force and frequency of contractions in an already contracting uterus (Fuchs et al 1981). It has been used traditionally for the induction and augmentation of labour

**Table 1.3** Factors that affect myometrial contractility

| Hormone/Factor | Mechanism of action |
| --- | --- |
| Oxytocin | Increases intracellular ionic calcium |
|  | Increases the synthesis and release of prostaglandins |
| Vasopressin | Increases the myometrial contractility by acting through its receptors |
| Relaxin | May increase prostaglandin production during labour |
| Corticotropin-releasing hormone | Increases the production of cortisol and may reduce 'progesterone block' |
| Adrenergic nerves |  |
| Alpha-1 | Increases calcium influx and increases and the contractility |
| Beta-2 | Increases cAMP and decreases the contractility |
| Prostaglandins |  |
| $PGE_2$ and $PGF_2\alpha$ | Increase calcium influx and increase the sensitivity of the myometrium to circulating oxytocin, resulting in an increase in both tonic tension and phasic contraction of the myometrium. |
| $PGI_2$ | Inhibits myometrial excitability and contractility |

(Roy and Arulkumaran 1991). At the cellular level, oxytocin appears to increase intracellular ionic calcium levels (Mironneau 1976; Soloff and Sweet 1982), leading to the amplification of both frequency and duration of electrical discharges from the myometrial cells. This effect is believed to be brought about by two specific mechanisms. First, the influx of calcium ions through specific agonist-operated ion channels, and second, the release of intracellular calcium ions from the sarcoplasmic reticulum, which is mediated by the second messenger, inositol triphosphate (IP3) (Schrey et al 1986, 1988) (Fig. 1.3).

Oxytocin also promotes the synthesis and release of prostaglandins ($PGE_2$ and $PGF_2\alpha$) from the uterine decidua that results in myometrial contractility (Fuchs et al 1984).

The effect of oxytocin on the uterus is marked in late pregnancy and during labour. In early pregnancy, the uterus remains insensitive to oxytocin even when large doses of it are administered. It is believed that the development of oxytocin receptors in the myometrium commences around the twentieth week of gestation. Thereafter, it remains unchanged until the onset of labour.

Contrary to earlier belief, it has been shown that there is no dramatic increase in the plasma concentration of oxytocin during late pregnancy or during the first and second

> Oxytocin also promotes the synthesis and release of prostaglandins ($PGE_2$ and $PGF_2\alpha$) from the uterine decidua that results in myometrial contractility.

stages in labour (Thornton et al 1988). There is no evidence to suggest that the levels of oxytocin are low in women with uterine inertia or incoordinate uterine action (Thornton et al 1992). Initially, these findings were quite unpalatable due to the widely held belief that oxytocin levels increased during labour. However, evidence suggests that though there was no absolute increase in the levels of oxytocin per se, the sensitivity of the myometrium to the circulating oxytocin increases with advancing gestation and peaks at parturition (Fuchs et al 1981).

> Sensitivity of the myometrium to the circulating oxytocin increases with advancing gestation and peaks at parturition.

A possible mechanism that is postulated for this increased myometrial sensitivity

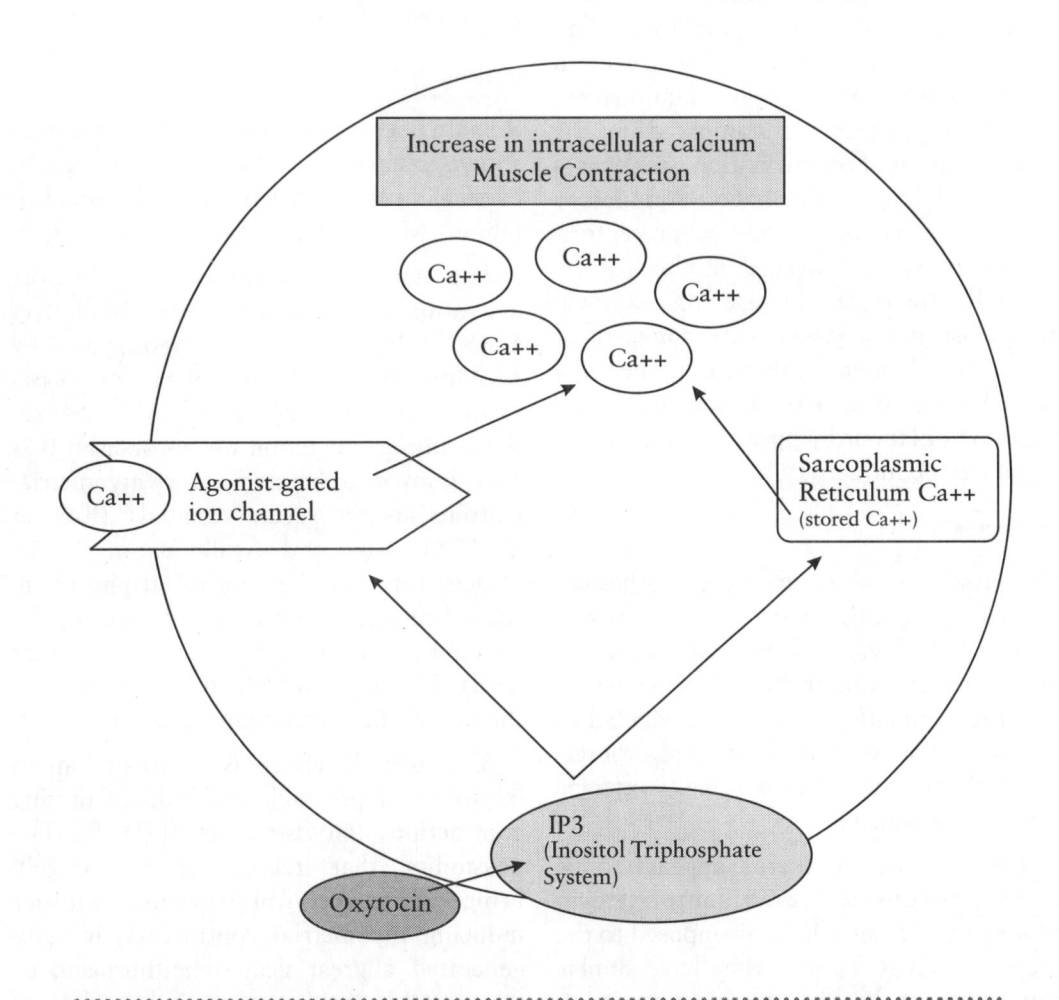

**Figure 1.3** Mechanism of action of oxytocin on the myometrial cell

to oxytocin is the lowering of the resting membrane potential in the myometrial cells towards term (Kao 1977). There are several factors that are believed to regulate the development of oxytocin receptors in the myometrium. These include estrogens that stimulate and progesterone that suppresses their development (Alexandrova and Soloff, 1980). It is not yet clear whether prostaglandins have any direct effect on the development of oxytocin receptors.

However, if one considers the clinical scenario whereby the amplitude and duration of uterine contractions are often higher when oxytocin is administered after prostaglandins as compared to the administration of oxytocin alone, it appears that prostaglandins may have a stimulatory effect on the synthesis of oxytocin receptors. Further research is needed in this regard. Recently, the effective use of oxytocin antagonists like atosiban in the management of preterm labour, further strengthen the view that oxytocin plays a vital role in the initiation of labour by positively influencing myometrial contractility.

### Vasopressin

Vasopressin is an octapeptide synthesised by the paraventricular and supraoptic nuclei of the hypothalamus and stored in the posterior pituitary gland. Due to its structural similarity to oxytocin, which also has similar sites of synthesis and storage, vasopressin has considerable oxytocic activities in humans.

The nonpregnant uterus appears to be more sensitive to vasopressin than to oxytocin (Embrey and Moir 1967), as opposed to the pregnant uterus. Though they have similar actions, oxytocin and vasopressin act on two different receptors (Guillon et al 1987). As described previously, the sensitivity of the myometrium to circulating oxytocin increases with advancing gestation and reaches its peak in labour. This is mainly due to an increase in the concentration of oxytocin receptors. In contrast, the density of vasopressin receptors peaks at 32 weeks of gestation (Fuchs et al 1984; Maggi et al 1990). It is not clear whether this finding has any practical significance. Further research is needed to find out whether vasopressin plays a role in the initiation or progression of preterm labour.

### Relaxin

Relaxin is a peptide hormone which has been shown to have some effect on the process of cervical ripening that precedes the onset of labour (MacLennan 1986).

Its main action appears to be the activation of collagenases (Von Malliot et al 1977). It has been well demonstrated by McMurty et al (1980) that human fibroblasts exhibit relaxin receptors and that relaxin has a mitogenic action on fibroblasts. It is also known to decrease the myometrial contractility in several animals (Roy et al 1984; Roy and Arulkumaran 1991). It acts through the inositol triphosphate second-messenger system, by decreasing the availability of intracellular ionic calcium levels. This in turn leads to a reduction of the myosin light chain kinase activity.

The overall effect is a reduction in oxytocin- or prostaglandin-induced uterine contractions (Goldsmith et al 1989). The possibility that relaxin can selectively bring about cervical ripening without inducing myometrial contraction, initially generated a great deal of enthusiasm, as this would enable us to induce labour without inappropriately stimulating the uterus in early labour. Subsequently, human recombinant relaxin in the form of a gel was made available and was subjected to various clinical trials. The results so far have been quite disappointing. Relaxin did not have any significant effect on the cervical score or the outcome of labour (Bell et al 1993). However, issues like optimum dosage and ideal route of administration need to be addressed by future research. It is believed that relaxin has a paracrine effect on amnion-inhibiting prostaglandin (PGE$_2$) production during pregnancy, facilitating its production during spontaneous labour. Some studies have shown that the vaginal application of purified porcine relaxin may facilitate cervical ripening, and hence, induction of labour (MacLennan et al 1980). In rats, relaxin infusions inhibit the secretion of oxytocin during labour and lactation (Jones and Summerlee 1986; O'Bryne et al 1986). However in humans, such an effect has not been demonstrated. Conversely, oxytocin infusions during pregnancies at term have not been found to have any effect on circulating relaxin concentrations (Hochman et al 1978). However, administration of prostaglandins (PGE$_2$) for the induction of second trimester abortion has been shown to increase the circulating levels of relaxin (Seki et al 1987).

It appears that relaxin does have a role in human parturition. The important question is whether it is essential for the onset of spontaneous or induced labour. It is well known that women with premature ovarian failure do not have any functional ovarian tissue, and hence, no relaxin in their circulation (Johnson et al 1991). Due to recent advances in assisted conception techniques, these women may become pregnant. Eddie et al (1990) have reported that the spontaneous onset of labour in women with premature ovarian failure is associated with successful cervical dilatation, though at a slower rate. Hence, it appears that unlike in rats, relaxin plays a facilitatory role in human labour and is not absolutely essential for its onset or progress.

## Other Peptides and Hormones

### Vasoactive intestinal peptide

Vasoactive intestinal polypeptide (VIP) is a neurotransmitter that is widely distributed in the gastrointestinal tract. It inhibits the contraction of smooth muscles and has vasodilatory properties opposing the actions of the cholinergic neurotransmitter, acetylcholine. More than twenty years ago, it was demonstrated that the nerves supplying the smooth muscles and the blood vessels in the uterine myometrium release VIP (Larsson et al 1977; Ottensen et al 1980). Further, it was found to dilate the blood vessels and inhibit uterine contractions in a dose-dependent manner (Ottensen et al 1980; Clarke et al 1981). The role of VIP on human parturition is not yet fully defined.

### Prolactin

Prolactin is a glycoprotein secreted by the anterior pituitary gland and it plays an important role in lactation. During pregnancy, prolactin levels do increase but it does not appear to have any systemic effects in humans. In animals, it has been found to influence maternal behaviour after birth. However, it is believed to play a paracrine

> Relaxin plays a facilitatory role in human labour and is not absolutely essential for its onset or progress.

role in human parturition, though the exact mechanism is largely unknown. It has been positively localised in the amnion as well as in the decidua (Bryant-Greenwood et al 1987).

It has been suggested that cervical prolactin could be used in the prediction of preterm delivery (O'Brien et al 1994). Subsequent studies have questioned this and found cervical ß-hCG to be more predictive of preterm delivery than cervical prolactin (Guvenal et al 2001).

**Corticotropin-releasing hormone (CRH)**

Corticotropin-releasing hormone (CRH) has been shown to increase the contractile response of the myometrium to circulating oxytocin (Quartero et al 1992), as well as the oxytocin induced prostaglandin production from the fetal membranes and placenta in in-vitro studies (Jones and Challis 1989). It is also well known that the hypothalamo–pituitary–adrenal axis plays a fundamental role in parturition in sheep, but it is believed to play a less important role in human parturition. However, maternal plasma levels of CRH increase exponentially during the second half of pregnancy, peaking at delivery. Also, high concentration of CRH has been detected in the umbilical cord plasma and amniotic fluid at term (Campbell et al 1987; Sasaki et al 1987; Goland et al 1986). Further, Laatikannen et al (1988) have shown that CRH levels do increase in the amniotic fluid in the third trimester. All these data suggest that CRH may be important for human parturition as well. In preterm labour, elevated levels of CRH have been reported (Frim et al 1988).

The source of this increased CRH appears to be the placenta and not the maternal or fetal hypothalamus. Genetic studies have elucidated the mRNA for CRH in the placental cells and the concentration of this mRNA parallels the increase in the plasma corticotropin-releasing hormone (Frim et al 1988). Also, umbilical venous plasma has a higher concentration of CRH compared to umbilical arterial plasma, suggesting that it is the placenta and not the fetus that is the major site of production (Goland et al 1986). Subsequently, Jones et al (1989) demonstrated that CRH level is higher in spontaneous labour than after an elective cesarean section and that stress acting through corticosteroids enhances its production.

Progesterone was found to inhibit it. There is consensus now that CRH does not have any direct effect on the myometrium. However, in vitro studies have shown that it enhances both the oxytocin induced prostaglandin production in the fetal membranes and the placenta as well as the contractile response of the myometrium to oxytocin itself (Jones et al 1989; Quartero et al 1992).

In human parturition, so far there has been no evidence to suggest that the fetal hypothalamo–pituitary–adrenal axis plays a direct role in the initiation or progression of labour. Extensive research has shown that the affinity of the myometrial receptors to circulating CRH increases dramatically at term (Hillhouse et al 1993). Moreover, as the pregnancy advances, the concentration of corticotropin-binding globulin (CBG), which is responsible for limiting the biological activity of CRH, falls. In practical terms, both these changes would result in an increase in the sensitivity of the myometrium to CRH and an increase in the levels of biologically active, free CRH levels, respectively. Evidence is also accumulating to suggest that CRH may stimulate the fetal hypothalamo–pituitary–adrenal axis, leading to an enhanced production of fetal cortisol (Riley and Challis 1991). This may cause a reduction in the synthesis of progesterone by the feto-placental unit and may serve to remove the 'progesterone block'. This is an exciting concept, which needs to be explored by further research.

## Role of the Autonomic Nervous System

The human uterus has a rich supply of both the adrenergic and cholinergic nerve fibres. Despite this, it appears that the autonomic nervous system does not play a major role in the initiation or progression of myometrial contractions.

### Adrenergic stimulation

Both alpha and beta adrenoceptors have been demonstrated in the human myometrium and stimulation of these receptors result, respectively, in myometrial contraction and relaxation (Roy and Arulkumaran 1991). Sex steroids modify the effects. Estrogen causes a reduction in the myometrial sensitivity to beta-agonist induced relaxation, making the myometrium more excitable. This effect is antagonised by progesterone.

The adrenergic system is composed of four receptors. These are alpha-1, alpha-2, beta-1 and beta-2. Both alpha and beta receptors act through second-messenger systems via G proteins (or GTP binding proteins) in the cell membrane. Stimulation of beta-1 and beta-2 receptors increases the intracellular cyclic adenosine monophosphate (cAMP) by the activation of the enzyme, adenyl cyclase. This enzyme converts adenosine triphosphate (ATP) to cAMP, which is responsible for a variety of intracellular events including phosphorylation reactions. Stimulation of alpha-2 receptor has an exactly opposite action and inhibits the production of cAMP. Alpha-1 receptors mediate their actions through a different second messenger, the inositol triphosphate system (IP3), and when stimulated, alter the intracellular ionic calcium levels.

In the light of our knowledge that the autonomic nervous system appears non-essential for human parturition, it is not surprising that studies so far have resulted in conflicting reports. A decrease in the beta-adrenoceptor activity (Litime et al 1989) as well as 'no change' in the concentration of beta-receptors (Dattel et al 1986) have been reported. Despite this ambiguity, beta-agonists are still being used in the management of preterm labour as they have been found to decrease the proportion of women delivering within 48 hours of the commencement of therapy.

Spatling et al (1989) have reported that continuous infusion of beta-agonists results in the down-regulation of their receptors and that the pulsatile administration may be more effective. This may partly explain why there is a wide variation in their clinical efficacy. Also, the number of alpha- and beta-receptors and hence their ratio in the uterine myometrium at various gestations is different. Therefore, women with predominant beta-adrenoceptor dominance are more likely to respond to tocolytic therapy with beta-agonists compared to those with alpha-adrenoceptor dominance. In vitro studies by Story et al (1989) showed that the administration of adrenaline and high concentration of isoproterenol (both of which are nonspecific adrenergic stimulants) caused excitable effects on human myometrial tissue at term, whereas forskolin, which directly activates adenyl cyclase (hence, the synthesis of cAMP) causes myometrial relaxation. This study further strengthens the postulate that the differential receptor concentrations on the myometrium are responsible for the inconsistent clinical effects of beta-sympathomimetics.

## Cholinergic system

The uterine myometrium being a smooth muscle, shows a typical contractile response to acetylcholine, which is the main neurotransmitter in the cholinergic system. Levels of acetylcholine remain unchanged during pregnancy and labour.

This is in contrast to the adrenergic neurotransmitters, which show a progressive reduction throughout the pregnancy. Although intravenous acetylcholine induces labour at term very effectively, its systemic side effects make it unacceptable for induction of labour.

## Role of Prostaglandins

Ever since their discovery, prostaglandins have been implicated in a wide variety of body functions. Prostaglandin F2-alpha (PGF$_2\alpha$) has a predominant effect on the uterine myometrium, whereas prostaglandins E2 and I2 (PGE$_2$, PGI$_2$) have their main effect on the cervix.

Prostaglandins F and E types have been used to induce myometrial contractions of the human pregnant uterus, both in vivo and in vitro. Unlike oxytocin which is ineffective in causing myometrial contractions in early pregnancy, prostaglandins are capable of inducing myometrial contractions at all gestational ages. Contrary to the early refractoriness and subsequent increase in the sensitivity of the myometrium to circulating oxytocin during the second half of pregnancy, no such refractory period exists for prostaglandins. Hence, they are widely used in the termination of pregnancy at all gestational ages. Conversely, human parturition can be delayed to some extent by the administration of antiprostaglandins such as indomethacin (Creasy 1990). This knowledge has been employed in the management of preterm labour to inhibit uterine contractions.

> Unlike oxytocin, the myometrium is sensitive to prostaglandins throughout pregnancy. Hence, they are widely used in the termination of pregnancy at all gestational ages.

Evidence so far has been overwhelming to indicate that prostaglandins are the 'final common pathway' in the onset and progression of human parturition. During the course of spontaneous labour, both prostaglandins (Hillier et al 1974; Keirse 1979) and their metabolites (Mitchel et al 1978; Brennecke et al 1985; Johnston et al 1993) have been found to increase in the peripheral circulation.

> Prostaglandins are the 'final common pathway' in the onset and progression of human parturition.

There is also a differential response according to the type of prostaglandins.

PGE$_2$ metabolites peak prior to the onset of established labour, whereas PGF$_2\alpha$ metabolites peak during labour and correlate directly with the duration of labour (Johnston et al 1993). In dysfunctional labour, this increase in the PGF$_2\alpha$ metabolites does not occur, indicating that it plays an important role in uterine contractility in labour. As we have mentioned before, PGE$_2$ has a predominant effect on the cervix, whereas PGF$_2\alpha$ has an effect on the myometrium. The biochemical detection of metabolites of PGE$_2$ before PGF$_2\alpha$ fits well into the clinical picture, where cervical ripening occurs prior to the onset of uterine contractions. Indeed, plasma concentrations of PGE$_2$ metabolites correlate well with the cervical score. Further, Greer et al (1990) have shown that following the administration of PGE$_2$ for induction of labour, there is an associated increase in the production of PGF$_2\alpha$ as well. This increase coincides with the onset of uterine contractions.

Like for oxytocin, the sensitivity of the myometrium to prostaglandins increases at term due to an increase in the number of myometrial receptors (Hertelendy and Molnar 1990). Both PGE$_2$ and PGF$_2\alpha$ can increase the sensitivity of the myometrium to circulating oxytocin by increasing the production of oxytocin receptors. These stimulatory prostaglandins are produced by the amnion and the decidua.

During pregnancy, the myometrium produces prostacyclin (PGI$_2$), which has an inhibitory effect on uterine contractility (Christensen and Green 1983). Progesterone blocks the synthesis of prostaglandins by the amnion and the decidua, whereas both estrogen and oxytocin increase its synthesis. Figure 1.4 shows the prostaglandin synthetic pathway.

## Mechanism of Action of Prostaglandins

Muscle physiology consists of three important concepts: phasic contraction, tonic tension and relaxation. Phasic contraction is intermittent and may last for

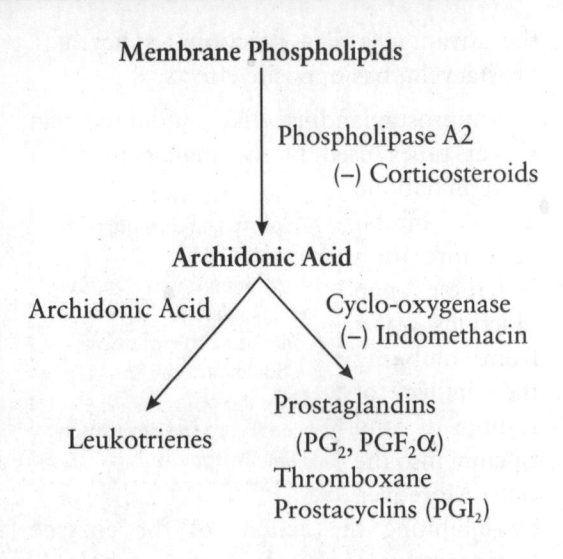

**Membrane Phospholipids**
↓ Phospholipase A2
(–) Corticosteroids
↓
**Archidonic Acid**

Archidonic Acid ↙   ↘ Cyclo-oxygenase
                              (–) Indomethacin
Leukotrienes     Prostaglandins
                         (PG$_2$, PGF$_2\alpha$)
                         Thromboxane
                         Prostacyclins (PGI$_2$)

**Figure 1.4** Prostaglandin synthetic pathway

a short or a long period of time, whereas tonic tension is fairly constant, lasting for prolonged periods. At the myometrial cellular level, prostaglandins have been found to induce both phasic contractions as well as tonic tension with superimposed phasic contractions (Chamley and Parkington 1984). In practical terms, they increase both the resting tone of the uterine myometrium as well as the amplitude and duration of the myometrial contractions.

At a molecular level, phasic contractions are due to the influx of sodium ions into the myometrial cell, whereas tonic tension is due the increased availability of intracellular calcium. Both these processes are affected by prostaglandins (Reiner and Marshall 1976).

Prostaglandins also induce the formation of gap junctions between the myometrial cells, which help in the development of coordinated myometrial action, giving the advantages of a functional syncytium. Prostacyclin has opposite effects.

Antiprostaglandins like indomethacin are at times used in the management of preterm labour. They inhibit the formation of these gap junctions, apart from inhibiting the influx of sodium and calcium into the cells. Moreover, by inhibiting the actions of the enzyme 'cyclooxygenase', they divert the arachidonic acid metabolism through the 'lipo-oxygenase' pathway. This leads to the production of leukotrienes instead of prostaglandins. Leukotrienes have minimum direct effect on human myometrial contractility.

> Antiprostaglandins prevent contractions by
> - inhibiting the formation of gap junctions
> - inhibiting the influx of sodium and calcium into the cells
> - leading to the production of leukotrienes

## Cervical Ripening

The cervix has to play a dual role in human reproduction. During pregnancy, it should remain firm and closed allowing the fetus to grow in utero until functional maturity is attained. During labour, it should soften and dilate, allowing the fetus to pass through the birth canal. The process by which the cervix becomes soft, compliant and partially dilated is termed 'cervical ripening'. This is a fundamental process that must occur, if parturition is to progress smoothly. Cervical ripening is thought to be due to a combination of biochemical, endocrine, mechanical, and possibly, inflammatory events. It is

> Cervical ripening is thought to be due to a combination of biochemical, endocrine, mechanical and inflammatory events.

believed that the increasing myometrial contractility, in the form of Braxton Hicks contractions, seen with advancing gestation plays a vital role in the effacement of the cervix, prior to the actual commencement of labour (Table 1.4).

**Table 1.4** Factors that affect cervical ripening

| Factor | Mechanism of action |
|---|---|
| Changes in ground substance (glycosaminoglycans) | Increase water content of the cervix and cause 'scattering and dispersion' of collagen. Increase formation of immature collagen |
| Enzymes and inflammatory mediators (elastase, collagenase etc.) | Increase collagen breakdown and remodelling |

Structurally, the cervix is mainly composed of collagen as opposed to the myometrium, which predominantly consists of smooth muscle. There are four types of collagen in the human body, these are types I, II, III and IV. The cervix is predominantly composed of types I (66 per cent) and III (33 per cent). The firmness of the cervix in the non-pregnant state is mainly due to the properties of these collagen fibrils, which are bound together tightly in the form of bundles. These bundles in turn are embedded in ground substance consisting of proteoglycans. As the name implies, the proteoglycans are made of a central core of proteins which are linked to glycosaminoglycans, which are repeating disaccharide units composed of a hexosamine (glucosamine or galactosamine)

> The cervix is predominantly composed of types I (66 per cent) and III (33 per cent) collagen.

## Physiopharmacology of Labour

and a uronic acid (glucuronic acid or idurionic acid) residue.

In the cervix, the main glycosaminoglycans are dermatan sulphate and chondroitin sulphate, both of which are highly negatively charged and hydrophobic. Hence, they repel water and are responsible for the firmness of the cervix. Moreover, by interacting with the central protein core as well as among themselves, glycosaminoglycans facilitate the optimum orientation of the collagen fibrils, enhancing the mechanical strength of the cervix.

It is well recognised that the cervix loses its firmness in late pregnancy and becomes soft and compliant. During labour it further loses its elasticity, viscosity and plasticity. These changes can be attributed to the changes that are taking place at the molecular level with regard to the glycosaminoglycans. Towards term, the glycosaminoglycan concentration of the cervix alters and the dermatan and chondroitin sulphates are replaced by hyaluronic acid, which has different physiochemical properties. Hyaluronic acid is hydrophilic and imbibes water. Accumulation of water within the substance of the cervix destabilises the collagen fibrils, contributing to cervical ripening (Figure 1.5). Indeed, it has been shown that the water content of the human cervix increases from 80 per cent in the non-pregnant state, to 86 per cent in late pregnancy (Liggins 1978; Uldbjerg et al 1983). This increase in the water content also decreases the effective concentration of collagen in the cervix, though the total content of collagen

```
┌─────────────────────────────────┐
│ Dermatan/chondroitin            │
│ sulphate (hydrophobic)          │
└────────────────┬────────────────┘
                 ↓
┌─────────────────────────────────┐
│ Replaced by hyaluronic acid     │
│ (hydrophilic)                   │
└────────────────┬────────────────┘
                 ↓
┌─────────────────────────────────┐
│ Imbibes water – 'soft'          │
└────────────────┬────────────────┘
                 ↓
┌─────────────────────────────────┐
│ Destabilises collagen fibrils   │
│ (decreases mechanical strength) │
└────────────────┬────────────────┘
                 ↓
┌─────────────────────────────────┐
│ Soft compliant cervix           │
│ 'cervical ripening'             │
└─────────────────────────────────┘
```

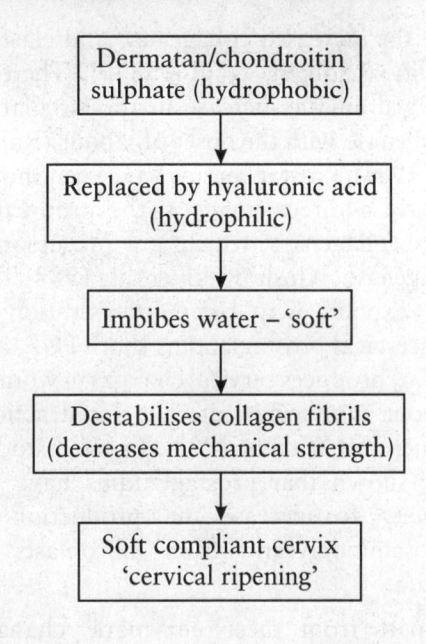

**Figure 1.5** Changes responsible for cervical ripening

increases at term. Further, the accumulation of water in between the collagen fibrils has a scattering or dispersing effect, resulting in reduced mechanical strength.

The change in the glycosaminoglycan composition is just one aspect of cervical ripening with various enzymes which also promote collagen remodelling. Collagenase is an enzyme that breaks down collagen types I, II and III and is produced by both the fibroblasts and the leukocytes. Leukocyte elastase is another enzyme that can break down elastin, collagen and proteoglycans. It is produced by macrophages, neutrophils and eosinophils. The levels of both these enzymes are found to increase with advancing gestation and are associated with progressive decline in the concentration of cervical collagen (Uldbjerg et al 1983). The levels of partially degraded soluble collagen concentration increase in tandem

> Hyaluronic acid contributes to accumulation of water within the substance of the cervix, which destabilises the collagen fibrils, contributing to cervical ripening

with the increased collagenase and elastase activity (Uldbjerg et al 1983b). There is also a dramatic increase in the circulating collagenase with the onset of labour (Rajabi et al 1984). Prostaglandins have been shown to have a direct effect on the production of procollagenase, which is a precursor of collagenase (Goshowaki et al 1988). This may explain why the administration of intracervical prostaglandins (both $PGE_2$ and $PGF_2\alpha$) produces cervical changes in women, without inducing uterine contractions (Hillier and Walters 1982). In vitro studies have shown that prostaglandins have the capacity to increase the production of glycosaminoglycans from fibroblasts in culture.

Apart from these enzymatic changes, there is also a process of cervical remodelling that takes place with advancing gestation. The mature collagen, which has many cross-links that are responsible for its tensile strength, is replaced by an immature collagen, which has few such cross-links. Functionally, the newly formed immature collagen is much weaker and is easily broken down during labour. The impact of these changes in the physical properties of collagen on the progress of labour has been well demonstrated. Granstrom et al (1991) have shown that the insufficient remodelling of collagen during pregnancy is an independent factor that results in prolonged labour. In their study, the collagenolytic activity in women with normal and prolonged labour did not show any significant difference. Therefore, abnormal remodelling of collagen may contribute to dysfunctional labour.

> Abnormal remodelling of collagen may contribute to dysfunctional labour.

It has been long recognised that sex steroids (estrogens and progesterone) have an 'opposing effect' on the cervix during pregnancy. Progesterone is believed to prevent cervical ripening during pregnancy. There is no direct evidence for this action, although the progesterone antagonist, mifepristone, has been found to cause cervical ripening in women undergoing termination of pregnancy. Therefore, indirectly, it can be deduced that progesterone may be responsible for maintaining the firmness of the cervix during pregnancy. However, it is not clear whether mifepristone causes cervical ripening directly or through the blockage of progesterone receptors.

As far as estrogens are concerned, research so far has provided conflicting evidence. Some studies have shown 'cervical ripening' in response to estrogens. However, others did not show any significant change. Thus, as far as the effect of sex steroids on cervical ripening is concerned, research has not provided any clear-cut answer. Considering the large amounts of estrogens and progesterone that are produced during the course of normal pregnancy, it does not seem unreasonable to expect that they may at least have an indirect effect in either stimulating or inhibiting the process of cervical ripening.

As previously discussed, the polypeptide hormone, relaxin, has been studied with regard to its effect on the cervix. Earlier studies reported that the concentration of relaxin in the human cervix increases towards late pregnancy. Relaxin, when applied locally, induced cervical ripening in most cases (MacLennan et al 1980). Subsequently, it has been found that relaxin also increases the production and secretion of collagenases from the amnion (Koay et al 1983). Relaxin has a dual action on the arachidonic acid pathway. It suppresses prostaglandin E$_2$ (PGE$_2$) production during pregnancy, but stimulates its production during spontaneous labour. It appears that this stimulation of prostaglandins during late pregnancy and during labour is its main mechanism of action. MacLennan et al (1980) showed that when relaxin and prostaglandins were administered together for cervical ripening, there was no additive effect, but when individually administered, relaxin was as effective as vaginal prostaglandins in causing cervical ripening. This suggests that the action of relaxin may be mediated through prostaglandin synthesis.

Based on current evidence, both prostaglandins and relaxins appear to play a key role in the process of cervical ripening. Activation of collagenases and modification of gene expression for relaxin in the amnion and the decidua should be areas of future research.

## Onset of Labour

We have so far discussed the mechanisms involved in cervical ripening and myometrial contractility. Prelabour changes, which start a few weeks before the actual commencement of labour, are a significant period in human parturition. The cervix gets ready to allow the passage of the products of conception and the myometrium gets prepared to begin effective uterine contractions to expel the same. The main question is, 'What ignites the "spark" that initiates labour?' Is it a signal from the mother, the fetus or both? Or, is it an external signal that is hitherto unknown to us? Ferguson's reflex refers to the pressure exerted on the cervix by the presenting part, which stimulates nerve endings in the cervical canal. This local reflex aids in cervix dilatation through a neuro-hormonal reflex. Ferguson's reflex is thought to play a role in the release of prostaglandins and oxytocin during labour. It is unclear whether this reflex has any role in the initiation of labour.

In human parturition, no dramatic changes in any hormones have been detected. Parturition in sheep is directly related to the maturation of the fetal hypothalamo–pituitary–adrenal axis (Challis and Brooks 1989), which results in increasing levels of corticotropin-releasing hormone (CRH), adrenocorticotropic hormone (ACTH) and fetal cortisol, respectively. Fetal cortisol, in turn, stimulates the formation of placental 17-alpha hydroxylase, which is involved in the conversion of progesterone to estrogen. Progesterone is essential for keeping the uterus quiescent during pregnancy in most mammals (Thornburn and Challis 1979). Hence, the reduction of progesterone may herald the removal of this 'progesterone block'. Moreover, the relative excess of estrogen reduces the threshold of myometrial contraction and induces a cascade of events leading to cervical ripening. Estrogen is also implicated in the production of prostaglandins, with the resultant formation of myometrial gap junctions and oxytocin receptors. In summary, there is an enhancement of myometrial contractility and cervical ripening that 'jumpstarts' labour.

Csapo (1961) first proposed the progesterone block theory to explain

> Ferguson's reflex refers to the pressure exerted on the cervix by the presenting part, which stimulates nerve endings in the cervical canal.

the onset of labour. According to him, labour was initiated when the delicate balance between the myometrial relaxant (progesterone) and myometrial stimulant (estrogen) was altered in favour of the latter. However, Thornburn and Challis (1979) demonstrated that the peripheral plasma levels of estrogen and progesterone do not change significantly immediately preceding labour, either at term or preterm. This was confirmed by the estimation of levels of estrogen and progesterone in uterine arterial and venous blood which revealed that there were no significant changes prior to labour (Davidson et al 1987). This points to the fact that there may not be a significant degree of conversion of progesterone to estrogen at the commencement of human labour. This generated a great deal of scepticism about the progesterone block theory of Csapo, especially after Lewis et al (1987) showed that there were no significant changes in the concentration of estradiol and progesterone in the saliva of pregnant women before, during or after spontaneous labour.

Recently, the interest in this progesterone block theory has resurfaced following the use of antiprogestogens as effective abortifacients. Mifepristone increases myometrial sensitivity to prostaglandins and induces cervical ripening. Although this may be attributed to an unknown mechanism at the molecular level (i.e. a direct action rather than due to blockage of progesterone receptors), it does indicate that progesterone may play a vital role in the initiation of human labour. It may be that there is a change in the level of progesterone at the cellular level which is not picked up by tests used to detect changes in the plasma or salivary concentrations of progesterone. Alternatively, there may be changes occurring at the level of the progesterone receptors, such as down-regulation. This may result in a suboptimal action of progesterone, even though its actual concentration is not altered. The possibility of an endogenous antiprogestogen, which is similar to mifepristone that is produced prior to the onset of labour, has also been considered.

Another possible mechanism is the modulation of estrogen and progesterone synthesis at the level of the fetal membranes. Mitchell et al (1987) argued that such an alteration of the estrogen and progesterone ratio occurring locally may not be detected by measurements of these hormone levels in the peripheral circulation. They also demonstrated that human amnion, chorion and decidua are capable of producing estrogen and progesterone from sulphated precursors. Further, the activity of the enzyme steroid sulphohydrase, was found to be increased in the chorion after spontaneous labour (Mitchell et al 1987). Although studies so far have not been able to show any significant changes in the plasma levels of estrogen and progesterone prior to labour, it seems clear that progesterone inhibits and estrogen stimulates the synthesis of prostaglandins (Abel and Baird 1980). However, it was later demonstrated by studies in chorion laevae cells that it was glucocorticoids and not progesterone that inhibited prostaglandin synthesis.

This may explain why mifepristone acts as a very efficient abortifacient, as it has a significant antiglucocorticoid activity. This may contribute to the reduction of the prostaglandin block by glucocorticoids.

Estrogen decreases the resting membrane potential of the myometrial cells and increases their excitability, whereas progesterone has an opposite effect (Garfield and Hayashi 1980). Recently, Petrocelli and Lye (1993) reported that estrogen stimulates the production of mRNA coding for connexin-43, which is a gap junction protein. Progesterone was found to inhibit this action. Current knowledge shows that estrogens and progesterone have opposing actions on the myometrium and cause uterine stimulation and relaxation, respectively. Further research is needed to determine whether they play a significant role in the onset of labour and the underlying mechanism.

## Prostaglandins

It is widely believed that prostaglandins constitute the 'final common pathway' responsible for the onset of labour. They are potent agents and can cause both myometrial contractions as well as cervical ripening. An increase in the levels of prostaglandins at the onset of labour has been demonstrated in all mammals, including humans. Levels of prostaglandins and their metabolites have been found to increase in the amniotic fluid in advanced labour. Therefore, it could be deduced that they are essential for the onset of labour.

Arachidonic acid (a precursor of prostaglandins) is stored mainly in the amnion, and prostaglandin synthesis has been demonstrated in the amnion with the commencement of labour. In order to initiate labour, the prostaglandins synthesised in the amnion should act in a paracrine fashion to stimulate the cervix, decidua and myometrium. To do so, they have to cross the chorion to reach its target tissues. The amnion appears to be a natural barrier to prostaglandins, as it contains the enzyme prostaglandin dehydrogenase that breaks down prostaglandins. It may be an inherent protective mechanism against preterm labour. Sceptics argue that prostaglandins could not reach their target tissues in the active form due to the presence of this enzyme in the chorion and hence, they could not play a significant role in the onset of labour. Cheung et al (1990) showed by immunocytochemical studies that most of the cells in the chorion, lacked the enzyme prostaglandin dehydrogenase. Therefore, prostaglandins may diffuse through these cells, which act as a safe passage to reach their target tissues. It is not yet clear whether the fetus sends any signal to increase the production of prostaglandins by the amnion or to decrease the expression of prostaglandin dehydrogenase or both, prior to the onset of labour.

Surprisingly, there have been no significant changes in the endogenous capacity to form prostaglandins by uterine tissues at the onset of labour (Fuchs et al 1984). However, the activity of prostaglandins was found to increase with the onset of labour. Subsequently, an endogenous inhibitor of prostaglandin synthesis (EIPS) has been detected in the amniotic fluid and the withdrawal of this inhibitory EIPS at term may explain the increase in the activity of prostaglandins observed with the onset of labour. Indeed, Saed et al (1982) demonstrated that amniotic fluid EIPS decreases towards term and particularly in labour. Apart from the amnion, the decidua also takes part in the production of prostaglandins and shows an increase in its production during labour (Skinner and Challis 1985). Possibly, the fetal signals act through the amnion and the maternal signals through the decidua to increase the synthesis of prostaglandins prior to and during labour.

So far, we have not determined the exact trigger to the onset of human parturition. It has been suggested that the fetus may excrete certain stimulatory factors in its urine, stimulating the amnion at term (Strickland et al 1983). These include platelet activating factors, epidermal growth factor, transforming growth factor-alpha, as well as various interleukins. Paradoxically, decidua can also exert an inhibitory effect on the production of prostaglandins by the fetal membranes, by secreting prolactin (Tyson et al 1985). This may explain why the separation of membranes from the decidua may induce labour. Possibly, this inhibitory effect of decidual prolactin on the amnion is removed, leading to the production of prostaglandins, culminating in labour.

> The exact trigger to the onset of human parturition has not been determined so far.

## Oxytocin

There is no doubt that oxytocin increases the amplitude and duration of myometrial contractions. Its role in the onset of labour, however, remains controversial, as studies have failed to show any increase in the oxytocin level at or prior to the commencement of labour (Vasicka et al 1978). Recent studies have demonstrated an increase in the oxytocin receptors in the myometrium (Fuchs et al 1984), increasing the sensitivity of the myometrium to circulating oxytocin. Subsequently, Miller et al (1993) have shown that oxytocin is locally synthesised by the decidua and may act in a paracrine manner to stimulate the myometrium. Several factors may influence this local production, notably inflammatory mediators such as cytokines. This may explain the onset of preterm labour in the presence of chorioamnionitis. A relative increase in the local estrogen to progesterone ratio has also been found to increase the decidual oxytocin production (Richard and Zingg 1990). The case for oxytocin playing a positive role in the onset of labour, was strengthened with the use of oxytocin antagonist 'atosiban' to inhibit preterm labour (Goodwin et al 1994).

> Inflammatory mediators such as cytokines may lead to the local production of oxytocin which may explain the onset of preterm labour in the presence of chorioamnionitis

Studies have shown that the concentration of oxytocin receptors is higher in early labour when compared to advanced labour, indicating that oxytocin is important for the onset of labour (Maggi et al 1990). Conversely, it has been suggested that increasing levels of oxytocin result in a down-regulation of its own receptors. This may well explain why despite such an increase in the secretion of oxytocin with advancing labour, the receptor levels decrease. Indeed, Bossman et al (1994) reported that women who received oxytocin infusion for longer than three hours had a lower concentration of oxytocin receptors compared to those who had a shorter treatment (or a lower total dose). This may imply that a higher concentration of oxytocin is essential for the initiation of labour and with increasing levels there is a mechanism of down-regulation, preventing uterine hyperstimulation and its sequelae. Augmentation of labour with very high doses of oxytocin may not necessarily bring about the desired outcome, as the down-regulation of oxytocin receptors may, in fact, decrease its overall pharmacological effect.

Thus, it appears that oxytocin is less important as a myometrial stimulant in advanced labour as compared to early labour. There is insufficient evidence to suggest that fetal oxytocin plays a significant role in the onset of labour.

## Relationship between Oxytocin and Prostaglandins

It is widely accepted that oxytocin and prostaglandins play a dual and synergistic role in human parturition. In a review in 1984, Fuchs et al reported that oxytocin acts on its receptors in the myometrium and the decidua to stimulate myometrial contractions and prostaglandin synthesis. Likewise, prostaglandins act on the cervix to bring about cervical ripening and dilatation and on the myometrium to potentiate the oxytocin induced myometrial contractions. This exemplifies the fact that there must be synergy between oxytocin and prostaglandins at the level of decidua and the myometrium if the labour is to progress smoothly. There is evidence to suggest that the increase in prostaglandin F metabolites in oxytocin-induced labour has its origin in the decidua and not in the amnion. This idea is further strengthened by our knowledge that atosiban acts as an oxytocin antagonist by blocking the oxytocin receptors in the decidua and not in the myometrium (Ivanisevic et al 1989); its clinical effectiveness may be due to the suppression of prostaglandin synthesis at the decidua.

The onset of labour heralds an increase in the local estrogen to progesterone ratio that induces the synthesis of oxytocin by the decidua as well as an increased expression of oxytocin receptors in the myometrium. Increasing oxytocin levels may then stimulate the synthesis and release of prostaglandins from the fetal membranes and the decidua, which in turn enhances further release of oxytocin (Fig. 1.6). Once this positive feed back loop is established, labour becomes an autonomous process with oxytocin and prostaglandins stimulating myometrial contractility and prostaglandins acting independently on the cervix to cause cervical ripening. Oxytocin appears to be the major stimulus for the initiation of labour, whereas prostaglandin $F_2\alpha$ is responsible for the progression of labour (Fuchs 1981; 1984).

> Oxytocin appears to be the major stimulus for the initiation of labour, whereas prostaglandin $F_2\alpha$ is responsible for the progression of labour

## Role of other Hormones

Relaxin is believed to play a minor role in the onset and progression of labour. It is generally accepted that relaxin interacts with oxytocin, prostaglandins, as well as the mechanical forces of labour. It has a negative effect on myometrial contractility

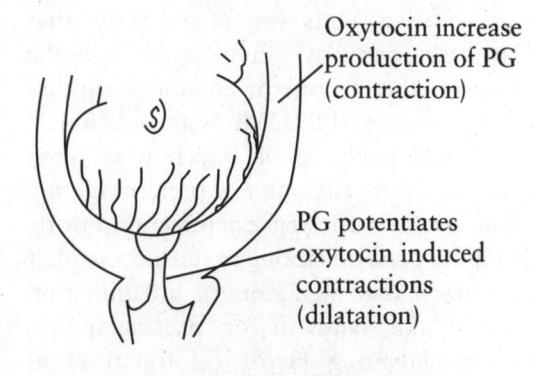

Oxytocin increase production of PG (contraction)

PG potentiates oxytocin induced contractions (dilatation)

**Figure 1.6** Synergistic relationship between oxytocin and prostaglandins (PG)

and may be involved in the process of cervical ripening.

Vasopressin has a structural similarity with oxytocin. The non-pregnant uterus responds more to vasopressin than to oxytocin, while the pregnant uterus at term is more sensitive to oxytocin than to vasopressin. Similar to the oxytocin receptors, vasopressin receptors increase in the decidua with progressive gestation. However, their overall concentration in the decidua is about half that of oxytocin receptors (Ivanisevic et al 1989). There is evidence to indicate that oxytocin and vasopressin may act on each other's receptors and atosiban blocks both oxytocin and vasopressin receptors (Ivanisevic et al 1989). Despite these findings, there is no clear evidence to indicate that vasopressin has a major role in the initiation and progression of labour. There is also no evidence to indicate that levels of corticotropin-releasing hormone (CRH) and fetal cortisol show a dramatic increase at the onset of labour.

## The Role of Inflammatory Mediators

Interest in the role of inflammatory mediators was aroused with the observation that chorioamnionitis was associated with the onset of labour. Preterm prelabour rupture of membranes (PPROM) with subclinical or clinical evidence of infection is often associated with the onset of preterm labour. Moreover, in the presence of infection, efforts to inhibit preterm labour are unsuccessful. It is believed that mediators of inflammation act via the synthesis of prostaglandins. Platelet-activating factor (Hoffman et al 1990), interleukins (especially IL-6) and tumour necrosis factor (TNF) have been implicated in the onset of preterm labour (Romero et al 1989). All these mediators have been found in high concentrations in the amniotic fluid at the onset of labour. It is also an interesting hypothesis that platelet activating factor (PAF), which is a marker of fetal lung maturity, may be secreted by the fetus once functional maturity is achieved to induce labour. Another attractive hypothesis is the local withdrawal of the immunosuppressive agents, which are responsible for the fetal allograft survival in utero, prior to the onset of labour. These include progesterone, human chorionic gonadotropin (hCG) and human chorionic somatomammotropin (hCS), all of which are produced in high concentrations by the feto-placental unit during pregnancy. These local immunosuppressive agents keep the cytotoxic lymphocytes responsible for allograft rejection at bay. Hence, removal of this block would increase the activity of cytotoxic lymphocytes, leading to the rejection of the fetal allograft, thereby initiating labour. Indeed, studies have shown that lymphocyte cytotoxicity is increased at the time of onset of term or preterm labour (Szekenes-Bartho et al 1986).

## Physiopharmacology of Labour: Clinical Applications

Application of the knowledge of physiopharmacology of labour is essential to optimise maternal and fetal outcome. Pharmacological agents are used in the management of preterm labour (Chandraharan and Arulkumaran 2005), postdate pregnancy (induction of labour), slow progress of labour (augmentation of labour), and postpartum hemorrhage. Use of medications to rapidly abolish uterine contractions in emergency situations (i.e. acute tocolysis) may help improve the outcome in several obstetric emergencies such as cord prolapse, uterine hyperstimulation and undiagnosed breech presentation (Chandraharan and Arulkumaran 2005).

## Recent Developments

Plasminogen activation cascade has been proposed to play an important role in the onset of labour. Activated plasminogen (i.e. plasmin) is implicated with a variety of connective tissue remodelling events including fetal membrane rupture and placental separation. In 1998, Tsatas et al reported an up-regulation of the concentration of urokinase plasminogen activator receptor (UPAR) in the amnion with the onset of labour. This is believed to localise the active plasminogen activator at the cell surface, thereby increasing the proteolytic activity in the fetal membranes. This may contribute to the rupture of membranes. Also, there has been evidence with regard to local 'functional progesterone withdrawal'. A nuclear transcription factor has been isolated (nuclear factor-kappa B or NF-kappa B), which negatively interacts with progesterone receptors and increases the expression of type-2 cyclooxygenase (COX-2) enzyme. Alport et al (2001) have reported an increase in the activity of this enzyme during labour, which may contribute to an increase in the production of prostaglandins as well as functional progesterone withdrawal.

The role of hyaluronidase for cervical ripening or induction of labour remains uncertain (Kavanagh et al 2001). Like cervical connective tissue remodelling, there has also been considerable interest in the remodelling of uterine connective tissue at term and at the onset of labour. Hjelm et al (2002) have recently reported a considerable remodelling of uterine connective tissue, with significant changes in the content of proteoglycans. These changes are believed to be essential for normal myometrial contractions during labour. Further, it has also been reported that uterine myometrium in vitro was more sensitive to arginine-vasopressin than to oxytocin, but there is no increase in the expression of myometrial vasopressin V1, a receptor mRNA, after the onset of labour (Thornton et al 2002). As the cervix is composed of predominantly connective tissue, most of the studies concentrated on connective tissue remodelling. Research is in progress to identify the role of cervical smooth muscle on the process of labour. Cervical smooth muscle activity has been correlated to the duration of the latent phase but not to the active phase. Frequent cervical contractions are not associated with a longer latent phase (Pajntar et al 2001).

## Conclusion

Labour is the most perilous journey a woman has to undertake. The physiology of labour itself appears to be as complex as the processes and the mechanisms involved. Unlike in sheep, the various regulatory factors that affect the onset of human labour are largely unknown. Human labour does not involve a simple 'on–off' mechanism, but needs considerable preparation during the process of prelabour. Cervical ripening with an increase in the formation of gap junctions and an increase in myometrial contractility, lay the groundwork. To date, we do not understand what exactly triggers the onset of labour; is it the fetus or the mother or both? Research in this millennium may answer these questions and may help us to institute more effective care during problem labour.

# References

Abel MH and DT Baird. 1980. The effects of 17 B estradiol and progesterone on prostaglandin production by human endometrium maintained in organ culture. *Endocrinology* May; 106 (5):1599–606.

Alexandrova M and MA Soloff. 1980. Oxytocin receptors and parturition I: Control of oxytocin receptor concentration in rat myometrium at term. *Endocrinology* 106:730–35.

Alport VC, D Pierber, DM Slater et al. 2001. Human labour is associated with nuclear factor Kappa-B activity, which mediated cyclo-oxygenase 2 expression and is involved with functional progesterone withdrawal. *Mol Hum Reprod* 7(6):581–6.

Balducci J, B Risek, NB Gilula et al. 1992. Gap junction formation in the human myometrium: A key to preterm labour? *Am J Obstet Gynecol* 168:1609–15.

Bell RJ, M Permezel, AH MacLennan, C Hughes, D Healy and S Bremecke. 1993. A randomised double blind placebo controlled trial of the safety of the vaginal recombinant human relaxin for cervical ripening. *Obstet Gynecol* 82:328–33.

Bossmar T, M Akerlund, G Fantoni et al. 1994. Receptors for and myometrial responses to oxytocin and vasopressin in preterm and term human pregnancy: effects of oxytocin antagonist atosiban. *Am J Obstet Gynecol* Dec; 171 (6):1634–42.

Brennecke SP, BM Castle, LM Demers, AC Turnbull. 1985. Maternal plasma prostaglandin E2 metabolite levels during human pregnancy and parturition. *Br J Obstet Gynaecol* 92 (4):345–9.

Bryant-Greenwood GD, MCP Rees, AC Turnbull. 1987. Immunohistochemical localisation of relaxin, prolactin and prostaglandin synthase in human amnion, chorion and decidua. *J Endocrinol* 114:491–96.

Campbell EA, EA Linton, CDA Wolfe et al. 1987. Plasma corticotropin releasing hormone concentration during pregnancy and parturition. *J Clin Endocrinol Metab* 64:1054–59.

Challis BR and AN Brooks. 1989. Maturation and activation of hypothalamo-pituitary adrenal functionin fetal sheep. *Endocr Res* May; 10 (2):182–204.

Chamley WA and HC Parkington. 1984. Relaxin inhibits the plateau component of the action potential in the circular myometrium of rat. *J Physiol (Lond)* 353:51–65.

Chandraharan E and S Arulkumaran. 2005. Recent advances in the management of Preterm Labour. Review Article. *J Obstet Gynecol India* Vol. 55, No. 2: March/April 118–24.

Chandraharan E and S Arulkumaran. 2005. Acute Tocolysis. Review Article. *Curr Opin Obstet Gynecol* 17: 151–6.

Cheung PY, JC Walton, HH Tai, SC Riley, JR Challis. 1990. Immunocytochemical distribution and localization of 15-hydroxy prostaglandin dehydrogenase in human fetal membranes. Decidua and placenta. *Am J Obstet Gynecol* Nov; 163 (5):1445–9.

Chow L and SJ Lye. 1994. Expression of the gap junction protein 'connexin-43' is increased in the human myometrium towards term and with the onset of labour. *Am J Obstet Gynecol* 170:788–95.

Christensen NJ and K Green. 1983. Bioconversion of arachidonic acid in human pregnant reproductive tissues. *Biochem Med* 30:162.

Clarke KE, EG Mills, SJ Stys and AC Seeds. 1981. Effects of vasoactive polypeptides on uterine vasculature. *Am J Obstet Gynecol* 139:182–88.

Cole WC and RE Garfield. 1986. Evidence for physiological regulation for myometrial gap junction permeability. *Am J Physiol* 251:C411–20.

Cole WC and RE Garfield. 1988. Effects of calcium ionophore A23187 and calmodulin inhibitors on intracellular communication in rat myometrium. *Biol Reprod* 38:55–62.

Creasy R. 1990. Preterm inhibition of myometrial contractility: Clinical considerations. In

*Uterine contractility*, ed RE Garfield, 371–80. Massachusetts: Serono symposia.

Csapo AI. 1961. The onset of labour. *Lancet* Aug 5; 2 (7197); 277080.

Dalton BJ, F Lam, JM Roberts. 1986. Failure to demonstrate a decrease in beta adrenergic receptor concentration or agonist effeicay in term or preterm human parturition. *Am J Obstet Gynecol* 154:450–6.

Dattel BJ, F Lam, JM Roberts. 1986. Failure to demonstrate decreased beta-adrenergic receptor concentration or decreased agonist efficacy in term or preterm human parturition. *Am J Obstet Gynecol* Feb; 154 (2) 450–6.

Davidson BJ, RD Murray, JR Challis, GJ Valenzuela. 1987. Estrogen, progesterone, prolactin, prostaglandin E2, prostaglandin F2 alpha, prostaglandin F1 alpha gradients across the uterus in women in labour and not in labour. *Am J Obstet Gynecol* Jul; 157 (1):54–8.

Eddie LW, IT Cameron, JF Leeton, DL Healy, P Renou. 1990. Ovarian relaxin is not essential for dilatation of the cervix. *Lancet* I:243.

Embrey MP and JC Moir. 1967. A comparison of the oxytocic effects of the synthetic vasopressin and oxytocin. *J Obstet Gynecol Br Cwlth* 74:648–52.

Frim D, R Emanuel, B Robinson et al. 1988. Characterisation and gestational regulation of the corticotropin-releasing hormone messenger RNA in human placenta. *J Clin Invest* 82:287–92.

Fuchs AR, F Fuchs, P Husslein, MS Soloff. 1984. Oxytocin receptors in pregnant human uterus. *Am J Obstet Gynecol* 150:734–41.

Fuchs AR, P Husslein, F Fuchs. 1981. Oxytocin and initiation of human parturition, II. Stimulation of prostaglandin production in human decidua by oxytocin. *Am J Obstet Gynecol* Nov 15;141:(6) 694–7.

Fuchs AR. 1981. Oxytocin and oxytocin receptors: maternal signal for parturition. In *Uterine contractility*, ed RE Garfield, 177–190. Massachusetts: Serono symposia.

Garfield RE and RH Hayashi. 1980. Presence of gap junctions in the myometrium of women in various stages of menstruation. *Am J Obstet Gynecol* 138:569–74.

Garfield RE and RH Hayashi. 1981. Appearance of gap junctions in the myometrium in women during labour. *Am J Obstet Gynecol* 140:254–60.

Garfield RE, RH Hayashi, MJK Harper. 1987. In vitro studies on the control of human myometrial gap junctions. *Int J Gynaecol Obstet* 25:241–48.

Goland RS, SL Warrralow, RI Stark, LS Brown, AG Frantz. 1986. High levels of CRH immunoreactivity in the maternal and fetal plasma during pregnancy. *J Clin Endocrinol Metab* 63:1199–203.

Goldsmith LT, JH Skurnick, AS Wojtezuk et al. 1989. The antagonist effect of oxytocin and relaxin on rat uterine segment contractility. *Am J Obstet Gynecol* 161:1644–49.

Goodwin TM, R Paul, H Silver et.al. 1994. The effect of oxytocin antagonist atosiban on preterm uterine activity in the human. *Am J Obstet Gynecol* Feb;170 (2):474–8.

Goshowaki H, A Ito, Y Mori. 1988. Effects of prostaglandins in the production of collagenase by rabbit uterine fibroblasts. *Prostaglandins* July 36 (1); 107–14.

Granstrom L, G Ekman, A Malmstrom. 1991. Insufficient remodelling of uterine connective tissue in women with protracted labour. *Br J Obstet Gynaecol* Dec; 98 (12); 1212–16.

Greer IA, M McLaren, AA Calder. 1990. Plasma prostaglandin E2 and prostaglandin F 2a metabolite levels following the vaginal administration of PGE2 for induction of labour. *Acta Obstet et Gynecol Scand* 69:621–66.

Guillon G, MN Ballestre, JM Roberts, SP Bottari. 1987. Oxytocin and vasopressin: distinct receptors in the myometrium. *J Clin Endocrinol Metab* 64:1129–35.

Guvenal T, E Kantas, T Erselcan, Y Culhaogku, A Celtin. 2001. Beta-human gonadotropin and prolactin assays in cervico-vaginal secretions as a predictor of preterm delivery. *Int J Gynaecol Obstet* 75(3):229–34.

Hertelendy F and M Molnar. 1990. Mode of action of prostaglandins on the myometrial cells. In *Uterine contractility*, ed RE Garfield, 221–36. Massachusetts: Serono symposia.

Hillhouse EW, N Milton, D Grammatopoulous, HWP Quartero. 1993. The identification of the human myometrial corticotropin releasing hormone receptor that increases in affinity during pregnancy. *J Clin Endocrinol Metab* 76:736–41.

Hillier K, AA Calder, MP Embrey. 1974. Concentration of prostaglandin F2a in amniotic fluid and plasma in spontaneous and induced labour. *J Obstet Gynecol Brit Emp* 81:257–63.

Hillier K and RM Walters. 1982. Collagen solubility and tensile properties of the rat uterine cervix in late pregnancy; effects of arachidonic acid and prostaglandin F2 alpha. *J Endocrinol* Dec; 95 (3); 341–7.

Hjelm AM and K Barchan, A Malmstrom, GE Ekman-Ordeberg. 2002. Changes in the uterine proteoglycan distribution at term pregnancy and during labour. *Eur J Obstet Gynecol Reprod Biol* 100 (2):146–51.

Hochman J, G Weiss, BG Steinetz, EM O'Brian. 1978. Serum relaxin concentrations in prostaglandin and oxytocin induced labour in women. *Am J Obstet Gynecol* 130:473–74.

Huszar G and MP Walsh. 1989. Biochemistry of the myometrium and the cervix. In *Biology of the uterus*, ed R Wynn and W Jollie. 2nd ed., 355-402. New York: Plenum Medical.

Ivanisevic M, Behrens O, Helmer H, Demarest K, Fuchs AR. 1989. Vasopressin receptors in human pregnant myometrium and decidua; interactions with oxytocin and vasopressin agonists and antagonists. *Am J Obstet Gynecol* Dec; 161 (6):1637–43.

Johnson MR, H Abdalla, ACJ Allman et al. 1991. Relaxin levels in ovum donation pregnancies. *Fert Steril* 56:59–61.

Johnston TA, IA Greer, RW Kelly, AA Calder. 1993. Plasma prostaglandin metabolite concentration in normal and dysfunctional labour. *Br J Obstet Gynecol* 100:483.

Jones SA and JRG Challis. 1989. Local stimulation of prostaglandin production by corticotropin releasing hormone in fetal membranes and the placenta. *Biochem Biophys Res Commun* 159:964–70.

Jones SA and AJS Summerlee. 1986. Relaxin acts centrally to inhibit oxytocin release during parturition: An effect that is reversed by naloxone. *J Endocrinol* 111:99–102.

Kao CY. 1977. Electrical properties of uterine smooth muscle. In *Biology of uterus*, ed RM Wynn and W Jollie. 2nd ed. New York: Plenum Medical: 423–96

Kavanagh J, AJ Kelly, J Thomas. 2001. Hyaluronidase for cervical priming and induction of labour. *Cochrane Database Syst Rev* 2001(2): CD003097.

Keirse MJNC. 1979. Endogenous prostaglandins in human parturition. In *Human Parturition*, ed ABM Andersen, JBGravenhorst. 101–4. The Hague: Leiden University Press.

Koay TS, CK Too, FC Greenwood, Bryant-Greenwood GD. 1983. Relaxin stimulates collagenase and plasminogen activator secretion by dispersed human amnion and chorion cells in vitro. *J Clin Endocrinol Metabol* Jun 56 (6):1332–4.

Laatikainen TJ, IJ Raisanen, KR Salmiren. 1988. Corticotropin releasing hormone in amniotic fluid during gestation and labour and in relation to fetal lung maturtion. *Am J Obstet Gynecol* 159:891–95.

Larsson LI, J Fahrenkray, OB Schaffalitzky de Muckdell. 1977. Vasoactive intestinal polypeptide occurs in the nerves in the female genital tract. *Science* 197:1374–75.

Liggins GC. 1978. Ripening of the cervix. *Semin Perinatol* Jul 2 (3); 261–271.

Litime MH, G Pointis, M Breunller et al. 1989. Disappearance of Beta adrenergic response of the human myometrial adenylate cyclase at the end of pregnancy. *J Clin Endocrinol Metab* 69:1–6.

MacLennan AH. 1986. Cervical ripening and the induction of labour by vaginal prostaglandin F2a and relaxin. In *Cervix in pregnancy and labour: Clinical and biochemical investigations*, ed DA Ellwood and ABM Anderson, 187–96. Edinburgh: Churchill Livingstone.

MacLennan AH, RC Green, GD Bryant-Greenwood, FC Greenwood, RF Seamark. 1980. Ripening of the human cervix and the induction of labour by purified relaxin. *Lancet* 1:220–23.

Maggi M, P Del-Carlo, G Fantoni et al. 1990. Human myometrium contains and responds to VI vasopressin receptors as well as oxytocin receptors. *J Clin Endocrinol Metab* 70: 1142–54.

McMurty JP, GL Floersheim, GD Bryant-Greenwood. 1980. Characterisation of binding of 125 I-labelled succinylated porcine relaxin in human and mouse fibroblats. *J Reprod Fert* 58:43–9.

Miller FD, R Chibbar, BF Mitchell. 1993. Synthesis of oxytocin in amnion, chorion and decidua; a potential paracrine role for oxytocin in the onset of human parturition. *Regul Pept* Apr 29; 45 (1–2):247–51.

Mironneau J. 1976. Effects of oxytocin of ionic currents underlying rhythmic activity and contraction in uterine smooth muscle. *Pfugers Arch* 3363:113–18.

Mitchell MD, JD Brunt, AR Wilkinson, AC Turnbull. 1978. Prostanoids in blood for neonatal resuscitation. *Lancet* Dec 23–30; 2 (8104–5):1382–3.

Mitchell BF, JR Challis, L Lukhash. 1987. Progesterone synthesis by human amnion, chorion and decidua at term. *Am J Obstet Gynecol* Aug; 157 (2):349–53.

O'Brian KT, L Eltringham, G Clarke, AJS Summerlee. 1986. Effects of porcine relaxin on oxytocin release from neurohypophysis in the anaesthetised lactating rat. *J Endocrinol* 109:393–97.

O'Brien JM, GH Peeler, DW Pitts et al. 1994. Cervico-vaginal prolactin: a marker for spontaneous preterm delivery. *Am J Obstet Gynecol* 171(4):1107–11.

Osa T,T Ogasawara, S Kato. 1983. Effects of magnesium, oxytocin and PGF on the generation 2 alpha and propagation of excitation in the longitudinal muscle of rat myometrium during late pregnancy. *Jap J Physiol* 33:51–67.

Ottensen B, G Wagner, J Farenkrug. 1980. Vasoactive intestinal polypeptide (VIP) inhibits prostaglandin F2a induced activity of the rabbit myometrium Aq. *Prostaglandins* Mar; 19 (3):427–35.

Pajntar M, B Leskosek, D Rudel, I Verdenik. 2001. Contribution of cervical smooth muscle activity to the duration of latent and active phases of labour. *Br J Obstet Gynecol* 108(5):533–8.

Petrocelli T, and SJ Lye. 1993. Regulation of transcripters encoding the myometrial Gap junction protein connexion -43 by estrogen and progesterone. *Endocrinology* July; 133 (1):284–90.

Quartero HWP, G Srivasta, B Gillham. 1992. Role for cyclic adenosine monophosphate in the synergistic interaction between oxytocin and corticotropin releasing hormone in isolated human gestational myometrium. *J Clin Endocrinol Metab* 36:141–5.

Rajabi M and JF Woessner. 1984. Rise in serum levels of P2 peptidase , an enzyme involved in collagen breakdown in human pregnancy and labour. *Am J Obstet Gynecol* Dec; 150 (7): 821–6.

Reiner O and JM Marshall. 1976. Action of PGF2 alpha on the uterus of the pregnant rat. *Naunyn Schmeidbergs Arch Pharmacol* 292 (3):243–50.

Richard S and HH Zingg. 1990. The human oxytocin gene promoter is regulated by estrogens. *J Biol Chem* Apr 15; 265 (11):6098–103.

Riley SC and JRG Challis. 1991. CRH production by the placenta and the fetal membranes. *Placenta* 12:105–119.

Romero R, M Sirtori, E Oyarzun et al. 1989. Infection and labour. Prevalence, microbiology and clinical significance of intra-amniotic infection in women with preterm labour and intact membranes. *Am J Obstet Gynaecol* Sept; 161 (3):817–24.

Roy AC, SR Kottegoda, SS Ratnam. 1984. Relaxin and reproduction. *Sing J Obstet Gynecol* 15:65–9.

Roy AC and S Arulkumaran. 1991. Pharmacology of parturition. *Ann Acad Med Singapore* 20:71–7.

Saeed SA, DM Strickland, DC Young, A Dang, MD Mitchell. 1982. Inhibition of prostaglandin synthesis by human amniotic fluid: acute reduction in inhibitory activity of amniotic fluid obtained during labour. *J Clin Endocrinol Metab* Oct; 55 (4); 801–3.

Saito Y, H Sakamoto, NJ MacLusky, J Naffij. 1985. Correlation between gap junctions and sex steroid receptors in the myometrial cells of pregnant and postpartum rats. *Am J Obstet Gynecol* 151:805–12.

Sasaki A, O Shinkawa, AN Margioris et al. 1987. Immunoreactive CRH in human plasma during pregnancy, labour and delivery. *J Clin Endocrinol Metab* 64:224.

Schrey P, PA Cornford, AM Read, PJ Steer. 1988. A role for phosphoinositide hydrolysis in humanuterine smooth muscle during parturition. *Am J Obstet Gynecol* 159:964–70.

Schrey P, AM Read, PJ Steer. 1986. Oxytocin and vasopressin stimulate inositol triphosphosphate production in human gestational myometrium and decidual cells. *Bioscience Reprod* 6: 613–19.

Seki K,T Uesato, K Kato. 1987. Serum relaxin concentration in women following the administration of 16,16, dimethyl-trans delta 2 prostaglandin I methyl ester during early pregnancy. *Prostaglandins* 33:739–42.

Soloff MS and P Sweet. 1982. Oxytocin inhibition of (calcium-magnesium) ATP-ase in rat myometrial plasma membranes. *J Biol Chem* 257:10687–93.

Spatling L, F Fallenstein, H Scneider, J Danus. 1989. Bolus tocolysis: Treatment of preterm labour with pulsatile administration of a beta adrenergic agonist. *Am J Obstet Gynecol* 160:713–17.

Story ME, S Hall, SP Ziccona, JP Paulin. 1989. Effects of adrenalin, isoprenalin and forskolin on pregnant human myometrium. *Clin Exp Pharmacol Physiol* 15:701–13.

Thornburn GD and JR Challis. 1979. Endocrine control of parturition. *Physiol Res* Oct; 59 (4):863–918.

Strickland DM, SA Saeed, ML Casey, MD Mitchell. 1983. Stimulation of prostaglandin bio-synthesis by urine of the human fetus may serve as a trigger for parturition. *Science* Apr 29; 220 (4):521–2.

Szekeres-Bartho J, P Varga, AS Pasca. 1986. Immunologic factors contributing to the initiation of labor –lymphocyte reactivity in term and threatened preterm delivery. *Am J Obstet Gynecol* Jul; 155 (1):108–12.

Thornton S, PJ Baldwin, PA Harris et al. 2002. The role of arginine vasopressin in human labour: Functional studies, fetal production and localisation of V1a receptor mRNA. *Br J Obstet Gynecol* 109(1):57–62.

Thornton S, JM Davison, PM Bayllis. 1988. Plasma oxytocin during the third stage of labour: Comparison of natural and active management. *BMJ* 297:167–69.

Thornton S, JM Davison, PM Bayllis. 1992. Plasma oxytocin during the first and second stages of spontaneous human labour. *Acta Endocrinologica* 126:425–29.

Tsatas D, MS Baker, EK Moses, GE Rice. 1998. Gene expression of plasminogen activation cascade components in human term gestational tissues with labour onset. *Mol Hum Reprod* 4(1): 101–6.

Tyson JE, JA Coshen, NH Dublin. 1985. Inhibition of fetal membrane prostaglandin production by prolactin; relative importance in inhibition of labour. *Am J Obstet Gynecol* Apr 15; 151 (8):1032–8.

Uldgberg N, G Ekman, A Malmstrom, K Olsson, U Umsten. 1983. Ripening of the human uterine cervix related to changes in collagenolytic activity. *Am J Obstet Gynecol* Nov 15; 47 (6): 662–6.

Vascika A, P Kumaresan, GS Han, M Kumaresan. 1978. Plasma oxytocin in initiation of labour. *Am J Obstet Gynecol* Feb 1; 130 (3): 263–73.

Von Malliot K, M Weiss, M Nagelschmidt, HJ Struck. 1977. Relaxin and cervical dilatation during parturition. *Archive fur Gynakologie* 223: 323–34.

Wolfs GMJA and M Van Leuwan. 1979. Electromyographic observation on the human uterus during labour. *Acta Obstet Gynecol Scand* supplement 90:1–61.

# CHAPTER 2

# THE MANAGEMENT OF THE FIRST STAGE OF LABOUR

*Daisy Nirmal, David I Fraser and Sambit Mukhopadhyay*

The management of spontaneous labour remains an important issue both in the developing and the developed world. In the developing world, prolonged and often neglected labour is associated with high levels of mortality and morbidity because of lack of appropriate healthcare, in particular, antibiotics and the surgical facilities to perform a cesarean section. The causes of death and morbidity include obstructed labour, sepsis, rupture of the uterus and postpartum hemorrhage (Rao 1992). In the developed world, the increasing cesarean section (CS) rate for dystocia or difficult labour contributes at least a third to the overall CS rate, and almost 70 per cent of those women who have a CS in their first labour request an elective CS in subsequent pregnancies (Thomas and Paranjothy 2001). CS leads to increased maternal morbidity as well as mortality, especially when it is performed as an emergency procedure (Murphy 1998; Bewley and Cockburn 2002). Further, the long-term risks of cesarean section have been reported, including an increased risk of placenta previa (Nielsen et al 1989) and ectopic pregnancy (Hemminki and Merilainen 1996). Delivery by cesarean section in the first pregnancy could increase the risk of unexplained stillbirth in the second. In women with one previous cesarean section delivery, the rate of unexplained antepartum stillbirth at or after 39 weeks gestation is about double the risk of stillbirth or neonatal death from intrapartum uterine rupture (Smith et al 2003). Maternal and fetal morbidity and mortality due to prolonged labour and CS for dystocia may be reduced by the proper management of poor progress in labour, especially the first stage of labour.

## Normal Labour

The precise definition of normal labour is the spontaneous onset of regular painful uterine contractions associated with the effacement and dilatation of the cervix and descent of the presenting part, with or without a 'show' or ruptured membranes. This process culminates in the birth of a healthy baby followed by expulsion of the placenta and membranes. In most cases, the outcome can be predicted prospectively by observing the progress of cervical dilatation and descent of the presenting part. Although labour is a dynamic, continuous process, it is normally divided into three functional stages for the purpose of management: the first, second and third stage of labour.

The basis for the scientific study of the progress of labour was developed by Friedman (1954), who described the labour progress of 100 consecutive primigravid women in spontaneous labour at term. The progress was presented graphically by plotting the rate of cervical dilatation against time. The resulting graph of cervical dilatation forms the basis of the modern partogram, a pictorial representation of the key events in labour presented chronologically on a single page. The maternal and fetal parameters recorded include cervical dilatation, the level of the presenting part (in fifths of the fetal head palpable above the pelvic brim, rather than the station which relates the level of the head to the ischial spines and is measured in cm above or below), the fetal heart rate (FHR), the frequency and duration of uterine contractions and the colour and quantity of amniotic fluid. Other maternal parameters include temperature, pulse, blood pressure and drugs used. This pictorial documentation of labour facilitates the early recognition of poor progress. Plotting of the cervical dilatation at regular intervals also enables prediction of the time of onset of the second stage of labour.

## Nomograms of Cervical Dilatation

The rate of cervical dilatation in labour has been studied in various ethnic groups in different countries (Philpott 1972; O'Driscoll et al 1973; Studd 1973; Ilancheran et al 1977). The nomograms derived show similar rates of cervical dilatation in the different ethnic groups and comparative studies have confirmed that any differences in ethnicity have little influence on the rate of cervical dilatation (Duignan et al 1975), or on uterine activity in spontaneous normal labour (Arulkumaran et al 1989a).

> Differences in ethnicity have little influence on the rate of cervical dilatation or on uterine activity in spontaneous normal labour.

Observations during the first stage of labour (defined from the time of admission to the labour ward to full dilatation of the cervix) show that the rate of cervical dilatation is composed of two phases. Following a slow 'latent' phase of labour during which the length of the cervix shortens from 3 cm to less than 0.5 cm (effacement) and dilates to 3 cm, there is a faster 'active phase', when the cervix dilates from 3 cm to full dilatation (conventionally taken as 10 cm because of the presenting diameters of the well-flexed vertex presentation of 9.5 × 9.5 cm, although in reality it refers to a situation when no cervix is palpable). In order to identify women at risk of prolonged labour, a line of acceptable progress is drawn on the partogram, i.e. the *alert line*. If the rate of cervical dilatation falls to the right of this line, progress is deemed unsatisfactory. The line of acceptable progress has conventionally been based on the slowest tenth percentile rate of cervical dilatation

> **Latent phase**: The length of the cervix shortens from 3 cm to less than 0.5 cm and dilates to 3 cm.
>
> **Active phase**: The cervix dilates from 3 cm to full dilatation.

> The latent phase may last for up to eight hours in nulliparas and up to six hours in multiparas.

observed in women who progress without intervention and deliver normally; in other words, 1 cm per hour. However, a certain grace period is given before intervention and is based on a line drawn parallel and one to four hours to the right of this (*action line*). Accordingly, the proportion of labours deemed to have unsatisfactory progress needing intervention can vary from 5 per cent to 50 per cent. In the presence of good contractions (at least > 2 in 10 minutes, lasting > 40 seconds), the latent phase may last for up to eight hours in nulliparas and up to six hours in multiparas. During the peak of the active phase of labour, the cervix dilates at a rate of 1 cm per hour in both nulliparas and multiparas (Hendricks et al 1970). Multiparas appear to dilate faster because they have shorter labours overall; not only do they have a shorter latent phase resulting in a more advanced cervical dilatation on admission, they have an increased rate of progress as full dilatation approaches. Construction of nomograms of anticipated normal progress or 'alert' lines with the addition of 'action' lines to the right of this, reduces the likelihood of prolonged labour being overlooked and is of considerable diagnostic and educational value (Fig. 2.1).

## Diagnosis of Labour

The accurate diagnosis of labour at term may be difficult, and can be even more difficult in those labouring before term. If the contractions are painful and regular and if the cervix is > 3 cm dilated (in other words, in the active phase), there is little difficulty in diagnosing labour. However, if the patient is in the latent phase of labour, it may be necessary to perform two examinations at least two hours apart (and preferably done by the same examiner), in order to detect any progressive cervical change and diagnose labour.

## Prelabour

This is the period of a few weeks before active labour, during which time increased uterine activity is noticed. It leads to the softening of the cervix, expansion of the isthmus and supravaginal cervix allowing formation of the lower segment. In the final days of prelabour, the mean cervical dilatation in nulliparas is 1.8 cm and 2.2 cm in multiparas (Hendricks et al 1970).

## 'False' or 'Spurious' Labour

Uterine contractions without effacement and dilatation of the cervix occur in the third trimester. They are usually termed Braxton-Hicks contractions and are painless. These contractions may become more frequent and painful without affecting cervical changes of effacement and dilatation and may abate spontaneously. Clinical experience is that this is more likely to occur in multiparas. Differentiating points between false and true labour are shown in Table 2.1.

Good antecedents for 'natural' or 'physiological' labour and childbirth are antepartum education that eliminates fear and anxieties about labour, regular exercise to promote relaxation, muscle control and breathing without hyperventilation throughout labour. In addition, the importance of one-to-one attention from a skilled professional attendant throughout labour to comfort the mother and give her constant reassurance has been stressed time and time again.

In the 1960s, a protocol for the active management of labour was established in

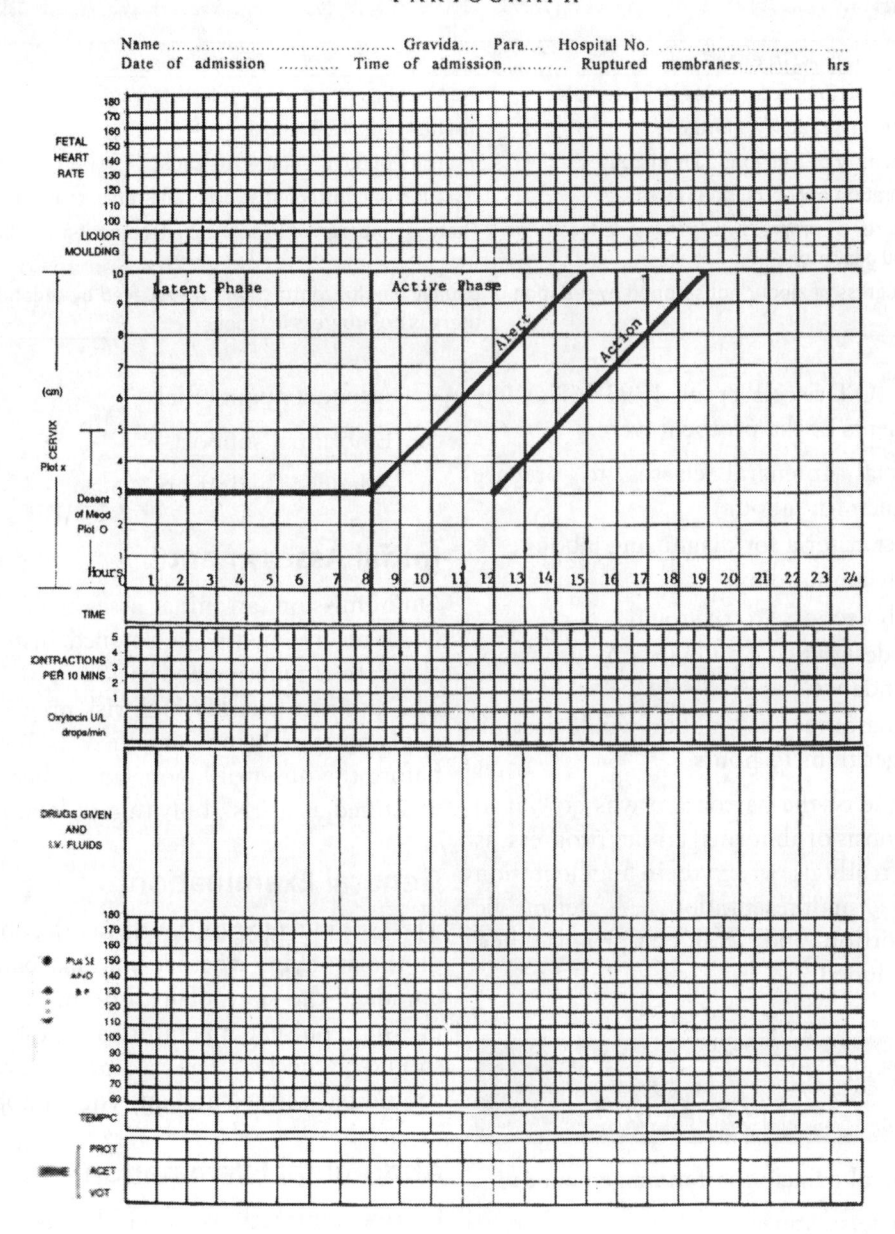

**Figure 2.1** WHO partograph showing alert and action lines in the latent and active phase of labour. Cervical dilatation, descent of head, fetal parameters (FHR, colour of liquor, caput and moulding), maternal parameters (pulse, blood pressure, results of urine tests and drugs used) can be entered.

**Table 2.1** Differences between true and false Labour

|   | True labour | False labour |
|---|---|---|
| 1. | Contractions occur at regular intervals | Contractions occur at irregular intervals |
| 2. | Interval gradually shortens | Interval remains irregular |
| 3. | Intensity of pain gradually increases | Intensity of pain remains the same |
| 4. | Duration of contractions increases | Duration of contractions varies and tends to become less |
| 5. | There is progressive cervical effacement and dilatation | There is no progress in cervical effacement and dilatation |
| 6. | Progress of labour not stopped by sedation | Usually painful contractions are relieved by sedation and there is no progress in labour |

Dublin (O'Driscoll et al 1993). The key components of the protocol were:
- Special antenatal classes to prepare women for labour
- Strict criteria for diagnosing labour
- Early amniotomy
- Early recourse to oxytocin
- A designated midwife in constant attendance
- A guarantee that labour would last no longer than 12 hours

The use of the partogram was crucial to the diagnosis of abnormal labour progress, as was the ready use of oxytocin augmentation once malpresentation, fetopelvic disproportion and fetal compromise had been excluded.

## Management of the First Stage of Labour

The general principles of management are:
1. Initial assessment
2. Observation and intervention if labour becomes abnormal
3. Close monitoring of the fetal and maternal condition
4. Adequate pain relief
5. Emotional support
6. Adequate hydration

### Initial Assessment

On admission, an initial assessment should be done by eliciting a detailed history, by clinical examination and basic investigations. The aim is to identify high-risk pregnancies: a proportion being identified as high-risk before the onset of labour and others being identified as at-risk only during labour.

### General Examination

This should include the general condition of the woman, whether she has pallor or jaundice; the state of hydration, her blood pressure, pulse, temperature and respiration should be checked. The cardiovascular status should be assessed and any edema noted.

### Abdominal Examination

Uterine contractions should be assessed by palpation, with relevance to their frequency and duration over a 10-minute period (Fig. 2.2). The fundal height should be measured to identify babies that may be significantly above or below the average

## The Management of the First Stage of Labour

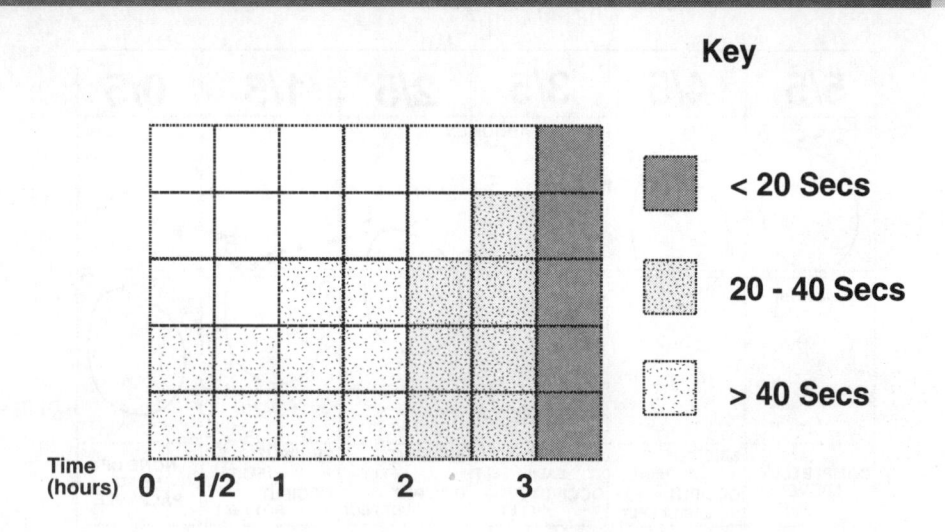

**Key**

▨ < 20 Secs

▦ 20 - 40 Secs

░ > 40 Secs

Time (hours)   0   1/2   1   2   3

**Figure 2.2** Quantification of uterine contractions by clinical palpation. Frequency per 10 min is recorded by shading the equivalent number of boxes. The type of shading indicates the duration of each contraction.

birthweight, and the level of the presenting part should be noted. The level of the head should be estimated in 'fifths' of head palpable above the pelvic brim (Fig. 2.3) because it excludes variation due to excessive caput and moulding and also variation produced by different depths of pelvis. It is easily reproducible. The fetal heart rate should be auscultated after a contraction for a minimum period of one minute, and at least every 15 minutes in the first stage and every five minutes in the second stage of labour (RCOG 2001a).

> The fetal heart rate should be auscultated
> - after a contraction for a minimum period of one minute
> - at least every 15 minutes in the first stage
> - every five minutes in the second stage of labour

### Vaginal Examination

The following points should be noted during vaginal examination:

- Any abnormal discharge from the vagina; evidence of ruptured membranes
- The colour and quantity of any amniotic fluid and whether it is clear, bloodstained or contains meconium
- Consistency, position, effacement and dilatation of the cervix
- The presenting part in relation to the ischial spines and caput or moulding of the head (station)
- The position of the presenting part
- The bony pelvis should be assessed with regard to its adequacy for childbirth

### Investigations

The urine should be examined for protein, ketones and sugar. Some commercial urinalysis 'stix' will also test for leukocytes, nitrites and blood. Their presence may signify a urinary tract infection. If it has not been checked recently, blood should be tested for hemoglobin and grouped and typed.

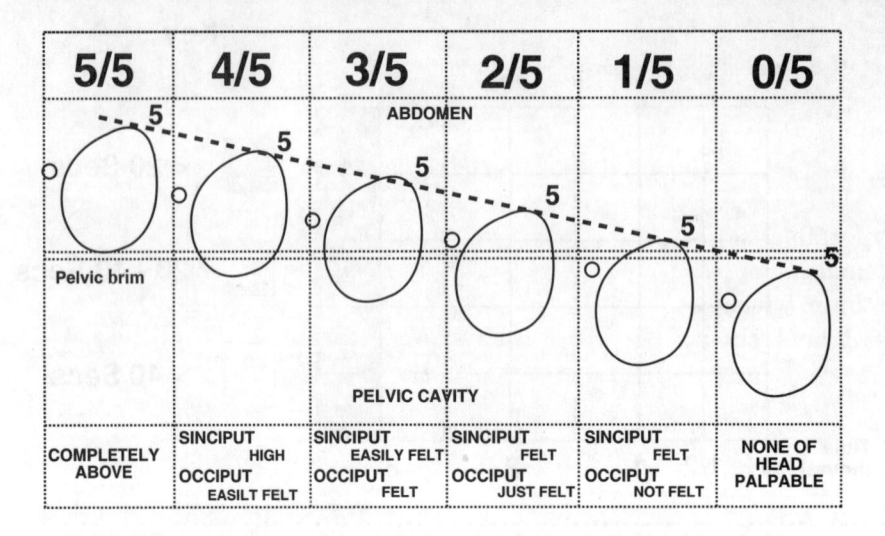

|  5/5  |  4/5  |  3/5  |  2/5  |  1/5  |  0/5  |
|---|---|---|---|---|---|
| COMPLETELY ABOVE | SINCIPUT HIGH / OCCIPUT EASILY FELT | SINCIPUT EASILY FELT / OCCIPUT FELT | SINCIPUT FELT / OCCIPUT JUST FELT | SINCIPUT FELT / OCCIPUT NOT FELT | NONE OF HEAD PALPABLE |

**Figure 2.3** Clinical estimation of descent of head in fifths palpable above the pelvic brim

Oral intake is often restricted in labour to reduce the risk of gastric aspiration and Mendelson's syndrome should general anesthesia be required. Fasting does not guarantee that the stomach will be empty but lowers the pH of the residual gastric fluid and contributes to dehydration and ketosis, necessitating intravenous rehydration. In order to reduce the chances of ketosis, many units in the UK now allow low risk women in normal labour to have oral fluids and an increasing number also permit low-residue solid food. Allowing women to eat in labour prevents the development of ketosis; it significantly increases residual gastric volume and is more likely to be associated with vomiting (Scrutton et al 1999). Isotonic high-calorie drinks might maintain nutrition and hydration, while minimising gastric volume.

> Low-risk women in normal labour may be allowed to have oral fluids. This avoids dehydration and ketosis.

In developing countries, many women are admitted to hospital with prolonged labour or with obstructed labour. They need to be rehydrated. Intravenous antibiotics may be necessary. Five per cent dextrose is used commonly, but it is best to give normal saline or Hartman's solution, to maintain a more physiological fluid and electrolyte balance. This may also help to avoid water intoxication if intravenous oxytocin is used over a long period in high dose.

> In prolonged labour or obstructed labour, rehydration is best accomplished with saline or Hartman's solution.

## Mobility and Posture in Labour

It is preferable not to confine the mother to bed in early labour. She may prefer ambulation or sitting in a chair and there is some evidence that an upright posture may increase the pelvic diameters and assist descent of the fetal head. Although many women prefer to be ambulatory early in labour, few remain upright for long and most will wish to lie down as labour progresses. In bed, she may assume the position that is most comfortable: sitting, reclining or the lateral recumbent position. Other than the dorsal position, which can cause aortocaval compression and should be discouraged, the actual position the mother chooses is probably unimportant, since there is no effect on the mode of delivery or analgesia requirement (MacLennan et al 1994; Bloom et al 1998).

## Use of Analgesia and Anesthesia

Analgesia or anesthesia is initiated on the basis of discomfort and pain. The type of analgesia to be used and the dose and frequency of administration are based to a considerable degree on the anticipated interval of time to delivery, the woman's preference, the availability of different modalities of pain relief and the experience of the medical attendants.

In the UK, the four most widely used forms of pain relief for labour are transcutaneous electronic nerve stimulation (TENS), nitrous oxide (Entonox), intramuscular narcotics (e.g.pethidine) and epidural analgesia.

A brief description of some analgesic and anesthetic agents is given below; a more detailed account is given in Chapter 3, on Pain Relief in Labour.

### Systemic analgesia

These include:

a. Sedatives and hypnotics: butobarbitone and phenobarbitone

b. Tranquilisers: phenothiazines (promazine, chlorpromazine, promethazine), diazepam and meprobamate

c. Narcotic analgesia: pethidine hydrochloride, pentazocine or morphine

> There is insufficient evidence to recommend one type of narcotic analgesia over another.

Newer drugs include salbuphine and butarphanol.

The narcotic drugs usually last for 2–4 hours and tend to be more effective as sedatives rather than as analgesics. At the moment, there is insufficient evidence to recommend one type of narcotic analgesia over another (Elbourne and Wiseman 2002).

### Inhalational analgesia

The most commonly used agent is Entonox a 50:50 mixture of nitrous oxide and oxygen. Other agents include flurane and trichloroethylene.

### Local analgesia

These drugs produce a temporary block of pain impulses along the appropriate nerves. The most commonly used drugs are lignocaine and bupivicain, although new combinations and admixtures are being developed.

The following blocks are used in obstetrics:

a. Perineal infiltration prior to performing an episiotomy

b. A pudendal block prior to outlet instrumental deliveries

c. A caudal block prior to instrumental deliveries

d. A lumbar epidural

The anesthetic technique that provides the greatest pain relief in labour is the epidural block. It provides segmental anesthesia, which works in all stages of labour. It has the additional advantage that cesarean sections or manual removal of the placenta can be performed without additional anesthesia. However, skilled and trained personnel are required to administer epidural anesthesia. Further, epidural anesthesia is associated with longer second stage of labour and an increased incidence of malposition, leading to higher rates of instrumental delivery (Howell 2002).

> Epidural block provides the greatest pain relief in labour but requires skilled and trained personnel for administration.

## Meconium

Meconium may be demonstrated in the fetal gut in the first trimester, but in utero passage is rare before 34 weeks. The incidence of meconium staining of the amniotic fluid (MSAF) increases as term approaches and may reflect fetal gut maturity (Becker et al 1940). The incidence of meconium passage in labour also increases with gestational age, and is much more common in post-date pregnancies, with a reported incidence of 44 per cent at delivery (Knox et al 1979). However, the passage of meconium in labour may have a more sinister explanation and an association between meconium passage in utero and poor neonatal outcome was recognised by Aristotle.

The appearance of fresh meconium in labour should prompt a search for evidence to confirm fetal well-being, such as fetal heart rate monitoring or fetal scalp blood sampling. This is particularly true for thick meconium, since this implies that there is little liquor to dilute the meconium, and this itself may indicate placental problems before the onset of labour. Thin meconium, on the other hand, is thin because it has been diluted in an adequate volume of liquor. In the presence of a normal fetal heart rate, meconium staining of the amniotic fluid is not an indication for immediate delivery or fetal blood sampling, especially if it is thin staining. However, if the heart rate becomes pathological in association with thick fresh meconium, early delivery should be considered, particularly in high-risk pregnancies.

> Thin meconium, in the presence of a normal fetal heart rate, is not an indication for immediate delivery or fetal blood sampling.

## Diagnosis of Poor Progress of Labour

Progress in labour is confirmed by observing the progressive effacement and dilatation of the cervix and the descent of the presenting part. The frequency and duration of uterine contractions is also recorded on the partogram. The maternal condition is monitored by observing the pulse, blood pressure, temperature and hydration at regular intervals throughout the labour. In addition, the use of anesthetic or oxytocic drugs should be recorded.

Fetal monitoring is by observation of the fetal heart rate at regular intervals. A gradual increase in the baseline FHR or prolonged bradycardias are non-reassuring signs. The character of the amniotic fluid is also important. Thick (grade 3) meconium with scanty fluid or fresh passage of meconium in labour, or the absence of amniotic fluid at the time of membrane rupture is also suggestive of possible hypoxia.

The use of a partogram for the management of labour facilitates the early detection of abnormal labour progress and identifies those women most likely to require intervention (WHO 1994). This can be used at all levels of obstetric care by basic care providers who have been trained to assess cervical dilatation. When used properly, it helps to detect abnormal labour progress promptly, allowing timely intervention.

In a WHO multicentre trial in southeast Asia involving over 35,000 women, the introduction of the partograph as part of an agreed labour management protocol was associated with a reduction in prolonged labour (from 6.4 to 3.4 per cent) and the proportion of labours requiring augmentation (from 20.7 to 9.1 per cent). The cesarean section rates also fell from 9.9 to 8.3 per cent and intrapartum stillbirths from 0.5 to 0.3 per cent. There were also improvements in fetal and maternal morbidity in both nulliparous and multiparous women (WHO 1994).

The term *dystocia* or difficult labour refers to poor progress of labour and is diagnosed when the rate of cervical dilatation is slower than anticipated. When a woman is admitted in the active phase of labour, the cervical dilatation can be plotted on the partogram and an expected progress or alert line can be constructed, usually corresponding to 1 cm per hour. Another line, the action line, can be added one to four hours to the right of the alert line and parallel to it. Alternatively, a commercially available stencil may be used to add the alert line.

The outcome of spontaneous labours has been studied and three distinct patterns of abnormal progress described (Studd et al 1975; Cardozo et al 1982; Gibb et al 1982). These are:

- Prolonged latent phase
- Primary dysfunctional labour and
- Secondary arrest of cervical dilatation

The latent phase is usually considered prolonged if it is more than eight hours in a nullipara and six hours in a multipara. Once established in the active phase of labour, primary dysfunctional labour is diagnosed when the progress falls to the right of the nomogram. If labour progresses normally in the early active phase but the cervix fails to dilate or dilates slowly thereafter, secondary arrest of cervical dilatation is diagnosed (Fig. 2.4). More than one of these abnormal labour patterns may occur in the same patient, since they frequently share a common etiology.

> The latent phase is usually considered prolonged if it is more than eight hours in a nullipara and six hours in a multipara.

> Secondary arrest of cervical dilatation: Labour progresses normally in the early active phase but the cervix fails to dilate or dilates slowly.

The use of the partogram with the anticipated progress line for an individual patient annotated allows the prompt recognition of abnormal cervical progress. The descent of the presenting part as a proportion of the presenting part (expressed as fifths) palpable abdominally is also an integral component of the partogram, and it too is plotted at each review. A poor rate of descent may also be an indication of developing mechanical problems in the labour. Poor progress has

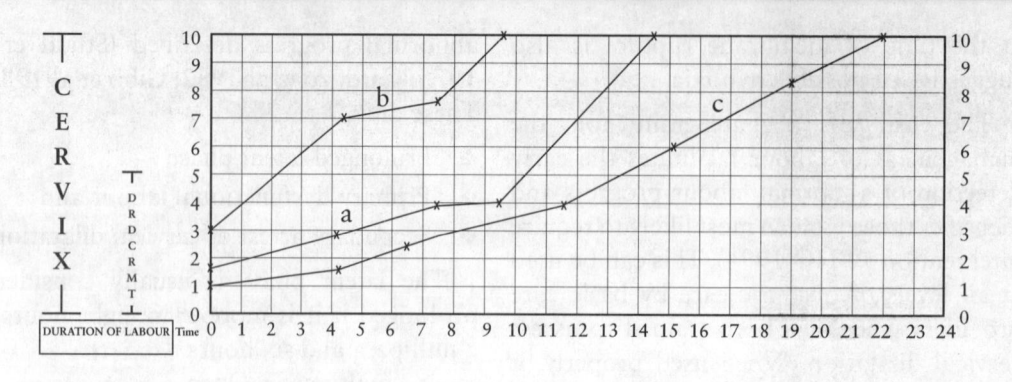

**Figure 2.4** Various forms of dysfunctional labour: (a) prolonged latent phase (b) secondary arrest of labour (c) prolonged latent phase and primary dysfunctional labour

conventionally been related to the three Ps, namely:

- Powers – the adequacy of the uterine contractions
- Passages – the resistance of the birth canal
- Passenger – relating to the size, position, degree of flexion, etc. of the baby

A fourth 'P' can be added to these, namely, poor practice.

Poor progress in labour does not identify the specific cause (that is, fault with the powers, passage or passenger) since these are frequently interrelated.

Primary dysfunctional labour (PDL) is the commonest abnormality of the first stage of labour, occurring in up to 25 per cent of spontaneous primigravid labours (Cardozo et al 1982), and 8 per cent of multiparas (Gibb et al 1982). The commonest cause is inadequate uterine activity. Secondary arrest of cervical dilatation (SACD) is much less common than the above, and is said to affect 6 per cent of nulliparas, and only 2 per cent of multiparas.

Although the commonest cause of SACD (especially in nulliparas) is still inefficient uterine activity, disproportion is far more likely to be the explanation than with PDL. However, secondary arrest does not always indicate cephalopelvic disproportion, as inadequate uterine contractions can be corrected, resulting in spontaneous vaginal delivery (Arulkumaran et al 1987). Nevertheless, a diagnosis of secondary arrest (especially in a multiparous woman) should prompt a search for obvious problems in the passenger (for example, hydrocephalus, brow presentation, undiagnosed shoulder presentation, large baby) and the passages (for example, a congenitally small pelvis, a deformed pelvis due to an accident or masses in the pelvis). Unfavourable pelvic diameters are a cause of cephalopelvic

> Secondary arrest of descent may be an indication of developing mechanical problems in the labour.

> Secondary arrest of cervical dilatation especially in nulliparas is commonly due to:
> - inefficient uterine activity
> - cephalopelvic disproportion

disproportion, but less common in the developed world, where better nutritional standards usually prevail. However, the fetus is more commonly the cause of relative disproportion by presenting a larger diameter of the vertex due to a malposition or deflexion, or both. In such cases, the dystocia may be overcome if the flexion and rotation to an occipito-anterior position can be encouraged by efficient uterine contractions.

## Management Options

## Augmentation

### Indications

Prolonged labour is associated with high rates of maternal infection, obstructed labour, uterine rupture and postpartum hemorrhage which may all end in maternal mortality.

> Prolonged labour may be associated with:
> - maternal infection
> - obstructed labour
> - uterine rupture
> - postpartum hemorrhage

In many areas of the developing world, it remains a common axiom 'not to allow the sun to set twice on a woman in labour', in order to prevent such tragic outcomes. Philpott (1972) in Africa, O'Driscoll et al (1973) in Dublin, and Studd (1973) in the UK all advocated and popularised the concept of augmentation to reduce the incidence of prolonged labour.

The active management of labour was based on the principle of anticipating and identifying that there may be a problem and then taking action. Increasing the uterine power, which was the common problem, is one of the many components of the policy of active management. It also helped to overcome any borderline disproportion by promoting flexion, rotation and moulding in vertex presentation.

The other components of active management included one-to-one midwifery care, reassurance, pain relief, hydration and fetomaternal surveillance. It was designed to prevent prolonged labour in nulliparas, and was also proposed as an approach to reduce the CS rate.

In the 1980s, the CS rate of the National Maternity Hospital in Dublin was only 4.8 per cent, nearly a third of the rates observed in units from the USA. Despite this difference, the neonatal mortality rate in Ireland was similar to that in the United States. Based on randomised control studies, it appears that active management of labour shortens the length of labour without affecting the rate of cesarean section or maternal or fetal morbidity (Lopez-Zeno et al 1992; Frigoletto et al 1995; Sadler et al 2000). Experience with active management as practised by the Dublin school demonstrated that 98 per cent of labours did not extend beyond 12 hours from the time of onset of labour (O'Driscoll et al 1984). Which particular component of the 'active management' protocol is most important remains contentious, though companionship in labour and continuity of care during pregnancy and childbirth does seem to be particularly helpful (Hodnett 2002).

The decision to augment labour should be governed by the rate of cervical dilatation based on the partogram; minor degrees of disproportion due to malposition and poor flexion of the head may be overcome by oxytocin infusion. Gross disproportion or malpresentation should be excluded. More forceful uterine contractions cause flexion at the atlanto-occipital joint and reduce the presenting diameter. This allows rotation of the occiput from a posterior to an anterior position. The increased force of contraction also helps moulding (a sign of mechanical compression), reduces the presenting diameter of the head and helps to increase the pelvic dimensions due to the descending head widening the sacroiliac and symphysis pubic joints.

*Moulding* is a process whereby the parietal, occipital and frontal bones of the skull first come together (moulding +). This is followed by one parietal bone going under the other and the occipital and frontal bones going below the parietal bones. Gentle digital pressure is adequate to reduce the overlapping of the bones (moulding ++). As mechanical compression increases, the moulding becomes more severe (moulding +++) and digital pressure will no longer restore the overlapping bones to their original position. *Caput* is the soft tissue swelling caused by the edema of the scalp that develops as the fetal head descends in the pelvis. The degree of caput increases in prolonged labour, though it is a less reliable sign of mechanical obstruction than moulding.

> **Moulding +**
> - parietal, occipital and frontal bones of the skull come together
>
> **Moulding ++**
> - overlapping of the bones occurs but gentle digital pressure is adequate to reduce the overlapping of the bones
>
> **Moulding +++**
> - moulding becomes more severe and digital pressure will not reduce the overlapping of the bones

## When to Augment Labour

The mechanical 'efficiency' of uterine contractions should be defined in terms of their clinical effect, which is the progress of cervical dilatation and descent of the head, and not in relation to the magnitude of uterine contractions.

Labour progress is observed with a wide range of uterine activity in both nulliparas and multiparas (Gibb et al 1984; O'Driscoll et al 1993). The more rapid the rate of progress for a given level of uterine activity, the more 'efficient' the contractions. It is important to recognise the difference between inefficient uterine activity and 'incoordinate' contractions. Inefficiency is the failure of the uterus to work in such a way that the labour progress is normal. Poor uterine activity can be demonstrated when cervimetric progress is abnormal even in the absence of disproportion or malposition (although both of these often coexist with inefficient uterine activity). Incoordinate uterine action is a descriptive term for the tocographic tracings (Figs. 2.5 and 2.6). Most records of uterine contractions will show some degree of irregularity, but they need not necessarily be associated with abnormal labour progress. Therefore the decision to augment labour should be governed primarily by the dynamic effects of the uterine activity, i.e., by the rate of cervical dilatation after disproportion and malpresentation have been excluded. The issue of whether oxytocin augmentation is

> Inefficient uterine contractions:
> - failure of labour to progress (dilatation or descent)
>
> Incoordinate uterine action
> - descriptive term for abnormal contractions on the tocographic tracings

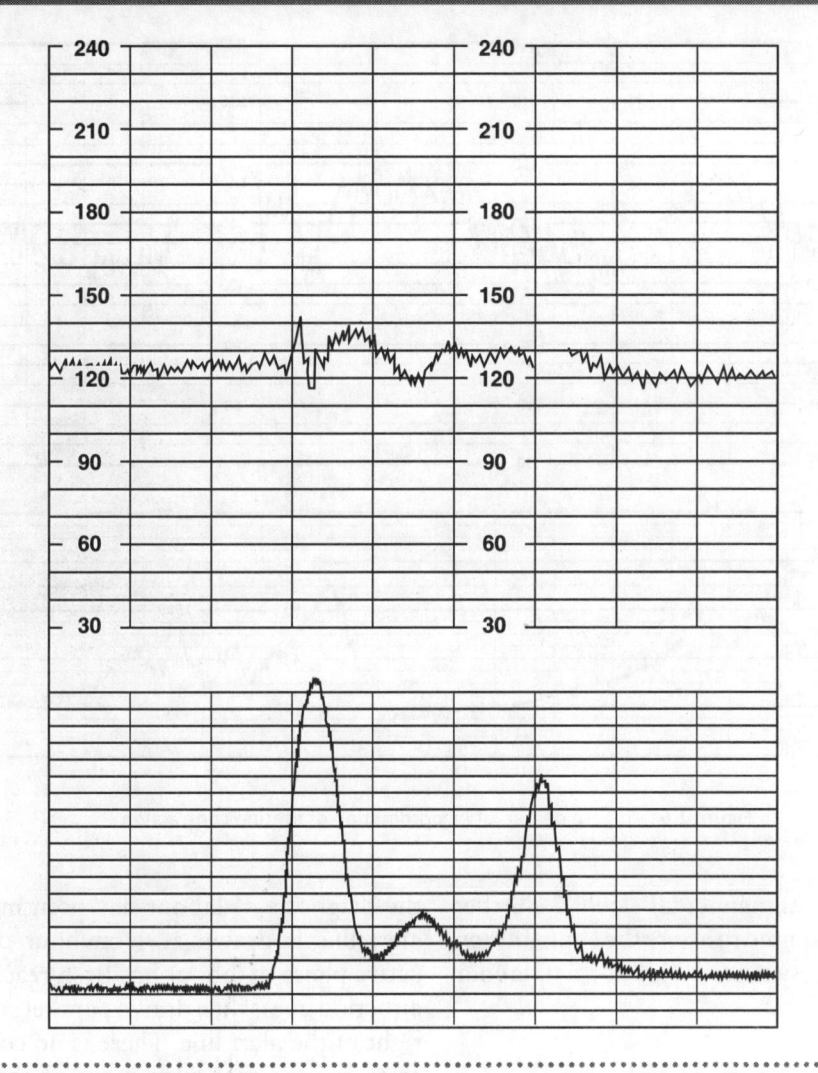

**Figure 2.5** Mild degree of incoordination of uterine contractions

appropriate in the presence of slow progress but apparently normal contractions, as demonstrated by intrauterine pressure measurement, needs further elucidation.

Traditionally, the active management of labour has sought to improve the outcome by enhancing the uterine contractions with oxytocin. However, a significant proportion of labours augmented for abnormal progress still result in cesarean section, implying that other factors are important. A recent in vivo study suggested that cervical smooth muscle activity contributed to the duration of the latent phase (Pajntar et al 2001). Other researchers have drawn attention to the importance of the head-to-cervix relationship, linking this to the intrauterine pressures developed during labour (Gough

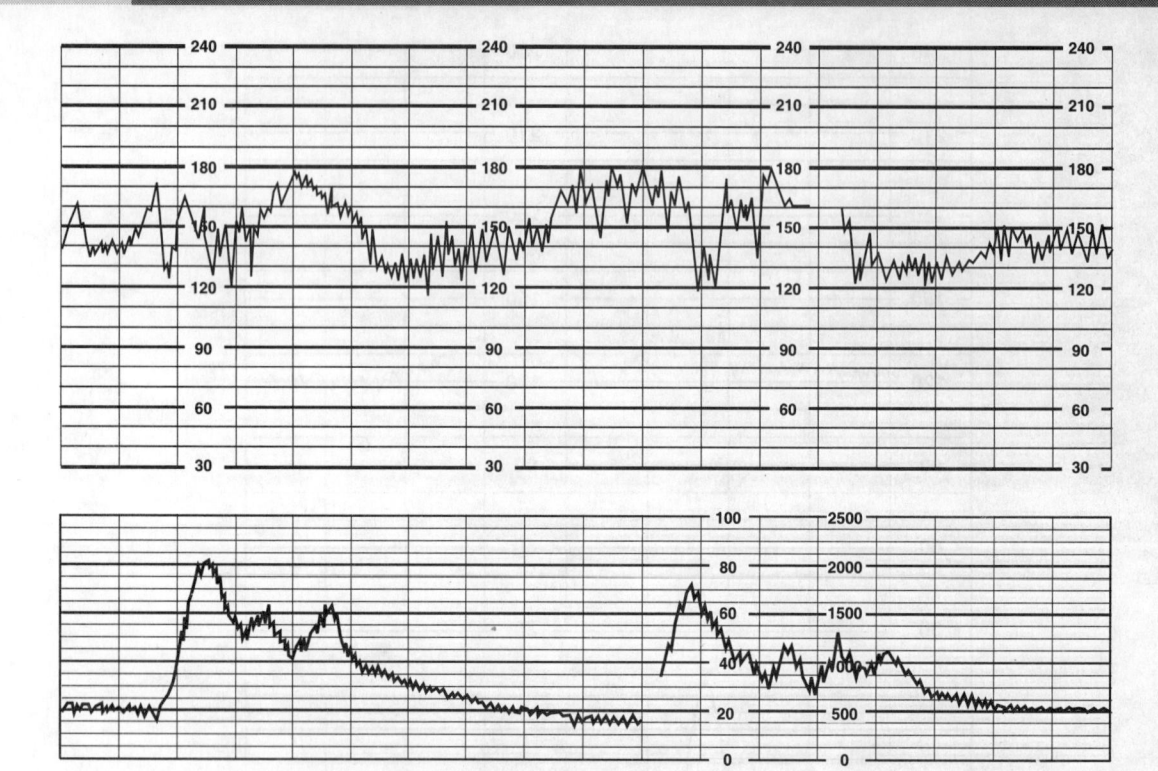

Figure 2.6 Severe degree of incoordination of uterine contraction

et al 1990; Allman et al 1996). Further research is required to assess the contribution of cervical resistance to abnormal labour progress.

## Practical Aspects of Labour Management

The diagnosis of active labour is dependent on a careful cervical assessment to define dilatation, effacement, consistency, position and station of the head. These are more important than 'soft' indicators such as regular contractions, show, or even amniotic membrane rupture.

On admission, the cervical dilatation should be plotted on the partogram, provided the diagnosis of labour has been made. An alert line is drawn at 1 cm/hour once the active phase of labour has been reached and an action line is then drawn parallel and to the right of the alert line. There is no consensus as to the 'correct' placement of the action line, whether it should be 1, 2, 3 or 4 hours to the right of the alert line, and different centres use different intervals. Modifying factors include the level of nursing and medical care available for the supervision of labour once oxytocin has been commenced, the risk of complications associated with prolonged labour (likely to be higher in the more disadvantaged communities) and social factors. For example, in many of the developed countries, there is a consumer demand for 'natural childbirth', which generally means avoiding all intervention unless it becomes unavoidable.

The actual presence of the action line on the partogram is more important than the precise time interval between it and the alert line. Its presence prompts action if labour progress falls to the right of that projected line. When action is needed, amniotomy alone may suffice to correct slow progress in some cases (see below), although oxytocin will be necessary if poor progress is maintained after amniotomy.

## Augmentation in the Latent Phase of Labour

The duration of the latent phase of labour varies widely and is a period when the diagnosis of labour can be difficult. Appreciable proportions of women have painful contractions for long periods in the latent phase with little cervical change. These contractions may subside and labour may fail to establish, leading to a sense of disappointment, frustration, and frequently, demoralisation. Despite this, the management of the latent phase, once maternal and fetal well-being has been confirmed, consists of explanation, reassurance, hydration, nutrition and ambulation.

> Management of the latent phase:
> • explanation
> • reassurance
> • hydration
> • nutrition
> • ambulation

The mainstay of management of the prolonged latent phase is to avoid unnecessary intervention. The decision to augment in the latent phase should be based on clear medical or obstetric indications, since augmentation with an unfavourable cervix is associated with a high risk of cesarean section. However, when the woman has been experiencing frequent, painful but apparently fruitless contractions for a long time, some action has to be taken. In these circumstances, augmentation may be appropriate.

> Augmentation in the latent phase, with an unfavourable cervix, is associated with a high risk of cesarean section and so should be avoided.

## Augmentation in the Active Phase of Labour

The decision to augment labour in the active phase is based on the observed progress of labour from the time the active phase is diagnosed. Most women are admitted in the active phase with cervical dilatation > 3 cm. The expected progress line or 'alert line' can be drawn at 1 cm/hour on the partogram.

O'Driscoll et al (1993) augment labour when the progress is to the right of this alert line, whereas most advocate augmentation only when the progress has deviated to the right of the 'action line' drawn one to four hours parallel to the alert line.

By allowing a 'period of grace', fewer women will require augmentation: 55 per cent of nulliparas with no period of grace (O'Driscoll et al 1973) compared to 19 per cent of women given a two hour period of grace (Arulkumaran et al 1987). Both methods of management yield comparable results, although prompt intervention does decrease the duration of labour and may be more appropriate when labour ward staffing is adequate and/or when bed strength is limited.

For women in favour of 'natural childbirth' who hope to avoid intervention, the action line may be drawn three or four hours to the right of the alert line, since the obstetric outcomes are similar. The WHO study with the action line drawn three hours to the right of the alert line showed a reduction in prolonged labour and cesarean section rates (WHO 1994).

> When the action line is drawn three hours to the right of the alert line, there is a reduction in prolonged labour and cesarean section rates (WHO 1994).

## Role of Artificial Rupture of the Membranes (ARM)

Artificial rupture of the membranes need not be performed as a routine. Once the active phase has started, that is, when the cervix is dilated more than 3 cm, the membranes may be ruptured and such a policy of early amniotomy leads to a reduction, on average, of between one and two hours in the duration of labour, and also to a reduction in the incidence of dystocia (Fraser et al 2002). However, it does not lower the rate of cesarean section or operative vaginal deliveries and a policy of routine amniotomy is not normally recommended (The UK Amniotomy Group 1994).

> Early amniotomy leads to:
> - reduction in the duration of labour
> - reduction in the incidence of dystocia

When ARM is not routinely performed, there are some occasions when it is indicated:

- ❖ To enhance uterine contractions when labour progress is abnormal
- ❖ To assess the volume and nature of the liquor in a high-risk labour, especially if the fetal heart rate pattern is abnormal
- ❖ To attach a fetal scalp electrode to get a better fetal heart rate trace or insert an intrauterine pressure catheter or
- ❖ When the patient specifically requests it.

ARM does have some drawbacks. When the presenting part is high there is a chance of cord prolapse, and if labour becomes unduly prolonged, the risk of infection is increased. Further, there is also an increased rate of fetal heart rate abnormalities (Goffinet et al 1997).

## Oxytocin Dosage and Time Increment Schedules

Oxytocin receptors in the uterus increase during pregnancy and labour, so that the uterus may be sensitive to very small doses of administered oxytocin (Fuchs et al 1984). The drug is best titrated in an arithmetical or geometric manner starting from a low dose. Oxytocin is often administered by gravity fed drips, which are unreliable and potentially unsafe. Overdosage may lead to uterine hyperstimulation and fetal distress, while a suboptimal dose may lead to failure to progress in labour, resulting in unnecessary intervention. The dangers of uncontrolled infusions to the fetus (Liston and Campbell 1974) and to the mother (Daw 1973) are well documented. Ideally, intravenous oxytocin should be administered using a peristaltic infusion pump.

Published protocols vary widely in terms of the oxytocin dilution, the starting dose and the rate of increase. Frequently, the protocols used for the induction of labour have been adapted for augmentation of labour, although the scientific validity of this has not been adequately tested. Early recommendations were based on in vitro pharmacological studies in which the half-life of oxytocin was thought to be 3-4 minutes (Fuchs and Fuchs 1984). However, in vivo studies suggest that the half-life of oxytocin is, in fact, 10-15 minutes (Seitchik et al 1984). Continuous intravenous infusion of oxytocin also shows first-order kinetics, with a progressive stepwise increase. With every increase in infusion rate, a steady plasma concentration is reached 40-60 minutes after the alteration of an infusion. A shorter increment interval results in the dose being increased before maximum plasma levels are reached. These findings, together with medicolegal concerns following cases of uterine hyperstimulation with oxytocin have prompted a closer study of the various oxytocin regimens.

In their recent guideline on 'Induction of Labour', The Royal College of Obstetricians and Gynaecologists recommended the regimen given in table 2.2 (RCOG 2001b).

## Achievement of Optimal Uterine Activity

There remains a dearth of literature regarding the level of uterine activity that should be produced by oxytocin titration to produce a good obstetric outcome. It has been suggested that the use of intrauterine pressure catheters may identify those who are most likely to need a cesarean section for failure to progress (Reddi et al 1988). It is known that active contraction area measurements using an intrauterine pressure catheter correlate better with the rate of cervical dilatation than the frequency or amplitude of contractions. Despite this, there is little evidence that using an intrauterine pressure catheter to measure uterine activity or using oxytocin titration to achieve a preset active contraction area profile is associated with a better obstetric outcome in augmented labours, compared with an oxytocin infusion titrated against

**Table 2.2** RCOG guidelines for induction of labour (2001)

| Time after starting (min) | Oxytocin dose (mU/min) | Volume infused (ml/hour) Dilution 30 IU Oxytocin in 500 ml normal saline | Volume infused (ml/hour) Dilution 10 IU Oxytocin in 500 ml normal saline |
|---|---|---|---|
| 0 | 1 | 1 | 3 |
| 30 | 2 | 2 | 6 |
| 60 | 4 | 4 | 12 |
| 90 | 8 | 8 | 24 |
| 120 | 12 | 12 | 36 |
| 150 | 16 | 16 | 48 |
| 180 | 20 | 20 | 60 |
| 210 | 24 | 24 | 72 |
| 240 | 28 | 28 | 84 |
| 270 | 32 | 32 | 96 |

the frequency of contractions (Arulkumaran et al 1989b).

In most centres, facilities to monitor the uterine activity with pressure catheters are not available. The uterine activity has to be judged clinically, on the basis of the frequency and duration of the palpated contractions. In a prospective study of women in whom disproportion had been excluded, two-thirds of women who failed to progress had two or fewer contractions in 10 minutes, while the remaining third had an 'optimal' contraction frequency of one in 3 minutes, over a period of four hours. In the latter group, oxytocin titration to achieve a contraction frequency of four in 10 minutes with each contraction lasting > 40 seconds was associated with the vaginal delivery of babies in good condition in 96 per cent (Arulkumaran et al 1991). This suggests that three contractions in 10 minutes is an appropriate target uterine activity with oxytocin titration, but if there is no progress with this frequency of contractions, the oxytocin dose may be increased to achieve a frequency of four or five in 10 minutes, provided the fetal heart rate is normal.

> Three contractions in 10 minutes is an appropriate target uterine activity with oxytocin titration.

## The Measurement of Uterine Contractions

The frequency of contractions can be assessed by either external or internal tocography. Some centres use intrauterine pressure catheters when oxytocin is administered because they feel that hyperstimulation of the uterus can be identified early and the oxytocin infusion rate adjusted accordingly, in the hope that this will improve the neonatal outcome. However, excessively frequent contractions can also be identified by external tocography. A prospective randomised study did not show a better obstetric outcome when intrauterine catheters were used in augmented labour, compared with external tocography (Chua et al 1990). Therefore, in a busy clinical practice, it is far easier, less invasive, cheaper and perfectly appropriate to assess uterine contractions using external tocography. On the other hand, in certain high-risk cases (such as pregnancies complicated by intrauterine growth restriction, or in those practices where medicolegal concerns are important), there are theoretical advantages to using intrauterine pressure catheters. In addition, internal tocography can be valuable in very obese women, where external tocography is less reliable. This is a particular benefit, given the increased rates of dysfunctional labour in overweight women (Johnson et al 1992).

The use of intrauterine pressure catheters has also been recommended in women with a previous cesarean section who are being augmented for poor labour progress. A sudden decline in uterine activity may indicate scar rupture, which may or may not be associated with scar pain, vaginal bleeding or maternal collapse (Beckley et al 1991; Arulkumaran et al 1992). Overall, there is limited place for intrauterine pressure measurement outside a research setting.

## Duration of Augmentation

There is general agreement that the use of the partogram and oxytocic augmentation for the management of abnormal labour progress is valuable. However, there is far less consensus regarding how long augmentation should continue before performing a

> A period of eight hours of augmentation with adequate monitoring, in the absence of gross disproportion, should result in the majority of nulliparous and multiparous women delivering vaginally with little risk of intrauterine hypoxia or birth injury.

cesarean section for 'failure to progress'. A period of eight hours of augmentation with adequate monitoring in the absence of gross disproportion should result in the majority of nulliparous and multiparous women delivering vaginally, with little risk of intrauterine hypoxia or birth injury. It is doubtful whether more than eight hours of augmentation in the presence of poor progress will result in greater number of vaginal deliveries without compromise to the fetus (Arulkumaran et al 1987). Fetal and maternal surveillance and monitoring of the progress of labour is important to avoid iatrogenic morbidity.

## Augmentation in Special Circumstances

### Multiparas

Caution must be exercised in augmenting multiparas, especially grand multiparas, where the cause of poor progress is more likely to be due to unrecognised disproportion than inadequate uterine activity. Augmentation in such situations might lead to uterine rupture, and the decision to augment under these circumstances should be made by a senior member of the obstetric team. In these women, if progress is abnormal despite

> Failure to progress despite augmentation is more likely to be due to disproportion in multiparas.

adequate spontaneous contractions, it may be better to observe them for a few more hours than to use oxytocin. Caution should also be exercised when augmentation is undertaken for failure to progress in the late first stage of labour (> 7 cm cervical dilatation), since a prolonged deceleration phase at the end of the first stage may herald shoulder dystocia. A prolonged period of augmentation should be avoided. Failure to progress despite augmentation is more likely to be due to disproportion in multiparas and an early decision should be taken as to the most appropriate mode of delivery.

### Previous cesarean section

The issue of vaginal birth after cesarean section (VBAC) remains highly contentious.

In 1918, Craigin introduced the concept of 'once a cesarean always a cesarean' when referring to a classical uterine incision. Throughout the remainder of the twentieth century, the medical pendulum swung back in favour of encouraging a trial of labour in the majority of women, assuming this was a safer alternative for them (and their babies) than an elective cesarean section. However, it is clear that for women who have had a previous cesarean section, major maternal complications are twice as likely among those having a trial of labour as compared to those undergoing an elective cesarean section. The additional burden of risk is largely borne by those women whose trial of labour ends in an emergency repeat cesarean section. Regardless of this, the overall risk of maternal morbidity was 8 per cent (McMahon et al 1996).

More recently, the results of a retrospective study of the risk of uterine scar rupture during labour were reported (Lydon-Rochelle et al 2001). The overall risk of scar

> In women with a previous cesarean scar, prostaglandin induction compared with non-prostaglandin induction is associated with statistically significant uterine rupture risk and a higher risk of perinatal death from uterine rupture.

rupture was 4.5:1000 but the risk was much higher for those induced without prostaglandins (7.7:1000), and as high as 24.5:1000 among women following prostaglandin induction of labour. Unfortunately, subset analysis to quantify the risk of scar rupture following augmentation of a spontaneous labour was not performed.

In a large prospective observational study, the risks of uterine rupture/10,000 VBAC (vaginal birth after cesarean section) deliveries were 102, 87 and 36/10,000 for induced, augmented and spontaneous labours, respectively (Landon et al 2004). This compares with an overall risk of scar rupture of 2/10,000 in women with an unscarred uterus whether the labour is induced, augmented or spontaneous (Ofir et al 2003). In an analysis of data collected from Scotland, prostaglandin induction compared with non-prostaglandin induction was associated with statistically significant uterine rupture risk (87/10,000 versus 29/10,000) and a higher risk of perinatal death from uterine rupture (11.2/10,000 versus 4.5/10,000). This compares with 6/10,000 risk of perinatal death in women with an unscarred uterus induced by prostaglandins identified by a Cochrane review (Kelly et al 2006).

Obviously, what constitutes an 'acceptable' level of risk to one group of patients will be completely unacceptable to others. The mode of delivery following a previous cesarean section should be discussed with each affected woman in the antenatal period.

### Breech

The most appropriate mode of delivery of the term breech is also the subject of much debate. The Term Breech Trial has recently reported its findings and noted a significantly lower risk of neonatal mortality or morbidity in those babies delivered by planned cesarean section, compared with those allocated to planned vaginal delivery, without any additional maternal morbidity (Hannah et al 2000). The evidence presented was so conclusive that an accompanying editorial suggested there was no longer any room left for disagreement about the delivery of the term breech. Cesarean section was the most appropriate mode (Lumley 2000). The benefit of cesarean section was greatest in those countries where the perinatal mortality rates (PMR) were low, where the numbers needed to treat (NNT) was 7. In countries with a high PMR, the NNT was 39. In other words, the resource implications of the NNT are greatest in those countries with fewer resources, a factor that may restrict the implementation of the study findings.

When vaginal delivery is attempted, dysfunctional labour is more in breech presentation (or any other malpresentation) than in cephalic presentation. If augmentation is carried out in the presence of breech presentation, it should be performed cautiously. Satisfactory results have been reported provided a low threshold for cesarean section is adopted if there is no progress in the first four hours of augmentation (Arulkumaran et al 1989c).

> Augmentation should be performed cautiously in the presence of breech presentation.

## Malposition

### Genuine cephalopelvic disproportion and relative disproportion due to malposition

If labour progress is abnormal, despite adequate augmentation, mechanical factors that may contribute to disproportion must be considered. Disproportion may be diagnosed when two-fifths or more of the head is palpable abdominally. Vaginal examination may reveal an edematous cervix that is loosely applied to the presenting part and gross moulding. Further, deflexion or malposition of the head may be identified with the maximal diameter of the head still high in the pelvis. A cardiotocographic tracing may show either early or variable decelerations, suggestive of head compression. Meconium-stained amniotic fluid sometimes appears for the first time. These signs are indicative of absolute cephalopelvic disproportion if the occiput is anterior with a well-flexed vertex presentation. A relative disproportion is one due to malposition of the head which is deflexed with the occiput felt laterally or posteriorly. Diagnosis of disproportion at full dilatation may be difficult. Fetal weight, the proportion of the head palpable abdominally, the degree of caput and moulding, the station and position of the presenting part must be carefully assessed. The descent of the head with contraction and bearing down effort may give additional clues to the degree of mechanical obstruction.

> Disproportion may be diagnosed when
> - two-fifths or more of the head is palpable abdominally
> - there is an edematous cervix that is loosely applied to the presenting part
> - there is gross moulding
> - there are early/variable decelerations on the CTG

In relative cephalopelvic disproportion due to malposition, the degree of flexion is unsatisfactory and the larger occipito-frontal (11 cm) diameter presents instead of the suboccipto-bregmatic (9.5 cm) diameter that presents in a well-flexed occipito-anterior position. The distinction between 'absolute' and 'relative' cephalopelvic disproportion may be useful in deciding whether to offer trial of labour or elective cesarean section in subsequent pregnancies. A patient who has a cesarean section for disproportion due to malposition and a deflexed head in her first pregnancy may well have a normal delivery in her subsequent labour if the head flexes and is in an occipito-anterior position. Thus, 67–77 per cent of women allowed a trial of labour following a previous cesarean section for failure to progress due to 'disproportion', will deliver vaginally in their subsequent pregnancy (Phelan et al 1987; Flamm et al 1994).

> A large percentage of women allowed a trial of labour following a previous cesarean section for failure to progress due to 'disproportion', will deliver vaginally in their subsequent pregnancy.

## Pelvimetry

Pelvimetry has been used to predict obstetric outcome for over 60 years, although there is now considerable debate regarding its use. Traditionally, pelvimetry was performed radiographically, but newer techniques such as CT or MRI pelvimetry, are accurate and safer.

In the majority of cases of failure to progress in labour, the relative contribution made by the passenger and the passages is difficult to evaluate. X-ray pelvimetry will accurately measure bony landmarks of the pelvis, but the dynamic nature of labour continuously alters the pelvic dimensions and the presenting part by flexion, rotation and moulding. Hence, static measurements are of little value in such situations.

The evidence from the literature is that antenatal pelvimetry is of no value in primigravid women with a cephalic presentation, except possibly in rare circumstances, such as a previous pelvic fracture (Varner et al 1980; Pattinson 2002). In a woman with a cephalic presentation, unless there is gross disproportion, a well-conducted trial of labour is the best test of the adequacy of the pelvis.

Finally, it has been suggested that x-ray pelvimetry in the puerperium following a cesarean section for dystocia, cephalopelvic disproportion or failure to progress may allow the selection of patients for whom a trial of labour in a subsequent pregnancy would be appropriate (Mathelier 1996). The value of x-ray pelvimetry in the antenatal period to predict suitability for a trial of labour in women with one previous cesarean section was assessed in a prospective controlled trial (Thubisi et al 1993). The authors concluded that antenatal pelvimetry did not predict the likelihood of vaginal delivery and was unnecessary. There is little evidence to support the routine use of pelvimetry for assessment for term breech vaginal delivery or vaginal birth after cesarean section (RCOG 2001c).

> Antenatal pelvimetry does not predict the likelihood of vaginal delivery and is unnecessary.

## Conclusion

Labour is a natural physiological phenomenon leading to childbirth. Many women have the rewarding experience of a safe vaginal birth of a healthy baby, while a small proportion continue to die of the complications of prolonged labour and its sequelae.

In an attempt to minimise the risks of adverse outcomes, obstetric interventions in labour have become more common. However, a perception of the widespread use of what are seen as unnecessary interventions has caused a degree of scepticism among women and some clinicians. These concerns, expressed by the general public in recent years, are perfectly valid and will continue to increase if obstetric practice is not continually scrutinised and subjected to rigorous scientific evaluation wherever possible.

This is one of the many challenges currently faced by those with an interest in the welfare of pregnant and labouring women and their babies.

# References

Allman ACJ, ESG Genevier, MR Johnson, PJ Steer. 1996. Head-to-cervix force: an important physiological variable in labour. *Br J Obstet Gynaecol* 103:763–68.

Arulkumaran S, CH Koh, I Ingemarsson, SS Ratnam. 1987. Augmentation of labour. Mode of delivery related to cervimetric progress. *Aust NZ J Obstet Gynecol* 27:304–308.

Arulkumaran S, DMF Gibb, S Chau, Piara Singh, SS Ratnam. 1989a. Ethnic influences on uterine activity in spontaneous labour. *Br J Obstet Gynaecol* 96:1203–1206.

Arulkumaran S, M Yang, I Ingemarsson, Piara Singh, SS Ratnam. 1989b. Augmentation of labour. Does oxytocin titration to achieve preset active contraction area values produce better obstetric outcome? *Asia Oceania J Obstet Gynecol* 15:333–37.

Arulkumaran S, AS Thavarash, I Ingemarsson, SS Ratnam. 1989c. An alternative approach to assisted vaginal breech delivery. *Asia Oceania J Obstet Gynecol* 15:47–51.

Arulkumaran S, S Chua, TM Chua, M Yang, Piara Singh, SS Ratnam. 1991. Uterine activity in dysfunctional labour and target uterine activity to be aimed at with oxytocin titration. *Asia Oceania J Obstet Gynecol* 17:101–106.

Arulkumaran S, S Chua, SS Ratnam. 1992. Symptoms and signs with scar rupture: Value of uterine activity measurements. *Aust NZ J Obstet Gynecol* 32:208–212.

Becker RF, WF Windle, EE Barth, MD Schulz. 1940. Fetal swallowing, gastro-intestinal activity and defecation in amnio. *Surg Gynecol Obstet* 70:603–614.

Beckley S, H Gee, JR Newton. 1991. Scar rupture in labour after previous lower segment cesarean section: The role of uterine activity measurement. *Br J Obstet Gynaecol* 98:265–69.

Bewley S, II Cockburn. 2002. The unfacts of 'request' cesarean section. *Br J Obstet Gynaecol* 109:597–605.

Bloom SL, DD McIntire, MA Kelly et al. 1998. Lack of effect of walking on labour and delivery. *N Eng J Med* 339:76–79.

Cardozo LD, DMF Gibb, JWW Studd, RV Vasant, DJ Cooper. 1982. Predictive value of cervimetric labour patterns in primigravidae. *Br J Obstet Gynaecol* 89:33–38.

Chua S, A Kurup, S Arulkumaran, SS Ratnam. Augmentation of labour. 1990. Does internal tocography result in better obstetric outcome than external tocography? *Obstet Gynecol* 76:164–67.

Daw E. 1973. Oxytocin induced rupture of the primigravid uterus. *J Obstet Gynecol Br Cwlth* 80:374–75.

Duignan NM, JWW Studd, AO Hughes. 1975. Characteristics of labour in different racial groups. *Br J Obstet Gynaecol* 82:593–601.

Elbourne D, RA Wiseman. 2002. Types of intra-muscular labour opioids for maternal pain relief in labour (Cochrane Review). In *The Cochrane Library*, Issue 2. Oxford: Update Software.

Flamm BL, JR Goings, Y Liu, G Wolde-Tsadik. 1994. Elective repeat cesarean delivery versus trial of labor: A prospective multicenter study. *Obstet Gynecol* 83:927–32.

Fraser WD, I Krauss, G Brisson-Carrol, J Thornton, G Breart. 2002. Amniotomy for shortening spontaneous labour (Cochrane Review). In *The Cochrane Library*, Issue 2. Oxford: Update Software.

Friedman EA. 1954. The graphic analysis of labor. *Am J Obstet Gynecol* 68:1568–75.

Frigoletto FD, E Lieberman, JM Lang et al. 1995. A clinical trial of active management of labor. *N Eng J Med* 333:745–50.

Fuchs AR and F Fuchs. 1984. Endocrinology of human parturition: A review. *Br J Obstet Gynaecol* 91:948–67.

Fuchs AR, F Fuchs, P Husslein, MS Soloff. 1984. Oxytocin receptors in the human uterus during pregnancy and parturition. *Am J Obstet Gynecol* 150:734–41.

Gibb DMF, LD Cardozo, JWW Studd, AL Magos, DJ Cooper. 1982. Outcome of spontaneous labour in multigravidae. *Br J Obstet Gynaecol* 89:708–711.

Gibb DMF, S Arulkumaran, KC Lun, SS Ratnam. 1984. Characteristics of uterine activity in nulliparous labour. *Br J Obstet Gynaecol* 91:220–27.

Goffinet F, W Fraser, S Marcoux et al for the Amniotomy Study Group. 1997. Early amniotomy increases the frequency of fetal heart abnormalities. *Br J Obstet Gynaecol* 104: 548–53.

Gough GW, NJ Randall, ES Genevier, IA Sutherland, PJ Steer. 1990. Head to cervix pressure and their relationship to the outcome of labour. *Obstet Gynecol* 75:613–18.

Hannah ME, WJ Hannah, SA Hewson et al. 2000. Planned cesarean section versus planned vaginal birth for breech presentation at term: a randomised multicentre trial. *Lancet* 356:1375–83.

Hemminki E and L Merilainen. 1996. Long term effects of cesarean section: ectopic pregnancies and placental problems. *Am J Obstet Gynecol* 174:1569–74.

Hendricks CH, WE Brenner, G Kraus. 1970. Normal cervical dilatation patterns in late pregnancy and labor. *Am J Obstet Gynecol* 106:1065–82.

Hodnett ED. 2002. Continuity of caregivers for care during pregnancy and childbirth (Cochrane Review). In *The Cochrane Library*, Issue 2. Oxford: Update Software.

Howell CJ. 2002. Epidural versus non-epidural analgesia for pain relief in labour (Cochrane Review). In *The Cochrane Library*, Issue 2. Oxford: Update Software.

Ilancheran A, SM Lim, SS Ratnam. 1977. Nomograms of cervical dilatation in labour. *Sing J Obstet Gynecol* 8:69–73.

Johnson JWC, JA Longmate, B Frentzen. 1992. Excessive maternal weight and pregnancy outcome. *Am J Obstet Gynecol* 167:353–72.

Knox GE, JF Huddleston, CE Flowers. 1979. The management of prolonged pregnancy: Results of a prospective randomized trial. *Am J Obstet Gynecol* 134:376–80.

Kelly AJ, J Kavanagh, J Thomas. 2006. Vaginal prostaglandin ($PGE_2$ AND F2 a) for induction of labour at term. *Cochrane database syst review* CD 003101

Landon MB, Hauth JC, Leveno KJ et al. 2004. Maternal and perinatal outcomes associated with a trial of labour after caesarean section. *N Engl J Med*; 351: 2581–9.

Liston WA and AJ Campbell. 1974. Dangers of oxytocin induced labour to the fetus. *BMJ* iii: 606– 607.

Lopez-Zeno JA, AM Peaceman, JA Adashek, ML Socol. 1992. A controlled trial of a program for the active management of labor. *N Eng J Med* 326:450–54.

Lumley J. 2000. Any room left for disagreement about assisting breech births at term? *Lancet* 356:1368– 69.

Lydon-Rochelle M, VL Holt, TR Easterling, DP Martin. 2001. Risk of uterine rupture during labor among women with a prior cesarean section. *N Eng J Med* 345:3–8.

MacLennan AH, C Crowther, R Derham. 1994. Does the opportunity to ambulate in labour confer any advantage or disadvantage? *J Matern Fetal Invest* 3:43–48.

Mathelier AC. 1996. Radiopelvimetry after cesarean section. *J Reprod Med* 41:427–30.

McMahon MJ, ER Luter, WA Bowes, AF Olshan. 1996. Comparison of a trial of labour with an elective second cesarean section. *N Eng J Med* 335:689–95.

Murphy KW. 1998. Reducing the complications of cesarean section. In *Recent Advances in Obstetrics and Gynaecology* ed J Bonnar, vol. 20, 141–52. Edinburgh: Churchill Livingstone.

Nielsen TF, H Hagberg, U Ljungblad. 1989. Placenta praevia and antepartum haemorrhage after previous cesarean section. *Gynecol Obstet Invest* 27: 88–90.

O'Driscoll K, JM Stronge, M Minogue. 1973. *BMJ* iii:135–38.

O'Driscoll K, M Foley, D MacDonald. 1984. Active management of labour as an alternative to cesarean section for dystocia. *Obstet Gynecol* 63:485–90.

O'Driscoll K, D Meagher, P Boylan. 1993. *Active Management of Labor*. 3rd ed. Mosby: Year Book Europe Limited.

Pajntar M, B Leskosek, D Rudel, I Verdenik. 2001. Contribution of cervical smooth muscle activity to the duration of latent and active phases of labour. *Br J Obstet Gynaecol* 108:533–38.

Ofir K, E Sheiner, A Levy et al 2003. Uterine rupture: risk factors and pregnancy outcome. *Am J Obstet Gynecol*: 189:1042-6

Pattinson RC. 2002. Pelvimetry for fetal cephalic presentation at term (Cochrane Review). In: *The Cochrane Library*, Issue 2 Oxford: Update Software.

Phelan JP, SL Clark, F Diaz, RH Paul. 1987. Vaginal birth after cesarean. *Am J Obstet Gynecol* 157:1510–15.

Philpott RH. 1972. Graphic records in labour. BMJ iv: 163–65.

Rageth JC, C Juzi, H Grossenbacher. 1999. Delivery after previous cesarean section: a risk evaluation. *Obstet Gynecol* 93:332–37.

Rao KB. 1992 Obstructed labour. In *Obstetrics and Gynaecology for Postgraduates*, vol.1, ed SS Ratnam, K Bhasker Rao, S Arulkumaran. Madras: Orient Longman.

RCOG Clinical Effectiveness Support Unit 2001a. *The Use of Electronic Fetal Monitoring*. Evidence-based Clinical Guideline Number 8, May 2001a. London: RCOG Press.

RCOG Clinical *Effectiveness Support Unit. Induction of labour*. June 2001b. London: RCOG Press.

RCOG Guideline No. 14. *Pelvimetry*. 2001c. London: RCOG Press.

Reddi K, SR Kambaran, PA Philpott. 1988. Intrauterine pressure studies in multigravid patients in spontaneous labour. Effect of oxytocin augmentation in delayed first stage. *Br J Obstet Gynaecol* 95:771–77.

Sadler LC, T Davison, LME McCowan 2000. A randomised controlled trial and meta-analysis of active management of labour. *Br J Obstet Gynaecol* 107:909–915.

Scrutton MJL, GA Metcalfe, C Lowy, PT Seed, G O'Sullivan. 1999. Eating in labour. *Anaesthesia* 54:329–34.

Seitchik J, J Amico, AG Robinson et al. 1984. Oxytocin augmentation of dysfunctional labour IV. Oxytocin pharmacokinetics. *Am J Obstet Gynecol* 150:225–32.

Studd JWW. 1973. Partograms and nomograms in the management of primigravid labour. *BMJ* IV: 451–55.

Studd J, DR Clegg, RR Saunders, AO Hughes. 1975. Identification of high risk labours by labour nomogram. *BMJ* ii:545–47.

Smith GCS, Pell PJ, Bobbie R .2003. Caesarean section and risk of unexplained stillbirth in subsequent pregnancy. The *Lancet* volume 362, issue 9398, 1779-1784

The UK Amniotomy Group. 1994. A multicentre randomised trial of amniotomy in spontaneous first labour at term. *Br J Obstet Gynaecol* 101:307–309.

Thomas J and S Paranjothy. 2001. Royal College of Obstetricians and Gynaecologists. Clinical Effectiveness Support Unit. *The National Sentinel Cesarean Section Audit Report*. London: RCOG Press.

Thubisi M, A Ebrahim, J Moodley, PM Shweni. 1993. Vaginal delivery after previous cesarean section: Is x-ray pelvimetry necessary? *Br J Obstet Gynaecol* 100:421–424.

Varner MW, DP Cruickshank, RL Berkowitz. 1980. X-ray pelvimetry in clinical obstetrics. *Obstet Gynecol* 56:296–300.

World Health Organization. 1994 *Maternal Health and Safe Motherhood Programme*. www.who.org

World Health Organization. 1994 Partograph in management of labour. *Lancet* 343:1399–1401

# CHAPTER 3

# PAIN RELIEF IN LABOUR

*Sunil T Pandya*

Pain relief in labour has always been associated with controversies. Misinterpretation of biblical scripture ('In sorrow thou shalt bring forth children') and religious taboos resulted in centuries of denial of pain relief, as clergy insisted that suffering in labour was consistent with divine intent (Cohen et al 1996). Fifteenth-century midwives were burned at the stake for offering pain relief during labour.

The modern era of obstetric analgesia began in 1847, when James Young Simpson, a Scottish obstetrician, administered ether to a woman with a deformed rickety pelvis during childbirth. The etherisation of labour was strongly criticised by Charles D. Meigs, a well-known obstetrician from Philadelphia, who believed in the concept of 'no-drug labour'; he hypothesised that, 'Labour pain has a purpose, uterine pain is inseparable from contractions and any drug that abolishes pain will alter contractions'. Simpson proposed that, 'Medical men may oppose for a time the super-induction of anesthesia in parturition, but they will oppose it in vain; for certainly our patients themselves will force use of it upon the profession. The whole question is, even now, one merely of time.'

The time came in 1853 and 1857, when John Snow (1853) administered chloroform to Britain's Queen Victoria during the birth of her eighth and ninth child, thus putting an end to the controversy to a large extent. The queen being the head of church, the religious taboos associated with pain relief in labour also resolved to an extent. By 1860, consumer demand for it rapidly ascended to the highest levels of society, especially in women belonging to the upper socio-economic class. Analgesia for childbirth soon became part of medical practice, by public acclaim.

Nonetheless, concerned about the possible adverse effects of using ether for relieving labour pain, Simpson wrote, 'It will be necessary to ascertain anesthesia's precise effect, both upon the action of the uterus and on the abdominal muscles, and its influence, if any, upon the child'. This quote is remarkable, given that today, more than a century and a half later, the possible effects of anesthesia on the progress of labour and on the neonate continue to concern anesthesiologists, obstetricians and patients.

## Does a parturient in labour need pain relief?

The experience of pain during labour is a complex and subjective interaction of multiple physiologic, psychological and socio-cultural factors on a woman's individual interpretation of labour stimuli (Donald et al 2002). The severity of labour pain has been previously recognised by Melzack (1984), who used a questionnaire developed to assess the intensity and emotional impact of pain (McGill pain rating index). It was observed that among nulliparous women with no prepared childbirth training, labour pain was rated to be as painful as digit amputation without anesthesia (Figure 3.1).

The ability of a woman or her obstetrician to predict her reaction to labour pains is limited. Ideally, a choice of pain relief methods should be offered to all women.

The physiological impact of labour pain on various systems is seen secondary to the release of catecholamine in response to pain.

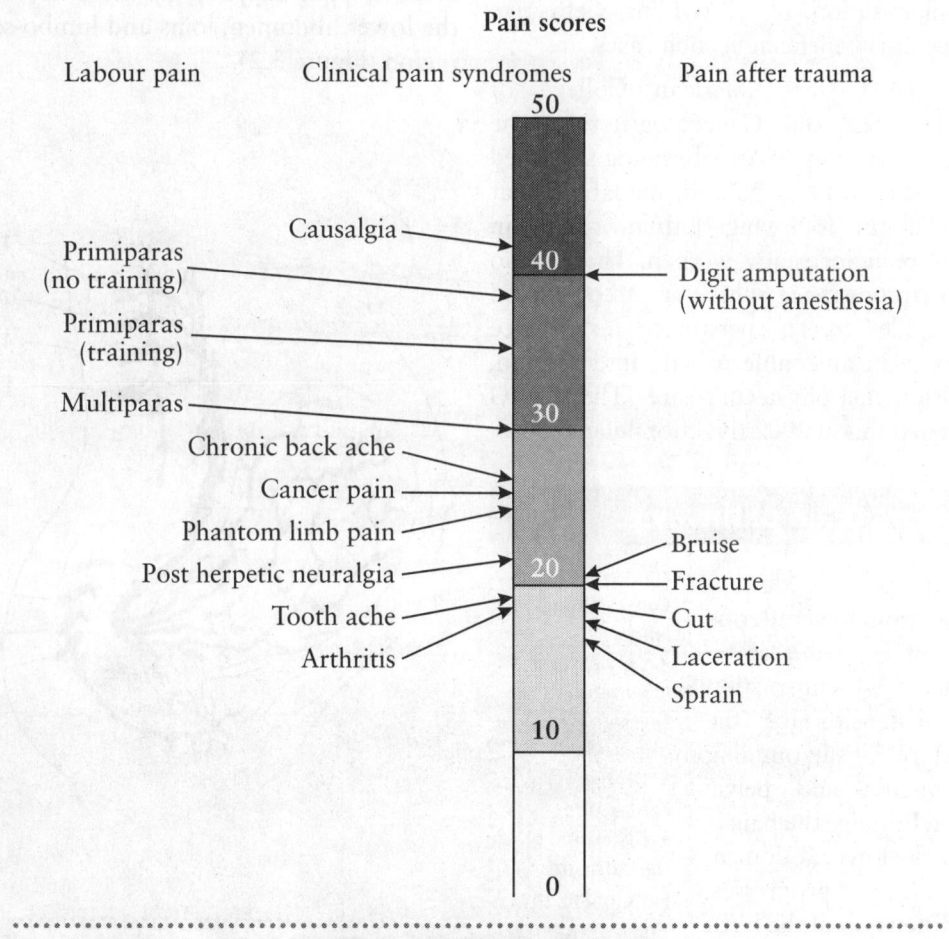

**Pain scores**

| Labour pain | Clinical pain syndromes | | Pain after trauma |
|---|---|---|---|
| | | 50 | |
| Primiparas (no training) | Causalgia | 40 | Digit amputation (without anesthesia) |
| Primiparas (training) | | | |
| Multiparas | | 30 | |
| | Chronic back ache | | |
| | Cancer pain | | |
| | Phantom limb pain | | Bruise |
| | Post herpetic neuralgia | 20 | Fracture |
| | Tooth ache | | Cut |
| | Arthritis | | Laceration |
| | | | Sprain |
| | | 10 | |
| | | 0 | |

**Figure 3.1** McGill pain rating index

This results in tachycardia, hypertension, increased cardiac output, and increased oxygen consumption. Hyperventilation–hypoventilation–apnea cycles during peak uterine contraction lead to carbon dioxide washout, causing hypocarbia and apnea. In addition, the pain during labour causes respiratory alkalosis and fetal acidemia. All these changes are well tolerated by healthy parturients and their fetuses (with normal uteroplacental perfusion); however, when maternal or fetal disease or compromise is observed, significant cardiopulmonary alterations may lead to maternal or fetal decompensation. Providing effective analgesia is beneficial in such cases.

In 1992, the American College of Obstetricians and Gynecologists and the American Society of Anesthesiologists issued a joint statement on pain during labour that included the following: 'Labour results in severe pain for many women. There is no other circumstance where it is considered acceptable for a person to experience severe pain amenable to safe intervention, while under a physician's care.' The ACOG reiterated this in 2002 (Practice Bulletin 36).

## Pain pathways

Labour pain is due to cervical and lower uterine segment dilatation, uterine contraction and distension of the structures surrounding the vagina and pelvic outlet. Initially, the pain is felt in the lower abdomen, but as labour progresses, the distension of the birth canal by the descending fetal part causes pain in the back, perineum and thigh.

> Causes of pain in labour
> • Cervical and lower uterine segment distension
> • Uterine contraction
> • Distension of the structures surrounding the vagina and pelvic outlet

## First stage pain

Afferent impulses from the uterus and cervix are transmitted via the Aδ and C fibres which travel with sympathetic nerves via the hypogastric plexus to enter the lumbar and lower thoracic parts of the sympathetic chain. Central connection to the spinal cord is via the dorsal root ganglion and lateral division of the posterior roots of T10-L1. Labour pains are therefore referred to the areas of skin supplied by these nerves i.e. the lower abdomen, loins and lumbo-sacral region (Figure 3.2).

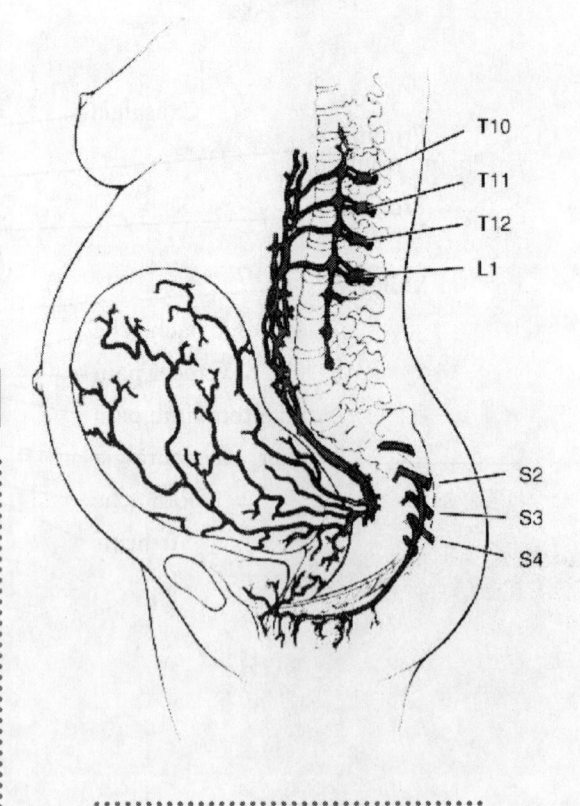

**Figure 3.2** Labour pain pathways

## Second stage pain

Afferent transmission from the vagina and pelvic outlet is also via Aδ and C fibres, but with the parasympathetic bundle in the pudendal nerves (S2, 3, 4). There is also a minor contribution from the ilio-inguinal, genito-femoral and the perforating branch of the posterior cutaneous nerve of the thigh.

It is important to appreciate that pain-sensitive structures in the pelvis are also involved, that is, the adnexae, the pelvic parietal peritoneum, bladder, urethra, rectum and the roots of the lumbar plexus. Therefore, the anesthesia must cover the dermatomes from L2 to S5. However, pain relief is not a simple matter of blocking pain from T10 to L1 dermatomes for the first stage and S2, 3, 4 dermatomes for the second stage of labour.

First stage pain is visceral pain, best relieved by a narcotic analgesic, while second stage pain is somatic in nature, best relieved by a local anesthetic. Thus, neuraxial analgesic techniques that use combinations of local anesthetic and narcotic in low doses are considered the most versatile techniques of pain relief in labour.

## Methods of pain relief

There are several methods of providing intrapartum pain relief (Figure 3.3). Women

### Methods of pain relief in labour

**Nonpharmacologic methods**
- Continuous support in labour
- Touch & massage
- TENS
- Intradermal sterile water injections
- Water bath
- Upright posture
- Acupuncture / Acupressure
- Hypnosis

**Pharmacologic methods**

Systemic opioids:
- Pethidine
- Fentanyl
- Remifentanil
- Butorphanol
- Tramadol

Inhalational Methods:
- Entonox - PCIA
- Sevox - PCIA

**Regional anesthetic techniques**

Neuraxial Techniques:
- CLE
- CSEA
- SA
- CSA

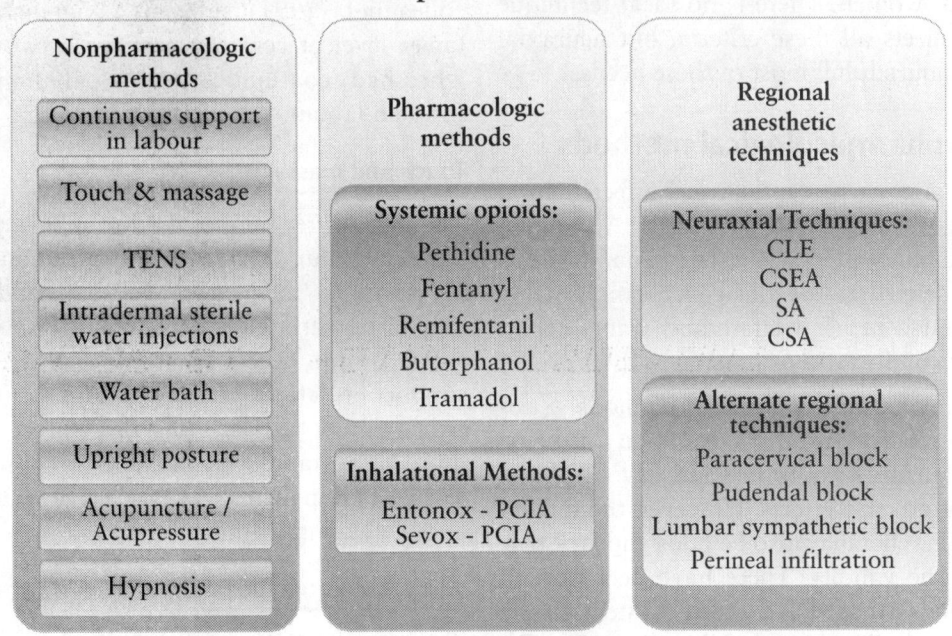

Alternate regional techniques:
- Paracervical block
- Pudendal block
- Lumbar sympathetic block
- Perineal infiltration

**TENS:** Transcutaneous electrical nerve stimulation; **PCIA:** Patient controlled inhalational analgesia; **Sevox:** Sevoflurane with oxygen; **CLE:** Continuous lumbar epidural; **CSEA:** Combined spinal epidural analgesia; **SA:** Spinal analgesia; **CSA:** Continuous spinal analgesia

Figure 3.3 Methods of pain relief in labour

vary in their needs and desire for pain relief during labour, with some aiming for natural childbirth with no pain relief and others wishing to employ some form of analgesia. The amount of pain relief does not necessarily equate with maternal satisfaction (Hodnett 2002). Preparation in childbirth classes plays an important role in pain management. Pain relieving interventions can be made easier and safer by reinforcing what has been taught in the childbirth classes.

Ideally, a good labour analgesia technique should significantly reduce the pain of labour without interfering with the progress of labour and the mode of delivery. Further, it should be free from any adverse effects on mother and fetus and should be useful for all women. There is no ideal technique that meets all these criteria, but neuraxial techniques fulfill most of these needs.

## Nonpharmacological methods

Pain and its perception, are affected by a woman's fears and anxieties. A woman in labour will perceive less pain if she is confident that the obstetric team is truly interested in her welfare and wants her to be as comfortable as possible.

Nonpharmacological methods of pain relief have the advantage of being inexpensive, easy to use and devoid of any major adverse effects. However, the quality of pain relief may also be poor and lack true scientific validity. There have been several methods that have been systematically reviewed (Penny and O'Hara 2002). The common nonpharmacologic methods that are practiced are as follows:

- Continuous labour support
- Touch and massage
- Warm water baths
- Vertical maternal position
- Transcutaneous electrical nerve stimulation (TENS)
- Acupuncture
- Hypnosis

### Continuous labour support

Continuous labour support is essential to a satisfying childbirth experience. Typically, the parturient's husband or friend provides this support. One study noted decreased maternal anxiety and medication requirements (Henneborm and Cogan 1975). Emotional support provided by doulas or trained individuals, also has a positive effect on pain in labour. Kennel and colleagues (1991) showed a significantly lower level of cesarean sections in women who had continuous emotional support through labour.

### Touch and massage

The various techniques used to relieve pain during labour include effleurage, counter pressure to alleviate back discomfort, reassuring patting or light stroking. Though there is not much scientific evidence to support its effect on labour and delivery pain, it may reduce some discomfort and more importantly, it transmits a sense of caring. This in turn fosters a sense of security and well-being (Minnich 2004).

### Vertical maternal position

It seems logical to allow the labouring woman to adopt the position that she is most comfortable in, while in labour (Figure 3.4). Several authors have studied the effect of various postures on pain perception and the outcome of labour (Gardosi et al 1989;

Melzack et al 1991; Bloom et al; 1998). The vertical maternal posture (sitting, standing, walking, squatting) has been compared to the horizontal position (supine and lateral). The use of birthing chairs and the squatting position has also been studied. The results are contradictory. Bloom and colleagues (1998) found that walking did not have any effect on labour and delivery.

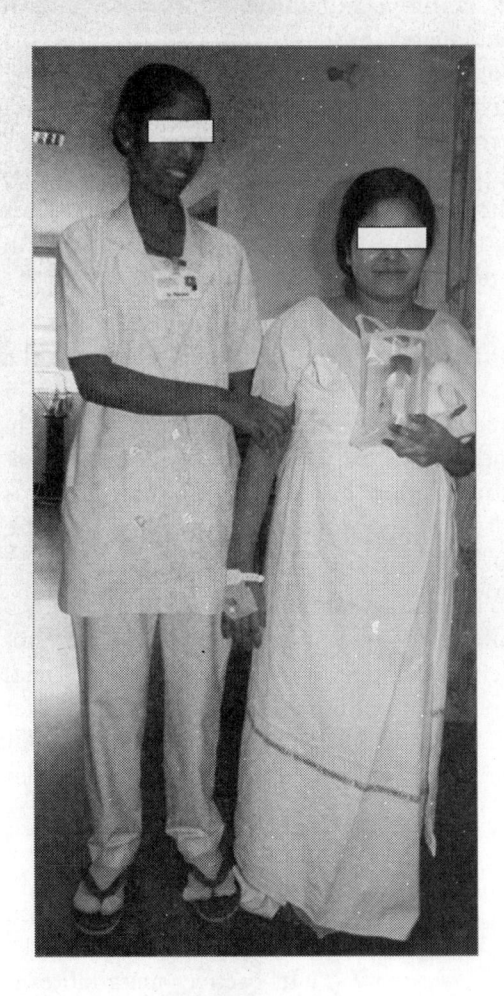

**Figure 3.4** Ambulation during labour. The patient is accompanied by a responsible labour ward nurse

### Transcutaneous electrical nerve stimulation (TENS)

Transcutaneous electrical nerve stimulation (TENS) involves transmission of low voltage current to the skin via wide surface electrodes. The placement of surface electrodes is over the lumbo-sacral regions. This method is non-invasive and has no harmful effects on the fetus. A systematic review by Dowswell and colleagues (2009) showed that overall, there was little difference in pain ratings between TENS and control groups, although women receiving TENS were less likely to report severe pain. Where TENS was used as an adjunct to epidural analgesia there was no evidence that it reduced pain. There was no consistent evidence that TENS had any impact on interventions and outcomes in labour. There was little information on outcomes for mothers and babies.

> There is no consistent evidence that TENS has any impact on interventions and outcomes in labour.

### Acupuncture

Use of acupuncture requires trained personnel. There is no standardisation of acupuncture points for relief of labour pain. Small studies (Skilnand et al 2002; Ramnero et al 2002) have shown acupuncture to reduce labour pain and shorten the duration of labour. However, larger studies are required to reach definite conclusions.

### Hypnosis

Hypnosis requires special training in the antepartum period and is time consuming. It requires the presence of a trained hypnotherapist during labour and it offers no clear benefit. Large, high-quality studies are required, if the potentially advantageous risk/benefit profile of hypnosis in the obstetric population is to be clearly elucidated. However, at present, it seems unlikely that it will attain widespread use during childbirth.

## Parenteral agents

### Systemic opioids

Systemic opioids have been used since the 1840s and pethidine (mepiridine) is the most widely used medication for labour analgesia. Bricker and Lavender (2002), in a systematic review, stated that if women opt for systemic analgesia, no strong preference for any of the opioids can be recommended. Pethidine is the most commonly used opioid worldwide. Pethidine has the advantage that most physicians are familiar with its use and side effects. They found no convincing research evidence to show that alternative opioids are better (Table 3.1).

> Pethidine is the most commonly used opioid worldwide, and although there are concerns about its potential maternal, fetal and neonatal side effects, it still is the most cost-effective opioid available for labour analgesia.

Systemic opioids can cause maternal side effects like nausea, vomiting, sedation, dysphoria, delayed gastric emptying and respiratory depression. They also have the potential of causing neonatal respiratory depression. Opioids may cause decreased variability of the fetal heart rate. Neonatal respiratory depression depends on the dose and timing of opioid administration.

### Pethidine

Pethidine (meperidine), an opioid agonist, is the most frequently used opioid worldwide (Bricker and Lavender 2002). The recommended dose for labour is 1–2 mg per kg body weight, repeated every 4–6 hourly. The onset of action is within 45 minutes after intramuscular (IM) administration. It is often administered along with an antiemetic, as nausea is one of the most common side effects. Ondansetron, 4 mg, given slowly intravenously (IV) is preferred. Promethazine is not a preferred antiemetic as it potentiates sedation and may compromise the upper airway, especially in individuals whose airway is already compromised as in preeclampsia and obesity.

Pethidine crosses the placenta by passive diffusion and equilibrates within the maternal and fetal compartments within 6 minutes. It is relatively contraindicated in mothers with liver disease, as its metabolite norpethidine has a very long half-life. It is also not recommended in women who are on antidepressants.

Neonatal complications relate to the total dose administered and dose-to-delivery interval. The maximum fetal uptake of pethidine occurs 2–3 hours after maternal intramuscular administration. Studies have shown that infants born within this interval have an increased risk of respiratory depression (Belfrage et al 1981). Its active metabolite is associated with neonatal respiratory depression and neurobehavioural changes.

> Infants born within 2–3 hours after IM administration of pethidine have an increased risk of respiratory depression.

**Table 3.1** Commonly used opioids and their important characteristics.

| Drug | Dose | Onset | Duration | Remarks |
|---|---|---|---|---|
| *Systemic Opioids for Labour Analgesia* ||||| 
| Pethidine | 1–2 mg per Kg IM<br>25–50 mg slow IV | 40–45 min IM<br>5–10 min IV | 2–3 hrs | Need to combine with anti-emetic to reduce nausea. Its active metabolite, norpethidine has a long half-life, it should be avoided in hepatic disease. Max. neonatal depression 1–4 hrs after dose |
| Tramadol | 1–2 mg per Kg IM or slow IV | 10–15 min IM | 2–3 hrs | Cause nausea, vomiting and giddiness. Rapid IV bolus can cause seizures. Has less sedation and respiratory depression compared to other opioids |
| Fentanyl | 0.5–1 micrograms per Kg IV or 1–2 micrograms IM | 2–3 min IV<br>10 min IM | 30–60 minutes | Usually administered by PCA or continuous infusion. Has less neonatal respiratory depression |
| Butorphanol | 1–2 mg IV/IM | 5–10 min IV<br>10–30 min IM | 3–4 hrs | It is more sedative. Opioid agonist/antagonist, has ceiling effect of respiratory depression |
| Pentazocine | 20–40 mg IV/IM | 2–3 min IV<br>5–20 min IM | 2–3 hrs | Causes dysphoria, tachycardia and hypertensive response, opioid agonist/antagonist |

IV- Intravenous, IM – Intramuscular, PCA – Patient controlled analgesia

Adapted from: Chestnut's *Obstetric Anesthesia: Principles and Practice*; eds Chestnut D, Polley S L, Tsen CL, Wong AC

Pethidine's effect on the progress of labour is contentious. Sosa and co-workers (2004), in a randomised controlled trial, concluded that pethidine should not be administered in parturients with cervical dystocia. They found that pethidine (100 mg IV) did not affect operative delivery rates in women at term with singleton gestations requiring oxytocin because of 'dystocia' at 4–6 cm. Pethidine worsened neonatal outcomes compared to placebo.

> Pethidine does not facilitate cervical dilatation in cervical dystocia and worsens neonatal outcomes when given for that indication.

### Morphine

Morphine was very popular historically during childbirth to provide 'twilight sleep', along with scopolamine. Currently, morphine usage in labour is not recommended as it causes excessive sedation and both maternal and neonatal respiratory depression.

### Fentanyl

Fentanyl is a highly lipid soluble synthetic opioid with analgesic potency 100 times that of morphine and 800 times that of pethidine (Chestnut et al 2009). Its rapid onset of action (within 2–3 minutes after intravenous administration) with short duration of action and with no major metabolites makes it superior for labour analgesia. It readily crosses the placenta, but in doses of 1 μm per kg body weight, it has no effect on the Apgar scores or neurobehavioral scores at 2 and 24 hours (Rayburn et al 1989). It can be administered in boluses of 25–50 μm every hour or as a continuous infusion of 0.25 μm per kg per hour. Because of its pharmacokinetics and pharmacodynamics, it is also suitable for patient-controlled intravenous analgesia (PCA). Compared to pethidine, it is superior in terms of better pain scores when used in labouring parturients. However, it does not relieve the pain completely, like all other narcotics. A need for cross over to superior neuraxial techniques like epidural analgesia is frequently noted (Chestnut et al 2009).

### Tramadol

Tramadol is a pethidine-like synthetic opioid having low affinity for mu receptors. Its potency is 10 per cent that of morphine. It causes no clinically significant respiratory depression at usual doses of 1–2 mg per kg body weight. Onset of action is within 10 minutes after intramuscular administration and the effect lasts for approximately 2–3 hours. Claahsen-van der Grinten et al (2005) demonstrated high placental permeability for tramadol. However, neonates possess complete hepatic capacity to metabolise tramadol. Kenkin and colleagues (2003) found no significant difference between women receiving pethidine or tramadol, when compared for duration of labour and Apgar scores. However, they found that pethidine seemed to be a better alternative than tramadol in obstetric analgesia because of its superiority in analgesic efficacy and low incidence of maternal side effects.

### Butorphanol

Butorphanol is an opioid with agonist–antagonist properties that resemble those of pentazocine. It offers analgesia with sedation. It is five times as potent as morphine and 40 times as potent as pethidine. The dose of butorphanol is 1 to 2 mg intramuscularly. Butorphanol at a dose of 2 mg produces respiratory depression, similar to that with morphine 10 mg or pethidine 70 mg. Butarphanol and pethidine should not be given contiguously, since butraphanol antagonises the narcotic action of pethidine. It is not used frequently for labour analgesia, as it produces excessive sedation.

### Remifentanil

Remifentanil is an ultra-short acting synthetic potent opioid. It has a rapid onset of action and is readily metabolised by plasma and tissue esterases to an inactive metabolite. The half-life is 6 minutes, thus allowing effective analgesia for consecutive uterine contractions (Chestnut et al 2009). It readily crosses the placenta, but is extensively metabolised by the fetus. Because of its pharmacokinetic profile, this agent has an advantage over other opioids for patient-controlled intravenous analgesia (PCA).

The recommended dose of remifentanil is an intravenous bolus of 20 μm with a lock-out interval of 3 minutes on the PCA pump. In a comparative study, Douma et al (2009) concluded that the efficacy of patient-controlled pethidine, fentanyl, and remifentanil for labour analgesia varied from mild to moderate. Remifentanil PCA provided better analgesia than pethidine and fentanyl PCA, but only during the first hour of treatment. In all groups, pain scores returned to pre-treatment values within 3 h after the initiation of treatment. In another study by D'Onofrio and colleagues (2009) on the efficacy and safety of intravenous infusion of remifentanil in 205 parturients, remifentanil was administered as a continuous infusion. The initial infusion of 0.025 µm per kg per minute was increased in a stepwise manner to a maximum dose of 0.15 µm per kg per minute. The maternal side effects were minimal and no fetal or neonatal side effects were noted.

Most studies concluded that maternal monitoring during intravenous PCA with remifentanil should be one-to-one, as maternal hypoventilation is more common and there are more episodes of oxygen saturation falling to <94 per cent on pulse oximetry. However, it is a promising solution in women requesting labour analgesia, when neuraxial techniques are contraindicated.

### Opioid antagonists

Naloxone is the opioid antagonist of choice for reversing the neonatal effects of maternal opioid administration. It should be noted that there is no benefit to maternal administration of naloxone during labour or just before delivery. It is best to administer it directly to the newborn if there is any neonatal respiratory depression. The dose of naloxone for reversing neonatal respiratory depression is 0.1 ml per kg. Administration of naloxone is not recommended during primary steps of neonatal resuscitation. The preferred route of administration is intravenous. Intramuscular route is acceptable if intravenous access is not available, although the absorption is delayed. Endotracheal administration of naloxone is not recommended. Naloxone may precipitate a withdrawal in the newborn of the opioid-dependent mother (Chestnut et al 2009).

For reversing maternal respiratory depression, the dose is 0.4 mg intravenously. It should be noted that it also reverses the analgesic action. The half-life of naloxone is short and repeat administration may be required if the duration of action of the narcotic is longer.

> Naloxone at a dose of 0.1 mg kilogram intravenously will reverse neonatal respiratory depression due to opioids.

## Inhalational methods

Inhalational labour analgesia involves inhalation of subanesthetic concentrations of agents with the mother remaining awake and her protective laryngeal reflexes intact. The only inhalational agent that has survived the test of time is nitrous oxide, which is administered as a 50:50 mixture of oxygen and nitrous oxide (Entonox). Other agents that have been tried in recent years are sevoflurane (Sevox), isoflurane and enflurane, which are volatile anesthetic agents.

### Entonox

Entonox, a mixture of 50 per cent oxygen and 50 per cent nitrous oxide, can provide analgesia for labour, but in a systematic review it was not found to be a potent labour analgesic (Rosen, 2002). Thirty per cent to 40 per cent of mothers report little or no benefit. It is administered through a demand valve via a mouth piece or face mask and the assembly should deliver a peak inspiratory flow of at least 25 L per minute. The mother's cooperation is required to achieve the maximum benefit. Inhalation should begin from the very beginning of the uterine contraction and should continue until the contraction ends. Entonox does not interfere with uterine activity and neonatal Apgar scores. However, a combination of pethidine or other opioids and nitrous oxide has been reported to cause maternal respiratory depression and hypoxemic episodes.

Entonox inhalation may be useful in places where neuraxial techniques are not practiced, and in parturients with a short labour.

## Regional analgesia in labour

Central neuraxial techniques (continuous lumbar epidural or combined spinal–epidural)) are the gold standard techniques for relief of labour pain and are, by far, the most effective methods of labour analgesia. These are the only techniques that relieve both the visceral pain (first stage pain) and somatic pain (second stage pain) effectively. These techniques require thoughtful preparation and meticulous attention to ensure maternal and fetal safety. Current practice advocates use of ambulatory or mobile epidurals using low dose mixtures of local anesthetics and lipophilic narcotic analgesic.

> Neuraxial analgesia (epidural) is the most effective form of intrapartum analgesia currently available.

Regional anesthetic technique can be classified as follows:

### Neuraxial techniques

Epidural analgesia
Combined spinal–epidural analgesia
Spinal analgesia
Continuous spinal analgesia

### Alternate regional analgesia techniques

Pudendal block
Paracervical block
Lumbar sympathetic block
Perineal infiltration

### Indications for neuraxial techniques are:

- Maternal request
- Hypertensive disorders of pregnancy
- Co-morbid medical diseases
- Multifetal pregnancy
- Trial of labour: After cesarean section (TOLAC) or Vaginal Birth After Cesarean section (VBAC)
- Prolonged labour
- Presumed fetal compromise
- Mothers with anticipated difficult airway and likely operative delivery
- Obesity and or anticipated shoulder dystocia
- Intrauterine fetal demise (IUFD)

### Contraindications for neuraxial techniques:

- Maternal refusal
- Coagulopathy and thrombocytopenia (severe preeclampsia, IUFD of long duration etc.)
- Local infection or systemic sepsis
- Inadequate staffing and facilities

## Continuous lumbar epidural analgesia and combined spinal-epidural analgesia (CSEA)

Epidural analgesia is the most versatile method of labour analgesia currently available and its use has increased dramatically in the last 20 years, especially in developed countries and a few dedicated centres in India. When compared to other techniques, satisfaction of birth experience is greater with these techniques (Figure 3.5a and 3.5b).

**Basic pre-requisites before administering an epidural or CSEA:**

- Informed consent.
- Pre-anesthetic assessment and examination of back.
- Resuscitation equipment and emergency drugs
- Maternal and fetal monitoring:
  - Blood pressure monitoring during initiation of epidural and every five minutes for the first 20 to 30 minutes after every dose is mandatory.
  - With intrathecal and epidural narcotic, monitoring for respiratory depression is also important.
  - NICE guidelines recommend that continuous electronic fetal monitoring should be employed during the establishment of epidural analgesia.
- Correction of hypovolemia/hydration: Hydration is not mandatory before epidural, but any hypovolemia should be corrected with Ringer's lactate solution or normal saline. Dextrose-containing solutions are best avoided, unless the patient is on an insulin regimen.

CSEA is not a routinely practiced technique. It involves a sequential epidural–spinal technique. (Figure 3.6 a & b). The epidural space is identified in the conventional way and through it a long spinal needle is passed into the subarachnoid space. The drug is then instilled into it. This is followed by threading and fixation of the epidural catheter, in the usual manner.

It is indicated in:

- Very early labour, where an intrathecal narcotic suffices, thus avoiding local anesthetic, so that there is no motor blockade
- Advanced labour, where immediate pain relief is obtained
- Obese individuals, as it complements the epidural technique.

Spinal anesthesia for labour pain (Gamlin and Lyons 1997) and continuous spinal anesthetic techniques (Valerie et al 2008) are not routinely recommended.

## Drugs used for epidural

Current practice advocates a low dose mixture of local anesthetic with a lipophilic narcotic (Hart et al 2003). The commonly used local anesthetic agents are bupivacaine and newer agents like ropivacaine and levo-bupivacaine. Bupivacaine is most economical and is as effective as the newer ones (Atienzar et al 2008). The concentrations of bupivacaine recommended are 0.0625 per cent to 0.1 per cent, both for activation of the epidural analgesia and for maintenance.

Bupivacaine is usually mixed with a lipophilic narcotic like fentanyl or sufentanil. Fentanyl is more economical and causes less respiratory depression. The concentration recommended is 2 mcg per ml. The volume

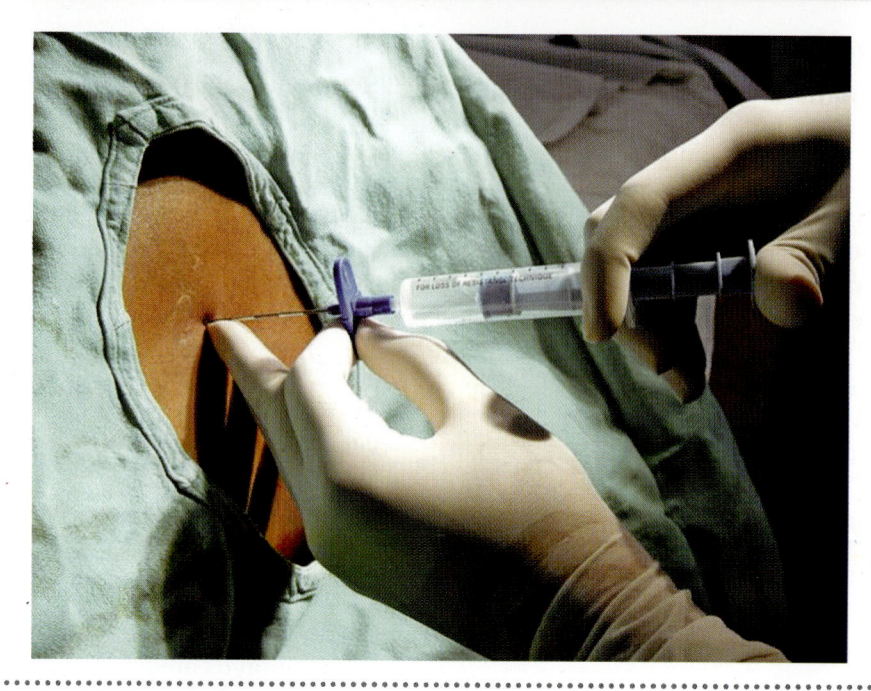

**Figure 3.5a** Loss of resistance technique with saline to identify the epidural space

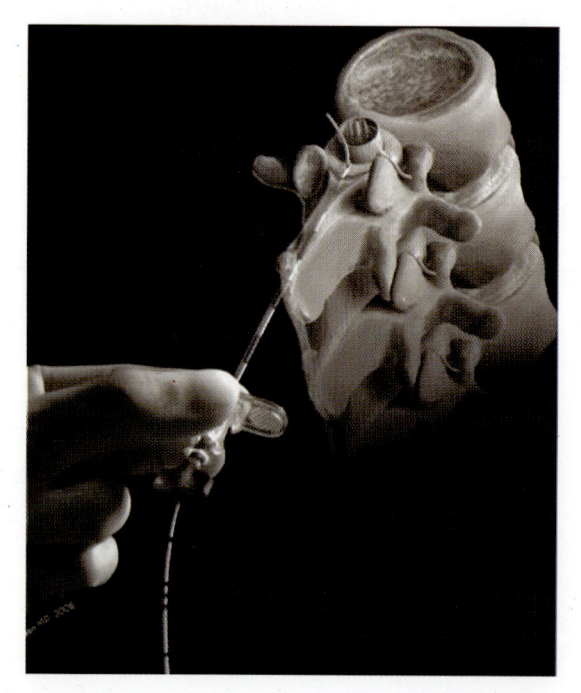

**Figure 3.5b** Cross section of vertebra with thecal sac showing placement of epidural catheter in the epidural space. (Modified from Chestnut's Obstetric anaesthesia, 4th edition, Mosby Elsevier, 2009; 12.238)

Pain Relief in Labour | 69

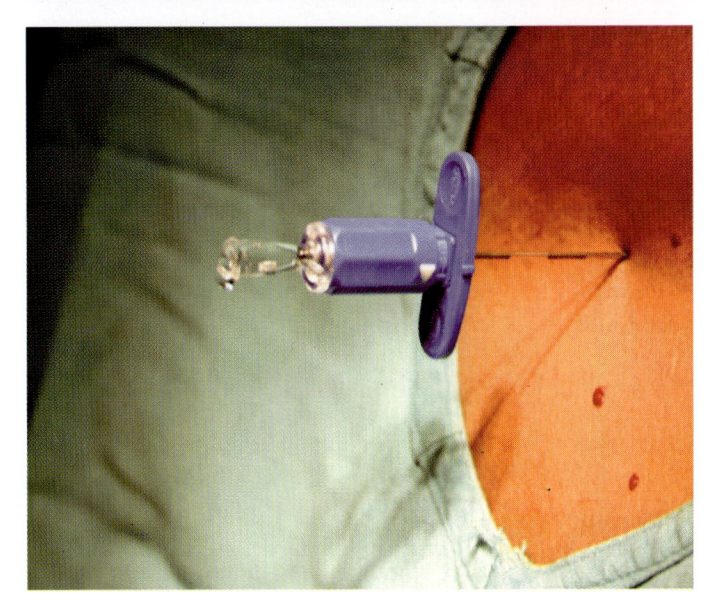

**Figure 3.6a** Sequential combined spinal epidural technique. After the identification of the epidural space in the usual way, a 27g pencil tip spinal needle is introduced through the epidural needle till it reaches the subarachnoid space and the spinal needle is locked over the epidural needle. Clear CSF is seen at the hub of the spinal needle through which the drug is administered. The Spinal needle is then removed and the epidural catheter is threaded the usual way

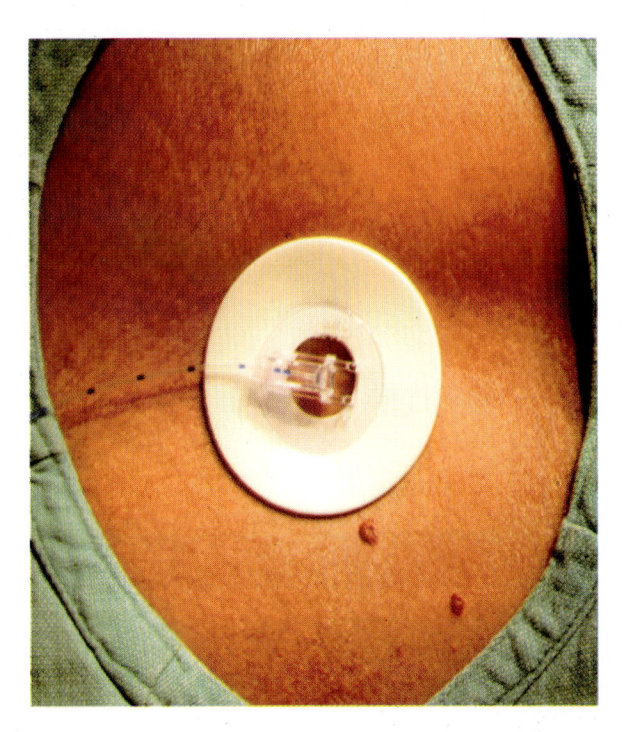

**Figure 3.6b** Epidural catheter fixation with a fixing device to prevent catheter migration

of epidural dose required is between 15 to 20 ml given during initiation and maintenance of the epidural block.

For CSEA, the intrathecal narcotics recommended are Fentanyl 20 to 25 mcg or sufentanil 5 to 10 mcg. Once the analgesic effect of the intrathecal narcotic is about to wear off, usually within 90–120 minutes, the epidural catheter can be activated and maintained in the usual way.

## Maintenance of regional analgesia during labour

This is achieved by one of the following methods:

- Manual intermittent boluses, usually administered by midwives.
- Continuous epidural infusion, not an ideal technique, as even the low dose mixture produces significant motor blockade and the need for breakthrough top-ups is more.
- Patient controlled epidural analgesia (PCEA) (Figure 3.7), is being increasingly used in several units. The maternal satisfaction is superior with PCEA as the woman has more control over her level of analgesia.

### Epidural and cesarean section rate

A systematic review by Leighton and Halpern, (2002) concluded that epidural analgesia does not increase the incidence of cesarean sections. Similarly, Liu and Sia (2004) found that epidural analgesia using low concentration infusions of bupivacaine

> Epidural analgesia does not increase the incidence of cesarean sections.

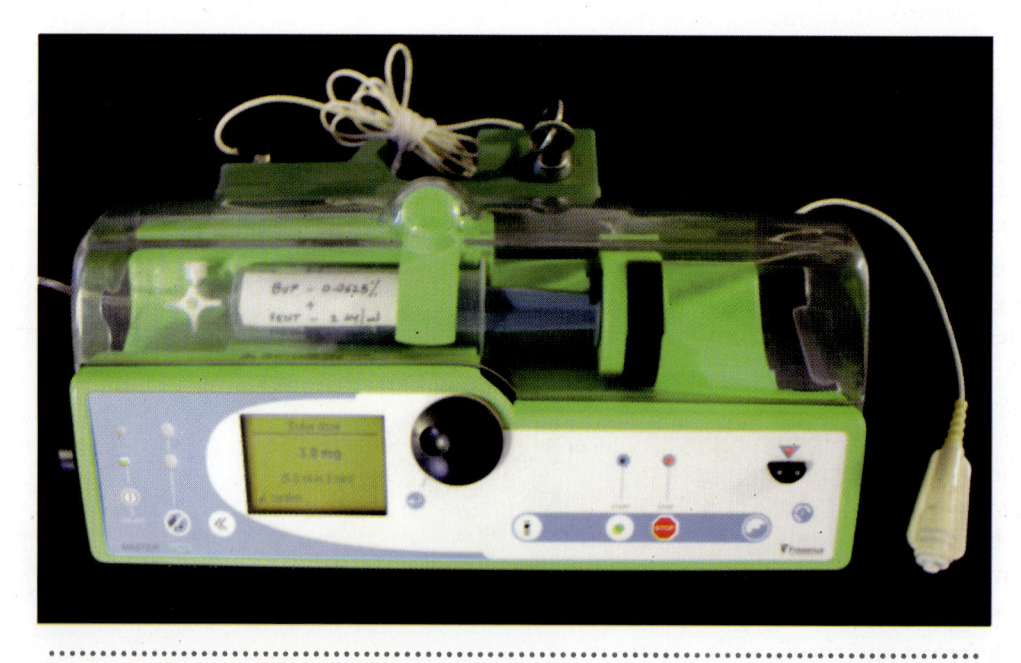

**Figure 3.7** Patient controlled epidural analgesia (PCEA) programmable pump. It offers superior maternal satisfaction.

# Pain Relief in Labour

is unlikely to increase the risk of cesarean section.

## Epidural analgesia: effect on duration of labour and instrumental deliveries

Prolongation of second stage of labour, fetal malposition and loss of the bearing-down reflex and the urge to push are generally considered indications for applying an instrument for facilitating delivery. In a systematic review, Lieberman and O'Donaghue (2002) found sufficient evidence to conclude that epidural is associated with a lower rate of spontaneous vaginal delivery, a higher rate of instrumental vaginal delivery and longer labour, particularly in nulliparous women. Liu and Sia (2004) also found that epidural analgesia increases the risk of instrumental vaginal delivery. However, in another systematic review (Leighton and Halpern 2002), there was no increase in the rate of instrumental delivery for dystocia.

> Epidural is associated with a lower rate of spontaneous vaginal delivery, a higher rate of instrumental vaginal delivery and longer labour, particularly in nulliparous women.

Epidural analgesia prolongs the second stage by about 15 minutes, but does not affect the neonatal outcome (Lieberman and O'Donaghue 2002). Although women receiving epidural analgesia had a longer second stage of labour, they had better pain relief (Liu and Sia 2004). Women who use this form of pain relief are at increased risk of having an instrumental delivery (Anim-Somuah et al 2005).

The practice of discontinuing epidurals is widespread and the size of the reduction in instrumental delivery rate could be clinically important. However, there is insufficient evidence to support the hypothesis that discontinuing epidural analgesia late in labour reduces the rate of instrumental delivery. There is evidence that it increases the rate of inadequate pain relief in the second stage of labour. Larger studies are required to determine whether discontinuing epidurals late in labour decreases instrumental delivery (Torvaldsen et al 2004).

## Timing of epidural analgesia

In 2000, the American Congress of Obstetricians and Gynecologists had recommended that obstetric practitioners should delay the administration of epidural analgesia in nulliparous women until the cervical dilatation reached at least 4–5 cm (ACOG 2000). In 2006, the ACOG rescinded that statement and reaffirmed the opinion it published jointly with the American Society of Anesthesiologists, in which the following statement was articulated: 'Labour causes severe pain for many women. There is no other circumstance where it is considered acceptable for an individual to experience untreated severe pain, amenable to safe intervention, while under a physician's care. In the absence of a medical contraindication, maternal request is a sufficient medical indication for pain relief during labour.'

> Epidural given early in labour does not increase the incidence of cervical dystocia or the cesarean section rate, and it should not be delayed to achieve an arbitrary cervical dilation of 5 cm.

Wong et al (2005) published a randomised clinical trial and concluded that epidural given early in labour does not increase the incidence of cervical dystocia or the cesarean section rate, and it should not be delayed to achieve an arbitrary cervical dilation of 5 cm.

### Epidural analgesia and fetal heart rate

Epidural analgesia can decrease beat-to-beat variability and can cause transient bradycardia, especially with an intrathecal narcotic. However, this is much less compared to pethidine. Hill and colleagues (2003) found no deleterious effects on the fetal heart rate as compared to intravenous pethidine. More importantly, epidural analgesia has no effect on the Apgar score. Studies have shown that cord pH is better in babies delivered under epidural compared to general anesthesia (Reynolds et al 2002; Sendag et al 1999).

## Complications and side effects of regional analgesia

### Hypotension

Epidurally injected anesthetics block the preganglionic autonomic fibres. This results in vasodilatation and reduction in systemic vascular resistance and a consequent fall in blood pressure. Maternal hypotension may lead to fetal heart rate abnormalities. In normal pregnant women, this complication is best treated with rapid infusion of 500 to 1000 ml of crystalloid solution. Pre-loading with crystalloid solution and maintaining a lateral position (Danilenko-Dixon et al 1996), may minimise the risk of hypotension.

> Pre-loading with crystalloid solution and maintaining a lateral position may minimise the risk of hypotension following epidural.

Despite these precautions, about one-third of women may develop hypotension after epidural analgesia (Sharma et al 1997).

### Accidental dural puncture and postdural puncture headache

The incidence of this complication is between 0.2 to 2 per cent. The incidence is less in dedicated units. It is secondary to inadvertent advancement of the epidural needle beyond the epidural space. Breaching the dura results in leakage of cerebrospinal fluid producing low-pressure headache. Classically, the headache is postural in nature, that is, it subsides on lying down and aggravates when the patient adopts an upright posture. The headache usually occurs 24 to 48 hours after epidural and is severe in 65–70 per cent of patients. Often, these patients require an epidural blood patch by an experienced anesthetist. Milder headaches may respond to oral caffeine and paracetamol tablets.

### Backache

Several studies have shown that epidural labour analgesia per se does not result in persistent postpartum backache. Anim-Somuah and colleagues (2005) reviewed the Cochrane database and concluded that the incidence of long-term backache was similar between women receiving epidural analgesia during labour and those who did not. Short-term local tenderness (3–7 days) may be seen in about 30 per cent of mothers, especially if there was technical difficulty and multiple attempts to place the

> Epidural does not increase the incidence of persistent postpartum back pain.

epidural catheter. Proper positioning and an experienced anesthetist can minimise this side effect.

### Bladder dysfunction

Although bladder dysfunction is seen postpartum in a small percentage of women due to several reasons, epidural can be a contributory factor. Mothers receiving epidural narcotic and local anesthetic can have difficulty in voiding urine. Bladder distension may not be recognised by these mothers, resulting in an over-distended bladder which may lead to postpartum bladder dysfunction. Checking for bladder distension and encouraging women in labour to void urine best prevents this problem. They can be offered a bed pan or a urinary catheter may be used to empty the bladder, if the duration of labour is prolonged beyond 6 hours.

### Maternal pyrexia

Several studies have shown that epidural analgesia may result in intrapartum fever in some women (Leighton et al 2002). Lieberman and O'Donaghue (2002) found the incidence of intrapartum fever associated with epidural analgesia to be 10–15 per cent above the baseline rate. With maternal pyrexia, the temperature rise in general is never above $1^0$ C and may be observed in women with prolonged labour. Always rule out and treat any underlying cause if the temperature rise is more than $1^0$ C. Irrespective of the cause, any pyrexia during the intrapartum period needs to be aggressively treated with hydration, antipyretics and other appropriate measures. Intrapartum pyrexia due to epidural does not warrant evaluation for neonatal sepsis.

### Miscellaneous complications

Other potential side effects of epidural analgesia are shivering, pruritus, and delayed gastric emptying.

Unintended intravascular local anesthetic toxicity and total spinal blockade (due to inadvertent intrathecal injection of local anesthetic) are rare and can best be avoided by adopting strict protocols and risk management strategies.

## Alternate regional analgesic techniques

Paracervical block, lumbar sympathetic block, pudendal block and perineal infiltration have been tried for relief of labour pain. These techniques do not relieve the pain completely and are not devoid of adverse effects. Paracervical block and lumbar sympathetic blocks are helpful in relieving the first stage pain, while pudendal block relieves the pelvic floor pain seen during the second stage. Perineal infiltration is helpful for episiotomy pain. The recommended drug for these blocks is 1% lignocaine, with or without adrenaline. The common complications of these techniques are:

- Parametrial hematoma
- Vasovagal syncope
- Fetal bradycardia which may be worrisome
- Systemic local anesthetic toxicity
- Laceration of vaginal mucosa
- Hypotension, especially with lumbar sympathetic block
- Parametrial, retropsoal or subgluteal abscess
- Needle stick injury to the physician

## References

ACOG committee opinion No. 339, 2006. Analgesia and Cesarean Delivery rates. *Obstet Gynecol*; 107:1487–1488.

ACOG Committee Opinion No. 339 (Reaffirmed, 2008). 2006. Analgesia and cesarean delivery rates. American College of Obstetricians and Gynecologists. *Obstet Gynecol* 107:1487–8.

American College of Obstetricians and Gynecologists: Practice Bulletin 36. 2002. Obstetric analgesia and anesthesia. *Obstet Gynecol* 100:177–191

Anim-Somuah M, Smyth R, Howell C. 2005. Epidural versus non-epidural or no analgesia in labour. *Cochrane Database Syst Rev*. Oct 19;(4): CD000331

Atienzar MC, Ma. Palanca J, Torres F, Borras R, Gil S, Esteve I, 2008. A randomized comparison of levobupivacaine, bupivacaine and ropivacaine with fentanyl, for labor analgesia; *International Journal of Obstetric Anesthesia;* 17, 106–111

American College of Obstetricians and Gynecologists. 2000. *Evaluation of cesarean delivery*. Washington, DC: ACOG;.

Belfrage P, Boreus LO, Hartvig P, et al. 1981. Neonatal depression after obstetrical analgesia with pethidine: The role of the injection-delivery time interval and of the plasma concentrations of pethidine and norpethidine. *Acta Obstet Gynecol Scand*: 60:43–9.

Bloom SL, McIntyre DD, Kelley MA et al. 1998. Lack of effect of walking on labor and delivery. *N Engl J Med*. 339:76-9

Bricker L and T Lavender 2002. Parenteral opioids for labor pain relief: A systematic review. *Am J Obstet Gynecol*. 186:S94,

Camille Le Ray, François A, François G, William F, October 2009. When to stop pushing: effects of duration of second-stage expulsion efforts on maternal and neonatal outcomes in nulliparous women with epidural analgesia. *American Journal of Obstetrics and Gynecology*; 201:4;361,e1–7

Chestnut DH et al. 2009. *Obstetric anesthesia: Principles and practice*; ed Polley S L, Tsen CL, Wong AC, 405–501. Mosby Elsevier.

Claahsen-van der Grinten HL, Verbruggen I, van den Berg PP, et al. 2005. Different pharmacokinetics of tramadol in mothers treated for labour pain and in their neonates. *Eur J Clin Pharmacol*; 61:523-9.

Cohen J. Doctor James Young Simpson, Rabbi Abraham De Sola, and Genesis, 1996. Chapter 3, verse 16. *Obstet Gynecol*; 88:895-8

Danilenko-Dixon DR, Tefft L, Haydon B et al. 1996. The effect of maternal position on cardiac output with epidural analgesia in labor. *Am J Obstet Gynecol* 174:332,

Donald C, Maureen P, Fredric D, David Hopkins P, Lieberman, Mayberry L, Judith P, et al, 2002. *Am J Obstet Gynecol*; Supplement to Vol, 186:5, S1–S15.

D'Onofrio P, Novelli AMM, Mecacci F, and Scarselli G; December 1, 2009. The Efficacy and Safety of Continuous Intravenous Administration of Remifentanil for Birth Pain Relief: An Open Study of 205 Parturients *Anesth. Analog*; 109(6): 1922–24.

Douma MR, Verwey RA, Kam-Endtz CE, Van der Linden PD, Stienstra R; 2009. Obstetric analgesia: A comparison of patient-controlled meperidine, remifentanil, and fentanyl in labour *Br. J. Anaesth*, 104:2, 209

Dowswell T, Bedwell C, Lavender T, Neilson JP. 2009. Transcutaneous electrical nerve stimulation (TENS) for pain relief in labour. *Cochrane Database of Systematic Reviews*, Issue 2.

Gamlin FMC and G Lyons. 1997. Spinal analgesia in labour, *International J Obstetric Anaesthesia*; 6:3;161–172

Gardosi J, Sylvester S, Lynch C. 1989. Alternative positions in second stage of labour: A randomized contolled trial. *Br J Obstet Gynaecol*. 96:1290–6

Hart EM, Ahmed N and Buggy DJ, Jan 2003. Comparison of Bupivacaine 0.25% V/s Low dose mixtures: Impact study; *International Journal of Obst. Anesthesia;* 12:1;4–8.

Hill JB, Alexander JM, Sharma SK, McIntire DD, Leveno KJ. 2003. A comparison of the effects of epidural and meperidine analgesia during labor on fetal heart rate. *Obstet Gynecol.* Aug;102(2):333–7.

Henneborm WJ, Cogan R, 1975. The effect of husband participation on reported pain and probability of medication during labour and birth, *J Psychosom Res.* 19:215–22.

Hodnett ED, 2002. Pain and women's satisfaction with the experience of childbirth: a systematic review, *Am J Obstet Gynecol.* 186: s160–72.

Howell CJ, Kidd C, Roberts W et al. 2001. A RCT of epidural compared with non-epidural analgesia in labour. *BJOG*; Jan 108:27–33

Kenkin HL, Keskin EA, Avsar AF, et al. 2003. Pethidine versus tramadol for pain relief during labor. *Int J Gynaecol Obstet.* 82:11–6.

Kennell J, Klaus M, McGrath S et al. 1991. Continuous emotional support during labor in a US hospital: A randomized controlled trial. *JAMA* 265:2197.

Lieberman E, O'Donoghue C, 2002. Unintended effects of epidural analgesia during labor: A systematic review, *Am J Obstec Gynecol* supplement186:5;S31–68

Liu EHC and ATH Sia. 2004. Rates of caesarean section and instrumental vaginal delivery in nulliparous women after low concentration epidural infusions or opioid analgesia:systematic review. *BMJ.* June 12; 328(7453):1410.

Leighton BL, Stephen Halpern H, 2002. The effect of epidural analgesia on labor, maternal and neonatal outcomes: A systematic review; *Am J Obstec Gynecol supplement*;186:5;S69–77

Maduska AL, Haghassemali M. 1978. A double-blind comparison of butorphanol and meperidine in labor: Maternal pain relief and effect on the newborn. *Can Anaesth Soc J*; 25:398–404.

Melzack R. 1984. The myth of painless childbirth. *Pain* 19:321.

Melzack R, Bélanger E, Lacroix, R. 1991. Labor pain: Effect of maternal position on front and back pain. *Journal of Pain and Symptom Management.* Vol 6. Issue 1. 476–480

Minnich ME. 2004. Childbirth Preparation and Nonpharmalogic Analgesia: in *Obstetric Anesthesia: Principles and Practice ed: Chestnut DH,* Elsevier Mosby

Penny P and MA O'Hara. 2002. Nonpharmacologic relief of pain during labor: Systemic reviews of five methods, *Am J Obstet Gynecol supplement,* 186:5;S131–519

Ramnero A, Hanson U, Kihlgren M. 2002. Acupuncture treatment during labour: A randomized controlled trial. *Br J Obstet Gynaecol* 109:637–44.

Rayburn W, Rathke A, Leuschen MP, et al. 1989. Fentanyl citrate analgesia during labor. *Am J Obstet Gynecol.* 161:202–6.

Reynolds F, Sharma SK, Seed PT. 2002. Analgesia in labour and fetal acid-base balance: A meta-analysis comparing epidural with systemic opioid analgesia. *Br J Obstet Gynaecol.* 109:1344.

Rosen MA. 2002. Nitrous oxide for relief of labor pain: A systematic review; *Am J Obstet Gynecol*; Supplement, 186:5;S110–30

Sendag F, Terek C et al. 1999. Comparison of Epidural and general anaesthesia for Elective CS, effect on APGAR and acid-base status. *Aust N Z J Obstet Gynecol*; 39:464–68

Sharma SK, Sidawi JE, Ramin SM, et al. 1997. Cesarean delivery: A randomized trial of epidural versus patient-controlled mepiridine analgesia during labor. *Anesthesiology* 87:487,

Simpson, JY. 1847. *Answer to the Religious Objections Advanced Against the Employment of Anesthetic Agents in Midwifery and Surgery.* Edinburgh

Skilnand E, Fossen D, Heiburg E. 2002. Acupuncture in the management of pain in labor. *Acta Obstet Gynecol Scand* 81:943–8.

Snow J. On administration of chloroform in during parturition. 1853. *Assoc Med J* 1:500–2.

Sosa CG, Balaguer E, Alonso JG, et al. 2004. Meperidine for dystocia during the first of labor: A randomized controlled trial. *Am J Obstet Gynaecol*; 191:1212–8.

Torvaldsen S, Roberts CL, Bell JC, Raynes-Greenow CH. 2004. Discontinuation of epidural analgesia late in labour for reducing the adverse delivery outcomes associated with epidural analgesia. *Cochrane Database Syst Rev*. Oct 18;(4): CD004457.

Valerie A. Arkoosh, Craig M. et al, 2008. A Randomized, Double-masked, Multicenter Comparison of the Safety of Continuous Intrathecal Labor Analgesia Using a 28-Gauge Catheter versus Continuous Epidural Labor Analgesia; *Anesthesiology*; 108:286–98

Wong CA, Scavone BM et al, 2005. The risk of Cesarean delivery in neuraxial analgesia given early vs. late in Labor; *NEJM*; 352: 655–65.

# CHAPTER 4

# CONSENT IN LABOUR

*Cleave Gass and Rehana Iqbal*

Consent is a topic of debate in both the ethical and legal arena. In most legal systems, it is the doctor's legal duty to seek consent from patients for treatment they might require. Only after consent has been obtained can treatment lawfully proceed, with a limited number of exceptions relating, for example, to life-saving emergency treatment. In the context of medical treatment there has been a move away from the paternalistic approach of 'doctor knows best' to a position of attempting to empower patients to make decisions about what they believe is in their best interests. Therefore, the role of doctors in this process has changed, in that they have to facilitate this decision-making process by providing information to patients to assist them to make an informed choice.

A fundamental principle when considering the validity of consent for treatment is respect for the patient's autonomy, and their right to decide whether or not to undergo any medical intervention. Morally however, it may be difficult for doctors not to instigate treatment when they believe there is benefit to the patient, but it is important to note that medical best interest is only a small component of overall best interests and the consequences of enforcing treatment on unwilling patients, thereby removing their autonomy, is worse than allowing refusal. It is recognised that adult patients have the right to refuse treatment even if this refusal is harmful to them. To treat without consent could result in a legal claim under battery.

> Adult patients have the right to refuse treatment even if this refusal is harmful to them. To treat without consent could result in a legal claim under battery.

## Introduction

In order to obtain a truly valid consent, three components are required: capacity, voluntariness and adequate information provision as to the general nature of the proposed procedure (Powers 2000). The first requirement, capacity, is necessary so that an individual is able to understand, retain and weigh the information provided to come to a decision and then communicate the decision made. These requirements for capacity were first legally recognised in the courts in the case of an adult refusing medically-recommended treatment (Re C

(Adult: Refusal of treatment) [1994] 1 All ER 819 (Fam Div).}. This legal definition of capacity has been given statutory recognition in the United Kingdom, following the Mental Capacity Act 2005 (MCA 2005). The second requirement is voluntariness. This implies that consent is given without coercion or pressure to accept or decline treatment. Lastly, for consent to be valid, adequate information must be provided in order that a decision to agree or refuse a proposed treatment can be made. This is influenced by the nature of the treatment, the risks and benefits, alternative treatments and the consequences of refusal. Whether these are ever possible to achieve or even present when obtaining consent from the labouring parturient is debatable.

In obstetrics, the need to obtain consent from women in labour has come to the forefront since the publication of *Changing Childbirth* in the United Kingdom (Changing Childbirth 1995), which aimed to make obstetrics and the entire birth process more women-centred. Arguably, although doctors have always had an obligation to give their patients detailed information prior to treatment, following the publication of this document, the importance of this duty has been reinforced. Therefore, doctors should ensure that women are given detailed information about the various treatment options that are available to them. Nationally, in the United Kingdom at least, the importance of obtaining consent has once again been emphasised by the publication of the Department of Health's *Guidelines Reference Guide to Consent for Examination or Treatment* (Reference Guide to Consent for Treatment 2000).

## Consenting women in labour

Women in labour present a particular group of patients in whom the obtaining of fully informed consent may be difficult, if not impossible, as some may temporarily lack the capacity to give consent, because of pain, fatigue or the effects of analgesia. Further, treatment decisions made by women in labour and their doctors are usually urgent and have consequences for both the mother and their child. However, to obtain consent beforehand prior to labour is the difficulty. This is clear from the following statement: it is difficult 'to form a theoretical opinion as to whether to have an epidural (for analgesia in labour) when one is pain-free as this is not in any way an informed decision' (Scott 1996). A further difficulty is that women in almost all situations tend to be vulnerable to discrimination and bias because of social, cultural and economic circumstances, so when seeking consent from women, it is important to remember that 'the principle of autonomy should emphasise the important role women must play in decision-making in respect to their health care' (FIGO Committee 2000).

> Obtaining of fully informed consent may be difficult in women in labour as some may temporarily lack the capacity to give consent, because of pain, fatigue or the effects of analgesia

## Informed consent

When considering consent issues in labour, the conflicts between the various theoretical models of 'informed' consent need to be considered. When seeking consent from a patient, a doctor is trying to involve that particular patient in the decision-making process by presenting her with a factual background, so that she can make a choice based on all the available information. It can be seen as a way of transferring power from the doctor to the patient and is an attempt at facilitating the patient's ability to maintain her individuality and autonomy, a fundamental aspect of human rights. However, there exists potential conflict between various theoretical models of consent, which may not always be easily resolvable (Alderson and Goodey 1998). Western medicine tends to assume a positivist concept of consent, this being defined by the need to distinguish factual concepts and then to define them by dichotomies e.g. competent/incompetent, informed/ignorant.

Consent can then be regarded as a commodity, something which doctors try to obtain from patients by giving them the available information, and then checking it against what they recall of the information that they have been given, in order to assess their ability to make an informed and conscious choice. It does not, however, take into account the reasons behind the choices patients may make, which can be influenced by a whole variety of external factors such as the patient's particular culturally determined worldview or by factors more immediate, such as the immense pain of labour. In this model of consent, 'social pressure and great anxiety and distress, are assumed to inhibit patients' ability to make independent, rational choices and so should be reduced or avoided if possible' (Alderson and Goodey 1998). Yet, this is the model generally used to assess the success of obtaining consent in labour, a state of great distress and anxiety for some women (Grancher et al 2000). Further, it has been questioned whether this minimalist approach to obtaining consent is always the most appropriate, and questions whether it could result in needless cruelty in the application of universal rules in the context of culturally different values which are subjective and cannot be accurately measured (Benatar and Benatar 1998).

## Theoretical Models of Consent

There are, however, different theoretical models involved in the process of obtaining consent, which should be considered when seeking it, as a certain model may well be more applicable in the particular circumstance. These theoretical models are constructed consent, functionalist consent, critical theory and postmodern choice, all of which may provide more appropriate theoretical models to consider when seeking consent in labour (Alderson and Goodey 1998).

## Constructed consent

In constructed consent, all social and personal influences are deemed equally valid; thus, it provides a theoretical framework of consent, which is regarded as a process rather than a specific event. The Department of Health's Guidelines in the United Kingdom on consent recognise this model stating that 'giving and obtaining consent is usually a process, not an on-off event. Patients can change their minds and withdraw consent at any time'. McHale and Fox explain this by noting that:

> ...a further important distinction to bear in mind is that between informed consent and informed choice. Even if a greater obligation had been imposed upon doctors to disclose the risks of a particular treatment, this would

frequently leave the patient only with a straightforward choice of whether to accept or reject a particular treatment. To make a fully informed choice, the patient must also be aware of a range of alternatives (McHale and Fox 1999).

However, the difficulties of utilising this model of consent in labour are two-fold. First, as decisions in labour are often required with some urgency, there may not have been time to establish the kind of rapport needed between the doctor and the woman in labour to create the relationship required to form a constructed consent. Second, the very essence of consent and autonomy may be blurred in the process of trying to determine all the variables influencing a particular choice, confusing the issue even further. However, this is the model that leading authorities on ethical issues in the provision of healthcare to women would espouse. The FIGO Report recognises that:

> ...when decisions regarding medical care are required, women should be provided with full information on the available management alternatives including the risks and benefits. Informing women and obtaining their input and consent, or dissent, should be a continuing process (The FIGO Committee 2000).

### Functionalist model of consent

In the functionalist model, consent is relegated to that of a token gesture or 'ceremony'. This represents consent obtained in order to transfer the onus of the risk of a particular procedure or aspect of research onto the patient, thus allowing the treatment to proceed without the danger of expensive litigation ensuing. The vast majority of instances of obtaining consent from patients in labour seem to equate to this functionalist model of consent. It becomes part of a checklist of duties to be performed, much the same as checking whether a particular patient has had their x-rays taken. An example of this is cited when a researcher quotes a consumer group representative as saying:

> ...my experience of talking to midwives about the issue of obtaining consent is that what quite a lot of midwives and other professionals understand by informed consent is that you tell parents what they should do and then they consent to that (Symon 2001).

This seems to represent a fairly typical model of obtaining consent, and although 'most doctors would not support extreme functionalism, in busy wards, clinics, and surgeries, consent tends to be treated as a simple or tedious formality' (Alderson and Goodey 1998).

### Critical Theory

Critical theory sees consent as the opposite. It is a form of protection for patients against doctors who have access to esoteric knowledge to which a patient has no special access. Thus, critical theory would regard consent not as 'one way medical information giving, but as an exchange of knowledge between doctor and patient so that together they can make more informed decisions'.

### Postmodern theories of consent

Lastly, postmodern theories would see consent as the right to choose whatever one wanted and to give one's own consent to treatment, regardless of its medical necessity, the patient being a consumer of healthcare, just as a political consumer might campaign for ethical care and the fair rationing of resources.

Much treatment is not for serious disease but for convenience, and even consent to major surgery like hysterectomy or spinal fusion may be influenced more by personal preferences than by clinical judgement (Alderson and Goodey 1998).

Arguably therefore, postmodern theories of consent perhaps best reveal the contradictions and confusion around the issues of consent and individual autonomy and rights in our society where there is such strong emphasis placed on choice and consumerism. It may be that:

> ...consent is a strong concept in being so versatile and durable, but it is vulnerable to conflicting interpretations and rejections as a worthless ideal... consent is too complex to be fully understood in any one theoretical model (Alderson and Goodey 1998).

There is, as noted earlier, an inherent difficulty in obtaining consent for a particular intervention prior to the event. This is exemplified, for instance, by the establishment of epidural analgesia, with its concomitant risks when a woman might be unable to anticipate the severity of the risks involved. This is acknowledged in Davies' statement that 'a first-time mother's optimistic anticipation of an easy labour is not to be discouraged, it has to be tempered with the acknowledgement that labour may well be much more painful than anticipated' (Davies 1996). The fact that capacity may be difficult to establish while a woman is in labour, makes the issue of obtaining valid consent for procedures performed during it even more complex. Further, it is well documented that recall of information given to women prior to labour in an effort to increase their ability to make an informed choice is extremely small, casting doubt on whether giving women information prior to their labour could realistically increase their ability to make an informed choice while in labour itself (Bowden et al 2001).

## Legal Standing of the Fetus

There are a number of compelling arguments for treatment despite the absence of consent, some of which may involve acting on behalf of the fetus. A consideration unique to pregnancy and the birth process is that a woman's rights to autonomy and bodily integrity may be sacrificed by misguided attempts at securing the well-being of her fetus. Calls for 'legal-personhood' to be attributed to the fetus need to be considered, especially in situations where a woman in labour withholds her consent to interventions, even though they may be beneficial to the fetus. In considering these arguments, it is worth considering first, the consequentialist argument that if the risks to the mother of having a medical intervention are minimal and the benefits to the unborn child are great, then surely to do nothing would be morally wrong.

For obvious reasons, it is more difficult to allow a fetus at term to die than in the earlier stages of the pregnancy, when the potential for independent life is not as developed. However, the consequences of enforcing treatment may be worse. Fear of this loss of autonomy could potentially lead to refusal to seek medical assistance during pregnancy and labour. There is an argument that by becoming pregnant and allowing pregnancy to come to term, the mother has accepted the responsibilities that this would entail, and by doing so, has in some way reduced her right to autonomy when that right conflicts with fetal well-being. This is a very slippery slope, in terms of argument. To support this could potentially require supporting prohibition of certain behaviours during pregnancy, such as smoking and alcohol consumption. Also, it could for instance, morally justify enforced renal donation by parents, if they have a child who so requires it. One could argue that morally, the fetus is a symbol of life, but it is not entitled to the same rights to life as the mother. All of these arguments look at the fetus' well-being and that of the mother separately. This perhaps reflects the way we medically manage these circumstances. In reality, a mother who has carried her unborn child to term is unlikely to make decisions without considering the fetus. Would it be morally wrong to prevent her making decisions about herself and her unborn child? Should seeking medical assistance obligate one to take the medical advice given?

A further difficulty in resolving this matter has been the paternalistic and misogynistic view held by the medical profession, and the tendency to use the fetus as reason for denying women the choice. Thomson observes:

> ...the medical profession constructed women who sought abortions as either ignorant, or evil 'rebellious women who had abandoned their maternal duties for selfish and personal ends'... This formulation reflects the historical perception of women as existing solely within the private sphere. Freedom to make educational or reproductive choices was seen as incompatible with the ideology of 'true womanhood', and the maternal ethic of care and responsibility (Thomson 1994).

There is a danger that this particular patriarchal view could be expanded not only to cover women's choices in obtaining abortions, but in other aspects of their choices, affecting their reproductive lives including those made while in labour itself.

## Court-enforced cesarean sections

The extent to which the law has supported the autonomy of women, including their right to consent to or refuse interventions in labour, can be understood by exploring the progression of the legal judgements in some enforced cesarean section cases, both in the United States and the United Kingdom. Arguably, the evolution of case law, particularly regarding the issue of court-enforced cesarean sections, has shown some progression towards the recognition of the ability of women to make informed choices while in labour.

In the case of Rochdale NHST v C, the courts found that C was not competent to make a decision due to a comment made in labour that 'I would rather die than have a cesarean section again'. In deciding this case, it was stated that in the circumstances of labour with the pain and emotional stress, a patient who seemed to be able to accept the inevitability of her own death was unable to weigh up considerations to make a valid decision about anything, surely still less one which involved her own life (Rochdale NHST v C [1997] 1 FLR 274). It is clear from this case that the principle of respect for autonomy was not overridden, but rather an impairment of capacity decided allowing medical intervention.

In the case of MB, a woman who was needle-phobic and refused cesarean section, the courts found her to lack capacity. Unlike the case above, it was felt that the needle-phobia impaired her capacity to give consent [Re MB (An Adult: Medical Treatment) [1997] 8 Med. LR 217]. The case of MB is particularly interesting in that it ruled that a woman in labour does have the capacity to give consent to and refuse cesarean section even if her life and the life of the unborn child is at risk. No concession was made for analgesics given. However, it did recognise that severe pain could impair capacity.

This recognition of capacity in labour and the maternal right to bodily integrity overriding any rights of the fetus is further reinforced in the case of St George's Healthcare NHS Trust v S. [St George's Healthcare NHS Trust v S. [1998] 3 All ER 673]. S was a 28-year-old woman, who due to an aversion to medical therapy presented for the first time at 36 weeks gestation with severe preeclampsia. She was informed that there was significant risk of death to her and the fetus, but declined treatment wanting to let nature take its course. A court declaration was successfully applied for and she underwent cesarean section despite her refusal. S subsequently successfully challenged the declaration. Although this case in ruling recognised the viable fetus as human, it stated that the fetus had no legal rights.

## Legal competence

Issues of legal competence should be considered with respect to the labouring parturient, including those of women under the age of legal competence, in order to examine to what extent their ability to give informed consent is recognised and protected. However, the assertion that 'no consent given in labour is ever fully valid' (Scott 1996) may well be justified. The analysis that 'there is a sense nonetheless that the prognosis for shared decision-making in obstetrics is grim' (Rhoden 1987) may well be true, given the inherent doubts surrounding competency in labour, the ambiguities surrounding the moral standing of the fetus and societal attitudes in some cultures towards women. The relatively new concept of birth-plans that state the explicit wishes of a woman concerning her labour should be considered, in conjunction with the guidance published by the Law Commission in the United Kingdom concerning advance directives. This may possibly represent a model whereby some guidance may be obtained as to a woman's choices before the event and to ensure better informed consent, as often the real world of medical decision-making bears little resemblance to the legal ideals espoused in the evolution of case law.

## Conclusion

What is certain is that treatment decisions in labour are challenging, and the consequences of consenting to treatment or not can have serious implications for both mother and fetus. When considering women's reproductive lives and the law, and questions of consent in labour particularly, there is also some disagreement as to whether the same criteria and theoretical models of consent should apply to obtaining it. Perhaps therefore, a different set of theoretical frameworks should be constructed, recognising the uniqueness of the situation, which may well be more appropriate. This argument can further be extended into the realm of women's lives generally based on their reproductive abilities.

Kay recognises the need to consider different models of gender-based equality when discussing this issue, accepting that pregnancy is a unique state in which perhaps different models and law should apply (Kay 1993). She observes that a woman and man have characteristics, which can be compared irrespective of their reproductive abilities. She refers to this as 'an assimilationist model of equality'. She further notes, however that there does have to be another model, which recognises a woman's unique position in pregnancy, and that models should be sought, upon which the differences are or can be made legally relevant.

This is further elucidated in Bridgeman and Millns' assertion that:

...in order to ensure equality of opportunity, the difference of being pregnant has to be acknowledged so that women are not disadvantaged as a consequence of their reproductive capabilities (Bridgeman and Millns 1998).

There would seem to be a danger, therefore, in assuming that the same models of consent should apply, irrespective of a person's reproductive status. Pregnancy is obviously unique and decisions taken during it are influenced by circumstances and situations not encountered elsewhere. When disagreements do arise, the involvement of appropriate healthcare professionals and legal teams may be necessary.

## References

Alderson P, Goodey C. 1998. Theories of consent. *BMJ* 317:1313–15

Bauman Z. 1998. *Life in fragments: Essays in postmodern morality*. 27 Oxford: Blackwell.

Benatar D and SR Benatar. 1998. Informed consent and research. *BMJ* 316:1008

Bowden M, A Brake, R Crombie, K Eagland, JS Thomas. 2001. Patient's recall of information given during the process of obtaining consent for regional anaesthesia. *Int J Obstet Anaesth* 10:238.

Bridgeman J, S Millns. 1998. *Feminist perspectives on law: Law's engagement with the female body*. London: Sweet and Maxwell.

Changing Childbirth. 1995. *Report of the Expert Maternity Group*. London: HMSO.

Davies AG. 1996. Ethics in obstetric anaesthesia. *Anaesthesia* 51:1182–93.

Grancher J, S Grice, J Dewan, J Eisenach. 2000. An evaluation of informed consent prior to epidural analgesia for labour and delivery. *Int J Obstet Anaesth* 9: 168–73.

Kay HH. 1993. Equality and difference: The case of pregnancy. In *Feminist Jurisprudence*, ed. P Smith. 27 Oxford: Oxford University Press.

McHale J, M Fox. 1999. *Health care law: Text and materials*. 354 London: Sweet and Maxwell.

Powers M J. 2000. Consent to treatment. <http://www.medneg.co.uk/consent to treatment.htm>

Reference Guide to Consent for Examination or Treatment. 2000. London: Department of Health.

Rhoden NK. 1987. Informed consent in obstetrics: Some special problems. *West New Eng Law Rev* 9(1):67–88.

Scott WE. 1996. Ethics in obstetric anaesthesia. *Anaesthesia* 51:717–18.

Symon A. 2001. *Obstetric litigation from A to Z*. 39 Salisbury: Mark Allen Publishing.

The FIGO Committee for the Ethical Aspects of Human Reproduction and Women's Health Recommendations on Ethical Issues in Obstetrics and Gynaecology. 2000. London: FIGO. www.figo.org

Thomson M. 1994. After Re S. *Med Law Rev* 2:141–42.

# CHAPTER 5

# INTRAPARTUM FETAL MONITORING

*Rohan D'Souza and Sabaratnam Arulkumaran*

With the onset of normal labour, a fetus embarks on the most perilous journey it will undertake in its lifetime. Although widely considered the best method of delivery for both mother and baby, a vaginal birth is not bereft of risks. Although the introduction of intrapartum fetal surveillance has not been able to make this journey any easier, it has certainly helped in making it much safer than it has ever been.

The main objective of intrapartum fetal monitoring is to identify the fetus at risk of an adverse outcome, based on our ability to understand how the fetus reacts to stress before it becomes compromised. Detection of impending intrapartum hypoxia/acidosis should enable obstetricians to undertake appropriate and timely interventions. Although a majority of congenital neurological handicaps are not related to intrapartum events, intrapartum hypoxia continues to be responsible for a proportion of these handicaps and for a significant number of perinatal deaths, even in the developed world. According to the most recent perinatal mortality report for England and Wales (CEMACH 2008), 260 stillbirths and 211 neonatal deaths in the last triennium were a direct result of intrapartum causes.

## Fetal Heart Rate Monitoring

Fetal heart rate (FHR) monitoring is the most commonly utilised method for the assessment of fetal well-being during labour, because the fetal heart is usually readily accessible to auscultation, even with basic equipment. This monitoring is performed either by intermittent auscultation (IA) or electronic fetal monitoring (EFM). While IA is limited to the length of time an attendant is physically able to apply a transducer to the maternal abdomen, EFM provides a continuous record of the FHR pattern over a desired length of time, usually on a two-channel chart, with FHR on the upper channel and the frequency, duration and amplitude of uterine contractions on the lower channel, constituting the cardiotocograph (CTG).

### Intermittent auscultation

Intermittent auscultation (IA) of the fetal heart rate in labour is done with a Pinard stethoscope or preferably with a handheld Doppler ultrasound fetal heart detector (Mahomed et al, 1994). Auscultation is best done for 60 seconds after a contraction, every 15 minutes in the first stage and every 5 minutes in the second stage of labour (ACOG 1995). Most maternity units however, have manpower difficulties which preclude the provision of the one-to-one care that IA requires (Morrison et al 1993; Kripke 1999; Penning and Garite 1999). Maintaining the required frequency of auscultation over several hours may be quite difficult to achieve, especially in obese mothers in whom fetal heart sounds may be muffled. Also, information on baseline variability is not possible and detection of late decelerations may not be reliable (Menticoglou and Harman 1999; Simpson et al 1999). However, when continuous CTG is not feasible or desirable, intrapartum monitoring can be done by IA and this is currently recommended in low-risk pregnancies and women delivering at home or in remote, rural locations. There is emerging evidence that there may be a role for IA in some high-risk pregnancies as well. A study in post-cesarean section pregnancies has suggested that IA may also be a safe mode of fetal surveillance as long as close monitoring is ensured (Madaan and Trivedi 2006).

A systematic review of recent trials comparing IA with EFM in low-risk pregnancies (Alfirevic et al 2006) has shown that women with IA were less likely to have cesarean sections and instrumental vaginal births for abnormal FHR patterns. However, these babies were more likely to have neonatal seizures and require admission to the neonatal unit. There was no difference in perinatal mortality or the subsequent incidence of cerebral palsy. The findings were similar even when both low- and high-risk pregnancies were included in the analysis.

> Auscultation is best done for 60 seconds after a contraction, every 15 minutes in the first stage and every 5 minutes in the second stage of labour

Based on recent evidence, The National Institute for Clinical Excellence (NICE 2007) has made the following recommendations with regard to intermittent fetal surveillance in labour:

1. IA of the FHR may be used for low-risk women in established labour in any birth setting.

2. Initial auscultation of the fetal heart should be done at first contact in early labour and at each further assessment undertaken, to determine whether labour has become established.

3. Once a woman is in established labour, IA of FHR after a contraction should be continued every 15 minutes during the first stage and every 5 minutes during the second stage for 60 seconds immediately after a contraction.

4. 'Moderate-level evidence' suggests that evidence of the superiority of the hand-held Doppler over the Pinard stethoscope was not robust enough to differentiate between the two techniques; therefore, either technique may be used for the purpose of IA.

5. Pregnancies being monitored by IA should be converted to continuous EFM if the following conditions are observed:
    - Meconium-stained liquor is significant
    - Abnormal FHR detected by IA (less than 110 beats per minute (bpm); greater than 160 bpm; any decelerations after a contraction)

- Maternal pyrexia (defined as 38.0 °C once or 37.5 °C on two occasions, 2 hours apart)
- Fresh bleeding in labour
- Oxytocin use for augmentation
- The woman's request

## Intermittent EFM

Intermittent EFM involves the use of the CTG at predetermined intervals during labour. The use of intermittent EFM has been compared with both IA as well as continuous EFM. The largest randomised trial of IA against EFM, consisting of over 12,000 patients showed no difference in the incidence of subsequent cerebral palsy, but showed a 55 per cent reduction in neonatal seizures in the EFM group (MacDonald et al 1985). A meta-analysis consisting of 58,855 cases revealed a similar reduction in neonatal seizures in the group monitored by EFM (Thacker et al 1995). Although EFM might not have prevented cerebral palsy, the recommendation was that the reduction in rates of neonatal seizures should promote its use over IA. EFM also reduces the risk of intrapartum fetal death from fetal hypoxia and prevents about one perinatal death per 1000 births (Vintzileos et al 1993, 1995).

In a study by Herbst and Ingemarsson (1994), the use of intermittent EFM for 15–30 minutes every second hour with IA in between during the first stage, was compared with the use of continuous EFM in the first stage of labour. Both groups had continuous EFM in the second stage of labour. Intermittent EFM (with stethoscope auscultation in between) was found to be as effective as continuous EFM in low-risk labours.

> EFM reduces the rate of neonatal seizures and also reduces the risk of intrapartum fetal death from fetal hypoxia. It has not been shown to reduce the risk of cerebral palsy.

### The admission cardiotocograph

The use of a 20-minute CTG on admission to the delivery suite as a screening test to identify the fetus at risk of intrapartum hypoxia has not been shown to improve neonatal outcome, although operative delivery rates remain unchanged (Impey et al 2003). Bix et al (2005) systematically reviewed three randomised trials and 11 observational studies assessing the prognostic value and effectiveness of the admission CTG compared with auscultation alone. They showed that women with admission CTG were more likely to have epidural analgesia, continuous EFM and fetal blood sampling (FBS). There was also borderline evidence that women with continuous EFM were more likely to have an instrumental birth and cesarean section compared with the auscultation group, although there was no evidence of differences in augmentation of labour, perinatal mortality or other neonatal morbidities. The routine use of the admission CTG is therefore not recommended.

## Continuous electronic fetal monitoring

Continuous EFM involves the use of a Doppler ultrasound transducer placed on the maternal abdomen or a fetal scalp electrode, after membranes have ruptured, to monitor the baby's heart rate. A pressure gauge transducer is also placed on the abdomen between the uterine fundus and the umbilicus to monitor uterine contractions. Both transducers are connected to a machine, which produces a two-channel recording on thermal paper available for interpretation and storage. This continuous recording of the FHR combined with a recording of uterine activity is called cardiotocography and is the most widely used method of intrapartum fetal surveillance in high-risk labour.

## The role of continuous electronic fetal monitoring in modern obstetrics

EFM has high sensitivity but its specificity is low (Mongelli et al 1997; Dildy 1999; Low et al 1999; Sweha et al 1999). A normal EFM pattern carries a predictive value of over 95 per cent for an Apgar score of 7 or greater, while an abnormal pattern carries a predictive value of about 50 per cent for an Apgar score of less than 7 (Banta and Thacker 1979). In general, abnormal FHR patterns for which cesarean or instrumental deliveries are undertaken are only associated with a 50 per cent chance of fetal acidosis (Tejani et al 1975; Banta and Thacker 1979).

The introduction of CTG into routine clinical practice in the 1960s was not preceded by large randomised trials to demonstrate its perceived benefits of reduction in perinatal mortality and long-term neurological handicap due to intrapartum hypoxia/acidosis. The widespread implementation of EFM does not appear to have brought about a reduction in cerebral palsy (Clark and Hankins 2003). In fact, it is now apparent that the main causes of congenital neurological handicap are more related to inherited and antenatal problems rather than intrapartum events (Steer and Danielian 1999; Huddleston 1999; Nelson 1999). The only consistently proven and clinically significant benefit from the routine use of continuous EFM compared with intermittent auscultation has been found to be the reduction of neonatal seizures, with an increase in cesarean sections and operative vaginal deliveries (Thacker et al 2001).

The clinical effectiveness of CTG is also reduced by variable and inconsistent interpretation, even among experts (Todros et al 1996; Bernades et al 1997; Ayres-de-Campos et al 1999), leading to inappropriate interventions for benign patterns and delayed or no intervention for abnormal patterns (Arulkumaran and Symonds 1999a). There is, therefore, a need for continuing education on CTG interpretation (Murray 1999; Arulkumaran and Symonds 1999b) to improve its value in clinical practice.

In view of the dubious performance of the CTG in randomised trials and the poor specificity of CTG patterns to correlate with subsequent injury in a specific way, the continued reliance on CTG by the medical profession is being lambasted on both medical and legal grounds (Lent 1999). EFM should be seen only as a screening test for intrapartum fetal hypoxia/acidosis (Low et al 1999; Berkus et al 1999); it is used in conjunction with other methods of intrapartum fetal surveillance, in order to avoid unnecessary operative intervention. The acceptable indications for the use of continuous EFM are given in Table 5.1.

Good practice would demand that the following measures be taken in order to optimise outcome and prevent litigation (D'Souza and Arulkumaran, 2009).

1. The patient's name, hospital number, date of birth, the date and time of the recording, pulse rate and temperature should always be checked and recorded before starting the actual recording.

**Table 5.1** Indications for the use of continuous EFM (Steer and Danielian 1999)

**Labour abnormalities**
- Induced labour
- Augmented labour
- Prolonged labour
- Prolonged rupture of membranes
- Regional analgesia
- Previous cesarean section
- Abnormal uterine activity

Suspected fetal distress in labour
- Meconium-staining of amniotic fluid
- Suspicious fetal heart trace on auscultation
- Abnormal FHR on admission CTG
- Vaginal bleeding in labour
- Intrauterine infection

**Fetal problems**
- Multiple pregnancies (all fetuses)
- Small fetus
- Preterm fetus
- Breech presentation
- Oligohydramnios
- Post-term pregnancy
- Rhesus isoimmunisation

**Maternal medical disease**
- Hypertension
- Diabetes
- Cardiac disease (especially cyanotic)
- Hemoglobinopathy
- Severe anemia
- Hyperthyroidism
- Collagen disease
- Renal disease

2. The clock on the CTG machine must always be checked. The time at the end of the trace must also be recorded.

3. If monitoring extends beyond one pack of paper, the packs should be labelled Part 1, 2, 3, etc. The timing and order of events is often crucial in Court and commonly disputed areas in cases of fetal compromise are the timing of intervention and what is an acceptable time delay from the time of decision-making to delivery.

4. The FHR should be auscultated by a Pinard's stethoscope or a Doppler device before commencing EFM to avoid the maternal pulse being recorded by the fetal monitor. A sudden, significant shift of baseline FHR during the course of the recording should prompt an immediate review of the CTG and a correlation between the recorded FHR and maternal pulse. Persistent signal loss should be investigated and should prompt the changing of the transducer, electrodes, connections and machine, if necessary. If these actions do not rectify the problem, IA should be performed and this should be documented in the medical records. The Courts will view an un-interpretable CTG with utmost suspicion and such a recording might jeopardise a successful defence.

5. All intrapartum events e.g. vaginal examination, FBS, siting of an epidural or an epidural top-up must be noted on the CTG.

6. Any member of staff who is asked to provide an opinion on a trace should note their findings on both the trace and the woman's medical records along with the date, time and signature.

7. Following birth, the healthcare professional should sign and note the date, time and mode of birth on the FHR trace.

8. Ideally, both tocograph and cardiograph tracings should be clearly recorded in a continuous manner. FHR pattern recognition should be in relationship to the uterine contractions.

9. A review of litigation cases found that around 30 per cent of traces were missing and that another 20 per cent could not be interpreted (Ennis and Vincent 1990). It has also been recommended that CTG should be kept for a minimum of 25 years. Electronic storage systems provide a robust system of storage and facilitate easy retrieval, research and audit. CTG tracings can be downloaded and stored online in powerful central servers. Other systems make use of write-once-read-many-times (WORM) optical disks that can archive 4000 cases, with an average of 8 hours of trace, along with the clinical data.

## CTG definitions and interpretation

The correct interpretation of the CTG requires the complete understanding of the features that have been described below and illustrated in Fig. 5.1.

### Baseline heart rate

This refers to the mean FHR when this is stable, excluding accelerations and decelerations, determined over a period of 5–10 minutes and expressed in beats per minute (bpm). A baseline rate between 110 and 160 bpm is regarded as 'normal'. NICE (2007) suggests that in the absence of infection, a baseline FHR of 160–179 bpm (moderate tachycardia) and 100–109 bpm (moderate bradycardia) is probably not associated with adverse neonatal outcome, in the presence of other reassuring FHR features. If there has been a rise in the baseline FHR, this needs further investigation.

> Baseline heart rate: Mean FHR when this is stable, excluding accelerations and decelerations, determined over a period of 5–10 minutes and expressed in beats per minute.

### Baseline variability (BLV)

This has been defined as the minor fluctuations in baseline FHR occurring at 3–5 cycles per minute and refers to the abrupt and usually chaotic changes of the interval between consecutive heart beats in the normal fetus. It is important to note that the appearance of variability will depend on physiological factors like the fetal sleep cycle, interventions and administration of certain medications and on technical factors, including whether the tracing is obtained from an internal or external transducer. Reduced BLV (<5 bpm) may be seen for up to 40 minutes and may represent a fetal sleep cycle. Although Spencer and Johnson (1986) showed that this could last up to 90 minutes, most guidelines would recommend a review of the whole case and appropriate intervention by this point.

> Baseline variability: The minor fluctuations in baseline FHR occurring at 3–5 cycles per minute

Samueloff et al (1994) showed that a cut-off of 5 bpm for amplitude and 5 cycles per minute for frequency maximises the sensitivity for detection of neonatal acidosis (cord artery pH<7.20) or 5-minute Apgar score of less than 7. Reduced BLV has been shown to be associated with an increased risk of cerebral palsy (Schifrin et al 1994; Shields and Schifrin 1988). Schifrin (2004) has emphasised that although most attention has been paid to the abnormalities associated with decreased variability, increased BLV is no more 'normal' than decreased BLV. Here again, the pattern and the evolution are important.

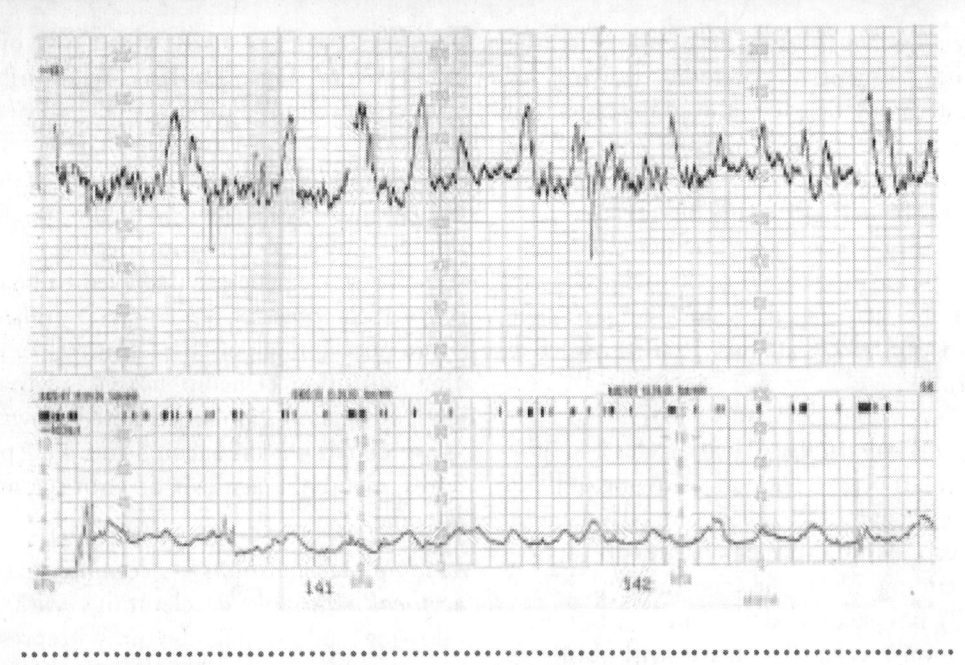

**Figure 5.1** Normal cardiotocograph

## Accelerations

It is defined as abrupt increases in the baseline FHR of more than 15 bpm and lasting over 15 seconds. The presence of accelerations is generally considered an indicator of good perinatal outcome. CTGs with more than two accelerations in a 20-minute window are called reactive traces and have a sensitivity of 97 per cent for an Apgar score greater than 7 at 5 minutes (Powell et al 1979; Krebs et al 1982). Accelerations are a very reassuring feature, so much so that neurological injuries seen with a reactive intrapartum FHR pattern are deemed to have occurred either in early pregnancy, as a consequence of birth trauma, or after birth (Schifrin 2004). With regard to accelerations, it is important to note that their incidence may be lower prior to 30 weeks, steadily increasing to term. Also, their size may be less than 15 bpm in the early preterm period.

> Accelerations: Abrupt increases in the baseline FHR of more than 15 bpm and lasting over 15 seconds.

## Cycling

CTG shows reactive segments with good variability (active sleep period) that alternates with segments of reduced variability and no or occasional accelerations (quiet sleep). Alternating segments of active and quiet epochs are termed cycling and are indicative of a fetus with a normal behavioural status.

## Decelerations

Various types of decelerations have been described, ranging from benign to highly suspicious varieties.

*Early decelerations*: These refer to the uniform, repetitive, periodic slowing of FHR with onset early in the contraction and return to baseline at the end of contraction. They generally do not drop to more than 40 beats from the baseline heart rate. These decelerations have been attributed to head compression and are not associated with metabolic acidosis or a low Apgar score (Krebs et al 1979; Cibils 1980; Low et al 1999).

*Late decelerations*: These refer to the uniform, repetitive, periodic slowing of FHR with onset at mid to end of contraction, nadir >20 seconds after the peak of the contraction and ending after the contraction. NICE (2007) has suggested that in the presence of a non-accelerative trace with baseline variability <5 bpm, the definition should include decelerations of <15 bpm. These represent a transient fall in partial pressure of oxygen (hypoxemia) below a certain threshold. There is an association between late decelerations and reduced Apgar scores at 5 minutes (Cibils 1975; Ellison et al 1991), metabolic acidosis (Krebs et al 1979; Low et al 1981), and marked increase in the odds of cerebral palsy, the risk of which is higher if both late decelerations and reduced variability are present (Nelson et al 1996). Late decelerations have a high sensitivity for predicting subsequent abnormal neurological examinations at 2, 4, 6, 9 and 12 months (Painter et al 1978). When accompanied by reduced BLV and the absence of accelerations, recurrent late decelerations are found to be associated with a low pH (<7.1) in >50% of cases (Sameshima and Ikenoue 2005).

*Variable decelerations – uncomplicated*: These refer to the variable, intermittent, periodic slowing of FHR with rapid onset and recovery (Fig 5.2). Time relationships with contraction cycles are variable and they may occur in isolation. They have a pre-shouldering followed by a sudden decline and quick recovery to the baseline, followed by another shouldering of the FHR. They are generally believed to be due to cord compression and may be relieved by re-positioning of the mother or by amnioinfusion. Uncomplicated variable decelerations are not consistently shown to be associated with reduced 5-minute Apgar scores, metabolic acidosis or poor neonatal outcome.

*Variable decelerations – complicated or 'atypical'*: Variable decelerations with the following additional features represent transient hypoxemia and are associated with poor adverse neonatal outcome when compared with FHR tracings with no decelerations or simple variable decelerations:

❖ Loss of primary or secondary rise in baseline rate
❖ Slow return to baseline FHR after the end of the contraction (late recovery)
❖ Prolonged increase of secondary rise in baseline (rebound tachycardia)
❖ Biphasic or 'combined' decelerations– variable followed by late component
❖ Loss of variability during deceleration
❖ Continuation of baseline heart rate at a lower level
❖ Decelerations with depth >60 beats and duration >60 seconds (Fig. 5.3).

*Prolonged decelerations*: NICE (2007) has categorised a drop in the FHR to less than 80 beats for less than 3 minutes as suspicious,

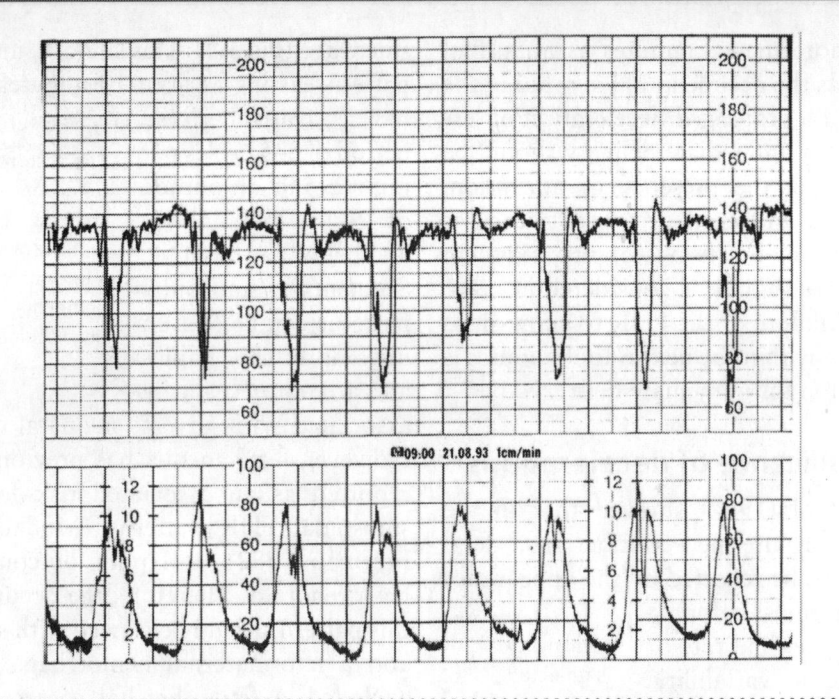

**Figure 5.2** Simple or uncomplicated variable decelerations

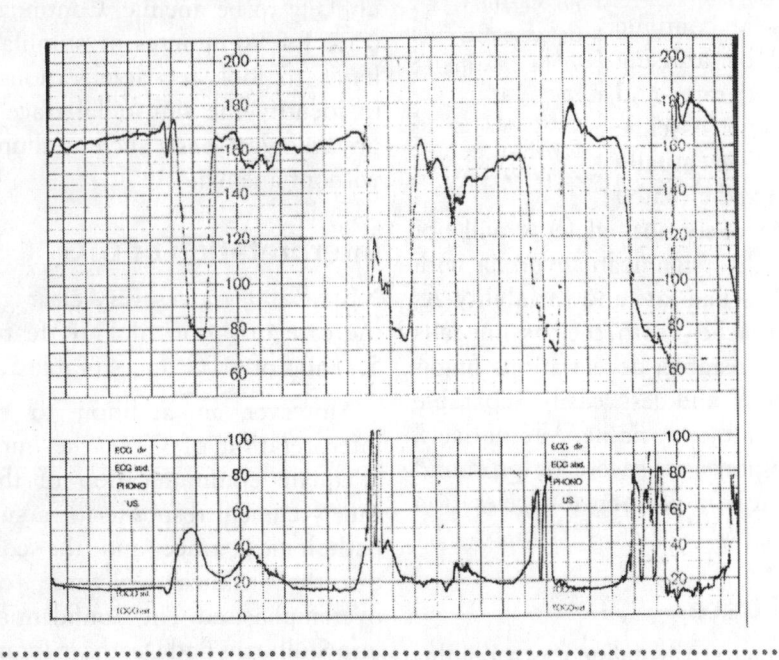

**Figure 5.3** Complicated or atypical variable decelerations with depth >60 beats, duration >60 seconds and reduced baseline variability

and for more than 3 minutes as abnormal (Fig 5.4), as the decline in pH is rapid in the presence of a prolonged deceleration of less than 80 bpm. Immediate delivery should be undertaken in the presence of abruption, scar rupture and cord prolapse. Measures such as altering position, stopping oxytocin and tocolysis should be considered in other cases, and failure of the FHR to show signs of recovery within the next 6 to 9 minutes is an indication for immediate delivery.

## The significance of decelerations

Murata et al (1982) showed that in the presence of uterine contractions, fetal hypoxia will be reflected by the appearance of decelerations before a rise in the baseline rate or a decrease in variability. With continued mild-to-moderate hypoxia, the decelerations continue accompanied by a rising baseline heart rate and a diminution in baseline variability, eventually leading to a fixed elevated rate. The previously normal fetus will not fail to respond to significant hypoxia with a change in baseline rate and variability. As the fetus approaches death, the baseline falls and becomes unstable; decelerations might be less obvious and less easily separable into type, i.e. late or variable. Alternatively, the initial response to severe or profound hypoxia might be a prolonged deceleration (bradycardia).

> Fetal hypoxia is reflected by the appearance of decelerations before a rise in the baseline rate or a decrease in variability.

## Sinusoidal trace

A sinusoidal pattern is defined as a regular oscillation of the baseline rate with markedly reduced baseline variability resembling a sine wave (Fig 5.5). This smooth, undulating pattern, lasting at least 10 minutes, usually has a relatively fixed period of 3–5 cycles per minute and amplitude of 5–15 bpm above and below the baseline. Segments of sinusoidal patterns can be seen in uncompromised babies and are not necessarily associated with adverse neonatal outcome. However, fetal anemia has previously been reported as an associated risk factor for sinusoidal FHR patterns (Modanlou and Freeman 1982), and poor outcomes have been reported. Therefore, the occurrence of this pattern should be viewed with suspicion and a feto-maternal hemorrhage must be excluded. A fetus that has a reactive CTG after the segment of sinusoidal pattern is unlikely to be anemic. Continuation of the trace for 90 minutes or stimulation of the fetus (to look for accelerations) will help to identify the sinusoidal trace that has a physiological basis such as thumb-sucking, without anemia.

> The occurrence of a sinusoidal pattern should be viewed with suspicion and a feto-maternal hemorrhage must be excluded.

## Interpretation of CTG

NICE (2007) gives very clear guidance on the categorisation of FHR features (Table 5.2) and of CTG traces (Table 5.3).

However, in addition to the correct interpretation of CTG, the importance of adequate communication of the findings, timely clinical response for a suspicious or pathological trace and the consideration of the clinical picture, cannot be overemphasised. The Confidential Enquiries into Stillbirths and Deaths in Infancy (CESDI 1997) found that 50 per cent of intrapartum deaths of babies over 1500 g with no

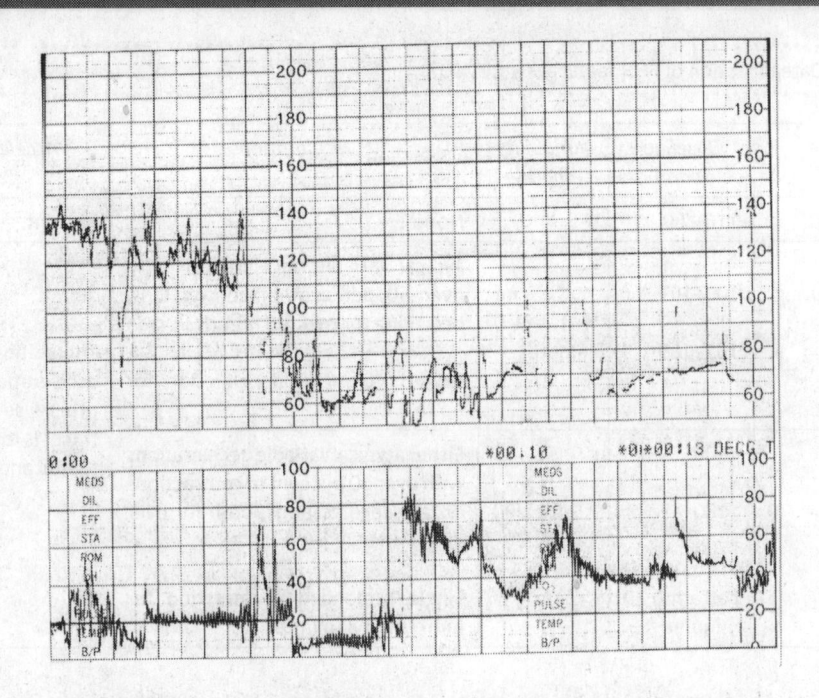

**Figure 5.4** Prolonged deceleration with a baseline rate <80 bpm for >3 mins

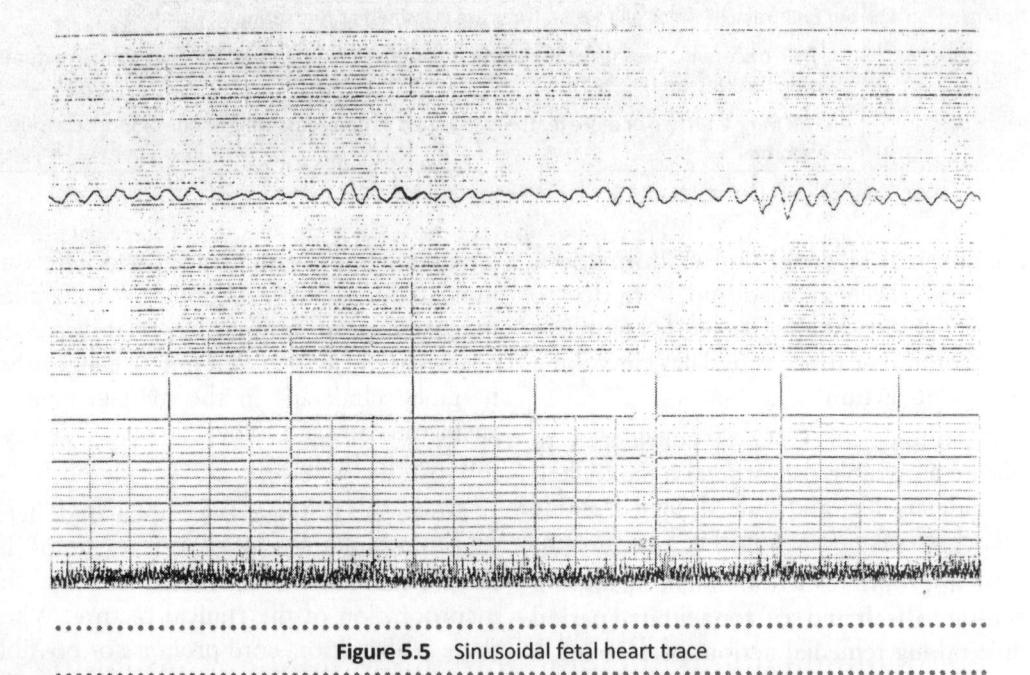

**Figure 5.5** Sinusoidal fetal heart trace

**Table 5.2** Categorisation of FHR features (NICE 2007)

| Feature | Baseline (bpm) | Variability (bpm) | Decelerations | Accelerations |
|---|---|---|---|---|
| Reassuring | 110-160 | ≥ 5 | None | Present |
| Non-reassuring | 100–109<br>161–180 | <5 for 40–90 minutes | Typical variable decelerations with over 50 per cent of contractions, occurring for over 90 minutes<br><br>Single prolonged deceleration for up to 3 minutes | The absence of accelerations with otherwise normal trace is of uncertain significance. |
| Abnormal | <100<br>>180<br>Sinusoidal pattern ≥ 10 minutes | <5 for >90 minutes | Either atypical variable decelerations with over 50 per cent of contractions or late decelerations, both for over 30 minutes<br><br>Single prolonged deceleration for more than 3 minutes | |

**Table 5.3** Categorisation of FHR traces (NICE 2007)

| Category | Definition |
|---|---|
| Normal: | An FHR trace in which all four features are classified as reassuring |
| Suspicious: | An FHR trace with one feature classified as non-reassuring and the remaining features classified as reassuring |
| Pathological: | An FHR trace with two or more features classified as non-reassuring or one or more classified as abnormal |

chromosomal or congenital malformations could have been avoided and were due to non-recognition of abnormal CTG patterns, poor communication and delay in taking appropriate action.

A pathological CTG is considered to indicate a possible risk of fetal hypoxia and it is indefensible, and indeed, unacceptable practice, to take no action (Fig 5.6).

An appropriate action might include a decision to 'wait and see' for a limited period while taking remedial action, performing a fetal scalp blood sampling (FBS) or effecting immediate delivery. Although the detailed management of intrapartum fetal distress is discussed in Chapter 7, a practice algorithm to guide clinicians in the management of suspicious and pathological traces has been outlined in Table 5.4.

However, it must be emphasised here, that interpretation of a CTG cannot be done in isolation and must involve the incorporation of the clinical picture. When there is abruption, cord prolapse or possible

## Intrapartum Fetal Monitoring

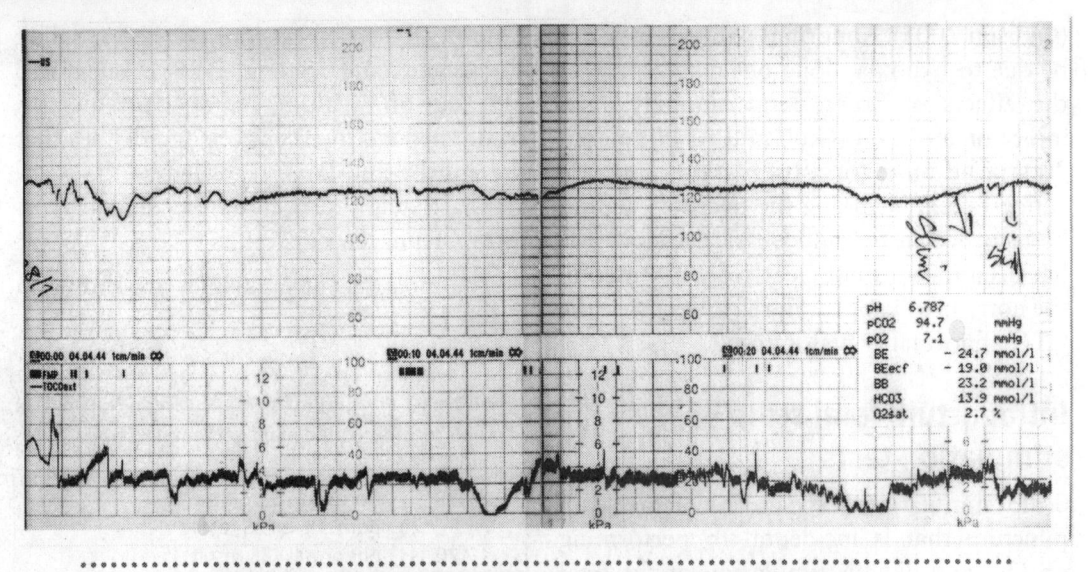

**Figure 5.6** Preterminal CTG pattern with absent baseline variability, no accelerations and shallow decelerations

**Table 5.4** Practice algorithm for the management of suspicious and pathological traces (NICE 2007)

- In cases where the CTG falls into the suspicious category, conservative measures should be used.
- In cases where the CTG falls into the pathological category, conservative measures should be used and fetal blood sampling performed where appropriate/feasible.
- In situations where fetal blood sampling is not possible or appropriate, delivery should be expedited.

scar rupture, a suboptimal CTG needs immediate intervention because these traces can suddenly change for the worse, resulting in a poor outcome (Gibb and Arulkumaran 2008). Fetal hypoxia and acidosis may develop faster with an abnormal trace when

> Fetal hypoxia and acidosis may develop faster with an abnormal trace when there is:
> - scanty thick meconium
> - intrauterine growth restriction
> - intrauterine infection with pyrexia
> - pre- or post-term labour

there is scanty thick meconium, intrauterine growth restriction, intrauterine infection with pyrexia and/or pre- or post-term labour (Williams and Arulkumaran 2004). In preterm fetuses (especially <34 weeks), hypoxia and acidosis can increase the likelihood of respiratory distress syndrome (Krasomski and Broniazczyk 1994), and may contribute to intra-ventricular hemorrhage (Lavrijsen et al 2005), warranting an early intervention in the presence of a pathological trace. Hypoxia can be made worse by oxytocin, epidural analgesia and difficult operative deliveries

(Okosun 2005). Abnormal patterns may not be due to hypoxia alone but may represent the effects of drugs, fetal anomaly, fetal injury or infection (Gibb and Arulkumaran 2008). The time of observation and the action taken, including the decision, should be recorded in the notes. If a decision that has been taken is not clearly documented in the notes it will appear in retrospect that the CTG abnormality was ignored.

## Intrapartum fetal scalp stimulation tests

Scalp stimulation tests include fetal scalp puncture that is incidental to performing an FBS and digital stimulation of the fetal scalp, which is performed by gentle digital stroking of the fetal scalp. A reassuring response is defined as an acceleration of the FHR. A meta-analysis of available data revealed observational evidence that response to digital stimulation of the fetal scalp is a good predictive test and response to fetal scalp puncture during FBS is a moderately predictive test for fetal acidemia (Skupski et al 2002). Based on the above findings, NICE (2007) has recommended that digital stimulation of the fetal scalp by the healthcare professional during a vaginal examination be considered as an adjunct with continuous EFM.

> Acceleration of the FHR, resulting from gentle digital stroking of the fetal scalp, is a reassuring response.

## Fetal Blood Sampling

### Fetal scalp pH

Fetal scalp blood sampling (FBS) during the first stage of labour was introduced by Saling in 1962 and was based on pH analysis. Empirically, based on some 80 cases, Saling (Bretscher and Saling 1967) suggested pH cut-off values, and consequently, recommended interventional guidelines that are still by-and-large regarded as the gold-standard with respect to the diagnosis of intrapartum fetal distress.

The most recent guidelines are shown in Table 5.5.

Table 5.5 Interpretation of FBS (scalp pH) results and recommended management (NICE 2007)

| | |
|---|---|
| ≥ 7.25 | Normal FBS result |
| 7.21–7.24 | Borderline FBS result |
| ≤ 7.20 | Abnormal FBS result |

- These results should be interpreted taking into account the previous pH measurement, the rate of progress in labour and the clinical features of the woman and baby.
- After an abnormal FBS result, consultant obstetric advice should be sought.
- After a normal FBS result, sampling should be repeated no more than 1 hour later if the FHR trace remains pathological, or sooner, if there are further abnormalities.
- After a borderline FBS result, sampling should be repeated no more than 30 minutes later if the FHR trace remains pathological, or sooner, if there are further abnormalities.
- The time taken to take a fetal blood sample needs to be considered when planning repeat samples.
- If the FHR trace remains unchanged and the FBS result is stable after the second test, a third/further sample may be deferred unless additional abnormalities develop on the trace.
- Where a third FBS is considered necessary, consultant obstetric opinion should be sought.

For FBS to be properly utilised, CTG interpretation has to be optimal and the attending obstetricians should be skilled at taking samples. Through a vaginal amnioscope, a capillary blood sample is taken from a small incision on the fetal scalp and analysed for indices of fetal acid–base status. FBS is an invasive procedure, requiring ruptured membranes and a sufficiently dilated cervix (minimum 3 cm). The scalp must be wiped clean and liquor excluded from the sample, as this will alter the pH towards alkalinity, potentially making an acidotic pH appear normal. The procedure is best performed in the left lateral position as the lithotomy position may lead to supine hypotension in the mother, producing further fetal acid–base compromise.

> FBS is an invasive procedure, requiring ruptured membranes and a sufficiently dilated cervix (minimum 3 cm).

During active labour, the integrity of the uteroplacental circulation and the frequency and intensity of uterine activity influence the fetal acid–base status. A normal fetus tolerates the effects of reduced placental blood flow during a normal contraction lasting about 60 seconds. If the uteroplacental circulation or fetus is compromised or uterine activity is excessive, there is an initial reduction in oxygen supply and an accumulation of $CO_2$ (respiratory acidosis). If the negative influence persists, anerobic respiration ensues, resulting in accumulation of lactic and pyruvic acids (metabolic acidosis). The speed of development of metabolic acidosis depends on the particular insult and the ability of the fetus to compensate. It has now been shown that respiratory acidemia ($CO_2$ accumulation) is harmless to the fetus, whereas metabolic acidemia (lactic acid accumulation) is associated with neonatal morbidity (Goldaber et al 1991; Low et al 1994; Andres et al 1999).

With regard to blood from the umbilical artery, where metabolic acidemia is usually regarded as pH <7.10–7.00, the acidemia is said to be moderate when the base deficit (BD) is >8 mmol/l, and severe when BD >12 mmol/l (Herbst et al 1997). Umbilical artery blood-measure of metabolic acidosis is the best indicator of tissue oxygen debt experienced by the fetus. Moderate and severe newborn complications have only been shown to occur in fetuses with an umbilical artery BD >12 mmol/l and the incidence was 10 per cent with BD 12–16 mmol/l (Low et al 1997). These umbilical artery BD values are often applied to FBS but have not been evaluated in clinical trials. Besides, no cut-off values are derived from FBS blood to fit with the higher pH values (<7.20) (Nordstrom 2004).

## Limitations of fetal scalp pH measurements

1. The procedural and technical difficulties in collecting sufficient quantity of blood for analysis and the need to repeatedly perform this invasive procedure make it rather unattractive for clinicians and women in labour. Also, facilities for performing FBS are not universally available.

2. Although acid–base machines have improved over the years, analysis can be compromised by air bubbles or clots in the blood sample; the machine might also be busy with its automatic calibrating system at the time for analysis. Blood sampling and pH analysis has been reported to fail in 20 per cent of cases (Westgren et al 1998)

3. On an average, the procedure takes 18 minutes to perform and therefore cannot be used in cases of acute fetal compromise (Tufnell et al 2006).

4. The result is valid only for a short period of time depending on the CTG pattern, and whether it persists or worsens. If the CTG does not improve, sampling may need to be repeated. If FBS has been performed on the same fetus up to three times and the CTG has not improved, delivery must be seriously considered unless progress in labour is rapid and spontaneous delivery is imminent.

5. Measurements may, however, be inaccurate in the presence of moderate to severe degrees of fetal scalp edema. Maternal hyperventilation leading to respiratory alkalosis can lead to a rise in the pH and obscure true fetal acidosis or produce a pH in excess of 7.4. Conversely, maternal ketoacidosis from prolonged labour may lead to an infusion acidemia in the fetus, with a low pH in the absence of hypoxia (Greene 1999). The true picture may be verified by checking maternal venous pH; a difference of more than 0.2 between the two samples should be regarded as an indication of true fetal acidosis.

6. FBS is inappropriate in certain clinical high-risk situations and in the presence of ominous CTG patterns, as ensuing acidosis can be rapid. These include prolonged bradycardia, cord prolapse, placental abruption and uterine scar dehiscence (Arulkumaran and Symonds 1999b). In these circumstances, performing an FBS would be a waste of valuable time.

7. NICE (2007) has recommended that the use of FBS be avoided in bleeding disorders such as hemophilia A and in women with certain maternal viral infections such as HIV, hepatitis B and herpes simplex. In the presence of abnormal FHR patterns in preterm labour (<34 weeks' gestation), the use of FBS may be associated with an increase in adverse neonatal outcome and an early delivery is advised.

8. Optimal interpretation of cord blood pH requires a paired sample from both umbilical artery and vein. The accuracy of calculated measures of metabolic acidosis is dependent upon the quality of pH and $pCO_2$ estimations (Low 2007).

## Fetal scalp lactate measurements

Nordstrom et al (1995) suggested that pre-acidemia is mainly of respiratory origin and the use of lactate in fetal surveillance might decrease the incidence of unnecessary interventions. It has recently been shown that lactate in umbilical cord arterial blood might be a more direct and more correct indicator of fetal asphyxia at delivery than pH (Gjerris et al 2008). The launch of reliable, handheld, microvolume devices in the 1990s has made the measurement of scalp blood lactate a clinical option. Maternal and fetal lactate concentrations increase with the duration of active bearing-down. It is estimated that fetal lactate increases by 1 mmol/l for every 30 minutes of maternal pushing; the corresponding value for the woman is 2 mmol/l (Nordstrom et al 2001). A lactate concentration of 4.8 mmol/l has been recommended as a cut-off value for intervention and the following guidelines (Table 5.6) have been recommended.

## Advantages of fetal scalp lactate measurements over fetal scalp pH

1. A randomised trial (Westgren et al 1998a) comparing these two measurements found lactate to be more favourable in

Table 5.6  Clinical guidelines for fetal scalp blood pH and lactate (using Lactate Pro™) (Kruger et al 1999).

|  | pH | Lactate (mmol/l) using Lactate Pro™ |
|---|---|---|
| Normal | > 7.25 | < 4.2 |
| Pre-acidemia/ pre-lactemia | 7.20–7.25 | 4.2–4.8 |
| Acidemia/ Lactemia | < 7.20 | > 4.8 |

clinical practice in terms of less sampling failure and reduced time from the decision to do a fetal scalp blood sample to the clinician receiving the result.

2. Although the trial was not large enough to allow correlation of neonatal outcome, there is retrospective data on fetal scalp blood pH and lactate analyses (Lactate Pro™), and neonatal outcome in cases with normal outcome and in cases with fetal distress (Nordstrom et al 1995; Kruger et al 1999).
3. A good correlation exists between lactate obtained at FBS close to delivery and cord arterial blood immediately after delivery (Kruger et al 1998).
4. The advantage of scalp lactate measurement is that a much smaller quantity of blood suffices (5μl) compared to pH measurements that require approximately 35 μl (Westgren et al 1998b).
5. Caput formation does not significantly alter the correlation between values obtained at FBS and values in the central fetal circulation (Nordstrom 2004).

At present, a large multi-centre randomised trial is in progress in Sweden to compare lactate and pH measurement for the clinical management of suspected fetal compromise. The main end-points of this study are metabolic acidemia or pH <7.00 in cord arterial blood at delivery.

## Fetal ECG Waveform Analysis

Fetal electrocardiographic surveillance involves computerised methods of analysing the ST and PR segments of fetal ECG.

### ST segment analysis

The ST waveform of the fetal ECG provides continuous information on the ability of the fetal heart muscle to respond to the stress of labour. An elevation of the ST segment and T wave, quantified by the ratio between the T wave and QRS amplitudes (T/QRS), identifies fetal heart muscle responding to hypoxia by a surge of stress hormones (catecholamines), which leads to utilisation of glycogen stored in the heart (an extra source of energy). ST segment depression can indicate a situation where the heart is not fully able to respond. The basis for ST waveform interpretation is given in Figure 5.7.

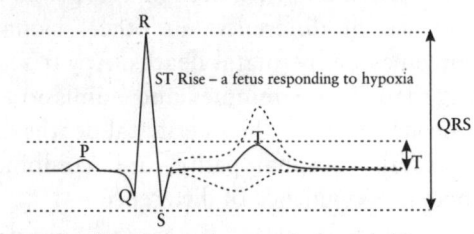

Figure 5.7  Principles of how to calculate the T/QRS ratio and the physiology behind different ST patterns. (Rosen 2004)

A special fetal monitoring device, STAN®, has been developed to allow detailed assessment of both fetal heart rate and ST waveform during labour after a standard fetal scalp electrode has been applied. The ST waveform changes are identified automatically and clinical action should be taken strictly according to the guidelines, which are based on extensive research.

## Summary of the pathophysiology of the ST waveform changes

The pathophysiology of ST waveform changes has been summarised in Table 5.7, while the clinical guidelines have been outlined in Table 5.8.

The most recent meta-analysis (NICE 2007) that includes a systematic review of ST analysis (Neilson 2005), as well as a recently published randomised trial (Ojala et al 2006) showed evidence that ST analysis significantly reduced the rate of instrumental vaginal birth and the need for FBS. There was no evidence of a difference in the CS rate and fetal acid–base status. There is evidence that ST analysis reduced the number of babies who developed neonatal encephalopathy and the number of babies with cord blood acidosis (pH less than 7.05, base excess less than −12 mmol/l), although there was no evidence of differences in other neonatal outcomes i.e. perinatal deaths, Apgar score less than 7 at 5 minutes and admission to a neonatal unit. When perinatal deaths and neonatal encephalopathy are combined, there is no evidence of difference.

In the light of current evidence, NICE (2007) concluded that ST analysis seems to add value to the use of EFM and reduces intervention, but recommended that another randomised trial be undertaken to consolidate these findings. The limitations identified were as follows.

1. Added cost
2. The use of fetal scalp electrodes
3. Additional staff training
4. If used when fetal heart rate abnormalities are already present, it may be necessary to perform FBS before using ST analysis.

## PR interval

Observational studies have shown that as the fetal heart slows, the PR interval lengthens and vice versa. Measurements of the PR/RR relation over short and long periods in labour have been studied.

*Conduction index (short-term measure):* This refers to the Pearson's correlation coefficient of the PR interval and FHR calculated over the previous 2·5 minutes and is a short-term measure. A persistently positive conduction index over 20 minutes is associated with an increased risk of acidemia (Murray 1992; van Wijngaarden et al 1996).

*Ratio index (long-term measure):* This is expressed as the percentage of time during labour in which the multiplied standard deviations of the PR interval and FHR exceed two positive standard deviations. A ratio index of more than 4 per cent was associated with the development of acidemia in the fetus (Mohajer et al 1994).

Although the use of PR intervals in intrapartum fetal surveillance has shown to reduce the rate of instrumental births (Luzietti et al 1997), a subsequent study (Strachan et al 2000) was deemed underpowered to show statistical differences in maternal and fetal outcomes.

**Table 5.7** Pathophysiology of ST-waveform changes (Rosen 2004)

- During hypoxia, a mature fetus reacts with an elevation of the ST segment and a progressive increase in T-wave height quantified by the ratio between the amplitude of the T-wave and the QRS complex.
- An increase in T/QRS emerges with the hypoxic stress that leads to myocardial glycogenolysis.
- This functional response to hypoxia appears well in advance of any signs of failing function of the CNS. The integrity of the CNS is maintained as long as there is adequate cerebral blood perfusion.
- ST depression with negative T-waves appears to provide information on a myocardium not fully responding to the hypoxic stress. Such a situation might emerge during the initial phase of hypoxia but also as the dominant pattern seen in fetuses exposed to long-term reduction of oxygen and nutritional supply and exposed to hypoxia. Endotoxin seems to play a role as well. The electrophysiological mechanism behind this is a situation of uncoordinated repolarization within the myocardial wall with prolonged repolarization in the endocardium.
- In fetuses suffering from infections, hypotension and anemia, persistently elevated ST waveforms were noted to precede intrauterine death.

**Table 5.8** STAN clinical guidelines: ST changes indicating clinical intervention if CTG is intermediary or abnormal (Rosen 2004)

| ST events | CTG classification | | |
|---|---|---|---|
| | *Intermediary* | *Abnormal* | *Pre-terminal* |
| Episodic T/QRS rise | Increase >0.15 from baseline | Increase >0.10 from baseline | Immediate delivery regardless of ST changes |
| Baseline T/QRS rise | Increase >0.10 from baseline | Increase >0.05 from baseline | |
| Biphasic ST: a component of the ST segment below the baseline | Continuous >5 minutes or >two episodes of coupled biphasic ST type 2 or 3 | Continuous >2 minutes or >one episode of coupled biphasic ST type 2 or 3 | |

## Fetal Pulse Oximetry (FPO)

FPO made its formal debut in the late 1980s, when investigators in the UK independently reported their initial experiences in measuring fetal oxygen saturation (FSpO$_2$) using cannibalised components of adult oximeters (Peat et al 1988; Gardosi et al 1989; Johnson et al 1989). Fetal oximetry essentially measures the oxygen saturation of hemoglobin by analysing the absorption patterns of red and near infra-red light using frequencies of 735 nm and 890 nm, respectively. Oxyhemoglobin absorbs more near infra-red light while deoxyhemoglobin absorbs more red light. A light emitting diode (LED) emits near infrared and red light sequentially and a photodetector measures the light that passes through unabsorbed. Percentage O$_2$ saturation is derived from measuring the unabsorbed light. The probe carries the LED and photodetector on either side of a body part, for example, finger (transmission mode) (Figure 5.8).

As there is no part of the fetus accessible in utero to which the transmission mode can be applied, modifications have been made to allow the LED and photodetector to be placed on the same side of a fetal part, for example, cheek (reflectance mode) (Figure 5.9).

Normal adult SpO$_2$ range is 95–100 per cent, while normal fetal range appears to be 30–70 per cent. SpO$_2$ < 30 per cent for over 10 minutes appears to be associated with acidosis (Seelbach-Gobel et al 1999) and may be of value when there are suspicious or abnormal FHR patterns. The 'critical threshold' of FSpO$_2$ – the level of fetal arterial oxygen saturation above which acidemia does not occur – has been set at 30 per cent, based on clinical observation of thousands of cases. Fetal vernix may impair sensor contact and hair may shunt light. Meconium staining of fetal skin, however, does not interfere with SpO$_2$ readings as its light absorption is non-pulsatile. The issues of sensor design, application to a fetal surface, calibration, threshold values and equipment safety have been resolved to a stage where FPO is now a realistic clinical monitoring modality. Application and use of currently available fetal pulse oximeter sensors have been shown to be easy to learn (Butterwegge 1998; Chua et al 1999). The SpO$_2$ values are displayed on a bedside unit, which can be connected through an interface in a CTG monitor, allowing concurrent recording on the CTG trace.

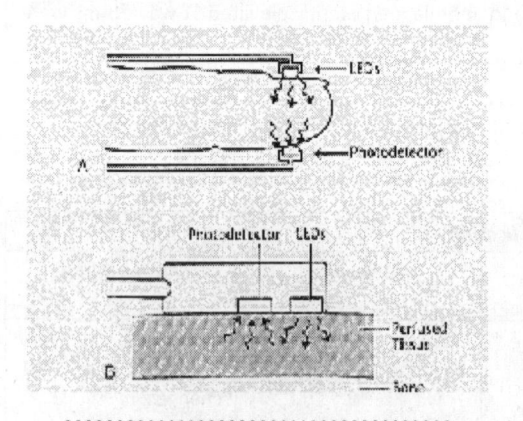

**Figure 5.8** Transmission (above) and reflectance (below) oximetry

The American multi-centre randomised trial (Garite et al 2000) was the first large-scale study to assess clinical utility of this new technology. Although FPO was found to reduce the cesarean section rate for non-reassuring CTG features by more than 50 per cent, the overall cesarean rates remained unchanged, questioning the overall benefit of this method of surveillance. The adoption of FPO in intrapartum surveillance has therefore not been endorsed because of concerns that its introduction would escalate the cost of medical care without necessarily improving clinical outcome (ACOG 2001, Liston et al 2002 a and b). The future of FPO depends largely on results of studies

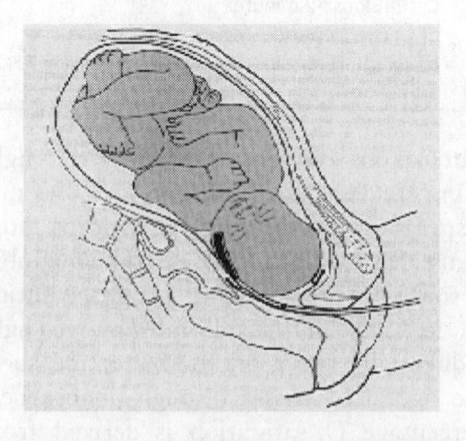

**Figure 5.9** FPO sensor applied to fetal cheek

that should show an impact of FPO as an adjunct to EFM to reduce cesarean rates without increasing the incidence of neonatal hypoxia at birth.

## Intrapartum Umbilical Artery Doppler Waveforms

Doppler sonographic measurements have been shown to predict fetal compromise throughout pregnancy (Hecher et al 1995) as well as during labour (Feinkind et al 1989). Umbilical artery (UA) and middle cerebral artery (MCA) Doppler waveform velocimetries have been studied because they reflect fetal blood flow most accurately, and consequently, oxygenation of the periphery and the cerebrum respectively (Meyberg et al 2000).

In the absence of FHR abnormalities, uterine contractions in labour have no effect on the UA pulsatility index (PI) (Fleischer et al 1987; Fairlie et al 1989). However, in the presence of late decelerations, increased UA systolic/diastolic (SD) ratios were observed and these were found to be associated with a higher incidence of meconium staining, cesarean rates for fetal distress, low Apgar scores and admission to the neonatal intensive care unit (Brar et al 1989; Damron et al 1994).

Recent studies indicate that in experienced hands, Doppler screening of fetal MCA waveforms during labour may be useful in the evaluation of intrapartum hypoxia in complicated pregnancies (Kassanos et al 2003). Although some studies suggest a strong correlation between Doppler velocimetry of the MCA and UA, fetal pulse oximetry and fetal morbidity (Siristatidis et al 2004), some others do not (Farrell et al 1999). A lot more research and validation would be required before fetal Doppler velocimetry can be clinically used for intrapartum surveillance.

## Near Infra-red Spectroscopy (NIRS)

The technique of near infra-red spectroscopy (NIRS) which allows measurement of change in the concentration of oxy/deoxy-hemoglobin in real time was first described by Jobsis (1977). As a detector of change in cerebral blood volume and tissue oxygenation following medical or physiological events, it offers unique possibilities of understanding the effects that events in labour have on cerebral oxygenation (Peebles et al 1992; Doyle et al 1993; Ramos-Santos et al 1993).

There has been considerable interest in this method of fetal surveillance since Vintzileos et al (2005) showed that fetal pulse-oxymetry (FPO) using NIRS is comparable to transvaginal FPO and recommended its use in a clinical setting. In fact, Kawamura et al (2007) hail NIRS as a non-invasive method for assessing placental oxygen dynamics on a real-time basis. However, NIRS has not been subjected to randomised trials and a recent Cochrane review concluded that there is currently insufficient evidence to assess its efficacy (Mozurkewich and Wolf 2000).

## Conclusion

The ultimate aim of intrapartum monitoring is to detect developing fetal hypoxia and acidosis, allowing for appropriate intervention. While the search for the perfect tool continues, the mainstay of intrapartum fetal surveillance is intermittent auscultation of the FHR in low-risk labour and continuous EFM in high-risk labour. While the measurement of fetal scalp pH is currently the most widely used adjunct, lactate measurements, computerised ECG waveform analysis and fetal pulse oximetry have recently undergone clinical evaluation to the extent that they are available for clinical use as adjuncts to continuous EFM in high-risk labour. Until a perfect method is devised to detect intrapartum hypoxia, the importance of the judicious use and the meticulous interpretation of the CTG will continue to dominate the science of fetal surveillance. A reminder of the following 'Clinical Pearls' (Arulkumaran et al 1995) would go a long way in avoiding litigation, while simultaneously ensuring an optimal obstetric outcome.

1. Accelerations and normal baseline variability are hallmarks of fetal health
2. Periods of decreased variability may represent fetal sleep
3. Hypoxic fetuses may have a normal baseline FHR of 110–160 bpm with no accelerations and baseline variability of <5 bpm for >40 min
4. In the presence of baseline variability <5 bpm, even shallow decelerations <15 bpm, are ominous in a non-reactive trace
5. Abruption, cord prolapse and scar rupture can give rise to acute hypoxia and should be suspected clinically
6. Hypoxia and acidosis may develop faster with an abnormal trace in patients with scanty, thick meconium, IUGR, intrauterine infection with pyrexia, and those who are pre- or post-term
7. In pre-term fetuses (especially <34 weeks), hypoxia and acidosis can aggravate RDS and may contribute to intraventricular hemorrhage and sequelae warranting early action in the presence of an abnormal trace
8. Hypoxia can be worsened by oxytocin, epidural analgesia and difficult operative deliveries
9. During labour, if decelerations are absent, asphyxia is unlikely
10. Abnormal patterns may represent effects of drugs, fetal anomaly or infection and not only hypoxia.

## References

Alfirevic Z, Devane D, Gyte GM. 2006. Continuous cardiotocography (CTG) as a form of electronic fetal monitoring (EFM) for fetal assessment during labour. *Cochrane Database of Systematic Reviews* (Online) 3:CD006066

American College of Obstetricians and Gynecologists 1995. Fetal heart rate patterns: monitoring, interpretation and management. *ACOG Technical Bulletin* no 207. Washington DC: American College of Obstetricians and Gynecologists.

American College of Obstetricians and Gynecologists. 2001. ACOG Committee Opinion. Number 258. Fetal Pulsoxymetry. *Obstet Gynecol*. 98:523–4

Andres RL, Saade G, Gilstrap LC, Wilkins I, Witlin A, Zlatnik F, et al. 1999. Association between umbilical blood gas parameters and neonatal morbidity and death in neonates with pathologic fetal acidemia. *American Journal of Obstetrics and Gynecology*. Oct;181(4):867-71.

Arulkumaran S, EM Symonds. 1999a. Intrapartum fetal monitoring – basic knowledge. *Obstet Gynecol*. 1(2):18–21.

Arulkumaran S, EM Symonds. 1999b. Intrapartum fetal monitoring – Medico-legal aspects. *Obstet Gynecol*. 1(2):23–26.

Arulkumaran S, I Ingermasson, S Montan, D Gibb, RH Paul, BS Schifrin, JAD Spencer et al. 1995. *Traces of you: Clinician's guide to fetal trace interpretation*. Boblingen: Hewlett Packard GmbH (5965-6246EN).

Ayres-de-Campos D, J Bernades, A Costa-Pereira, L Pereira-Leite. 1999. Inconsistencies in classification by experts of cardiotocograms and subsequent clinical decision. *Br J Obstet Gynecol*. 106:1307–10.

Banta HD, Thacker SB. 1979. *Costs and benefits to electronic fetal monitoring: A review of the literature*. Washington (DC): National Center for Health Service Research; DHEW Publication no. (PHS) 79: 3245.

Berkus MD, O Langer, A Samueloff, EMJ Xenakis, NT Field. 1999. Electronic fetal monitoring: That's reassuring. *Acta Obstet Gynecol Scand*. 78: 15–21.

Bernades J, A Costa-Pereira, D Ayres-de-Campos, HP van Geijn, L Pereira-Leite. 1997. Evaluation of inter-observer agreement of cardiotocograms. *Int J Gynecol Obstet*. 57:33–37.

Bix E, Reiner LM, Klovning A, Oian P. 2005. Prognostic value of the labour admission test and its effectiveness compared with auscultation only: a systematic review. *BJOG*. Dec;112(12):1595-604.

Brar HS, Platt LD, Paul R.H. 1989. Fetal umbilical velocity waveforms using Doppler ultrasonography in patient s with late decelerations. *Obstetrics and Gynecology*, 73, 363–366.

Bretscher J, Saling E. 1967. pH values in the human fetus during labor. *American Journal of Obstetrics and Gynecology* Apr 1;97(7): 906-11

Butterwegge M. 1998. Fetal pulse oximetry: From the first experimental studies of broad clinical use. An assessment of current status. *Zeitschrift fur Geburtshilfe und Neonatologie* 202(6):227–34.

Chua S, J Yam, K Razvi, SM Yeong and S Arulkumaran. 1999. Intrapartum fetal oxygen saturation monitoring in a busy labour ward. *Eur J Obstet Gynecol Reprod Biol* 82(2):185–89.

Cibils LA. 1975. Clinical significance of fetal heart rate patterns during labor. II. Late decelerations. *American Journal of Obstetrics and Gynecology*. Nov 1;123(5):473–94.

Cibils LA. 1980. Clinical significance of fetal heart rate patterns during labor. VI. Early decelerations. *American Journal of Obstetrics and Gynecology* Feb 1;136(3):392–8.

Clark SL, Hankins GD. 2003. Temporal and demographic trends in cerebral palsy–fact and fiction. *American Journal of Obstetrics and Gynecology*. Mar;188(3):628–33

Confidential Enquiry into Stillbirths and Deaths in Infancy. 1997. *Fourth Annual Report. Concentrating on intrapartum related deaths 1994–1995*. London: Maternal and Child Health Research Consortium.

Confidential Enquiry into Maternal and Child Health (CEMACH) Perinatal Mortality 2006: England, Wales and Northern Ireland. 2008. London: CEMACH

Damron DP, Chaffin DG, Anderson CF, Reed KL. 1994. Changes in umbilical arterial and venous blood flow velocity waveforms during late decelerations of the fetal heart rate. *Obstetrics and Gynecology*, 84, 1038–40.

Dildy GA. 1999. The physiologic and medical rationale for intrapartum fetal monitoring. *Biomed Instrument Technol* 33:144–51.

Doyle PM, O'Brien PMS, Wickramasinghe YABD, Houston R, Rolfe P. 1993. Transcerebral near infrared spectroscopy used to observe changes in fetal cerebral haemodynamics during labour. *J Perinat Med*.

D'Souza R, Arulkumaran S. 2009. Intrapartum fetal surveillance. In *Best Practice in Labour and Delivery*, ed Warren and Arulkumaran. 38–53 Cambridge: Cambridge University Press.

Ellison PH, Foster M, Sheridan-Pereira M, MacDonald D. 1991. Electronic fetal heart monitoring, auscultation, and neonatal outcome. *American Journal of Obstetrics and Gynecology*. May;164(5 Pt 1):1281–9

Ennis M, Vincent CA. 1990. Obstetric accidents: A review of 64 cases. *BMJ* (Clinical research ed. May 26; 300(6736):1365–7

Fairlie F. M., Lang G. D. and Sheldon C. D. 1989. Umbilical artery flow velocity waveforms in labour. *British Journal of Obstetric and Gynaecology*, 96, 151–7.

Farrell T, Chien PF, Gordon A. 1999. Intrapartum umbilical artery Doppler velocimetry as a predictor of adverse perinatal outcome: a systematic review. *Br J Obstet Gynaecol.* Aug; 106(8):783–92.

Feinkind L, Abulafia O, Delke I, Feldman J, Minkoff H. 1989. Screening with Doppler velocimetry in labor. *Am J Obstet Gynecol.* 161:765–770

Fleischer A, Anyaegbunam AA, Schulman H, Farmakides G, Randolph G. 1987. Uterine and umbilical artery velocimetry during normal labor . *American Journal of Obstetrics and Gynecolog y*, 157, 40–43.

Gardosi J, Carter M, Becket T. 1989. Continuous intrapartum monitoring of fetal oxygen saturation. *Lancet* Sep 16;2 (8664):692–3

Garite TJ, Dildy GA, H McNamara et al. 2000. A multicenter controlled trial of fetal pulse oximetry in the intrapartum management of nonreassuring fetal heart rate patterns. *Am J Obstet Gynecol* 183(5):1049–58.

Gibb D, Arulkumaran S, eds. 2008. *Fetal Monitoring in Practice*. 3rd ed: Churchill Livingstone;

Gjerris AC, Staer-Jensen J, Jorgensen JS, Bergholt T, Nickelsen C. 2008. Umbilical cord blood lactate: A valuable tool in the assessment of fetal metabolic acidosis. *European Journal of Obstetrics, Gynecology, and Reproductive Biology*. Jul;139(1):16–20

Goldaber KG, Gilstrap LC, 3rd, Leveno KJ, Dax JS, McIntire DD. 1991. Pathologic fetal acidemia. *Obstetrics and Gynecology*. Dec;78(6):1103–7.

Greene KR. 1999. Scalp blood gas analysis. *Obstet Gynecol Clin N Am* 26(4):641–57.

Hecher K, Campbell S, Doyle P, Harrington K, Nicolaides KH. 1995. Assessment of fetal compromise by Doppler ultrasound investigation of fetal circulation. *Circulation* 91:129–132

Herbst A, Ingemarsson I. 1994. Intermittent versus continuous electronic monitoring in labour: a randomised study. *British Journal of Obstetrics and Gynaecology* Aug;101(8):663–8

Herbst A, Thorngren-Jerneck K, Wu L, Ingemarsson I. 1997. Different types of acid-base changes at birth, fetal heart rate patterns, and infant outcome at 4 years of age. *Acta obstetricia et Gynecologica Scandinavica*. Nov;76 (10):953–8

Huddleston JF. 1999. Intrapartum fetal assessment. *Clin Perinatol*. 26(3):549–68.

Impey L, Reynolds M, MacQuillan K, Gates S, Murphy J, Sheil O. 2003. Admission cardiotocography: a randomised controlled trial. *Lancet*. Feb 8;361(9356):465–70.

Jobsis FF. 1977. Non-invasive infrared monitoring of cerebral and myocardial oxygen sufficiency and circulatory parameters. Science; 198:1264–6

Johnson N, Johnson VA, Bannister J, Lilford RJ. 1989. Measurement of fetal peripheral perfusion with a pulse oximeter. *Lancet*. Apr 22;1(8643):898.

Kassanos D, Siristatidis C, Vitoratos N, Salamalekis E, Creatsas G. 2003. The clinical significance of Doppler findings in fetal middle cerebral artery during labor. *Eur J Obstet Gynecol Reprod Biol*. Jul 1;109(1):45–50.

Kawamura T, kakogawa J, Takeuchi Y, Takani S, Kimura S, Nishiguchi T, Sugimura M, Sumimoto K, Kanayama N. 2007. Measurement of placental oxygenation by transabdominal near-infrared spectroscopy. *Am J Perinatol*. Mar;24(3):161–6.

Krasomski G, Broniarczyk D. 1994. The influence of perinatal asphyxia on the occurrence of respiratory distress syndrome in preterm labor. *Ginekologia polska*. Oct;65(10):547–52

Krebs HB, Petres RE, Dunn LJ, Jordaan HV, Segreti A. 1979. Intrapartum fetal heart rate monitoring. I. Classification and prognosis of fetal heart rate patterns. *American Journal of Obstetrics and Gynecology*. Apr 1;133(7):762–72.

Krebs HB, Petres RE, Dunn LJ, Smith PJ. 1982. Intrapartum fetal heart rate monitoring. VI. Prognostic significance of accelerations. *American Journal of Obstetrics and Gynecology*. Feb 1;142(3):297–305.

Kripke CC. 1999. Why are we using electronic fetal monitoring? *Am Fam Physician* 59(9):2421–22.

Kruger K, Kublickas M, Westgren M. 1998. Lactate in scalp and cord blood from fetuses with ominous fetal heart rate patterns. *Obstetrics and Gynecolog*. Dec;92(6):918–22.

Kruger K, Hallberg B, Blennow M, Kublickas M, Westgren M. 1999. Predictive value of fetal scalp blood lactate concentration and pH as markers of neurologic disability. *American Journal of Obstetrics and Gynecology*. Nov;181(5 Pt 1):1072–8

Lavrijsen SW, Uiterwaal CS, Stigter RH, de Vries LS, Visser GH, Groenendaal F. 2005. Severe umbilical cord acidemia and neurological outcome in preterm and full-term neonates. *Biology of the neonate*.;88(1):27–34

Lent M. 1999. The medical and legal risks of the electronic fetal monitor. *Stanford Law Review*. 51(4):807–37

Liston R, Crane J, Hamilton E, Hughes O, Kuling S, MacKinnon C, et al. 2002a. Fetal health surveillance in labour. *J Obstet Gynaecol Can*. Mar;24(3):250-76; quiz 77–80.

Liston R, Crane J, Hughes O, Kuling S, MacKinnon C, Milne K, et al. 2002b. Fetal health surveillance in labour. *J Obstet Gynaecol Can*. Apr;24(4): 342–55.

Low JA, Cox MJ, Karchmar EJ, McGrath MJ, Pancham SR, Piercy WN. 1981. The prediction of intrapartum fetal metabolic acidosis by fetal heart rate monitoring. *American Journal of Obstetrics and Gynecology*. Feb 1;139(3):299–305

Low JA, C Panagiotopoulos, EJ Derrick. 1994. Newborn complications after intrapartum asphyxia with metabolic acidosis in the term fetus. *Am J Obstet Gynecol* 170:1081–87.

Low JA, Lindsay BG, Derrick EJ. 1997. Threshold of metabolic acidosis associated with newborn complications. *American Journal of Obstetrics and Gynecology*. Dec;177(6):1391–4

Low JA, V Rahi and EJ Derrick. 1999. Predictive value of electronic fetal monitoring for intrapartum fetal asphyxia with metabolic acidosis. *Obstet Gynecol*. 93:285–91.

Low JA. 2007. Fetal Monitoring during Labour. In: DK E, editor. *Dewhurst's Textbook of Obstetrics & Gynaecology*: Blackwell Publishing. p. 56–62

Luzietti R, Erkkola R, Hasbargen U, *et al*. 1997. European Community Multicentre Trial "Fetal ECG Analysis During Labour": the P-R interval. *Journal of Perinatal Medicine* 25:27–34

MacDonald D, A Grant, M Sheridan-Pereira et al. 1985. The Dublin randomised controlled trial of intrapartum fetal heart rate monitoring. *Am J Obstet Gynecol*. 152:524–39.

Madaan M, Trivedi SS. 2006. Intrapartum electronic fetal monitoring vs. intermittent auscultation in postcesarean pregnancies. *International Journal of Gynaecology and Obstetrics*. Aug;94(2):123–5

Mahomed K, Nyoni R, Mulambo T, Kasule J, Jacobus E. 1994. Randomised controlled trial of intrapartum fetal heart rate monitoring. *BMJ* (Clinical research ed. Feb 19;308(6927):497–500

Menticoglou SM, CR Harman. 1999. Problems in the detection of intrapartum fetal asphyxia with intermittent auscultation. *Austr New Zeal J Obstet Gynaecol*. 39(2):218–22.

Meyberg R, Hendrik HJ, Ertan AK, Friedrich M, Schmidt W. 2000. The clinical significance of antenatal pathological Doppler findings in fetal MCA compared to umbilical artery and aorta. *Clin Exp Obstet Gynecol*. 27:2–5

Modanlou HD, Freeman RK. 1982. Sinusoidal fetal heart rate pattern: its definition and clinical significance. *American Journal of Obstetrics and Gynecology*. Apr 15;142(8):1033-8.

Mohajer MP, Sahota DS, Reed NN, Chang A, Symonds EM and James DK. 1994. Cumulative changes in the fetal electrocardiogram and biochemical indices of fetal hypoxia. *Eur J Obstet Gynecol Repod Biol* 55: 63–70

Mongelli M, TKH Chung, AMZ Chang. 1997. Intervention and benefit for conditions of very low prevalence. *Br J Obstet Gynecol*. 104:771–73.

Morrison JC, BF Chez, ID Davis et al. 1993. Intrapartum fetal heart rate assessment: Monitoring by auscultation or electronic means. *Am J Obstet Gynecol* 168:63–66.

Mozurkewich E, Wolf FM. 2000. Near-infrared spectroscopy for fetal assessment during labour. *Cochrane Database of Systematic Reviews* 2000, Issue 3. Art. No.: CD002254. DOI: 10.1002/14651858.CD002254

Murata Y, Martin CB, Jr., Ikenoue T, Hashimoto T, Taira S, Sagawa T, et al. 1982. Fetal heart rate accelerations and late decelerations during the course of intrauterine death in chronically catheterized rhesus monkeys. *American Journal of Obstetrics and Gynecology.* Sep 15;144(2):218–23

Murray HG. 1992. *Evaluation of the fetal electrocardiogram. [DM thesis]*, University of Nottingham, Nottingham.

Murray M. 1999. Certification in fetal heart monitoring: Is it really worth the additional effort and expense for perinatal nurses. *Am J Matern Child Nurs* 24(1):10.

National Institute for Clinical Excellence (NICE). 2007. *Intrapartum care: Care of healthy women and their babies during childbirth*. London: RCOG.

Neilson JP. 2005. Fetal electrocardiogram (ECG) for fetal monitoring during labour. (Cochrane Review). In: *Cochrane Database of Systematic Reviews*, Issue 4, 2005. Oxford

Nelson KB, Dambrosia JM, Ting TY, Grether JK. 1996. Uncertain value of electronic fetal monitoring in predicting cerebral palsy. *The New England Journal of Medicine*. Mar 7;334(10):613-8

Nelson KB. 1999. The neurologically impaired child and alleged malpractice at birth. *Neurol Clin*. 17(2):283–93.

Nordstrom L, I Ingermarsson, M Kublickas, B Persson, N Shimojo, M Westgren. 1995. Scalp blood lactate: A new test strip method for monitoring fetal well-being in labour. *Br J Obstet Gynaecol*. 102:894–99.

Nordstrom L, Achanna S, Naka K, Arulkumaran S. 2001. Fetal and maternal lactate increase during active second stage of labour. *BJOG* Mar;108(3):263–8

Nordstrom L. 2004. Fetal scalp and cord blood lactate. *Best Practice and Research*. Jun;18(3):467–76.

Ojala K, Vaarasmaki M, Makikallio K, et al. 2006. A comparison of intrapartum automated fetal electrocardiography and conventional cardiotocography – a randomised controlled study. *BJOG:*113(4):419–23.

Okosun H AS. Intrapartum Fetal Surveillance. *Current Obstetrics and Gynaecology*. 2005;15(1):18–24

Painter MJ, Depp R, O'Donoghue PD. Fetal heart rate patterns and development in the first year of life. *American Journal of Obstetrics and Gynecology*. 1978 Oct 1;132(3):271–7

Peat S, Booker M, Lanigan C, Ponte J. 1988. Continuous intrapartum measurement of fetal oxygen saturation. *Lancet*. Jul 23;2(8604):213.

Peebles DM, Edwards AD, Wyatt JS, et al. 1992. Effects of frequency of uterine contractions on human fetal cerebral oxyhaemoglobin concentration measured by near infrared spectroscopy. *Br J Obstet Gynaecol*;99:700

Penning S, Garite TJ. 1999. Management of fetal distress. *Obstet Gynecol Clin North Am* 26(2):259–74.

Powell OH, Melville A, MacKenna J. 1979. Fetal heart rate acceleration in labor: excellent prognostic indicator. *American Journal of Obstetrics and Gynecology*. May 1;134(1):36–8.

Ramos-Santos E, Devoe LD, Wakefield ML, Sherline DM, Methany WO. 1993. The effects of epidural anaesthesia on the Doppler velocimetry of umbilical and uterine arteries in normal and hypertensive patients during active term labour. *Obstets Gynecol*. 77(1):20–6

Rosen KG, Amer-Wahlin I, Luzietti R, Noren H. 2004. Fetal ECG waveform analysis. *Best Pract Res*. 485–514

Sameshima H, Ikenoue T. 2005. Predictive value of late decelerations for fetal acidemia in unselective low-risk pregnancies. *American Journal of Perinatology* Jan;22(1):19–23

Samueloff A, Langer O, Berkus M, Field N, Xenakis E, Ridgway L. 1994. Is fetal heart rate variability a good predictor of fetal outcome? *Acta Obstetricia et Gynecologica Scandinavica*. Jan;73(1):39–44.

Schifrin BS, Hamilton-Rubinstein T, Shields JR. 1994. Fetal heart rate patterns and the timing of fetal injury. *J Perinatol*. May-Jun;14(3):174–81.

Schifrin BS. 2004. The CTG and the timing and mechanism of fetal neurological injuries. *Best Practice and Research*. Jun;18(3):437–56

Seelbach-Gobel B, M Heupel, M Kuhnert and M Butterwegge. 1999. The prediction of fetal acidosis by means of intrapartum fetal oximetry. Am J Obstet Gynecol. 180: 73–81.

Shields JR, Schifrin BS. 1988. Perinatal antecedents of cerebral palsy. Obstetrics and Gynecology. Jun;71(6 Pt 1):899-905.

Simpson N, LW Oppenheimer, A Siren, O McDonald, D McDonald, A Dabrowski. 1999. Accuracy of strategies for monitoring fetal heart rate in labor. Am J Perinatol 16(4):167–73.

Siristatidis C, Salamalekis E, Kassanos D, Loghis C, Creatsas G. 2004. Evaluation of fetal intrapartum hypoxia by middle cerebral and umbilical artery Doppler velocimetry with simultaneous cardiotocography and pulse oximetry. Arch Gynecol Obstet. Dec;270(4):265–70)

Skupski DW, Rosenberg CR, Eglinton GS. 2002. Intrapartum fetal stimulation tests: a meta-analysis. Obstetrics and Gynecology. Jan; 99(1):129–34

Spencer JA, Johnson P. 1986. Fetal heart rate variability changes and fetal behavioural cycles during labour. British Journal of Obstetrics and Gynaecology. Apr;93(4):314–21.

Steer PJ and P Danielian. 1999. Fetal distress in labour. In High risk pregnancy – Management options, ed DK James, CP Weiner, B Gonik. 1121–49 London: WB Saunders.

Strachan BK, van Wijngaarden WJ, Sahota D et al. 2000. Cardiotocography only versus cardiotocography plus PR-interval analysis in intrapartum surveillance: a randomised, multicentre trial. Lancet 355:456–9.

Sweha A, TW Hacker and J Nuovo. 1999. Interpretation of fetal heart rate during labour. Am Fam Physician 59(9):2487–2500.

Tejani N, L Mann, A Bhakthavathsalan, RR Weiss. 1975. Correlation of fetal heart rate – uterine contraction patterns and fetal scalp pH. Obstet Gynecol. 46:392–96.

Thacker SB, DF Stroup, HB Peterson. 1995. Efficacy and safety of intrapartum electronic fetal monitoring: An update. Obstet Gynecol. 86: 613–620.

Thacker SB, Stroup D, Chang M. 2001. Continuous electronic heart rate monitoring for fetal assessment during labor. Cochrane Database of Systematic Reviews (Online). (2):CD000063

Todros T, CU Preve, C Plazzotta, M Biolcati and P Lombardo. 1996. Fetal heart tracings: observers versus computer assessment. Eur J Obstet Gynecol Reprod Biol 68:83–86.

Tuffnell D, Haw WL, Wilkinson K. 2006. How long does a fetal scalp blood sample take? BJOG. Mar;113(3):332–4

van Wijngaarden W, DS Sahota, DK James, T Farrell, W Mires et al. 1996. Improved intrapartum surveillance with PR interval analysis of the fetal electrocardiogram: A randomized trial showing a reduction in fetal blood sampling. Am J Obstet Gynecol. 174(4):1295–99.

Vintzileos AM, A Antsaklis, I Varvarigos et al. 1993. A randomised trial of intrapartum electronic fetal heart rate monitoring versus intermittent auscultation: A meta-analysis. Obstet Gynecol 85:149–155.

Vintzileos AM, Nioka S, Lake M, Li P, Luo Q, Chance B. 2005. Transabdominal fetal pulse oximetry with near-infrared spectroscopy. Am J Obstet Gynecol. Jan;192(1):129–33

Westgren M, Kruger K, Ek S, Grunevald C, Kublickas M, Naka K, et al. 1998. Lactate compared with pH analysis at fetal scalp blood sampling: a prospective randomised study. British Journal of Obstetrics and Gynaecology. Jan;105(1): 29–33.

Westgren M, K Kruger, S Ek, C Grunevald et al. 1998a. Lactate compared with pH analysis at fetal scalp blood sampling: A prospective randomised study. Br J Obstet Gynecol. 105:29–33.

Westgren M, M Kublickas and K Kruger. 1998b. Role of lactate measurements during labour. Obstet Gynecol Surv. 54(1):43–8.

Williams B, Arulkumaran S. 2004. Cardiotocography and medicolegal issues. Best Practice and Research. Jun;18(3):457–66

# CHAPTER 6

# UTERINE CONTRACTIONS

*Rohan D'Souza, Vivek Nama and Sabaratnam Arulkumaran*

In the absence of mechanical difficulties like feto-pelvic disproportion or fetal malposition, efficient uterine contractions and the expulsive efforts of the mother should result in an unassisted vaginal delivery. However, dysfunctional labour has been estimated to affect up to 21 per cent of primigravid labours (Selin et al 2008) and is the commonest cause of emergency cesarean sections (Thomas et al 2000). A systematic approach to the understanding of the pathophysiology of uterine contractions, the methods of measuring uterine activity, the recognition and correction of inadequate uterine activity and recent research into the subject would go a long way in reducing the high incidence of operative delivery and its associated health and economic implications.

## The physiology of uterine contractions

Embryologically, the uterus develops from fusion of the two mullerian ducts which explains the bilaterally symmetrical arrangement of its muscle fibres. The uterine myometrium is composed of smooth muscle cells, the myocytes, which are attached to elastin and collagen that provide support while simultaneously allowing the myocytes to contract and retract. Fluctuating membrane potential of the myocytes throughout pregnancy means that the uterine myometrium is far from quiescent. In fact, on bimanual examination, the uterus may be felt to be contracting from as early as the fourteenth week of pregnancy. However, these contractions are weak, arrhythmic and infrequent. It is only when later in pregnancy this sporadic activity becomes coordinated that they are able to bring about changes in the cervix.

Uterine contractions in early pregnancy are due to uncoordinated myogenic activity of individual uterine muscle fibres and are also probably due to increased estrogen secretion in pregnancy. Estrogen lowers the resting potential in the myocytes, thus making them more excitable; progesterone tends to raise the membrane potential making the uterus more quiescent. In late pregnancy, however, the action of progesterone on the estrogen-primed uterus leads to the coordinated uterine activity observed in late pregnancy, labour and the immediate puerperium, although its effect is mediated or influenced by oxytocin and prostaglandins among others. The coordination of myocyte activity is a result of formation of connexin gap junctions, which although present throughout pregnancy, become maximally expressed in labour.

The smooth muscle of the uterus has a number of advantages compared to the striated muscle of the body. First, it has a greater degree of shortening with contractions than striated muscle. A second advantage is that the force generated can be in any direction, in contrast to striated muscle, where the force exerted is along the axis of the fibres of the striated muscle. The arrangement of thick and thin muscle fibres in long random bundles is a further advantage in facilitating the shortening and force generating capacity of smooth muscle and enabling multidirectional force generation.

> Uterine smooth muscle has several advantages due to the arrangement of thick and thin muscle fibres in long random bundles:
> - a greater degree of shortening with contractions
> - the force generated can be in any direction

The interaction between actin and myosin is the key to muscle contraction. This interaction causes activation of ATPase leading to ATP hydrolysis, which in turn leads to phosphorylation of myosin and generation of the contractile force. The process of phosphorylation of myosin requires activation of the enzyme myosin light chain kinase and the latter is dependent on $Ca^{2+}$. Therefore, ion channels (sodium, calcium and potassium) that are present within the myometrium have a pivotal role in the regulation of myometrial activity by controlling the influx of calcium and thereby the intracytosolic calcium ion concentrations.

In paraplegic patients, the uterus contracts normally, albeit painlessly, leading to the assumption that the nervous system has a minor role in influencing uterine activity in labour. Sensory fibres via the sacral nerves reach the cervix and are responsible for pain on stretching the cervix, while the pain from the body of the uterus in association with uterine contractions is thought, among other causes, to be ischemic in origin and transmitted via the sympathetic system. The uterus has adrenergic, cholinergic and peptidergic innervation. Alpha-adrenoceptors in the uterus are responsive to adrenaline and noradrenaline and have an excitatory influence, while beta-adrenoceptors (which predominate throughout gestation) are inhibitory, being influenced by adrenaline and favour uterine quiescence.

## Parameters of uterine contractions – definitions

Uterine contractions generally start at the uterine fundus and then travel down the body of the uterus. They can be described in terms of the following parameters:

**Baseline tone** is the uterine pressure or tone between contractions. This is a reflection of atmospheric pressure, hydrostatic pressure and elastic recoil of the uterus and surrounding tissues (Steer 1993)

**Amplitude** is the maximum uterine pressure above the baseline tone.

**Frequency** is the number of contractions occurring over a 10-minute period.

**Duration** is the time in seconds where the uterine tone is above its baseline, i.e.

**Table 6.1** Units of uterine activity

| Unit | Description | Remarks |
|---|---|---|
| Montevideo unit (Caldeyro Barcia et al 1957) | Mean amplitude x mean frequency over 10 mins (initially described as intensity x frequency) | Ignores any contribution from the duration of contractions and the shape of the contractions |
| Alexandria unit (el-Sahwi et al 1967) | Montevideo unit x mean duration over 10 mins | No contributions taken from the shape of contractions. Incorporating the duration showed that longer contractions decreased the duration of labour |
| Uterine activity unit (UAU) (Miller et al 1976) | Area under the pressure curve (Torr-min) over 1 min minus 1UAU = 1 Torr min | Includes the contraction frequency, duration and amplitude and includes the baseline tone and hence not widely adopted |
| Uterine activity integral (UAI) or active contraction area (Steer et al 1984) | Active area under the pressure curve over 15 min (Intrauterine pressure minus the baseline pressure) | Measures active pressure including maternal efforts, especially in second stage |
| Mean active pressure (MAP) (Phillips and Calder 1987) | UAI divided by 900 (kPa), measuring over 1 second (15 min = 900 sec) | Independent of the duration of the integration period |
| Mean contraction active pressure (MCAP) (Phillips and Calder 1987) | UAI/total duration of contraction | When the integration period is with respect to one contraction |

the time between the onset and offset of a contraction.

**Relaxation time** is the time in seconds, between the end of one contraction and the beginning of the next.

## Quantification of uterine activity

The precise quantification of uterine activity has not led to improvement in fetal outcome or in cesarean section rates and may not really be required unless very high doses of oxytocin are being used. However, it assists in understanding and interpreting the tocogram and various units of quantification have been described as shown in Table 6.1.(Nama and Arulkumaran 2009).

The various parameters of uterine contractions are schematically represented in Figure 6.1.

The units of quantification of uterine activity, described in Table 6.1 do not take into account the 'shape' of contractions. The 'shape' of the contraction has been shown to be important in patients with dysfunctional labour. This 'shape' is measured by the F:R ration, where F (fall) is the time for a contraction to return to baseline from its peak and the R (rise) is the time for a contraction to rise to its peak (Bakker and van Geijn 2008). Although the evidence is not robust, an increased F:R ratio has been shown to be associated with a higher need for

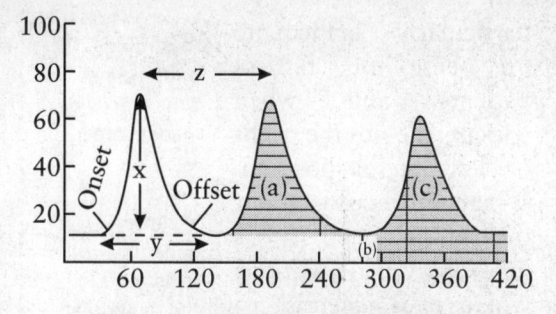

**Figure 6.1** Parameters of uterine contractions

X - active pressure or amplitude
Y - duration
Z - contraction interval related to frequency
(a) - active contraction area
(b) - basal tone
(c) - total contraction area

is reached. During this time, the fetus relies on the blood entrapped in the intervillous space as a reservoir for oxygenation. Monitoring of the frequency, duration and baseline tone of uterine contractions is imperative, especially in augmented or induced labours in order to prevent hyperstimulation and fetal hypoxia on the one hand, and dysfunctional labour on the other.

## Methods of Measurement

### Maternal perception of uterine activity

An intrauterine pressure of 15 mmHg from the baseline pressure is effective in producing cervical changes and is experienced as pain. However, the threshold of pain varies from woman to woman and may be influenced by parity and maternal weight (Cottrill et al 2004). The reliance on a parturient's assessment of frequency and duration of contractions may, therefore, not always be reliable.

> The threshold of pain varies from woman to woman and may be influenced by parity and maternal weight.

### Manual palpation of uterine contractions

Traditionally, uterine activity is assessed by abdominal palpation of contractions. The examining hand is placed between the umbilicus

> The duration of a contraction is from the time the contraction is felt abdominally to when the contraction passes, measured in seconds. However, the estimated duration may be less than the actual duration of the contraction.

cesarean delivery (Althaus et al 2006). Again, low amplitude, high-frequency contractions (tachysystole) may cause fetal compromise and still remain within the normal limits of these quantification methods. Hence, it has been suggested that even if the above units are used for quantification of uterine activity, it is mandatory to record frequency and duration of uterine contractions (Vanner and Gardosi 1996)

> Monitoring of the frequency, duration and baseline tone of uterine contractions is imperative, especially in augmented or induced labours, in order to prevent hyperstimulation and fetal hypoxia on the one hand and dysfunctional labour on the other.

### The importance of measuring uterine contractions

Uterine blood flow is minimal during the ascending phase of a uterine contraction, stabilising after the peak intensity of a contraction and uterine fundus and the duration and frequency of the uterine contractions is quantified over a 10-minute period (Arulkumaran and Lennox 1988). The duration of a contraction is from the time the contraction is felt abdominally to when the contraction passes, measured in seconds. Manual palpation of contractions is not influenced by a woman's position in labour, her parity or gestational age, but it must be remembered that since the first and last part of the contractions may not be palpable, the duration estimated may be less than the actual duration of the contraction (Gibb 1989). Although it gives little information about the intensity of the contractions or the basal pressure between contractions, it is adequate for management of labour in most circumstances (Arulkumaran and Ratnam 1987).

## External tocography

This involves the use of a transducer fastened to the maternal abdomen over or near the region of the uterine fundus. The transducer detects changes caused by uterine contractions in the anterio-posterior diameter of the abdomen. An on-line graphical record using such devices provides information on the duration and frequency and an approximation of the strength of contractions, as the latter will depend on the tightness of the elastic belt holding the transducer on the abdomen, maternal posture and the thickness of the abdominal wall (Steer 1993). Recording of uterine activity may be

> External monitoring is the mainstay of uterine activity measurement because of:
> • ease of use
> • less invasive nature
> • low cost
> • same clinical outcome as internal monitoring

particularly inadequate in obese or restless patients and when patients lie in the right or left lateral position. Where information about the uterine activity is inadequate or in situations where it is essential to quantify the strength of contraction and the basal uterine tone between contractions (e.g. previous uterine scar and augmentation with oxytocin) internal monitoring of uterine activity may be desirable. However, external tocography is used in most cases because of its non-invasive nature, easy application and low cost, with minimal discomfort for the mother. Cordless transducers are available allowing ambulation of women in labour or to have labour and birth under water.

> Recording of uterine activity may be inadequate in:
> • obese patients
> • restless patients
> • patients in the right or left lateral position

## Internal tocography

The first attempts at recording intrauterine pressures were made by Schatz in Germany in 1872, by inserting a rubber bag in the uterus under anesthesia and connecting it to a manometer (Allman and Steer 1993). Caldeyro-Barcia used the transabdominal method by introducing a catheter into the uterus and serially recorded intrauterine pressure throughout gestation. The transcervical approach was first used in 1952 by Williams and Stallworthy, who introduced a polythene catheter in the uterus through the vagina and cervix using a Drew-Smythe catheter. Developments of the original concept over time included smaller and more flexible catheters, which could be connected to electronic recording devices.

Currently, there are two main varieties of intrauterine pressure catheters (IUPC):

*fluid-filled* and *transducer-tipped*. Although small differences in pressure measurements have been noted between the same and different types of catheters in the same amniotic cavity (Knoke et al 1976; Steer et al 1978; Chua et al 1992), these differences have not been shown to make any difference to the management or outcome of labour, because it is the cumulative pressure over time rather than the minor variations in intrauterine pressure between contractions that has a bearing on labour outcome (Arulkumaran 1994). The active contraction area measured by intrauterine pressure catheters has a better correlation with the rate of cervical dilatation than the individual variables of frequency or amplitude of contractions. The titration of oxytocin, however, to achieve a preset active contraction area profile has not been shown to improve obstetric outcomes compared to titration to achieve a preset frequency of contractions (Arulkumaran et al 1989b).

> The titration of oxytocin to achieve a preset active contraction area profile has not been shown to improve obstetric outcomes compared to titration to achieve a preset frequency of contractions.

The advantages of internal tocography are that it is unaffected by maternal position, and is more comfortable for the patient, allowing for amnioinfusion if required (Nageotte 2003). It is now considered one of the most accurate ways of measuring uterine activity in labour, although a prospective RCT did not show a better outcome when IUPCs were used compared to external tocography in augmented labour (Chua et al 1990).

Internal tocography is invasive and is not bereft of risks, because it involves the rupture of membranes. The use of IUPCs in the extra-amniotic space has not been shown to provide comparable information to similar catheters inserted intra-amniotically when membranes are ruptured (Chua et al 1994). IUPCs may increase the risk of infection. There have been reports of uterine perforation, fetal hemorrhage due to puncture of a fetal vessel and placental abruption (Chan et al 1973; Nuttall 1978). Fluid-filled catheters require more frequent readjustment and have an increased tendency for artefact due to air bubbles, kinked cables and catheter occlusion by vernix, meconium, blood or fetal parts (Devoe et al 1989). These problems were overcome by the development of transducer-tipped catheters, where the tip lies in the amniotic cavity and the entire transmission passes electronically through the catheter and via a flexible extension cable to the contraction module of the fetal monitor.

Further developments in technology have resulted in fibreoptic catheters, dual-channel multifunctional uterine probes, balloon probes and single use (disposable) catheters that have a separate channel to allow sampling of the amniotic fluid as well as offering the potential to be used for amnioinfusion. The fact that they do not require complex manometry measurements makes them user friendly and simple to insert and use (Figure 6.2).

## Uterine Electromyography (EMG)

The uterine EMG is the result of electrical activity generated at the microscopic level. Measurements of uterine activity by trans-abdominal EMG are comparable to IUPC for measuring the strength of uterine contractions (Maul et al 2004). A typical uterine EMG system includes abdominal

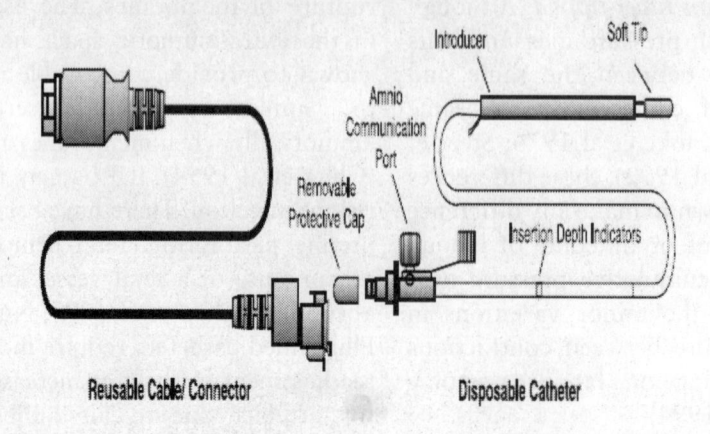

**Figure 6.2** Intrauterine catheter with amnioinfusion port

surface electrodes, electrical filters/amplifiers and acquisition and analysis hardware/software. The EMG waves can be analysed by a number of sophisticated mathematical methods in order to determine the extent of the electrochemical preparedness of the myometrium for labour and subsequent delivery. These measurements may even be used to measure the synchronisation and concordance of contractions (Jiang et al 2007).

## Comparison of various methods

In augmented (Chua et al 1990) or induced (Chia et al 1993) labour, no difference in cesarean section rates or neonatal morbidity was noted, whether monitored by external or internal tocography. There was good correlation between the two methods with respect to frequency and duration of contractions, even in the moderately obese (Miles et al 2001). The frequency and duration of contractions is of greater importance for adequate placental perfusion and the avoidance of fetal compromise rather than amplitude alone.

While IUPCs are limited by their invasiveness and the need for ruptured membranes, external uterine monitors are uncomfortable, often inaccurate and depend on the subjectivity of the examiner. However, external monitoring has remained the mainstay of uterine activity measurement because of the ease of use, less invasive nature, low cost and the same clinical outcome as internal monitoring.

## Uterine activity in normal labour

In most normal labours, contractions at the end of the first stage have a frequency of 3–5 in 10 minutes, amplitude of more than 50 mmHg and duration of approximately 60 seconds. In order to overcome dysfunctional

> There is no difference in cesarean section rates or neonatal morbidity whether labour is monitored by external or internal tocography.

labour, it has been suggested that a contraction frequency of 4–5 per 10 minutes, with a duration of 40 seconds (Arulkumaran 1994) and a relaxation time of 51 seconds in the first stage and 36 seconds in the second stage (Bakker et al 2007) is maintained. Any increase in contraction frequency and/or decrease in relaxation time may lower the umbilical artery pH.

> Usually, contractions at the end of the first stage have
> - a frequency of 3–5 in 10 minutes
> - an amplitude of more than 50 mmHg
> - a duration of approximately 60 seconds

## Excessive uterine activity

The commonest cause for excessive uterine activity is exogenous oxytocin administration, but it may also occur in spontaneous labour due to increased uterine sensitivity to oxytocin with advancing labour. The following definitions are commonly applied to describe excessive uterine activity.

**Polysystole:** The uterus contracts more than once every two minutes or a frequency of >5 in 10 minutes.

**Uterine hyperstimulation:** Polysystole occurs in response to oxytocin.

**Hypertonic uterine activity:** Rise in baseline pressure above 20 mmHg, but where the contractions do not merge.

**Tetanic uterine contractions:** Contractions lasting for three minutes or more. These are unusual in spontaneous labour but can be encountered in oxytocin-induced or augmented labours. Tetanic contractions are associated with hypertonic uterine activity, dramatic reduction of perfusion to the retroplacental blood pool and may precipitate FHR abnormalities, especially where the fetus has poor reserves.

Excessive uterine activity can be treated with the administration of subcutaneous terbutaline, with the discontinuation of oxytocin in case of induced or augmented labours. Pacheco et al (2006) showed that subcutaneous terbutaline can be used without discontinuation of oxytocin but the advantages of such an approach over the traditional approach of oxytocin discontinuation and terbutaline need to be evaluated.

> Management of tachysystole
> - Discontinue oxytocin
> - Administer 0.25 mg terbutaline subcutaneously

## Incoordinate uterine activity

Incoordinate uterine activity is not an uncommon finding, especially in primiparous labours. Uterine activity may be incoordinate in terms of frequency of contractions or duration/strength of the contractions or a combination of both, but a wide variation of incoordinate uterine activity is associated with normal progress in labour (Gibb et al 1984). Incoordinate uterine activity in itself is not an indication for the use of oxytocin unless they are found to be inefficient in terms of progress in labour. The use of oxytocin will not necessarily correct the incoordinate uterine activity but will make the contractions more efficient, thus improving the chances of an unassisted vaginal delivery.

**Factors affecting uterine activity may include maternal and fetal characteristics and are discussed overleaf:**

*Ethnicity:* Ethnic differences do not appear to influence uterine activity once other confounding variables such as parity, stature, uterine fibroids and fetal size have been accounted for (Arulkumaran 1989a).

*Obesity:* Obesity is associated with poor uterine contractility and dysfunctional labour (Zhang et al 2007). This may be due to a disruption of the signalling mechanisms by elevated cholesterol levels (Wray 2007).

*Myometrial hypoxia and intracellular acidosis:* Myometrial hypoxia can lead to myometrial lactic acidosis which in turn decreases uterine contractility, resulting in dysfunctional labour (Parratt et al 1995; Quenby et al 2004)

*Parity:* The uterus has to perform a given quantum of activity in labour to effect delivery and the total uterine activity is a reflection of the cervical and pelvic tissue resistance (Arulkumaran et al 1985). As seen in Figure 6.3, the parous uterus needs to expend significantly less effort to effect normal vaginal delivery than its nulliparous counterpart until the late first stage, suggesting that parity may have a greater influence on the resistance offered by the cervix than the pelvic tissues (Arulkumaran et al 1984).

*Fetal presentation:* Uterine activity does not appear to be affected by presentation (breech or vertex) when matched for fetal and maternal characteristics and stage of labour (Arulkumaran and Lennox 1988).

## Induced and augmented labours

Induction of labour is common practice in modern obstetrics with wide variation in rates between units within the same country. Where the cervix is favourable, artificial rupture of membranes and oxytocin infusion titrated to produce four contractions per ten minutes is the common method. Induction of labour with oxytocin has been shown to reduce the inter-contraction interval and increase the contraction regularity (Oppenheimer et al 2002), while augmentation with oxytocin has been shown to first increase the frequency of contractions followed by an increase in their amplitude, after which a stable phase is achieved (Steer et al 1985). Any further increase in oxytocin, however, increases the baseline tone and the frequency of contractions with a reduction in their amplitude, causing hyperstimulation. Gibb et al (1985) looked at titrating the oxytocin to achieve the fiftieth centile of uterine activity observed in spontaneous normal labour according to parity, but the outcome was no better than when oxytocin was titrated to produce four to five contractions in ten minutes, thus

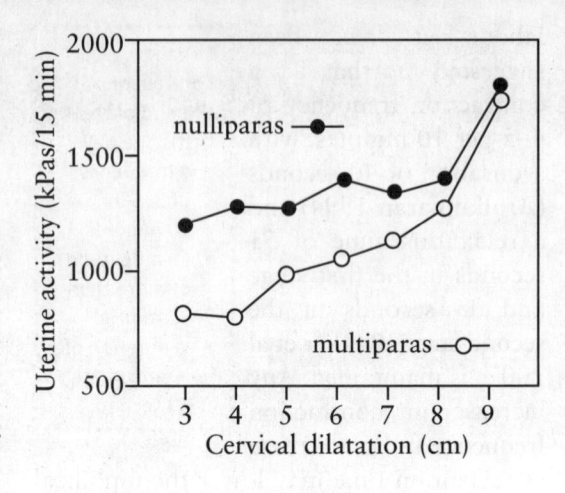

**Figure 6.3** Uterine activity in nulliparas and multiparas in the first stage of labour

indicating that quantification of uterine activity offered no advantage in induced labour over and above using frequency of uterine contraction to titrate oxytocin.

Crane et al (2001) showed that the induction or augmentation of labour using misoprostol is associated with a greater incidence of tachysystoles, while the use of dinoprostone is associated with hyperstimulation and also that repeated doses result in contraction abnormalities.

## Uterine activity in the presence of a cesarean section scar

In women with a previous cesarean section scar, the level of uterine activity depends upon whether they have had a previous vaginal delivery or at least laboured and reached the active phase of labour. Thus, women who had a cesarean section electively or in the latent phase of labour tend to exhibit higher levels of uterine activity compared to those with a previous vaginal delivery or when a cesarean section was performed in the active phase of labour (Arulkumaran et al 1989c). Women with a uterine scar who are augmented show higher levels of uterine activity compared to those who make normal progress and require no augmentation. Further, those women with a previous cesarean scar who are likely to deliver vaginally show satisfactory progress in the first few hours of augmentation compared to their counterparts who may need a cesarean section for poor progress (Silver and Gibbs 1987; Arulkumaran et al 1989c).

The main concern in the presence of a uterine scar is the possibility of scar rupture, which although rare may have devastating consequences for mother and baby. The classical signs of scar rupture (maternal hypotension, tachycardia and vaginal bleeding) occur late. There are conflicting opinions as to whether internal tocography may help in earlier identification of scar integrity, although it is unable to predict impending scar rupture. Rodriquez et al (1989) concluded that IUPCs were not of value in detecting early rupture of the uterus, while Beckley et al (1991) and Arulkumaran et al (1992) have shown that they may be helpful by demonstrating a fall in intrauterine pressure with a breach in the uterine scar (Figure 6.4).

The loss of intrauterine pressure may, however, not always be detectable if the catheter tip is located in an isolated pool of amniotic fluid, or indeed, in situations where there is an incomplete rupture of the scar with an intact peritoneum (Paul et al 1985). Reduction in uterine activity may be more easily detected and greater notice taken of, with internal tocography compared to external tocography, where a sudden reduction in uterine activity may be attributed to alteration of posture or loosening of the belt.

## Monitoring of uterine activity and medico-legal implications

Of labours requiring fetal scalp blood sampling, 50 per cent had a poor tocography recording for a quarter of the total monitoring time, indicating that more satisfactory recording is required. Medicolegal issues are commonly due to inadequate uterine contraction monitoring, cessation of monitoring of FHR or uterine contractions much earlier than the time of delivery, failure to recognise that the uterus is contracting more than five times in 10

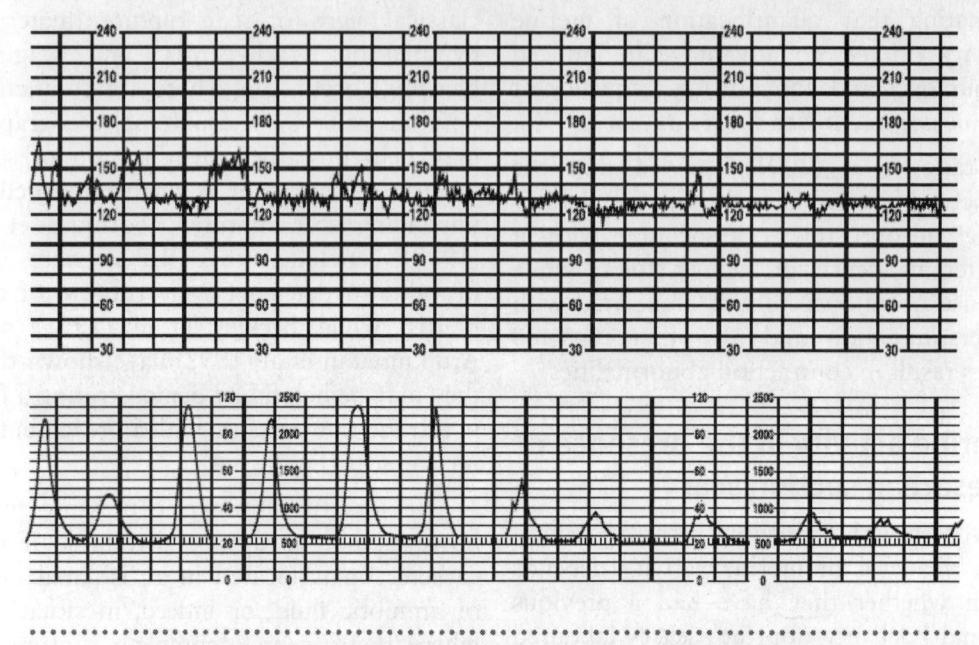

**Figure 6.4** Decline in uterine activity with loss of integrity of cesarean scar. Baseline pressure and frequency were not affected

minutes and pathological FHR patterns caused by uterine hyperstimulation. Hence, monitoring of uterine contractions is indispensable, especially with the use of oxytocin infusion. FIGO (1995) has provided guidelines on methods of uterine activity monitoring and their interpretation. Computer-assisted automated analysis of uterine activity along with FHR interpretation may aid the improvement of reporting criteria and clinical management of cases (Ayres-de Campos et al 2000).

## Conclusion

Monitoring of uterine activity is important in labour, more so where there is inadequate progress with the need for augmentation (with or without a previous uterine scar) and abnormalities in the fetal heart rate pattern. In general, external tocography provides adequate contraction-monitoring information. The use of internal catheter tip transducers offer no advantage in terms of improving outcome by trying to achieve predetermined levels of uterine activity over and above simply aiming for four to five contractions per 10 minutes, as detected by standard external transducers. There may be a role for the use of internal tocography in certain situations such as with oxytocin augmentation, especially when used in multiparous patients or in the presence of a uterine scar or when external monitoring is inadequate due to patient body habitus, restlessness or posture.

# References

Althaus JE, Petersen S, Driggers R, Cootauco A, Bienstock JL and Blakemore JA. 2006. Cephalopelvic disproportion is associated with an altered uterine contraction shape in the active phase of labor. *Am J Obstet Gynecol.* 195(3):739–42.

Allman AC and Steer PJ. 1993. Monitoring uterine activity. *Br J Hosp Med.* 49(9):649–53

Arulkumaran S, Gibb DMF, Lun KC, Heng SH, Ratnam SS. 1984. The effect of parity on uterine activity in labour. *Br J Obstet Gynecol.* 91:843–48.

Arulkumaran S, Gibb DMF, Ratnam SS, Heng SH, Lun KC. 1985. Total uterine activity in induced labour: An index of cervical and pelvic tissue resistance. *Br J Obstet Gynecol.* 92:693–97.

Arulkumaran S and Ratnam SS. 1987. Current trends in monitoring uterine contractions in labour. *Sri Lanka J Obstet Gynecol.* 13:114–27.

Arulkumaran S and Lennox C. 1988. *The partograph section II. A user's manual.* Geneva: WHO.

Arulkumaran S, Gibb DMF, Chua S, Singh P and Ratnam SS. 1989a. Ethnic influence on uterine activity in spontaneous normal labour. *Br J Obstet Gynaecol.* 06:1203–06.

Arulkumaran S, Yang M, Ingemarsson I, Singh P and Ratnam SS. 1989b. Augmentation of labour. Does quantification of active contraction area to guide oxytocin titration produce better obstetric outcome? *Asia Oceania J Obstet Gynecol* 15:47–51.

Arulkumaran S, Ingemarsson I and Ratnam SS. 1989c. Oxytocin augmentation in dysfunctional labour after previous caesarean section scar. *Br J Obstet Gynecol* 96:939–41.

Arulkumaran S, Chua S and Ratnam SS. 1992. Symptoms and signs of scar rupture – value of uterine activity measurement. *Austr NZ J Obstet Gynecol* 32:208–212.

Arulkumaran S. 1994. Uterine activity in labour. In *The Uterus*, ed T Chard, JG Grudzinskas, 356–77. Cambridge: Cambridge University Press.

Ayres-de Campos D, Bernardes J, Garrid A, Marques-de Sa J, Pereira-Leite L. 2000. SisPorto 2.0: A program for automated analysis of cardiotocograms. *J Matern Fetal Med* 9: 311–8

Bakker PC, Kurver PH, Kuik DJ and Van Geijn HP. 2007. Elevated uterine activity increases the risk of fetal acidosis at birth. *Am J Obstet Gynecol.* 196:311–6

Bakker PC, van Geijn HP. 2008. Uterine activity: Implications for the condition of the fetus. *J Perinat Med* 36:30–7

Beckley S, Gee H and Newton JR. 1991. Scar rupture in labour after previous lower uterine segment caesarean section: The role of uterine activity measurement. *Br J Obstet Gynaecol.* 98:265–9

Caldeyro-Barcia R, Sica-Blanco Y, Poseiro JJ, Gonzalez-Panizza V, Mendez-Bauer C, Fielitz C, Alvarez H, Pose SV and Hendricks CH. 1957. A quantitative study of synthetic oxytocin on the human uterus. *J Pharmacol Exp Ther.* 121: 18–31.

Chan WH, Paul RH and Teows J. 1973. Intrapartum fetal monitoring. Maternal and fetal morbidity and perinatal mortality. *Obstet Gynecol.* 41: 7–13.

Chia YT, Arulkumaran S, Soon SB, Norshida S and Ratnam SS. 1993. Induction of labour: does internal tocography result in better obstetric outcome than external tocography. *Aust NZ J Obstet Gynaecol.* 33:159–61

Chua S, Kurup A, Arulkumaran S and Ratnam SS. 1990. Augmentation of labour. Does internal tocography result in better obstetric outcome than external tocography? *Obstet Gynecol* 76:164–167.

Chua S, Arulkumaran S, Yang M, Ratnam SS and Steer PJ. 1992. The accuracy of catheter tip pressure transducers for measurement of intrauterine pressure in labour. *Br J Obstet Gynecol* 99: 186–89.

Chua S, Arulkumaran S, Yang M, Steer PJ and Ratnam SS. 1994. Intrauterine pressure: comparison of extra vs intraamniotic methods using a transducer tipped catheter. *Asia Oceania J Obstet Gynaecol* 20:35–8.

Cottrill HM, Barton JR, O'Brien JM, Rhea DL and Milligan DA. 2004. Factors influencing maternal perception of uterine contractions. *Am J Obstet Gynecol* 190:1455–7.

Crane JM, Young DC, Butt KD, Bennett KA and Hutchens D. 2001. Excessive uterine activity accompanying induced labor. *Obstet Gynecol* 97:926–31

Devoe LD, Gardner P, Dear C and Searle N. 1989. Monitoring intrauterine pressure during active labor. A prospective comparison of two methods. *J Reprod Med* 34:811–4

El-Sahwi S, Gaafar AA, Toppozada HK. 1967. A new unit for evaluation of uterine activity. *Am J Obstet Gynecol* 800: 900–3

FIGO Study Group on the Assessment of New Technology, International Federation of Gynecology and Obstetrics. 1995. Intrapartum surveillance: recommendations on current practice and overview of new developments. *Int J Gynaecol Obstet*. 49: 213–21

Gibb DMF, Arulkumaran S, Lun KC and Ratnam SS. 1984. Characteristics of uterine activity in nulliparous labour. *Br J Obstet Gynaecol*. 91: 220–27.

Gibb DMF, Arulkumaran S and Ratnam SS. 1985. A comparative study of the methods of oxytocin infusion for induction of labour. *Br J Obstet Gynecol*. 92:688–92.

Gibb DMF, ed. 1989. *Uterine activity in Labour*. Turnbridge Wells, Kent: Castle House Publications

Jiang W, Li G and Lin L. 2007. Uterine electromyogram tocography to represent synchronization of uterine contractions. *Int J Gynaecolo Obstet*. 97: 120–4.

Knoke JD, LL, Newman MRI and Roux JF. 1976. The accuracy of intrauterine pressure during labour. A statistical analysis. *Comp Biomed Res*. 9:177–86.

Maul H, Maner WL, Olson G, Saade GR and Garfield RE. 2004. Non-invasive transabdominal uterine electromyography correlates with the strength of intrauterine pressure and is predictive of labor and delivery. *J Matern Fetal Neonatal Med* 15:297–301.

Miles AM, Monga M and Richeson KS. 2001. Correlation of external and internal monitoring of uterine activity in a cohort of term patients. *Am J Perinatol*. 18(3):137–40.

Miller C, Yeh SY, Schifrin BS, Paul RH and Hon EH. 1976. Quantification of uterine activity in 100 primiparous patients. *Am J Obstet Gynecol* 124: 398–405.

Nageotte M, ed. 2003. *Uterine Contraction Monitoring*. 3$^{rd}$ ed. Philadephia: Lippincott Williams and Wilkins

Nama V and Arulkumaran S. 2009. Uterine contractions. In *Best Practice in Labour and Delivery*, ed R Warren and S Arulkumaran, 54–65. Cambridge: Cambridge University Press

Nuttall ID. 1978. Perforation of a placental fetal vessel by an intrauterine pressure catheter. *Br J Obstet Gynaecol*. 85:573–4

Oppenheimer LW, Bland ES and Dabrowski A et al. 2002. Uterine contraction pattern as a predictor of the mode of delivery. *J Perinatol*. 22:149–53.

Pacheco LD, Rosen MP, Gei AF, Saade GR and Hankins GD. 2006. Management of uterine hyperstimulation with concomitant use of oxytocin and terbutaline. *Am J Perinatol*. 23:377–80.

Parratt JR, Taggart MJ, Wray S. 1995. Changes in intracellular pH close to term and their possible significance to labour. *Pflugers Arch*. 430: 1012–4.

Paul RH, Phelan JP, Yeh, SH. 1985. Trial of labour in patient with a prior Caesarean birth. *Am J Obstet Gynecol*. 151:287–304.

Phillips GF and Calder AA. 1987. Units for the evaluation of uterine contractility. *Br J Obstet Gynaecol* 94:236–41.

Quenby S, Pierce SJ, Brigham S and Wray S. 2004. Dysfunctional labour and myometrial lactic acidosis. *Obstet Gynecol*. 103: 718–23.

Rodriquez MH, DT Masaki, JP Phelan and FG Diaz. 1989. Uterine rupture: Are intrauterine pressure catheters useful in diagnosis. *Am J Obstet Gynecol*. 161:666–69.

Selin L, Wallin G and Berg M. 2008. Dystocia in labour – risk factors, management and outcome: a retrospective observational study in a Swedish setting. *Acta Obstet Gynecol Scand*. 87:216–21.

Silver KR and Gibbs RS. 1987. Predictors of vaginal delivery in patients with a previous Caesarean section who require oxytocin. *Am J Obstet Gynecol*. 156:57–60.

Steer PJ, Carter MC, Gordon AJ and Beard RW. 1978. The use of catheter tip pressure transducers for the measurement of intrauterine pressure in labour. *Br J Obstet Gynecol*. 85:561–66.

Steer PJ, Carter MC and Beard RW. 1984. Normal levels of active contraction area in spontaneous labour. *Br J Obstet Gynaecol*. 91:211–9.

Steer PJ, Carter MC and Beard RW. 1985. The effect of oxytocin infusion on uterine activity levels in slow labour. *Br. J Obstet Gynaecol*. 92:1120–6.

Steer PJ. 1993. Standards in fetal monitoring – practical requirements for uterine activity measurement and recording. *Br J Obstet Gynaecol*. 100 (Suppl 9):32–6.

Thomas J, Callwood A and Paranjothy S. 2000. National Caesarean Section Audit: Ppdate. *Pract Midwife* 3(11):20.

Vanner T, Gardosi J. 1996. Intrapartum assessment of uterine activity. *Baillieres Clin Obstet Gynaecol*. 10:243–57.

Wray S. 2007. Insights into the uterus. *Exp Physiol*. 92:621–31.

Zhang J, Bricker L, Wray S and Quenby S. 2007. Poor uterine contractility in obese women. *Br J Obstet Gynaecol*. 114:343–8.

CHAPTER 7

# THE MANAGEMENT OF INTRAPARTUM FETAL DISTRESS

*Rohan D'Souza and Sabaratnam Arulkumaran*

Labour is rightly regarded as the most dangerous journey of a woman's life. In less developed countries, the perinatal morbidity and mortality from intrapartum events is still unacceptably high. The World Health Organisation (WHO) argues that intrapartum morbidity and mortality are largely avoidable with skilled care and, indeed, in the developed world, perinatal mortality has declined considerably over the last 50 years with good antenatal and intrapartum care. In 2005, the combined stillbirth and neonatal mortality rate had fallen to 8 per 1000 births with less than a tenth of these deaths caused by intrapartum events (CEMACH 2007). It must be remembered that although cesarean sections are becoming safer, they still have a higher morbidity and mortality rate when compared with a spontaneous vaginal birth for the mother, and must not be resorted to unless the benefits significantly outweigh the risks. Presumed fetal distress was the indication for 22 per cent of cesarean births in the UK (NCCWCH 2004). The challenge of modern obstetrics is to identify the fetus at risk of asphyxia without causing harm from unnecessary intervention for either the mother or the fetus. Although frequently used as an indication for operative intervention in labour, the precise definition of 'fetal distress' still eludes us.

## Terminology

**Fetal asphyxia:** Asphyxia is a Greek word that means 'without pulse'. Experimentally, asphyxia is defined as impaired respiratory gas exchange accompanied by the development of metabolic acidosis. In the clinical context, fetal asphyxia is progressive hypoxemia and hypercapnea with a significant metabolic acidemia.

**Fetal distress** is a term used to describe the situation where the clinician feels that the fetus is hypoxic or acidotic or is at risk of becoming so and the concern is significant enough to warrant intervention, usually in the form of operative delivery.

'Fetal distress' is not a diagnosis, but rather a concern or indication for delivery. The fact that most babies delivered for presumed fetal distress show little or no sign of compromise is a reflection of the vagueness of any definition applied to the term. However, it may be argued that action was taken before significant impairment

# The Management of Intrapartum Fetal Distress

occurred. Although widely used, the term 'fetal distress' is poorly defined and the underlying 'cause' for it is not always known even after delivery.

## Diagnosis

A majority of babies with suboptimal umbilical artery pH and base deficit have normal Apgar scores (Sykes et al 1982), and 80 per cent of depressed newborns have normal cord pH (Thorpe et al 1996), reflecting a discrepancy between biochemical parameters and immediate neonatal adaptation. Accurate identification of the baby that is getting 'distressed' as opposed to the baby that is coping with the 'stress' of labour is vital.

Contemporary obstetric practice lays great emphasis on fetal heart rate (FHR) monitoring as the main means of assessing fetal well-being in labour and this has been discussed in Chapter 5 on Intrapartum Fetal Monitoring. Whether done by intermittent auscultation or continuous electronic methods, FHR monitoring serves as a screening test for the detection of fetal hypoxia or acidosis. A normal FHR pattern is not difficult to define and is associated with a very low risk of fetal acidosis. Suspicious or abnormal FHR patterns are, however, associated with significant inter-observer variation in interpretation (Bernades et al 1997; Ayres-de-Campos et al 1999). However, it has been recognised that even significantly abnormal CTG patterns e.g. baseline tachycardia with late decelerations may be associated with only a 50 per cent risk of fetal acidosis on fetal blood sampling (FBS) (Beard et al 1971). Therefore, there is a significant risk of unnecessary operative intervention unless FHR monitoring is backed up by diagnostic testing, like fetal blood sampling (Wood et al 1981), or indeed, by newer methods like fetal pulse-oximetry or fetal ECG analysis which have been discussed in Chapter 5.

## Managing Fetal Distress

Strachnan (2009) identifies three key 'decision makers' in managing presumed fetal distress in labour:

1. The fetal reserve
2. The likely cause, and
3. The potential response to resuscitation

### The fetal reserve

Growth restriction, placental insufficiency and infections like chorioamnionitis can significantly lower the fetal reserve. Growth-restricted babies have reduced glycogen stores in the liver, which reduces their ability to cope with hypoxic insult. Conditions like preeclampsia, antepartum or intrapartum bleeding and post-maturity affect placental function and transfer, making hypoxia in labour more likely. Infections like chorioamnionitis increase the metabolic and oxygen requirement of the fetus, making it more likely to become hypoxic. Inflammatory cytokines compound the effects of hypoxia

> FHR monitoring serves as a screening test for the detection of fetal hypoxia or acidosis. Suspicious or abnormal FHR patterns are, however, associated with significant inter-observer variation in interpretation.

> Growth restriction, placental insufficiency and chorioamnionitis can significantly lower the fetal reserve.

on cell damage. In a Western Australian case-control study, these conditions were common findings in infants that developed neonatal encephalopathy (Badawi et al 1998). It is important therefore, to make an assessment of fetal reserve and this should ideally be done prior to labour by reviewing antenatal notes and a thorough obstetric examination. Unfortunately, half of the growth-restricted babies will still not be recognised before labour.

## The likely cause of fetal distress in labour

The commonest causes for fetal distress in labour include

1. Maternal position
2. Uterine contractions
3. Cord compression
4. Labour dystocia
5. Sudden dramatic events
    a. Cord prolapse
    b. Placental abruption
    c. Uterine rupture
    d. Vasa previa

The identification of the underlying cause aids in instituting the appropriate treatment to relieve the 'distress.'

### Maternal position

Aortocaval compression from the gravid uterus reduces the maternal uterine artery flow and reduces the pre-load to the mother's heart, reducing cardiac output. This can exacerbate fetal compromise. Aortocaval compression is seen most commonly in the supine position and less frequently in the standing and semi-recumbent positions and may also be associated with fetal occipito-posterior positions.

### Uterine contractions

Borell et al (1965) showed that the fetal exchange of oxygen and carbon dioxide with the maternal circulation is compromised by uterine contractions. At full dilatation of the cervix, the Ferguson reflex releases further oxytocin, increasing the frequency of contractions, thereby causing further compromise to gaseous exchange during the second stage. Although no changes are found in the 'passive second stage' (Piquard et al 1989), maternal pushing during the 'active second stage' further increases the risk of acidemia, with higher levels of lactic acid and carbon dioxide and increasing acidosis. Uterine hyperstimulation reduces the 'relaxation time' between contractions and therefore increases the risk of fetal hypoxia. It must be noted that a placenta that is already compromised will be more susceptible to the effect of uterine activity on the reduction of gaseous exchange.

> A placenta that is already compromised will be more susceptible to the effect of uterine activity on the reduction of gaseous exchange.

### Cord compression

The umbilical cord that delivers oxygenated blood to the fetus is prone to compression against fetal parts during contractions. Wharton's jelly in the cord is usually protective against

> The cords of growth-restricted babies have reduced Wharton's jelly as well as total and lumen vein areas and are more prone to compression and its consequences.

severe compression and normally grown fetuses do not tend to be affected except in the extremes of cord prolapse or entanglement. The cords of growth-restricted babies, however, have reduced Wharton's jelly as well as total and lumen vein areas (Gill and Jarjoura 1993) and are, therefore, more prone to compression and its consequences.

### Labour dystocia

Prolonged and obstructed labours eventually exhaust the fetus because of frequent contractions over a prolonged period of time, thereby resulting in FHR abnormalities and presumed fetal distress.

### Sudden dramatic events

- **Cord prolapse:** A prolapsed cord can get compressed between the pelvic brim and the fetal presenting part resulting in a sudden drop in the FHR.
- **Placental abruption:** The premature separation of the placenta is generally associated with continuous abdominal pain, a tonically contracted uterus, vaginal bleeding and abnormalities of FHR.
- **Uterine rupture:** Often, the earliest sign in cases of uterine rupture or scar dehiscence is an abnormality of the FHR. Other signs include the presence of pain between contractions, sudden cessation of contractions, a rise of the presenting part on abdominal palpation and vaginal bleeding.
- **Vasa previa:** Although rare, it must be considered in all cases of acute fetal distress. Since the blood lost is primarily fetal, it could be associated with high rates of fetal mortality. The diagnosis must be considered with any bleed after a spontaneous or artificial rupture of membranes that is accompanied by a sudden drop in the FHR. The CTG may show a characteristic sinusoidal pattern (Figure 7.1). Another pattern could be prolonged decelerations coinciding with membrane rupture.

## Resuscitatory Measures for CTG Abnormalities

Several resuscitatory interventions have been shown to be beneficial in the presence of FHR abnormalities. Often, a combination of these measures is required to effect 'intrauterine resuscitation' and these may produce long-lasting effects, allowing labour to continue, or short-term effects, allowing optimal arrangements to be made for operative delivery. These measures may, however, be underutilised in clinical practice (Hendrix et al 2000), either because of lack of facilities or supporting data.

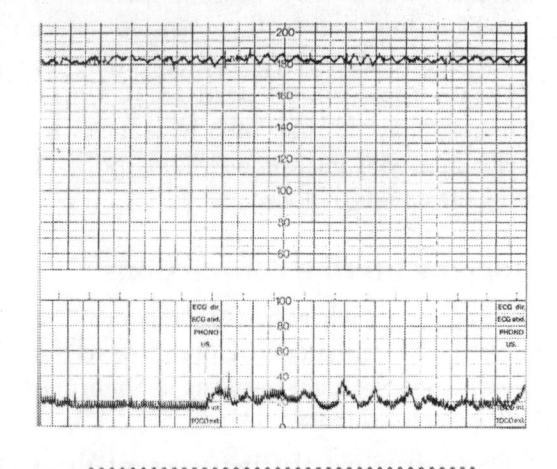

Figure 7.1 Sinusoidal fetal heart rate pattern

## Changing maternal position

As discussed earlier, the supine position adopted by many women in labour makes them vulnerable to aortocaval compression by the gravid uterus. Encouraging women to be ambulant for as long as possible minimises the incidence of supine hypotension and the resultant FHR abnormalities. When FHR abnormalities are detected with the parturient in a supine or semi-recumbent position, merely changing the maternal position to a left of right lateral position restores the venous return, uterine perfusion and often resolves the FHR abnormality. These are preferred to 15 degree tilts or the use of wedges, as the angle of tilt may be over-estimated or may not be adequate.

> Changing the maternal position to a left of right lateral position restores the venous return, uterine perfusion and often resolves the FHR abnormality

The effect of supine hypotension due to the compressive effect of the uterus, may be more pronounced in women with epidural analgesia which may cause a peripheral vasodilatation and a hypotensive effect (Thorpe and Breedlove 1996) leading to FHR abnormalities (Umstad et al 1993). This risk may be substantially reduced by preloading with intravenous fluids prior to siting the epidural block.

## Stopping uterine contractions

Contractions, whether spontaneous or induced, reduce maternal blood flow to the placental villous space resulting in abnormal FHR patterns (Figure 7.2).

Often, reducing the frequency of these contractions, thereby increasing the relaxation time between contractions, is sufficient to alleviate distress. If uterine hyperstimulation has occurred without the use of oxytocin, a tocolytic would need to be considered. In induced and augmented labours, the traditional management has been the administration of subcutaneous terbutaline with the discontinuation of oxytocin. Pacheco et al (2006) showed that subcutaneous terbutaline without discontinuation of oxytocin is more effective than the traditional approach of oxytocin discontinuation, but discontinuation of oxytocin followed, if necessary, with a tocolytic may be a better approach. In multiparous women with syntocinon, once labour is established, it is often possible to reduce or completely discontinue the infusion without any reduction of uterine activity.

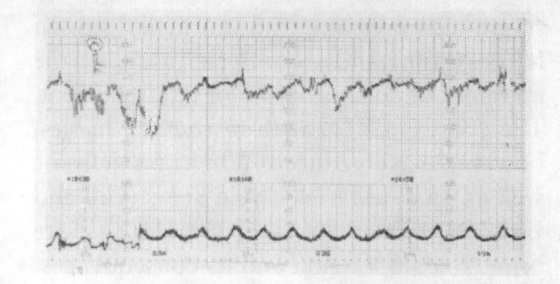

**Figure 7.2** Variable decelerations from uterine contractions occurring<5 in 10 minutes with syntocinon. These resolved on reducing the infusion rate.

## Tocolysis

Intravenous betamimetic drugs have been shown to be of benefit when FHR abnormalities are considered to be due to excessive uterine activity. The relief obtained may be temporary, but this allows time for appropriate delivery arrangements. Long-lasting relief may also be obtained, allowing labour to continue and a vaginal delivery achieved. The total bolus doses of tocolytic agent used in this situation are small compared to doses used to suppress preterm labour and therefore cause less severe side effects compared to those encountered from preterm tocolysis (Ingemarsson and Arulkumaran 1985).

Terbutaline is the tocolytic with most published data in situations of acute emergency. It is also better tolerated and easier to use when the indication is intrapartum FHR abnormality. In the past, this was administered as an *intravenous bolus of 250 μg terbutaline diluted in 5 ml of saline given over five minutes*. This produced a rapid effect within one or two minutes (Ingemarsson et al 1985), with the effect lasting about 17 minutes for spontaneous labour and about 15 minutes for augmented labour. NICE (2007) currently recommends *a subcutaneous dose of 250 μg*. Administered subcutaneously, the side-effects are negligible and the risk of post-partum hemorrhage is largely unfounded. In case this does occur, the action can be reversed with 1 mg propranolol, administered intravenously. Terbutaline is not effective in reducing uterine activity when given as an inhalation using a nebuliser (Kurup et al 1991).

Other agents with a tocolytic effect include glyceryl trinitrate (GTN), nifedipine, indomethacin, magnesium sulphate and atosiban, an oxytocin antagonist. Although nifedipine and atosiban are currently the recommended agents in threatened preterm labour, they have not been adequately evaluated for acute tocolysis. Atosiban has a favourable side effect profile (Moutquin et al 2000; Romero et al 2000) and its use as an acute tocolytic is currently being evaluated.

## Intravenous fluids

Maternal hypovolemia and hypotension can decrease the uteroplacental blood supply, thereby resulting in abnormal FHR patterns. It is for this reason that NICE recommends that the mother be assessed for signs of dehydration and/or hypotension when assessing a suspicious CTG in labour and treated appropriately with a bolus of 500 ml crystalloid (NICE 2007). Although this seems very logical, there are no randomised trials looking at the use of a fluid bolus for management of fetal distress, and caution must be exercised in patients with preeclampsia. Also, glucose-containing solutions should be avoided because of the potentially detrimental effects on the fetus, including increased fetal lactate and decreased fetal pH.

> Terbutaline is the tocolytic of choice and is given as a subcutaneous dose of 250 μg.

> Glucose-containing solutions should be avoided in labour because of the potentially detrimental effects on the fetus, including increased fetal lactate and decreased fetal pH.

## Amnioinfusion

The umbilical cord is prone to compression during uterine contractions when there is oligohydramnios. This manifests as variable decelerations, which if persistent may lead to hypoxia/acidosis. Maternal repositioning may relieve the pressure on the umbilical cord and resolve the FHR abnormalities. When maternal repositioning fails to resolve the problem, and when oligohydramnios is confirmed by ultrasound, the cord compression may be alleviated by amnioinfusion. This involves the instillation of warm saline or Ringer's lactate solution (Puder et al 1994; Washburne et al 1996; Pressman and Blakemore 1996) through a catheter into the uterine cavity. The volume infused depends on the degree of oligohydramnios determined by ultrasound assessment, e.g. 250 ml if the amniotic fluid index (AFI) is between 5 and 10 cm and 500 ml if the AFI is less than 5 cm (Ouzounian and Paul 1996). The aim is to maintain an AFI of 10 cm or more.

Amnioinfusion may be performed prophylactically when cord compression is anticipated, or therapeutically when FHR abnormalities have already occurred. A meta-analysis of prophylactic intrapartum amnioinfusion in 1533 women demonstrated lower rates of intrapartum FHR abnormalities, cesarean delivery, acidosis at birth and Apgar scores of less than seven at five minutes (Pitt et al 2000). The role of prophylactic amnioinfusion when there are no CTG abnormalities needs further evaluation. Trials have not shown any benefit of the use of amnioinfusion in the case of meconium-staining of liquor, to reduce the incidence of meconium aspiration syndrome (NCCWCH, 2007).

The benefit from a therapeutic procedure is, however, more established (Enkin et al 2000; Hofmeyr 2000d). When used therapeutically, apart from relieving FHR abnormalities, amnioinfusion reduces rates of operative delivery, both overall and for fetal distress (Owen et al 1990; Strong et al 1990). Rates of adverse neonatal outcome including meconium aspiration syndrome and maternal postpartum endometritis are also reduced. Rathor et al (2002) using 500 ml saline amnioinfusion in 200 women in labour at term with meconium-stained amniotic fluid found significant decrease in cesarean section rates, meconium at the level of the cords, improvement in one-minute Apgar scores and fewer admissions to the neonatal unit compared with controls.

> Therapeutic amnioinfusion relieves FHR abnormalities, reduces rates of operative delivery meconium aspiration syndrome and maternal postpartum endometritis.

Amnioinfusion has not been shown to have any statistically significant association with maternal or fetal adverse effects. Potential complications include uterine overdistension, cord prolapse and fatal amniotic fluid embolism. Wolfe et al (1998) reported a case of fatal maternal meningitis following amnioinfusion, but the trials so far reported have not been large enough to reveal uncommon but serious maternal complications (Ouzounian and Paul 1996; Enkin et al 2000; Hofmeyr 2000a,b). In particular, amniotic fluid embolism is rare and a significant association with amnioinfusion would only be derived from very large studies.

## Maternal oxygen administration

Oxygen administration to the mother for perceived fetal distress has been used for several decades on the premise that increased maternal oxygen saturation leads to increased fetal oxygen supply. The transfer of oxygen to the fetus is, however, dependent on perfusion of the placenta and the integrity of the feto-maternal interface rather than the oxygen saturation of maternal blood. Oxygen inhalation by the healthy mother increases the partial pressure of oxygen in the maternal blood and may confer some benefit, but not adequate to reverse FHR abnormalities in labour. There is currently not enough evidence to support the use of maternal oxygen therapy in the management of suspected fetal compromise (Hofmeyr 2000c).

There is some concern about the use of oxygen in growth-restricted fetuses (Harding et al 1992). In the animal model, oxygen supplementation restored fetal pO2 levels in moderately but not severely growth-restricted fetuses and fetal oxygenation was worse on discontinuation of oxygen therapy. This may be the cause of FHR abnormalities after discontinuation of maternal oxygen therapy in growth-restricted fetuses (Bekedam et al 1991). Raised cerebrovascular resistance has been demonstrated by Doppler velocimetry in response to maternal oxygen administration in hypoglycemic human fetuses (Arduini et al 1988). This effect potentially diverts much needed oxygen from the brain to peripheral tissues. Available information suggests that at least in growth-restricted fetuses, oxygen administration may cause more harm than good. It is therefore important that when oxygen is given to the mother for FHR abnormalities, it is done along with other resuscitatory measures such as maternal repositioning, hydration, and amnioinfusion. Delivery may need to be instituted if the FHR abnormality is severe and does not resolve or FBS reveals suboptimal parameters.

## Miscellaneous treatment

**Piracetam** is a derivative of gamma amino benzoic acid (GABA). It is thought to promote the metabolism of brain cells when they are hypoxic and has been used to prevent adverse effects of fetal distress. Results from some trials suggest that treatment with Piracetam reduces the duration of labour and improves neonatal outcome (Huaman et al 1983). A recent Cochrane review (Hofmeyr and Kulier 2002) concluded that there is currently inadequate evidence to support clinical use of Piracetam, except in the context of clinical trials.

**Pyridoxine** administered during labour is thought to reduce cord blood affinity for oxygen, allowing more oxygen to be released to tissues (Temesvari et al 1983). Although this approach has potential benefit, there is inadequate information to recommend its use in clinical practice.

## Management of Fetal Distress during Sudden Dramatic Events

Fetal distress caused by sudden dramatic labour events such as placental abruption, uterine rupture and vasa previa will not be reversed with intrauterine resuscitation. However, intrauterine resuscitation is rarely contra-indicated even when immediate delivery is planned, as it will optimise fetal oxygenation during the preparation for delivery.

In cases of cord prolapse, although the management is to deliver the fetus promptly, elevation of the presenting part above the pelvic brim will relieve cord compression. This can be achieved by digital displacement by keeping the hand in the vagina and lifting the head until delivery. Alternatively, a knee-elbow position or an exaggerated Sim's position can be used. Bladder filling with 500 ml of saline using a Foley catheter can also be useful. Tocolysis will help reduce compression of the cord from contractions.

The cord vessels can go into spasm when exposed to air, and hence, it should be reduced into the vagina to maintain the warmth and moisture content of the cord. If the FHR recovers, a rapid sequence spinal block can be used instead of a general anesthetic to effect delivery.

## Delivery of the fetus

When the FHR does not improve with any or all of the above measures, the only option is to expedite delivery, often by operative intervention. Equally, when the interventions have resulted in a normal CTG, there may be a case for continuing with conservative management. The only randomised trial conducted in 1959 was underpowered to study differences in perinatal mortality and it is unlikely that a similar study will be conducted within contemporary practice. Cochrane reviewers (Hofmeyr and Kulier 1998) concluded that there was too little evidence to show whether operative management is more beneficial than treating factors which may be causing the baby's distress.

Once a decision to deliver is made, the choice between a cesarean section and an operative vaginal delivery depends on the clinical situation. In cases of fetal distress, a baby has to be delivered within 30 minutes of decision making. The choice of anesthesia depends on the severity of suspected distress and the outcome of a discussion between the anesthetist and the mother. A rapid sequence spinal anesthetic can be used effectively within the 30-minute window, in most circumstances. On an average, the decision-to-delivery interval with a cesarean section tends to be between 30 and 40 minutes, while for operative vaginal delivery the interval is between 20 and 30 minutes. If it is deemed appropriate to deliver the baby vaginally, there appears to be no advantage of forceps over a vacuum in the presence of fetal distress and the decision to delivery time intervals are comparable. Although delivery in the room is generally considered quicker than delivering in theatres, this must be balanced against the risk of failure in the room, causing increased morbidity (Murphy and Koh 2007).

> In cases of fetal distress, a baby has to be delivered within 30 minutes of decision making.

## Medicolegal Implications of Fetal Distress

In the UK, substandard care was attributable to 75 per cent of intrapartum-related fetal deaths. The main issues identified were failure to recognise a problem, failure to act appropriately and the lack of effective communication. A similar survey of malpractice cases in Sweden identified neglecting to monitor fetal well-being, signs of fetal asphyxia, injudicious use of oxytocin and choosing the non-optimal mode of delivery as the most common events leading to litigation. The importance of 'high-velocity decision making' and effective communication between members of the obstetric team cannot be underestimated.

## Summary

Intrapartum fetal distress is a vague term in common use and it is usually inferred from abnormal FHR patterns. The degree of fetal compromise based on FHR abnormalities should be verified by other diagnostic modalities, namely, FBS or fetal ST wave form analysis. It is important to distinguish the fetus that is able to cope with the stresses of labour from the one that is in distress and requires emergency interventions. Assessing fetal reserve must take place early in labour and an attempt must be made to identify and to correct any underlying cause for fetal distress. Resuscitatory measures may be instituted for short or medium term effect, respectively, to allow optimal delivery arrangements or for labour to continue. Measures with beneficial effects include alteration of maternal position, tocolytic agents, cessation or reduction of oxytocin infusion, administration of intravenous fluids and amnioinfusion. Other measures for which benefit is not confirmed include maternal oxygen administration and fetal drug treatment. A decision to expedite delivery in the most appropriate manner at the most appropriate time should be communicated well and effected without delay in order to avoid poor outcome and consequent litigation.

## References

Arduini D, Rizzo G, Mancuso S and Romanini C. 1988. Short term effects of maternal oxygen administration on blood flow velocimetry waveforms in healthy and growth retarded fetuses. *Am J Obstet Gynecol*. 159:1077–80.

Ayres-de-Campos D, Bernades J, Costa-Pereira A, Pereira-leite L. 1999. Inconsistencies in classification by experts of cardiotocograms and subsequent clinical decision. *Br J Obstet Gynecol*. 106:1307–10.

Badawi N, Kurinczuk JJ, Keogh JM, Alessandri LM, O'Sullivan F, Burton PR, Pemberton PJ, Stanley FJ. 1998. Antepartum risk factors for newborn ecephalopathy: the Western Australian case-control study. *Br Med J* 317: 1549–53.

Beard RW, Filshie GM, Knight CA and Roberts GM. 1971. The significance of the changes in the continuous fetal heart rate in the first stage of labour. *J Obstet Gynecol Br C'wlth* 78:865–81.

Bekedam DJ, Muller EJH, Snidjers, RJM and Visser GHA. 1991. The effects of maternal hyperoxia on fetal breathing movements, body movements and heart rate variation in growth retarded fetuses. *Early Hum Dev*. 27:223–232.

Bernades J, Costa-Pereira A, Ayres-de-Campos, van Geijn HP, Pereira-Leite L. 1997. Evaluation of inter-observer agreement of cardiotocograms. *Int J Gynecol Obstet*. 57:33–37.

Borell U, Fernstrom I, Olsen L and Wiqvist N. 1965. Influence of uterine contrations on the uteroplacental blood flow at term. *Am J Obstet Gynecol*. 93:44–57.

Confidential Enquiry into Maternal and Child Health. 2007. *Perinatal Mortality 2005: England, Wales and Northern Ireland*. CEMACH: London.

Enkin M, Keirse MJNC, Neilson J, Crowther C, Duley L, Hodnett E and Hofmeyr J. 2000. Care of the fetus during labour. In *A guide to effective care in pregnancy and childbirth*. London: Oxford University Press.

Gill P and Jarjoura D. 1993. Wharton's jelly in the umbilical cord. A study of its quantitative variations and clinical correlates. *J Reprod Med* 38: 11–7.

Harding JE, Owens JA and Robinson JS. 1992. Should we try to supplement growth retarded fetuses? A cautionary tale. *Br J Obstet Gynecol*. 99:707–10.

Hendrix NW, Chauhan SP, Scardo JA, Ellings JM and Devoe LD. 2000. Managing non-reassuring fetal heart rate pattern before Cesarean delivery. Compliance with ACOG recommendations. *J Reprod Med*. 45(12):995–99.

Hofmeyr GJ and Kulier R. 1998. Operative versus conservative management for 'fetal distress' in labour. *Cochrane Database Syst Rev*. 1998(2): CD001065.

Hofmeyr GJ. 2000a. Amnioinfusion for meconium stained liquor. *Curr Opin Obstet Gynecol* 12(2):129–32.

Hofmeyr GJ. 2000b. Amnioinfusion for meconium-stained liquor in labour. *Cochrane Database of Systematic Reviews* (2):CD000014.

Hofmeyr GJ. 2000c. Maternal oxygen administration for fetal distress. *Cochrane Database of Systematic Reviews* (2):CD000136.

Hofmeyr GJ. 2000d. Prophylactic versus therapeutic amnioinfusion for oligohydramnios in labour. *Cochrane Database of Systematic Reviews* (2): CD000176.

Hofmeyr GJ, R Kulier. 2002. Piracetam for fetal distress in labour. *Cochrane Database of Systematic Reviews* (2):CD001064.

Huaman EJ, Hassoun R, Itahashi CM, Pereda GJ and Meija MA. 1983. Results obtained with piracetam in fetal distress during labour. *J Int Med Res* 11(3):129–36.

Ingemarsson I and Arulkumaran S. 1985. Beta-receptor agonists in current obstetric practice. In *Recent advances in perinatal medicine*, ed M Chiswick, vol. 2, pp 39–58. London: Churchill Livingstone.

Ingemarsson I, Arulkumaran S, Ratnam SS. 1985. Single injection of terbutaline in term labour II. Effect on uterine activity. *Am J Obstet Gynecol* 153:865–69.

Kurup A, Arulkumaran S, Tay D, Ingemarsson I, Ratnam SS. 1991. Can terbutaline be used as a nebuliser instead of intravenous injection for inhibition of uterine activity? *Gynecol Obstet Invest*. 32: 84–87.

Moutquin JM, Sherman D, Cohen D, Mohide PT, Hochner-Celnikier D, Fejgin M, Liston RM, Dansereau J, Mazor M, Shalev E, Boucher M, Glezerman M, Zimmer EZ and Rabinovici J. 2000. Double-blind, randomized, controlled trial of atosiban and ritodrine in the treatment of preterm labor: A multicenter effectiveness and safety study. *Am J Obstet Gynecol*. 182(5):1191–99.

Murphy DJ and Koh DK. 2007. Cohort study of the decision to delivery interval and neonatal outcome for emergency operative vaginal delivery. *Am J Obstet Gynecol*. 196: 145.e 1–7

National Collaborating Centre for Women's and Children's Health. 2004. Caesarean Section. Clinical Guideline. London.

National Institute For Clinical Excellence (NICE). 2007. *Intrapartum Care: Care of healthy women and their babies during childbirth*. London: RCOG Press.

Ouzounian JG and Paul RH. 1996. Clinical role of amnio-infusion. *Bailliére's Clin Obstet Gynecol*. 10:259–272.

Owen J, Henson BV and Hauth JC. 1990. A prospective randomised study of saline solution amnioinfusion. *Am J Obstet Gynecol*. 162:1146–49.

Pacheco LD, Rosen MP, Gei AF, Saade GR and Hankins GD. 2006. Management of uterine hyperstimulation with concomitant use of oxytocin and terbutaline. *Am J Perinatol*. 23 377–80.

Piquard F, Schaefer A, Hsiung R, Dellenbach P and Haberey P. 1989. Are there two biological parts in the second stage of labor? *Acta Obstet Gynecol Scand*. 68:713–8.

Pitt C, L Sanchez-Ramos, AM Kaunitz, F Gaudier. 2000. Prophylactic amnioinfusion for intrapartum oligohydramnios: A meta-analysis of randomized controlled trials. *Obstet Gynecol*. 95(5):861–66.

Pressman EK, KJ Blakemore. 1996. A prospective randomized trial of two solutions for intrapartum amnioinfusion: effects on fetal electrolytes, osmolality, and acid-base status. *Am J Obstet Gynecol*. 175(4):945–49.

Puder KS, Sorokin Y, Bottoms SF, Hallak M and Cotton DB. 1994. Amnioinfusion: does the choice of solution adversely affect neonatal electrolyte balance? *Obstet Gynecol*. 84:956–59.

Rathor AM, Singh R, Ramji S and Tripathi R. 2002. Randomised trial of amnioinfusion during labour with meconium stained amniotic fluid. *Br J Obstet Gynecol*. 109(1):17–20.

Romero R, Sibai BM, Sanchez-Ramos L, Valenzuela GJ, Veille JC, Tabor B, Perry KG, Varner M, Goodwin TM, Lane R, Smith J, Shangold G and Creasy GW L Sanchez-Ramos et al. 2000. An oxytocin receptor antagonist (atosiban) in the treatment of preterm labor: A randomized, double-blind, placebo-controlled trial with tocolytic rescue. *Am J Obstet Gynecol*. 182(5):1173–83.

Strachnan B. 2009. The management of intrapartum 'fetal distress'. In *Best Practice in Labour and*

*Delivery.* ed Warren R and Arulkmaran S. Cambridge: Cambridge University Press.

Strong TH, Hetzler G, Sarno AP and Paul RH. 1990. Prophylactic intrapartum amnioinfusion: A randomised clinical trial. *Am J Obstet Gynecol.* 162:1370–74.

Sykes GS, Molloy PM, Johnson P, Gu W, Ashworth F, Stirrat GM, Turnbull AC. 1982. Do Apgar scores indicate asphyxia? *Lancet* 1(8270): 494–95.

Temesvari P, Szilagyi I, Eck E and Boda D. 1983. Effects of an antenatal load of pyridoxine (vitamin B6) on the blood oxygen affinity and prolactin levels in newborn infants and their mothers. *Acta Paediatr Scand.* 72(4) 525–9.

Thorpe JA, Dildy GA, Yeomans ER, Meyer BA and Parisi VM. 1996. Umbilical cord blood gas analysis at delivery. *Am J Obstet Gynecol.* 175:517–22.

Thorpe JA and Breedlove G. 1996. Epidural analgesia in labor: An evaluation of risks and benefits. *Birth* 23(2):63–83.

Umstad MP, Ross A, Rushford DD and Permezel M. 1993. Epidural analgesia and fetal heart rate abnormalities. *Austr NZ J Obstet Gynecol.* 33(3):269–72.

Washburne JF, Chauhan SP, Magann EF, Rhodes PG, Naef III RW and Morrison JC. 1996. Neonatal electrolyte response to amnioinfusion with lactated Ringer's solution vs. normal saline. A prospective study. *J Reprod Med.* 41(10):741–44.

Wolfe RR, Norwick ML and Bofill JA. 1998. Fatal maternal beta-hemolytic group B streptococcal meningitis: a case report. *Am J Perinatol.* 15(11):597–600.

Wood C, Renou P, Oats J, Farrell E, Beischer N and Anderson I. 1981. A controlled trial of fetal heart rate monitoring in a low risk obstetric population. *Am J Obstet Gynecol.* 141:527–34.

# CHAPTER 8

# FLUID MANAGEMENT IN LABOUR

*W C Maina, David I Fraser and Sambit Mukhopadhyay*

Advances in obstetric care, prevention of infection, safer cesarean section and better surgical techniques, widespread availability of blood transfusion services and treatment of shock have all contributed to the reduction in maternal morbidity and mortality over the last four to five decades. While most pregnant mothers are young, healthy individuals and require minimal intervention or monitoring, some high-risk mothers will require specialised input and intensive monitoring. Ensuring correct fluid and electrolyte balance forms a basic component of intrapartum or perioperative care. It is important to realise the various physiological changes that occur during normal and abnormal pregnancy. These changes may indirectly influence fluid management during the intrapartum or immediate post-delivery period. One should also bear in mind that inappropriate fluid therapy to the mother may adversely affect the fetus intrapartum and the newborn in the immediate neonatal period.

Colloids, crystalloids and many drugs used in therapy cross the placenta readily and equilibrate with the fetal vascular compartment. As a result, volume, energy, hematological and electrolyte imbalance may occur with fluid administration. This chapter highlights the different aspects of fluid management in various medical and obstetric disorders of the mother.

## Physiological Considerations

The most important hemodynamic changes in the maternal circulation during pregnancy are the increase in cardiac output and blood volume and the fall in peripheral vascular resistance. Plasma volume, red cell mass and cardiac output increase during pregnancy. Plasma volume increases by 40 per cent and red cell mass increases by 20 to 30 per cent. This hypervolemia per se helps in combating the hazards of acute blood loss, which may cause

> Important hemodynamic changes in the maternal circulation during pregnancy are:
> - increase in cardiac output
> - increase in blood volume
> - fall in peripheral vascular resistance.

> The hypervolemia of pregnancy helps in combating the hazards of acute blood loss in the antenatal or postpartum period.

dramatic changes in the blood volume immediately after delivery. Pregnancies complicated by fetal growth restriction and preeclampsia are associated with relatively lower maternal cardiac output and relatively higher peripheral resistance than are pregnancies without these complications. As a result, the normal expansion of the intravascular volume is attenuated. These inadequate adaptive changes occurring in such pregnancies often make patients highly sensitive to hemodynamic instability, should there be excessive blood loss during the intrapartum or immediate postpartum period.

> Pregnancies complicated by fetal growth restriction and preeclampsia have:
> - lower maternal cardiac output
> - higher peripheral resistance
> - inadequate increase in intravascular volume

## Hydration in Labour

Fasting in labour has been an established practice since the 1940s. This is now under careful scrutiny and many units have now abandoned such a policy, allowing eating and drinking in normal labour. No increase in maternal mortality has been reported with this policy of allowing eating and drinking in labour (Ludka and Roberts 1993). Little is known about the differences in progress in labour, birth outcomes and neonatal status between mothers who consume food and/or fluids during labour and women who fast during labour (Sleutel and Golden 1999). Increased fluids improve skeletal muscle performance in prolonged exercise. A randomised controlled trial of the effect of increased intravenous hydration showed a lower incidence of prolonged labour and possibly less use of oxytocin in the group who received increased intravenous fluid as opposed to the group receiving limited fluids in labour (Garite et al 2000).

The risk of maternal aspiration in normal 'low-risk' labour is probably exaggerated. Only one study evaluated the probable risk of maternal mortality due to aspiration and estimated the risk at approximately seven in 10 million births (Sleutel and Golden 1999). A recent review of oral intake during labour concluded there was insufficient evidence on the relationship between fasting times for clear liquids and the risk of emesis or reflux or both or pulmonary aspiration during labour (ACOG 2009). Although there is some disagreement, most experts concur that oral intake of clear liquids during labour does not increase maternal complications. Examples of clear fluids include, but are not limited to, water, fruit juices without pulp, carbonated beverages, clear tea, black coffee and sports drinks.

> Oral intake of clear liquids during labour does not seem to increase the risk of
> - emesis
> - reflux
> - pulmonary aspiration during labour

A recent prospective observational study has revealed the association between high fluid intake during labour and the development of hyponatremia (Moen et al 2009). Almost 300 women were included in the study. They were allowed to drink freely in labour and blood samples were collected on admission and at delivery. Of the 61 women who had taken more than 2.5 litres of fluid, 16 (26 per cent) were found to have hyponatremia ≤ 130 mmol/L. In labours exceeding 8 to 10 hours, a fluid intake of 300 mL per hour was sufficient for the development of hyponatremia, indicating that tolerance to a water load is markedly diminished during labour. Women with the lowest concentration of plasma sodium also had prolonged second stage of labour, and were more often delivered instrumentally or by emergency cesarean section for failure to progress. In addition to these outcomes, hyponatremia is known to cause irritability, headaches, nausea and vomiting. Severe hyponatremia can cause cerebral edema and coma. Excessive fluid intake or administration should therefore be avoided where there is no clinical indication.

> High fluid intake during labour can lead to the development of hyponatraemia. Excessive fluid intake or administration should therefore be avoided where there is no clinical indication.

## Maternal Ketonuria

Maternal ketonuria is a common indication for fluid administration during labour. Increased energy consumption coupled with partial starvation gives rise to ketones in the blood (ketosis) and urine (ketonuria). Ketone bodies transport fat-derived energy from the liver to other organs to provide an alternative source of energy. They also cross the placenta. It is not clear whether ketosis during labour is a normal physiological response, or if women with ketosis require intervention. This uncertainty is reflected in differences in opinion and practice. A recent systematic review assessing the effects on maternal, fetal and neonatal outcomes of intravenous fluids or increased oral intake to women in labour for the treatment of ketosis compared with no intervention found no evidence on which to base practice (Toohill et al 2008).

Studies conducted in the late 1970s and mid-1980s focused on maternal biochemistry during or shortly after labour. Maternal ketonuria was thought to cause impaired myometrial function and dysfunctional labour (Dumouline and Foulkes 1984), although correction of ketonuria does not improve the progress of labour (Dahlenburgh et al 1980; Singh et al 1982). Treating ketonuria during labour with infusions of 10 per cent dextrose in water or excessive volumes of 5 per cent dextrose has been shown to be dangerous, causing hyponatremia in the mother (Evans et al 1986) and causing rebound hypoglycemia (Kenepp et al 1982) and hyponatremia (Tarnow-Mordi et al 1981) in the neonate. Hyponatremia in the newborn impairs erythrocyte membrane function. This alters the intracellular electrolyte content and pH, predisposing to hemolysis (Zeilder and Kim 1979), thus increasing bilirubin levels. An increased osmotic fragility (Arieff and Guisado 1976), impaired erythrocyte, leucocyte and neuronal functions were also noted by Kenepp et al (1980).

Morton et al (1985) compared the effects of one litre of either normal saline, Hartmann's solution, 5 per cent dextrose or 10 per cent dextrose in women in whom ketonuria was detected during the first stage of labour. They concluded that the rapid infusion of dextrose or Hartmann's solution produced significant elevation in blood lactate and pyruvate level and therefore recommended that normal saline be used. However, Piquard et al (1990) showed that the adverse events did not occur if the glucose infusion rate was restricted to 30 g per hour. If more than 500 mL of 5 per cent dextrose solution is required, it would be wiser to use fluids containing sodium (Spencer et al 1981).

# Role of Oral Carbohydrate Drinks

## Isotonic sports drink versus water

Sports drinks have become very popular in the last decade. Most contain mixtures of carbohydrates (such as glucose and dextrose), sodium, potassium and calcium, together with flavouring to make them more palatable.

The results of a study of the effect of one such sports drink on the outcome of labour were published by Kubli et al in 2002. In this study, 60 women at 37 weeks of gestation or greater were randomised in early labour (isotonic sports drink n=30; water only n=30). Women in the sports drink group were permitted to consume up to 500 mL in the first hour and then a further 500 mL every 3–4 hours. By the end of labour, plasma β-hydroxybutyrate and non-esterified fatty acids were significantly increased and the plasma glucose significantly decreased in the water-only group. There were no significant differences between the groups in gastric volume measured within 45 minutes of delivery, or in the volume vomited or number of vomiting episodes reported within one hour of birth or throughout labour. The mean calorific intake in the sports drink group was 47 kcal/h and zero in the water-only group. There was no difference between the two groups in duration of labour, use of oxytocin, use of epidural analgesia, mode of birth or neonatal outcome.

Thus, on the basis of this study, it appears that isotonic sport drinks prevent the ketosis of labour without the increase in gastric volumes and tendency to vomit seen in women who eat during labour.

## Carbohydrate solutions

A group of researchers in the Netherlands has conducted randomised controlled trials evaluating the effects of carbohydrate solutions versus placebo.

The first study involved 201 nulliparous women randomised at 2–4 cm cervical dilatation (carbohydrate solution n=102; placebo n=99) (Scheepers et al 2002a). The second trial involved 202 nulliparous women randomised at 8–10 cm dilatation (carbohydrate solution n=100; placebo n=102), (Scheepers et al 2004). The final study involved 100 nulliparous women randomised at 8–10 cm cervical dilatation (carbohydrate solution n=50; placebo n=50) (Scheepers et al 2002b).

In the first study, a high proportion of women had high-risk pregnancies (80 per cent of the carbohydrate and 82 per cent for the placebo – not statistically significant), presumably because in the Netherlands, women considered at low risk are delivered by independent midwives. The median total intake of the study solution was 300 ml in the placebo group and 400 ml in the carbohydrate group (P=0.04). The median total calorific intake by the placebo group during the study was 0 KJ and 802 KJ for the carbohydrate group (P < 0.001). There was no statistically significant difference in the need for augmentation or pain-relieving medication when women in the carbohydrate group were compared to women in the placebo group. While there was no significant difference between the carbohydrate and placebo groups for spontaneous birth or for instrumental birth, the cesarean section rate for the carbohydrate group (21 per cent) was significantly higher than that noted in the placebo group

(7 per cent). There were no significant differences in Apgar scores at 1 minute and 5 minutes or the arterial umbilical cord pH between the carbohydrate and placebo groups.

In the second study, the median intake was 200 mL in the placebo group and 200 mL in the carbohydrate group (p=0.42). There were no significant differences in spontaneous birth, instrumental birth, or cesarean section when the carbohydrate group was compared with the placebo group. No significant differences were observed in neonatal outcome. In addition when the two groups were compared, there were no significant differences in changes in glucose, lactate or plasma β-hydroxybutyrate. A significant decrease in free fatty acid levels was observed in the carbohydrate group. No significant differences were observed in cesarean section rates or neonatal outcome. The proportion of high-risk pregnancies in both groups was similar to that in the first study.

None of these studies reported on the incidence of vomiting, or volumes vomited.

In summary, these studies have demonstrated no evidence of difference in mode of birth, or fetal and neonatal acid–base balance between taking carbohydrate solution and placebo during labour. There appears to be no significant benefit in treating ketosis associated with labour. The National Institute for Health and Clinical Excellence (NICE 2007) recommends that women may drink in established labour and may be informed that isotonic drinks may be more beneficial than water.

> There appears to be no significant benefit in treating ketosis associated with labour.

## Common Indications for Intravenous Infusion in Labour

1. Use of regional anesthesia
2. Poor progress in labour
3. Diabetes
4. Special circumstances (see below)
5. Preeclampsia
6. Postpartum hemorrhage

## Regional Anesthesia

The chemical sympathectomy that follows epidural blockade can cause hypotension, especially if the mother is already hypovolemic. Reduced uterine blood flow from maternal hypotension may contribute to fetal heart rate changes. Intravenous fluid preloading may help to reduce maternal hypotension but using lower doses of local anesthetic, and opioid-only blocks, may reduce the need for preloading.

> Intravenous fluid preloading may help to reduce maternal hypotension caused by epidural analgesia.

In a randomised study, Kenepp et al (1982) concluded that the infusion of dextrose in normal saline gave no advantage over 5 per cent dextrose infusion and neither solution decreased the incidence of hypotension. They inferred that rapid infusions of dextrose are not advisable if delivery is not imminent and in diabetic patients, because they increase fetal insulin levels.

Hofmeyr et al (2004) conducted a systematic review to assess the effects of prophylactic intravenous fluid preloading before regional analgesia during labour on maternal and fetal well-being. Six studies with a total of 473 participants were included. In one epidural trial using high-dose local anesthetic, preloading with intravenous fluids was shown to counteract the hypotension which frequently follows traditional epidural analgesia (relative risk (RR) 0.07, 95 per cent confidence interval (CI) 0.01 to 0.53; 102 women). This trial was also associated with a reduction in fetal heart rate abnormalities (RR 0.36, 95% CI 0.16 to 0.83; 102 women); no differences were detected in other perinatal and maternal outcomes in this trial and another high-dose epidural trial. In the two epidural low-dose anesthetic trials, no significant difference in maternal hypotension was found (RR 073, 95% CI 0.36 to 1.48; 260 women), although they were underpowered to detect less than a very large effect. No significant differences were seen between groups in these trials for fetal heart rate abnormalities (RR 0.64, 95% CI 0.39 to 1.05; 233 women). In the two combined spinal/epidural (CSE) trials, no differences were reported between preloading and no preloading groups. In the spinal/opioid trial, the RR for hypotension was 0.89, 95 per cent CI 0.43 to 1.83 (40 women) and 0.70, 95 pe cent CI 0.36 to 1.37 for fetal heart rate abnormalities (32 women). In the opioid only study (30 women), there were no instances of hypotension or fetal heart rate abnormalities in either group. They concluded that preloading prior to traditional high-dose local anesthetic blocks may have some beneficial fetal and maternal effects in healthy women. Low-dose epidural and CSE analgesia techniques may reduce the need for preloading. The studies were too small to show whether preloading is beneficial for women having regional analgesia during labour using the low-dose local anesthetics or opioids.

A recent randomised trial (Tamilselvan et al 2009) has demonstrated that intravenous fluid preload in healthy women undergoing planned cesarean delivery under spinal anesthesia increases cardiac output and intravascular volume, but does not attenuate the hypotension associated with spinal anesthesia. This new evidence challenges the common practice of preloading with 500–1000 mL of crystalloid to limit the fall in blood pressure when the vascular compartment expands in response to a sympathetic blockade.

## Poor Progress in Labour

Poor progress of labour requiring augmentation with oxytocin infusion is by far the most common indication for the use of intravenous fluids. Hyperstimulation of the uterus may occur either as a result of high dosage or increased sensitivity of the uterus to oxytocin with the progress of labour. Other important properties of oxytocin to be considered are its antidiuretic, vasodilator and vasoconstrictor effects. Vasodilatation occurs primarily in the subcutaneous vessels and results in flushing, with vasoconstriction occurring primarily in the splanchnic bed and coronary arteries (Ajmal 2010). These cardiovascular changes can result in hypotension, tachycardia

> Low-dose epidural and combined spinal/epidural analgesia techniques may reduce the need for preloading.

> When oxytocin infusions are prolonged and the infusions approach 40 mV/minute, urinary output decreases significantly and potential exists for water intoxication

and myocardial ischemia (Svanstrom et al 2008). When oxytocin infusions are prolonged and the infusion approaches 40 mV/ minute, there is a dramatic drop in the urinary output and potential exists for water intoxication. Significant side effects are rare when oxytocin is properly diluted and administered by infusion pump. Allergic reactions, including anaphylaxis, can occur rarely and may be fatal. Derangements of neonatal biochemistry leading to neonatal seizures can occur in severe cases.

Prior to initiating oxytocin infusion, baseline vital signs (that is, temperature, pulse, respiration and blood pressure) and fetal and uterine status should be assessed. The use of continuous cardiotocographic monitoring permits the evaluation of the fetal heart rate and the frequency of uterine activity.

It has been a tradition in most obstetric units to use a glucose solution of 5 per cent strength for oxytocin infusion. An intravenous electrolyte-free solution significantly decreases maternal sodium levels and the concurrent use of oxytocin further reduces them (Spencer et al 1981). Cord sodium levels are reduced with the use of oxytocin and electrolyte-free solutions. When oxytocin is used for the induction of labour, more than 500 mL of fluid vehicle may be required; hence, the use of fluids containing sodium is advisable (Spencer et al 1981). Higher strength of oxytocin would limit the volume of infusion to the mother, but precise control of the infusion by a syringe or peristaltic infusion pump becomes mandatory to avoid uterine hyperstimulation, fetal compromise

> Sodium containing fluids are recommended for oxytocin infusion.

and the remote possibility of uterine rupture. Oxytocin-induced hyperstimulation of the uterus is one of the important causes of litigation. To avoid such problems, the ideal dose of oxytocin which would effect vaginal delivery in optimal time without fetal compromise should be infused. The medication sticker on the oxytocin solution should reflect the concentration of oxytocin used.

Most dosage schedules retain the original approach of escalating the dose until effective contractions are established and subsequently maintain this dose until delivery. In the majority, the desired frequency of uterine contractions can be achieved with doses less than 11mU/minute (Steer et al 1985; Arulkumaran et al 1985). In 2007, the National Institute for Health and Clinical Excellence recommended that when oxytocin is used, the time between increments of the dose should be no more frequent than every 30 minutes. Oxytocin should be increased until there are 4–5 contractions in 10 minutes.

Water intoxication is prevented by using balanced salt intravenous solutions, limiting the total dose of oxytocin, monitoring fluid intake and output and observing patients at risk for signs and symptoms of weakness, restlessness, nausea, vomiting, diarrhea, polyuria or oliguria and seizures.

In summary, infusion of oxytocin in accordance with recommended protocols will minimise the risk of harm to both the mother and her fetus while optimising the outcome of labour.

## Diabetes

Adequate control of maternal blood sugar levels immediately before and during labour is essential to prevent diabetic ketoacidosis in the mother and excessive fetal insulin secretion, causing subsequent hypoglycemia in the neonate. This is usually achieved with the administration of insulin infusion to maintain a tight blood glucose control (4–7 mmol/L). Table 8.1 illustrates the regimen used at the Norfolk and Norwich University Hospital (UK).

**Table 8.1** Suggested IV insulin sliding scale for use during labour (syringe pump, 50 units soluble insulin in 50 ml N saline)

| Current total daily insulin dose | Up to 40 units/ day | 41–60 units/ day | 61–90 units/ day | >91 units/ day |
|---|---|---|---|---|
| Capillary Glucose (mmol /l) | Infusion rate (units/ hr) | Infusion rate (units/ hr) | Infusion rate (units/ hr) | Infusion rate (units/ hr) |
| 0–3 | 0 | 0 | 0 | 0 |
| 3.1–6.9 | 1.0 | 1.5 | 2.0 | 2.0 |
| 7.0–8.9 | 1.5 | 2.0 | 3.0 | 4.0 |
| 9.0–10.9 | 2.0 | 3.0 | 4.0 | 5.0 |
| 11.0–15.0 | 3.0 | 4.0 | 5.0 | 6.0 |
| >15 | Call doctor | Call doctor | Call doctor | Call doctor |

❖ 1 litre 5% glucose + 20mmol/l KCL should be started at 100 mL/hour

❖ Check capillary blood glucose hourly

❖ For type 2 diabetes and gestational diabetes, commence insulin infusion if the blood glucose is >7 mmol/L

❖ The same regimen should be used for emergency and elective CS

❖ Check urea and electrolytes (U&E) 4–6 hourly

To prevent the development of hypoglycemia after delivery, glucose infusion should be continued and the administration of insulin discontinued. Further, insulin requirements would depend on the blood glucose level of the mother. Usually, the patient is commenced on her pre-pregnancy insulin regimen.

The use of oxytocin for induction or augmentation should follow appropriate protocols. When used concomitantly with insulin, oxytocin should be used in a separate intravenous bag and not with insulin. Two separate infusion control devices are necessary, one for the insulin-containing fluid and one for the oxytocin-containing fluid.

> When used concomitantly with insulin, oxytocin should be used in a separate intravenous bag and not with insulin.

Diabetic ketoacidosis (DKA) represents a state of acutely decompensated diabetes and is classified as mild, moderate or severe. Severe DKA is a life-threatening emergency; in order to optimise outcome, urgent assistance should be sought from the diabetic team. Immediate goals include clinical and biochemical assessment, replacement of insulin, fluids and electrolytes. The following protocol is used at the Norfolk and Norwich University Hospital (UK) (Tables 8.2 to 8.4).

### Initial treatment

❖ Actrapid insulin (Actrapid®), a short-acting insulin is given in 6u IV bolus and 1L 0.9% saline over 30 mins.

❖ If on insulin glargine (Lantus™) or detemir (Levemir™) as background insulin, continue Lantus/Levemir but discontinue short-acting insulin and use insulin scale A.

- If on insulatard (Insulatard®), a long-acting insulin, discontinue insulatard and short-acting insulin and use scale B.
- Call on the diabetes team urgently for ongoing management of patient.

Table 8.2  Insulin sliding scale for use in DKA

| Blood glucose (mmol/l) | Scale A Insulin (units/hour) | Scale B Insulin (units/hour) | Scale C Insulin (units/hour) |
|---|---|---|---|
| 0–4 | 0.5 | 0.5 | 0.5 |
| 4.1–7 | 1.5 | 2 | 2.5 |
| 7.1–9 | 2.0 | 2.5 | 3.0 |
| 9.1–11 | 3.0 | 3.5 | 4.0 |
| 11.1–14 | 4.0 | 5.0 | 6.0 |
| 14.1–17 | 5.0 | 6.0 | 8.0 |
| 17.1–22 | 6.0 | 8.0 | 10.0 |
| >22 | 8.0 | 10.0 | 10.0 |

If there are two consecutive readings >11 mmol/L, consider moving to higher dose scale (from A to B or B to C)

Table 8.3  Fluid replacement in DKA

| Fluid | Time period |
|---|---|
| 1L 0.9% saline | 30 mins |
| 1L 0.9% saline | 1 hour |
| 1L 0.9% saline | 2 hours |
| 1L 0.9% saline | 4 hours |
| 1L 0.9% saline | 6 hours |
| 1L 0.9% saline | 6 hours |

This is a guideline and fluid replacement will vary depending on level of dehydration at presentation.

Switch to 5% dextrose when capillary glucose <11 mmol/l

If acidosis/ketones not resolving consider increasing insulin dose and giving 10%–20% dextrose

Table 8.4  Potassium replacement in DKA

| Plasma potassium (mmol/l) | KCl to be added from 2nd litre of fluid onwards |
|---|---|
| < 3.5 | 40 mmol/l |
| 3.5–5.5 | 20 mmol/l |
| > 5.5 | Not required |

Invasive hemodynamic monitoring is preferable to monitor fluid replacement and to prevent shock from decreased intravascular volume or pulmonary edema from excessive fluid replacement.

## Preeclampsia and Hypertensive Disorders

Maternal blood volume increases progressively with increasing gestational age and is generally proportional to the size of the conceptus. In preeclampsia, the blood pressure is elevated, there is little if any increase in blood volume and plasma albumin is low (Studd et al 1970; Horne et al 1970). Renal leak of albumin occurs in preeclampsia and this effectively gives rise to low intravascular oncotic pressure, leading to loss of fluid from the vascular compartment. Volume expansion has been explored in severe cases in an attempt to lower blood pressure or improve placental and renal blood flow. However, there is insufficient data to recommend it (Duley 1992; Magee et al 1999). Also, it could be potentially dangerous as it can provoke circulatory overload and pulmonary edema.

The incidence of significant renal damage in preeclampsia is low. Regular fluid intake–output charts should be maintained in preeclampsia and renal function should be taken into consideration before initiating fluid therapy. Oliguria can occur with severe disease and may result from a number of underlying pathophysiological changes (Clark et al 1986). The first subset of patients is those in whom oliguria is secondary to intravascular volume depletion (e.g. hemorrhage). Hemodynamic monitoring in this subset characteristically demonstrates a low wedge pressure, moderately increased systemic vascular resistance, a low to normal cardiac output and hyperdynamic left ventricular function. Volume infusion will raise the pulmonary wedge pressure and cardiac output, decrease systemic vascular resistance and may increase the urinary output. A second group includes patients with isolated renal arterial spasm. These patients demonstrate persistent oliguria when the measured intravascular volume would normally be sufficient to perfuse the kidneys. Those in whom systemic vascular resistance is within the normal range can be managed with pharmacologic pre- and/or afterload reduction (e.g. use of diuretics). The third subset includes patients with increased vascular resistance, elevated wedge pressure and low cardiac output. Oliguria develops from vasospasm in preeclampsia with depressed left ventricular function and low cardiac output. Volume restriction and afterload reduction will be helpful in correcting oliguria in this group.

Preload refers to the initial myocardial muscle fibre length and is determined by intraventricular volume and pressure. As preload increases in a normal heart, the cardiac output increases. A higher preload than normal is required to maintain adequate cardiac output in a failing heart. Afterload refers to ventricular wall tension during systole and is dependent primarily on pulmonary and systemic vascular resistance. In a normal heart, there is an inverse relationship between afterload and cardiac output.

Sodium retention with an increase in total body sodium occurs in preeclampsia (Chesley 1966, Graves 2007), but sodium restriction and administration of sodium-free solutions are ineffective in mobilising edema. This is because of good compensatory capacity of the intrarenal regulation mechanism and humoral control of renin aldosterone system (Chesley 1978). Hyponatremia is a consequence of salt restriction or the use of diuretics. Arias (1984) advocates a 50 per cent correction of the sodium deficit by using a 3% sodium chloride solution. Full correction may not be advisable, as sodium excretion is delayed to twice the normal time in preeclamptic patients compared with normal pregnant women when hypertonic saline solution is infused (Chesley et al 1958).

Crystalloid solutions are the mainstay of fluid therapy in the preeclamptic patient even if the central oncotic pressure is low. Administration of colloid solutions can transiently elevate oncotic pressure, but may compound the problem by allowing the intravascular fluid into interstitial space through the damaged capillaries. Oxytocin infusion has been used to advantage without complications, despite its antidiuretic properties. Close monitoring of fluid intake and output must be undertaken in order to prevent an imbalance of hydrostatic and oncotic forces that can potentiate the occurrence of pulmonary edema.

> Crystalloid solutions are the mainstay of fluid therapy in the preeclamptic patient

It is important to strike a balance between overzealous administration of intravenous fluid (increasing the risk of pulmonary edema) and underperfusion, predisposing to oliguria and renal complications. The objective is to maintain a minimum urinary output of 100 mL/4 hours (an alternative output to 1 mL/kg body weight/hour). A fluid management regimen for severe preeclampsia is suggested below:

> In pre-eclamptic patients in labour, a minimum urinary output of 100 mL/4 hours should be maintained.

### Principles of fluid management in preeclampsia

1. Accurate recording of fluid balance (including delivery and postpartum)
2. Maintenance crystalloid infusion of Hartmann's 85 mL/h. For women who require postpartum oxytocin regimen, this can be safely given by diluting 20 units of oxytocin in 50 ml of Hartmann's solution and delivering this through a syringe driver set at 25 mL/h.
3. Selective monitoring of central venous pressure (CVP), hemorrhage, oliguria, significant fall in platelet count, liver tenderness
4. Selective colloid expansion in oliguria and low CVP.
5. Diuretics in pulmonary edema

If initial hematocrit <35 per cent (0.35), continue Hartmann's 85 mL/h.

If initial hematocrit >35 per cent (i.e. hemoconcentrated), give 500 mL colloid e.g. Gelofusine over 20 minutes and then continue Hartmann's solution at 85 mL/h.

Any oral intake should be subtracted from Hartmann's 85 mL/h.

Prior to epidural analgesia, give a preload of 500 mL Gelofusine and then continue the Hartmann's 85 mL/h

### Management of oliguria and CVP in preeclampsia

1. Oliguria is defined as <100 mL/4 hours
2. The anesthetist will set up and supervise the CVP
3. Initially manage expectantly
4. If it persists for a further 4 hours, consider fluid challenge
5. If CVP is less than 4 mmHg and oliguria persists, consider further fluid challenge
6. If CVP is >8 mmHg careful assessment for pulmonary edema (chest x-ray and oxygen saturation) should be made
7. CVP >4 mmHg and no pulmonary edema, manage expectantly and consider further fluid challenge
8. Consider dopamine infusion (5 µg/kg/min) to enhance renal blood flow with persistent oliguria
9. Involve renal physician if renal failure is suspected.

## Postpartum Hemorrhage (PPH)

Allowing for the physiological increase in pregnancy, total blood volume at term is approximately 100 mL/kg (Jansen et al 2005). A blood loss of more than 40 per cent of total blood volume (approximately 2800 ml) is generally regarded as 'life-threatening'. A blood loss of 500–1000 mL (in the absence of clinical signs of shock) should prompt basic measures of monitoring and 'readiness for resuscitation', whereas an estimated loss of more than 1000 mL (or a smaller loss associated with signs of shock) should prompt a full protocol of measures to resuscitate, monitor and arrest the bleeding (RCOG 2009).

In most situations where urgent resuscitation is needed, this usually involves intravenous fluids followed by blood transfusion. A maximum of 3.5 litres of fluid (up to 2 litres of warmed Hartmann's solution as rapidly as possible, followed by up to a further 1.5 litres of warmed colloid, if blood is still not available) should be infused while awaiting compatible blood (Scottish Obstetric Guidelines and Audit Project 1998). If there is delay in availability of crossmatched blood, group O, Rh D-negative blood should be administered. The alternative option would be to administer ABO and D compatible uncrossmatched blood. Monitoring such patients for disseminated intravascular coagulation is essential. The use of coagulation factors should be guided by coagulation studies (RCOG 2007). Intraoperative cell salvage can minimise the need for allogenic blood transfusion. In the UK, cell salvage is recommended for women in whom an intraoperative blood loss of more than 1500 mL is anticipated (RCOG 2007).

Whereas blood transfusion is a life-saving treatment, it is not without risk. Recipients may rarely develop transfusion-transmitted infection or immunological sequelae such as red cell alloimmunisation. The major risk of blood transfusion, however, occurs when an 'incorrect blood component' is transfused.

> - Blood loss of 500–1000 mL: basic measures of monitoring and 'readiness for resuscitation'
> - Loss of more than 1000 mL (or a smaller loss associated with signs of shock): a full protocol of measures to resuscitate, monitor and arrest the bleeding

> A maximum of 3.5 litres of fluid should be infused while awaiting compatible blood

## Hydration for Treatment of Preterm Labour

Stan et al (2002) conducted a systematic review to assess the efficacy of intravenous or oral hydration to avoid preterm birth in women with preterm labour. Two small randomised controlled studies with a total of 228 women revealed no advantage of intravenous hydration compared to bed rest alone. They concluded there was insufficient evidence for hydration in women with preterm labour to prevent preterm birth.

## Conclusion

Administration of fluids is a common intervention in labour. Sound knowledge of the physiological changes in the circulatory volume and the hemodynamic changes occurring in various disorders of pregnancy is essential in optimising maternal and fetal outcome. Moderate intake of clear fluids does not appear to cause significant maternal complications. However, excessive fluid intake is not recommended due to the risk of hyponatremia. Treating ketosis of labour in previously healthy women has not been shown to be beneficial. Most studies suggest that fluid preloading does not attenuate the hypotension associated with regional anesthesia. Oxytocin infusion is the commonest pharmacological intervention in labour. Adherence to recommended protocols is crucial in order to minimise the complications associated with its administration. Fluid management in women with diabetes, preeclampsia, major PPH and other complications of labour should be guided by reference to local or national guidelines.

# References

Ajmal M. 2010. Oxytocin at caesarean section-are we giving too much? *BJOG* 117;1:118–119.

American College of Obstetricians and Gynaecologists. 2009. Oral intake during labour. ACOG committee opinion no. 441. *Obstet Gynecol*. 114:117

Arieff AL, R Guisado. 1976. Effects on CNS of hyponatremic states. *Kidn Int*. 10: 104–109.

Arias F. 1984. Hypertension during pregnancy. In *High risk pregnancy and delivery*, ed F Arias. Toronto: Mosby.

Arulkumaran S, DMF Gibb, SS Ratnam, KC Lun, SH Heng. 1985. Total uterine activity in induced labour: Index of cervical and pelvic tissue resistance. *Br J Obstet Gynecol*. 92:693–97.

Chesley LC. 1966. Sodium retention and preeclampsia. *Am J Obstet Gynecol*. 95:127–32.

Chesley LC. 1978. *Hypertensive disorders in pregnancy*. New York: Appleton-Century Crofts, 215–21.

Chesley LV, C Valenti, H Rein. 1958. The excretion of sodium loads by nonpregnant and pregnant, normal hypertensive and preeclamptic women. *Metabolism* 7:575.

Clark SL, Greenspoon J, Aldahl D. 1986. Severe preeclampsia with persistent oliguria: Management of haemodynamic subsets. *Am J Obstet Gynecol*. 154:90–494.

Dahlenburg GW, RH Burnell, R Braybrook. 1980. The relation between cord serum and sodium levels in newborn infants and maternal intravenous therapy during labour. *Br J Obstet Gynecol*. 87:519–22.

Dumouline JG, J Foulkes. 1984. Commentary: Ketonuria during labour. *Br J Obstet Gynaecol*. 91:97–98.

Duley L. 1992. Plasma volume expansion in pregnancy-induced hypertension. In *Pregnancy and childbirth module*, ed MW Enkin, MJNC Keirse, JP Neilson. *Cochrane database of systematic reviews*, no. 05734. Cochrane updates on disc, 1994, issue 1. Oxford: Update software.

Evans SE, JS Crawford, ID Stevens, GM Durbin, H Daya. 1986. Fluid therapy for induced labour under epidural analgesia: Biochemical consequences for mother and infant. *Br J Obstet Gynecol*. 91:97–98.

Garite TJ, J Weeks, K Peters-Phair, C Pattillo, WR. Brewster 2000. A randomised controlled trial of the effect of increased intravenous hydration on the course of labour in nulliparous women. *Am J Obstet Gynecol*. 183:1544–48.

Graves SW. 2007. Sodium regulation, sodium pump function and sodium pump inhibitors in uncomplicated pregnancy and preeclampsia. *Front Biosc*. Jan 1;12:2438–46.

Hofmeyr G, Cyna A, Middleton P. 2004. Prophylactic intravenous preloading for regional analgesia in labour. *Cochrane Database Syst Rev*. Oct 18;(4): CD000175.

Horne CHW, PW Howie, RB Goudie. 1970. Serum alpha 2–macroglobulin, transferrin, albumin and IgG levels in preeclampsia. *J Clin Pathol* 23:514–18.

Jansen AJ, van Rhenen DJ, Steegers EA, Duvekot JJ. 2005. Postpartum haemorrhage and transfusion of blood and blood components. *Obstet Gynecol Surv*;60:663–71.

Kenepp NB, WC Shelly, S Kumar, CA Stanley, BB Gutsche. 1980. Effects on newborn of hydration with glucose in patients undergoing caesarean section with regional anaesthesia. *Lancet* 1:645.

Kenepp NB, WC Shelly, S Kumar, CA Stanley, BB Gutsche. 1982. Fetal and neonatal hazards of maternal hydration with 5% dextrose before caesarean section. *Lancet* 1:1150–52.

Kubli M, Scrutton MJ, Seed PT. 2002. An evaluation of isotonic 'sport drinks' during labour. *Anaesth Analg*. 94:404–8

Ludka LM, CC Roberts. 1993. Eating and drinking in labour. A literature review. *J Nurse Midwifery* 38:199–207.

Magee LA, MP Ornstein, P van Dadelszen. 1999. Management of hypertension in pregnancy. *BMJ* 318:1322–36.

National Institute for Health and of Clinical Excellence. 2007. Intrapartum care; care of healthy women and their babies during childbirth. London: NICE

Moen V, Brundin L, Rundgren M, Irestedt L. 2009. Hyponatraemia complicating labour-rare or unrecognised? A prospective observational study. *BJOG*. 116:552–561

Morton KE, MC Jackson, MDG Gillmer. 1985. A comparison of the effects of four intravenous solutions for the treatment of ketonuria during labour. *Br J Obstet Gynecol*. 92:473–79.

Piquard F, R Hsiunh, P Haberey. 1990. Does fetal acidosis develop with maternal glucose infusions in labour? *Obstet Gynecol*. 74:909–14.

Royal College of Obstetricians and Gynaecologists. 2009. Prevention and management of postpartum haemorrhage. Green-top Guideline No. 52.

Royal College of Obstetricians and Gynaecologists. 2007. Blood transfusion in obstetrics. Green-top Guideline No. 47.

Scheepers HCJ, Thans MCJ, de Jong PA, Essed GGM, Le Cassie S, Khanhai HHH. 2002a. A double-blind, randomised,placebo controlled study on the influence of carbohydrate solution intake during labour. *Br J Obstet Gynaecol*. 109:178–81.

Scheepers HCJ, de Jong PA, Essed GGM, Khanhai HHH. 2004. Carbohydrate solution intake during labour just before the start of the second stage: a double-blind study on metabolic effects and clinical outcomes. *Br J Obstet Gynaecol*. 111:1382–7.

Scheepers HCJ, Thans MCJ, de Jong PA, Essed GGM, Khanhai HHH. 2002b. The effects of oral carbohydrate administration on fetal acid base balance. *J Perinat Med*. 30:400–4.

Scottish Obstetric Guidelines and Audit Project. 1998. The Management of Obstetric Haemorrhage: A Clinical Practice Guideline for Professionals Involved in Maternity Care in Scotland. SPCERH Publication No. 6. Edinburgh: Scottish Programme for Clinical Effectiveness in Reproductive Health

Singh S, E Choo-Kang, JST Hall. 1982. Hazards of maternal hydration with 5% dextrose. *Lancet* ii: 335–36.

Sleutel M, SS Golden. 1999. Fasting in labor: Relic or requirement. *J Obstet Gynecol Neonat Nurs* 28:507–12.

Spencer SA, NP Mann, ML Smith, AMJ Wolfson, S Benson. 1981. The effects of intravenous therapy during labour on maternal and accord serum sodium levels. *Br J Obstet Gynecol*. 88:480–83.

Stan CM, Boulvain M, Pfister R, Hirsbrunner-Almagbaly P. 2002. Hydration for treatment of preterm labour. *Cochrane database of Syst. Rev.* issue 2. Art No.:CD003096. DOI: 10.1002/14651858.CD003096.

Steer PJ, MC Carter, K Choong, M Hanson, AJ Gordon, P Pradhan. 1985. A multicentric prospective controlled trial of induction of labour with an automated closed loop feedback controlled infusion system. *Br J Obstet Gynecol*. 92:1127–33.

Studd JWW, JD Blainey, DE Bailey. 1970. Serum protein changes in the preeclampsia-eclampsia syndrome. *J Obstet Gynecol Br Cwlth* 77:796–801.

Svanstrom M, Biber B, Hanes M, Johansson G, Naslund U, Balfors E. 2008. Signs of myocardial ischaemia after injection of oxytocin: a randomised double-blind comparison of oxytocin and methylergometrine during caesarean section. *Br J Anaesth*. 100:683-9.

Tamilselvan P, Fernando R, Bray H, Sòdhi M, Columb M. 2009. The effects of crystalloid and colloid preload on cardiac output in the parturient undergoing planned caesarean delivery under spinal anesthesia: a randomised trial. *Anesth Analg*. 109:1916–21.

Tarnow-Mordi WO, JC Shaw, D Liu, DA Garner, FV Flynn. 1981. Iatrogenic hyponatremia of the newborn due to maternal overload: A prospective study. *BMJ* 283:639–42.

Toohill J, Soong B, Flenady V. 2008. Interventions for ketosis during labour. *Cochrane Database Syst Rev*. Jul 16(3):CD004230

Zeilder RB, HD Kim. 1979. Effect of low electrolyte media on salt loss and haemolysis of mammalian red blood cells. *J Cell Physiol*. 100:551–61.

# CHAPTER 9

# MANAGEMENT OF SECOND STAGE OF LABOUR

*Pankaj Desai and Purvi Patel*

The second stage of labour is traditionally defined as the period from full dilatation of the cervix until delivery of the fetus. It is characterised by descent of the fetal presenting part in the pelvis.

It is a period of increased risk for the fetus (Menticoglou 1992; Piqaurd et al 1989), but there are very few evidence-based clinical practice guidelines for second stage management (Kadar et al 1986; Cheng et al 2004). Considerable controversy exists concerning the management aspects of the second stage of labour like second stage duration, timing and techniques of pushing, effect of epidural analgesia, fetal surveillance, role of episiotomy and instrumental vaginal delivery. Earlier, an arbitrary time limit was imposed on the second stage of labour; this was 60 minutes in the case of primigravidas and 30 minutes in the case of multigravidas. Several newer studies have challenged this concept and have shown that the duration of the second stage could be longer without any adverse effects on the mother or the fetus. This chapter discusses the diagnosis and management of second stage of labour and examines the evidence related to various management practices and the controversies associated with the management of the second stage.

## Mechanism of labour in second stage

In normal labour, descent of the presenting part should be progressive, although the rate of progress may be variable. Descent of the presenting part may begin in the first stage of labour as in primigravidas and it continues through the second stage of labour. In the majority of cases, the fetus enters the pelvis in the occipito-transverse position, descends through the pelvis and undergoes internal rotation at the level of the mid-pelvis into the occipito-anterior position. The descent of the presenting part and the level at which internal rotation takes place is dependent on the configuration of the sacrum, the size and prominence of the ischial spines, the degree of convergence of the pelvic side-walls and the sub-pubic angle. Internal rotation occurs at the level of the midpelvis in a gynecoid pelvis as against

> Pelvic anatomy plays a role in the mechanism of labour and can influence the duration of the second stage.

at the level of the perineum in a platypelloid pelvis. Posterior rotation leads to a face-to-pubis delivery in an anthropoid pelvis. Thus, the pelvic anatomy plays a role in the mechanism of labour and can influence the duration of the second stage.

## Normal physiology

Cervical dilatation in the late first stage and the distension of vagina in the second stage leads to the utero-pituitary reflex (Ferguson reflex) and results in a surge in oxytocin, inducing strong uterine contractions. The uterine contractility increases in frequency and duration. The contact of the presenting part with the pelvic floor results in an involuntary urge to bear down and push. Thus, maternal expulsive efforts are added to the uterine forces. Both these forces reduce the uteroplacental perfusion, ultimately reducing the oxygen delivery to the fetus. Fetal cerebral blood oxygenation reduces when the contraction intervals become less than 2 to 3 minutes apart. Healthy fetuses have compensatory mechanisms that are capable of coping with this, as long as the second stage is not unduly prolonged. Fetal acidosis in the second stage is, in normal circumstances, respiratory in origin, but a fetus that is unable to compensate for the reduced oxygen supply during the second stage, develops an added metabolic acidosis. The duration of the second stage should be recorded more appropriately as the *passive* and the *active* phases since the duration of the active phase may have three times more influence over the decline in fetal pH than the duration of the second stage as a whole.

> Ferguson reflex (the utero-pituitary reflex) is set off by cervical dilatation in the late first stage and the distension of vagina in the second stage and results in a surge in oxytocin, inducing strong uterine contractions.

## Phases of second stage of labour

As with the first stage, the second stage is divided into two phases, each with different clinical implications.

### Phase 1–Passive phase (Phase of descent, Pelvic phase)

The passive phase is from full cervical dilatation until the fetal head reaches the pelvic floor. Physiologically, this phase is more like an extension of the first stage, and its duration is subject to considerable individual variation, contributing significantly to the overall variability seen in the length of the second stage. The major portion of the fetal descent occurs in this phase.

> The passive phase is from full cervical dilatation until the fetal head reaches the pelvic floor.

### Phase 2–Active phase (Expulsive phase, Perineal phase)

The active phase is marked by the maternal urge to bear down. The mother can exhibit many signals indicating the transition into the active phase of the second stage of labour: change in facial expressions, words and actions, or in the way she squeezes her companion's hand (Enkin et al 2000; McKay and Roberts 1990). Clear signs of having moved into the active phase

> The active phase is marked by the maternal urge to bear down.

are breathing hard, powerful sounds, and an overwhelming urge to push.

## Diagnosis of the second stage of labour

Usually, the diagnosis of the second stage is made by a vaginal examination. Diagnosis of the onset of the second stage is subjective; the time of its occurrence is really unknown i.e. it may have already occurred prior to examination. However, if the presenting part is visible at the introitus, full cervical dilatation can be assumed. Some women feel the urge to bear down even before complete cervical dilatation. When the progress of labour leads one to believe that the cervix may not be fully dilated, cervical dilatation should be checked by vaginal examination. If the cervix is less than 8 cm dilated, the woman should be asked to adopt a comfortable position (for example, on her side) and try to resist the urge to push by using breathing techniques. Epidural analgesia may be given, if necessary.

## Latency from full cervical dilatation to pushing

When the onset of the second stage is diagnosed by full dilatation of the cervix, it is possible that the presenting part may still be above the ischial spines, which creates the problem of deciding how much time should be allowed for fetal descent. It also has to be decided when pushing should be encouraged, or more specifically, when the end of the 'latent' or fetal descent phase has occurred and the 'active' or physiological urge to bear down phase starts.

The PEOPLE (Pushing Early or Pushing Late with Epidural) trial (Fraser et al 2000) demonstrated that delaying maternal pushing for a maximum of two hours compared with immediate pushing at full cervical dilation in nulliparous women with epidural anesthesia was associated with a significant reduction in the incidence of difficult births (from 22.5 per cent to 17.8 per cent). The reduction in risk of difficult birth was most marked in women in whom the station was above +2 at the onset of the second stage and, particularly, when the position was other than occipito-anterior. Data on multiparous women are more limited, but Hansen et al (2002) found no difference in outcomes in multiparous women who waited for one hour before pushing. Overall, a policy of delayed rather than early pushing for women with epidural anesthesia reduces operative intervention at the expense of an increased duration of second stage. (Buxton et al 1988; Roberts 2003)

> A policy of delayed rather than early pushing for women with epidural anesthesia reduces operative intervention at the expense of an increased duration of second stage.

In relation to fetal outcome, a randomised controlled trial identified better fetal oxygen saturation when pushing was delayed for up to two hours. Simpson and James (2005) and Hansen et al (2002) reported fewer incidences of fetal heart rate decelerations in both primigravidas and multigravidas who waited before pushing. Fraser et al (2000) identified lower umbilical cord blood pH among infants in the delayed pushing group, but the authors felt that these results were of uncertain clinical significance. This finding contrasts with that of Piquard et al (1989), who reported that fetal acid–base status did not change during the passive phase of the second stage of labour in women without epidural anesthesia.

In nulliparous women with epidural anesthesia, waiting for up to two hours prior to the onset of pushing is appropriate if there is continued descent of the head and reassuring fetal and maternal status. It is recommended to wait two hours before pushing in all women with epidural anesthesia, who have no urge to push, or in whom the station of the presenting part was above +2, or who have a fetus in an occipito-posterior or occipito-transverse position. All women without epidural can commence pushing when the urge is present, if the cervix is >8 cm dilated.

## Duration of pushing

Time limits for the active (pushing) phase of the second stage cannot be stipulated because conclusive evidence is lacking. It is known, however, that the duration of active pushing is more important for the fetal and maternal condition than the total duration of the second stage of labour (Roberts 2003; Saunders et al 1992). The findings of the PEOPLE trial (Fraser et al 2000) related to nulliparous women with epidural anesthesia support a general consensus that waiting for up to two hours before pushing results in a reduction in the median duration of active pushing (from 110 minutes to 68 minutes) (Fraser et al 2000). Hansen et al (2002) and Brancato et al (2008) documented a similar finding. When the fetal heart rate is reassuring, Piquard et al (1989) found that the fetal scalp pH decreased slowly during the active pushing phase.

## Pushing techniques

The traditional pushing instruction is to take a deep breath, hold it for 15–20 seconds and exert downward pressure, long and hard, using the diaphragm and abdominal muscles. This is essentially a Valsalva manoeuvre. The action results in an increase in intrathoracic pressure, which leads to a reduction in venous return to the right atrium resulting in a reduction in maternal cardiac output that persists briefly after the breath is released. If, due to the supine position, there is also vena caval obstruction, there may be a reduction in uteroplacental perfusion. Bearing-down efforts also exacerbate aortic compression.

When undirected pushing is allowed, there is an average of four to five bearing-down efforts with each contraction, each with a duration of 4–6 seconds. Such efforts are often associated with an open rather than a closed glottis. Thus, women may make grunting noises while pushing as opposed to holding their breath. There is no time-related decline in fetal pH when this undirected pushing is used.

Studies support a spontaneous, mother-led approach to bearing-down in the second stage of labour, although it is associated with a slightly longer second stage (Enkin et al 2000; Yildirim and Beji 2008; Hansen 2009). Where spontaneous pushing does not result in progressive decent of the presenting part, a more directive approach may assist the mother to use her contractions more effectively.

## Total duration of second stage

The time limits and statistical norms for the duration of the stages of labour were established in 1954 by the American obstetrician, Emanuel A Friedman, in 'Friedman's curve of labour'. Friedman's research became the benchmark for assessing progress in labour. These normative guidelines generally have become prescriptive and have led to operative deliveries if the length of labour crosses some specific time threshold. However, more recently, this concept has been challenged and new evidence supports the theory that normal labour, both first and second stages, takes much longer than had been originally suggested by Friedman.

The length of the second stage varies according to the maternal positioning, position of the fetus, use of oxytocin augmentation, quality of the uterine contractions, pushing efforts of the woman and the type of analgesia used (Archie and Biswas 2003; Altman and Lydon-Rochelle 2006). The length of a normal second stage must be considered separately for nulliparas and multiparas, with and without epidural analgesia, as generally, epidural analgesia may double the length of a second stage.

> The length of the second stage varies according to:
> - maternal positioning
> - position of the fetus
> - use of oxytocin augmentation
> - quality of the uterine contractions
> - pushing efforts of the woman
> - type of analgesia used

## Nulliparous women

In a large study, Menticoglou et al (1995) found that 93 per cent of nulliparous women with epidural anesthesia delivered within four hours of full cervical dilatation. Of the 7 per cent of women whose second stage of labour exceeded four hours, less than one third achieved a spontaneous vaginal birth. There was no change in neonatal mortality or low cord pH at the time of birth when the second stage of labour lasted up to five hours.

Similarly, Myles and Santolaya (2003) and Hansen et al (2002) found no difference in neonatal outcomes if the second stage lasted more than four hours. However, maternal complications have been reported in association with a second stage longer than four hours, including postpartum hemorrhage, third and fourth degree lacerations, chorioamnionitis, operative vaginal births and cesarean sections (Cheng et al 2004; 2007). Contrary to this, Hansen et al (2002) found no adverse maternal outcomes when the second stage of labour lasted up to 4.9 hours in primigravidas with epidural anesthesia. Paterson et al (1992) found that 90 per cent of nulliparous women without epidural anesthesia were delivered within three hours. The adverse outcomes attributed to 'prolonged' second stage may be consequent upon underlying causative factors and not on the absolute duration (Sleep 1990).

Large retrospective studies (Saunders et al 1992; Janni et al 2002; Cheng et al 2004; Altman and Lydon-Rochelle 2006; Lu et al 2009) have concluded that although cases of second stage labour of up to three hours do not seem to carry undue risk to the fetus, women who remain in the second stage for this length of time suffer a higher rate of early morbidity (postpartum hemorrhage and infection), though this effect is less marked in women who deliver spontaneously. Increased maternal morbidity in women with prolonged second stage may be partially attributed to the higher rate of operative procedures and should not be solely based on the elapsed time after full dilatation (Janni et al 2002). This increase in risk needs to be weighed against the risk of instrumental delivery (Murphy 2001). The effect of prolonged second stage of labour on pelvic support and urinary and fecal continence requires further investigation. Extremely prolonged second stage (>4 hours) is associated with increased incidence of postpartum hemorrhage and cesarean section (Cheng et al 2004; Naime et al 2008)

There is no evidence to justify the imposition of arbitrary time limits on the length of the second stage (Caughey 2009; Rouse et al 2009). Maternal status, fetal status and the rate of descent of the presenting part should guide management. However, abnormal descent should be suspected with excessive duration of the second stage (i.e. more than two hours in primigravidas and more than one hour in multigravidas) (SOGC Clinical Practice Guidelines 1998).

> Abnormal descent should be suspected with a duration of the second stage > 2 hours in primigravidas and > 1 hour in multigravidas.

The American College of Obstetricians and Gynecologists (ACOG) guidelines (2003) define dystocia in nulliparous women as a second stage that lasts for more than three hours when regional anesthesia is used, and more than two hours when it is not. For multiparous women, the respective values are two hours and one hour.

Continuing the second stage beyond the following time limits may not be appropriate if there is slow or no progress despite oxytocin-augmented contractions. Extending these time limits may be appropriate if progress continues and spontaneous vaginal birth is imminent:

❖ Nulliparous women with epidural anesthesia: four hours.
❖ Nulliparous women without epidural anesthesia: three hours.
❖ Multiparous women with epidural anesthesia: three hours.
❖ Multiparous women without epidural anesthesia: two hours.

## Delayed descent in second stage

As per Friedman's curve, descent is expected to occur at the rate of 1 cm/hour in primigravidas and 2 cm/hour in multigravidas. However, maternal as well as fetal factors may affect the descent rate. Increasing maternal age, maternal obesity, maternal pelvic masses (fibroid, ovarian cyst, pelvic kidney), persistent occipito-posterior position, fetal weight of 4 kg or more are associated with prolonged second stage. Fenstein et al (2002) have identified nulliparity, fetal macrosomia, epidural analgesia, hydramnios, hypertensive disorders and gestational diabetes as the major risk factors for a prolonged second stage of labour.

> Prolonged second stage may occur with:
> • increasing maternal age
> • maternal obesity
> • maternal pelvic masses (fibroid, ovarian cyst, pelvic kidney)
> • persistent occipito-posterior position
> • fetal weight of 4 kg or more

If there is a delay in the second stage of labour, exclude a full bladder, cephalo-pelvic disproportion, malposition of the fetal head, e.g. occipito-posterior or occipito-transverse, or deflexed fetal head, inelastic perineal tissues, especially in the older primipara and inadequate uterine activity (Enkin et al 2000).

If the head is presenting, its relationship to the brim of the pelvis should be assessed. Abdominal palpation is a satisfactory way of gauging the descent of the presenting part (see Chapter 2, Figure 2.3) and may reduce the number of vaginal exams that are necessary. It is important to assess caput and moulding of the fetal head in addition to determining descent and position during vaginal examination, especially if progress is slow and cephalopelvic disproportion is suspected.

If the fetal head is engaged, the membranes are intact and descent is slow, a controlled rupture of the membranes may facilitate delivery. Failure of descent may be due to inadequate or incoordinate uterine contractions, malposition or malpresentation of the fetus or cephalopelvic disproportion. Malpresentation or minor degrees of cephalopelvic disproportion may sometimes be overcome by encouraging the mother to vary her position. Intravenous oxytocin can be used if contractions are inadequate.

> If the fetal head is engaged, the membranes are intact and descent is slow, a controlled rupture of the membranes may facilitate delivery.

## Oxytocin augmentation

Oxytocin infusion increases the frequency and amplitude of the uterine contractions. Oxytocin is generally used to treat uncomplicated delays in the second stage of labour as it can correct fetal malpositions and can enhance the fetal descent. Oxytocin administration can begin at any time during the second stage, particularly in nulliparous women with epidural anesthesia, or where contractions are assessed to be inadequate or there is lack of progress. Women who are already receiving oxytocin at the onset of the second stage should continue to receive it during the second stage. For primigravidas with epidural anesthesia, one randomised trial reported a reduction in instrumental birth rates when oxytocin was routinely initiated at the time of full cervical dilatation. (Saunders et al 1992)

## Maternal position in labour

It has been traditional practice for women to be positioned and to push in the horizontal, semi-Fowler's, or lithotomy position during the second stage of labour (Mayberry et al 2000). Use of these positions is often dictated by interventions such as epidural analgesia, electronic fetal monitoring, or intravenous lines that limit mobility. When the second stage is conducted with the mother in the dorsal position, progressive fetal acidosis can occur, but this does not occur when the second stage is conducted with the mother in a left lateral position, indicating aortocaval compression as an important contributory factor.

### Hemodynamic implications

Hemodynamic implications of aortocaval compression for uteroplacental circulation can be summarised as follows:

1. Aortic compression decreases uteroplacental circulation.
2. Obstruction of the inferior vena cava resulting in reduced right atrial filling pressures leads initially to a maternal

adaptive response of peripheral vasoconstriction. This mechanism has the potential to further impair uteroplacental circulation if it is part of a generalised vasoconstriction response.

3. If inferior vena cava obstruction is uncompensated or compensatory mechanisms are exceeded, then maternal hypotension ensues, thereby adversely affecting uteroplacental circulation.

4. Decrease in femoral arterial pressure occur more frequently than decreases in brachial arterial pressure in the supine position, and thus, the fetal consequences of aortocaval compression are likely to occur with greater frequency and severity than are the maternal consequences.

### Clinical implications

There is a time-related decrease in the fetal pH associated with the supine position during the second stage of labour, whereas with left lateral position, this decrease does not occur. Cardiac output is reduced by 17 per cent when the mother is in the supine position and 11 per cent for both the lithotomy position and the right lateral position, in comparison with the left lateral position. Thus, the left lateral position is preferable hemodynamically to the right. Studies of fetal heart rate (FHR) changes, fetal cerebral oxygenation and fetal pH confirmed the significant potential adverse fetal effects of supine positioning. As the uterine contractions exacerbate aortocaval compression, it is particularly important that the labouring woman does not adopt a supine position for any length of time, more so in second stage.

A meta-analysis (De Jonge et al 2004) identified that women pushing in the supine position had higher rates of instrumental deliveries and episiotomies, and more pain, than those using other positions. Use of upright or lateral position compared with supine or lithotomy position is associated with a shorter second stage of labour (5.4 minutes), fewer assisted deliveries, fewer episiotomies, fewer reports of severe pain and less abnormal fetal heart rate patterns (Gupta and Nikodem 2000).

> Women pushing in the supine position have higher rates of instrumental deliveries and episiotomies.

Simkin and Ancheta (2000) recommend various physiologic positions and identify contributing features unique to each position. They assert that positioning is a key primary intervention when lack of progress is identified in the second stage. Positional changes may cause constant subtle changes in the relationship of the pelvis to the fetus that may facilitate labour. Frequent changes in position may help when fetal malposition is identified, or to relieve back pain. Mayberry et al (2000) recommend squatting, semi-recumbency, standing, and upright kneeling to generate increased intra-abdominal pressure and increased anteroposterior and transverse diameters of the pelvic outlet, but this has not been confirmed by research.

The pros and cons of various non-supine positions are listed as below:

### Lying on the side:

Advantages: Fewer perineal lacerations because of greater control of the fetal head during childbirth, and greater relaxation and less tension of the perineal muscles.

Disadvantage: Need a person to help hold up the leg of the woman.

*Squatting*:
Advantages: Both the transverse and anterior–posterior diameter of the pelvic outlet are bigger. This results in less oxytocin stimulation, fewer mechanically assisted deliveries, fewer and less severe perineal lacerations (if the perineum was adequately supported), and fewer episiotomies.

Disadvantage: If used without adequate perineal support, can result in increased maternal injuries.

*Hands and knees*:
Advantages: Less perineal trauma, because gravity directs pressure away from the perineum, and at the same time, promotes fetal descent, and there is increased perineal elasticity in this position

Disadvantage: Wrist fatigue and tiring for the woman if used for long periods

*Sitting*:
Advantage: Shorter duration of second stage; increased bearing-down pressure.

Disadvantage: The use of birth chairs during second stage has been associated with increased incidence of postpartum hemorrhage. There is speculation that this may be related to perineal trauma exacerbated by obstructed venous return. A change in maternal position immediately after delivery may reduce this risk.

It is recommended that a woman may choose a position comfortable to her for delivery.

## Epidural analgesia and second stage management

Epidural analgesia can abolish the normal expulsive urges (Ferguson's reflex) that occur during the active phase of the second stage and that, combined with the decreased muscle tone of the anterior abdominal wall, makes pushing both less effective and misdirected, with the parturient tending to push more toward the symphysis than the rectum. The decrease in muscle tone of the pelvic floor may also inhibit or delay anterior rotation of the descending fetal head, resulting in an increased incidence of malrotation.

In contrast to the above, there is evidence to show that epidural analgesia may accelerate an already prolonged and exhausting labour and reduce the need for delivery by cesarean section for failure to progress. The provision of effective analgesia reduces the inhibitory effect of endogenous maternal catecholamines on uterine contractility, attenuates maternal acidosis and permits the mother to tolerate augmentation with oxytocin (Maltau and Anderson 1975; Schnider et al 1983; Desai et al 2006).

Though epidural analgesia is associated with an increased incidence of instrumental deliveries, progressively more dilute concentrations of local anesthetic agents reduce this increased incidence. The dose-sparing effect of opioid–local anesthetic combinations further adds to this reduction. Low- (as opposed to high-) concentration local anesthetic solutions appear to reduce the increased incidence of mid-cavity rotation forceps delivery. Increasing the duration of Phase 1 of the second stage with epidural usage can reduce the number of instrumental deliveries without compromising fetal outcome. When Phase 1 lasts beyond 3 hours there is increased maternal morbidity.

## Fetal monitoring during the second stage

In a normal second stage, fetal well-being can be monitored by intermittent auscultation at five-minute intervals in the active second stage. There may be difficulty in auscultation of the fetal heart sounds with fetal descent in the late second stage of labour. Continuous intrapartum electronic fetal monitoring is recommended when oxytocin is used for augmentation of labour or when auscultation is difficult or when there is an increased risk of fetal hypoxia due to risk factors (e.g. IUGR, thick meconium).

One should be aware of the various normal patterns of fetal heart that occur during the second stage, especially the active phase, so that unnecessary operative intervention can be avoided. FHR decelerations are common during the second stage and obstetricians should be able to differentiate between patterns that are benign or well tolerated by a healthy fetus and those that are indicative of progressive fetal hypoxia and require urgent delivery. Early decelerations indicate head compression whereas late decelerations indicate possibility of compromise to uteroplacental perfusion with onset of hypoxia, which can proceed to acidosis if it is allowed to persist for a long time. It has been noted that as long as the normal baseline and baseline variability are maintained, even when decelerations are present with each contraction, the fetal outcome is not compromised. Fetal heart rate patterns suggestive of progressive hypoxia are progressive tachycardia, progressive bradycardia, loss of variability and widening and deepening of decelerations. When there is doubt about fetal well-being and the delivery is not imminent, a fetal scalp pH or fetal scalp stimulation is indicated. Management may include left lateral position, oxygenation and reducing oxytocin infusion.

A fetal heart rate classification specific to the active second stage of labour was described by Melchior and Bernard (1991). It described five fetal heart rate patterns: from type 0 to type 4. A reduction in pH and a rise in lactate and pCO2 values occurred as one progressed from type 0 to type 4:

- Type 0: normal pattern of FHR
- Type 1: normal baseline FHR with decelerations and subsequent return to baseline level
- Type 2: rapid decrease in the baseline FHR resulting in prolonged bradycardia
- Type 3: onset of accelerations during each contraction while the baseline FHR is decreased to the level of bradycardia
- Type 4: initially, the FHR remains normal (single decelerations may occur) and later the FHR decreases, resulting in prolonged bradycardia.

The length of maternal bearing-down efforts were matched to the Melchior's classification pattern in a study which suggested optimal length of bearing-down efforts could be 30 minutes for type 0, 20 minutes for type 1 and 10 minutes for type 2, 3 or 4 (Dupuis and Simon 2008).

## Episiotomy

Routine episiotomy is not recommended. The postulated but not substantiated beneficial effects of episiotomy are a reduction in the likelihood of third degree perineal tears, preservation of the pelvic floor and perineal muscle leading to improved sexual function and a reduced risk of fecal and/or urinary incontinence, reduced risk of shoulder dystocia, easier repair and better healing of a straight clean incision rather than a laceration. The benefits postulated for the fetus are reduced asphyxia, cranial trauma, cerebral hemorrhage and mental retardation. There is no data available to support these claims. The presumed effect of episiotomy on shortening the second stage of labour has not been demonstrated. The adverse effects include: extension into the anal sphincter or the rectum, unsatisfactory anatomic results such as skin tags, asymmetry, or excessive narrowing of the introitus; vaginal prolapse; rectovaginal or anal fistulas; increased blood loss and hematoma; pain and edema; infection and dehiscence; and delayed return of sexual function.

A study of 1000 women randomised to restricted use of episiotomy and to liberal use of episiotomy revealed no clinically significant differences between the two groups in regard to postpartum perineal pain, dyspareunia and urinary incontinence at 10 days, three weeks and three years postpartum. There was no difference in fetal outcomes though fetal indications were the primary reason for episiotomy in the restricted group. Episiotomy does not prevent subsequent loss of pelvic floor strength. Current evidence supports a restricted use of episiotomy (Lai et al 2009).

Restrictive episiotomy policies appear to have a number of benefits compared to policies based on routine episiotomy. There is less posterior perineal trauma, less suturing and fewer complications, no difference for most pain measures and severe vaginal or perineal trauma, but there was an increased risk of anterior vaginal and labial trauma with restrictive episiotomy (Carroli and Mignini 2009). These results are similar for both mediolateral and midline episiotomy. This raises the possibility that episiotomy may have a more specific protective effect on the tissues around the bladder neck. There is no good evidence, however, that a liberal use of episiotomy is protective against urinary incontinence. In the three-year follow-up of a comparison of liberal with restricted use of episiotomy, rates and severity of incontinence were similar in the two trial groups.

Indications for episiotomy include any condition that places the woman at risk for perineal tearing, such as large-sized baby, preterm or growth-restricted fetus, anticipation of shoulder dystocia, fetal malpresentations and malpositions, instrumental delivery, fetal distress (to speed up the delivery) maternal exhaustion or distress, previous third degree tears or severe scarring of the perineum.

> Restrictive episiotomy policies result in:
> - less posterior perineal trauma
> - less suturing
> - fewer complications
> - no difference for most pain measures and severe vaginal or perineal trauma

> Indications for episiotomy:
> - large-sized baby
> - preterm or growth-restricted fetus
> - anticipation of shoulder dystocia
> - fetal malpresentations and malpositions
> - instrumental delivery
> - fetal distress to speed up the delivery
> - maternal exhaustion or distress
> - previous third degree tears or severe scarring of the perineum.

Median episiotomies are associated with higher risk of extension into the rectum and compromise of the external anal sphincter muscle. Mediolateral episiotomies are associated with greater postpartum pain, more blood loss, greater difficulty in repair, and more dyspareunia, especially when compared with spontaneous tears. Because of the potential for greater expansion of the pelvic floor with mediolateral episiotomy, this procedure may theoretically help lower the risk for incontinence, but data from studies have shown similar outcomes.

> Episiotomy
> - Median:
>   o risk of extension into the rectum
>   o compromise of the external anal sphincter
> - *Mediolateral:*
>   o greater postpartum pain
>   o more blood loss
>   o greater difficulty in repair
>   o more dyspareunia

## Care of the perineum

The aim should be to minimise any perineal trauma.

There are other issues, apart from episiotomy, which need attention to prevent perineal damage. The type of perineal lacerations and the manner in which they are repaired influence the long-term effects on perineal integrity. Forceps deliveries, occipito-posterior positions, babies weighing more than 4 kg and nulliparity are associated with more third degree perineal tears.

### Hands-on versus hands-poised

The hands-on method described by Ritgen in 1855, usually involves pressure on the infant's head upon crowning and support with the other hand of the perineum, with the aim of protecting against perineal lacerations. In the hands-poised method, the fetal head or perineum is not touched or supported by the delivering personnel. These two methods are associated with similar incidences of perineal or vaginal tears, but the hands-on method is associated with an increased incidence of episiotomy. A policy of hands-poised has also been supported by a quasi-randomised study, reporting less third-degree tears compared with hands-on.

### Prevention of perineal tears at vaginal delivery

Conducting the delivery of the fetal head in an uncontrolled and unhurried manner minimises perineal trauma and also reduces the need for episiotomy. Evidence does not support the use of perineal massage, lubricants and hot compresses to reduce the perineal tears.

Antenatal perineal massage to prevent perineal tears is recommended by some but evidence does not support this recommendation. In fact, it has been associated with an increase in the incidence of perineal tears. The maternal position at delivery may have some minor influence on the incidence and pattern of perineal tears: there are more tears with squatting and lithotomy positions. Ironing out (massaging the perineum) in the second stage is not recommended due to the fact that touch may be a disruptive distraction, and also, the increase in vascularity and edema in the tissues that are already at risk of trauma is counter-productive. In the only controlled comparison, no difference was found in the over-all risk of perineal trauma, although fewer women in the perineal massage group had a third or a fourth degree perineal tear.

## Pelvic floor

In a study on maternal morbidity at four months postpartum, 23 per cent had stress incontinence, 12 per cent had urge incontinence, 29 per cent had some urinary incontinence and 4 per cent had fecal incontinence. Maternal age and forceps-assisted delivery were risk factors for urinary incontinence (Baydock et al 2009). The factor most strongly associated with pelvic floor dysfunction following birth is instrumental delivery (Wheeler and Richter 2007). Therefore, maximising the chances of spontaneous vaginal birth during the second stage is desirable.

> Instrumental delivery is the factor most strongly associated with pelvic floor dysfunction following birth.

## Second stage partogram

Sizer et al (2000) described a second-stage partogram based on a system of scoring the descent and position of the fetal head and suggested using this system for studying progress in the second stage of labour and for predicting mode of delivery and obstetric outcome. In a prospective observational study, the position and station of the fetal head were observed and scored at diagnosis of the second stage of labour; an hour later, and then at 30 minute intervals until delivery was achieved. The score at diagnosis of the second stage of labour was assessed for its ability to predict eventual mode of delivery and duration of labour.

A nomogram was defined for nulliparas and multiparas and was used to define normal and abnormal progress in the second stage, associated factors in the first stage of labour, and mode of delivery. An increased total score at the onset of the second stage of labour was associated with an increased chance of spontaneous vaginal delivery, decreased chance of instrumental vaginal delivery, and emergency cesarean delivery. Abnormal progress as defined by the nomogram is associated with use of epidural anesthesia, induction of labour, augmentation, dystocia and increased incidence of operative delivery. No significant difference was found between normal and abnormal second stages of labour and fetal outcome as determined by APGAR scores. The second-stage partogram may offer an objective basis for management of the second stage of labour (Basu et al 2009). However, its use has to be further validated by other studies.

## Delayed second stage and operative delivery

The rate of operative vaginal delivery has remained fairly constant at 10 to 15 per cent (RCOG 2005). Although it is now generally well established that there are significant risks associated with rotational and mid-cavity deliveries (Chiswick and James 1979), there are low morbidity rates associated with most operative deliveries (Gei and Belfort 1999). It should also be remembered that cesarean section in the second stage of labour is not without considerable morbidity (Murphy et al 2001 and Villar et al 2007). The operators should use their skill and judgment to determine the best choice of instrument for the situation (NICE Guideline 2007). The RCOG (2005) currently advises that the vacuum extractor

> The vacuum extractor should be the first choice for instrumental delivery because it is associated with less maternal trauma.

should be the first choice. Although this can have a higher failure rate and increased risks of cephalhematoma, it has been shown to be associated with less maternal trauma (Johanson and Menon 1998; Johanson et al 1999; Fitzpatrick et al 2003).

Use of local anesthetic–opioid combination for epidurals and delayed pushing in primiparous women with an epidural will reduce the risk of rotational and mid-cavity deliveries (Schmitz and Meunier 2008). In primiparous women with epidural anesthesia, starting oxytocin in the second stage of labour can reduce the need for non-rotational forceps delivery. Use of upright positions can reduce instrumental deliveries (Roberts et al 2005). There is no evidence that discontinuing an epidural in the second stage of labour will decrease the risk of assisted delivery.

Operative vaginal delivery should not be attempted unless the criteria for safe delivery have been met. Operative vaginal delivery should be abandoned where there is no evidence of progressive descent with each pull or where delivery is not imminent following pulls of a correctly applied instrument by an experienced operator, over three contractions and bearing-down efforts. The use of sequential instruments is associated with an increased risk of trauma to the infant. However, the operator must balance the risks of a cesarean section following failed vacuum extraction with the risks of forceps delivery following failed vacuum extraction.

## Fundal pressure

The role of fundal pressure during second stage is controversial. Much of the data about maternal–fetal injuries related to fundal pressure are not published for medical–legal reasons; however, anecdotal reports suggest that these risks exist. (Simpson and Knox 2001; Merhi and Awonuga 2005) Fundal pressure during birth can cause damage to uterine and abdominal tissue, and is extremely painful to the mother.

## Prophylactic interventions

Prophylactic intrapartum maternal oxygenation in the second stage of labour is associated with more frequent, low (<7.20) cord blood pH values than the control group. There are no other statistically significant differences between the groups (Fawole and Hofmeyr 2003). There is no evidence to support the prophylactic use of betamimetics during the second stage of labour (Hofmeyr and Kulier 1996).

## Delivery

In the active phase of second stage, the head advances with each uterine contraction and then recedes as the uterus relaxes. The perineum thins out under the pressure of the head. With further descent, the occiput hinges under the symphysis pubis. With further descent, the largest diameter of the fetal head passes through the vulva after crowning. The head is born by extension after which it restitutes due to the untwisting of the fetal neck. The delivery of the head should be unhurried and gentle. Either gentle support of the perineum or a 'hands-off' approach, with verbal coaching and encouragement, can be used.

After the delivery of the head, the shoulders rotate internally. The head should be supported as it restitutes and rotates externally. Mucus is aspirated from the mouth and throat and nuchal cord should be checked for. If the cord is loose around the neck, it can either be left alone or slipped over the head easily. If not, it must be clamped doubly and then cut and unwound. Once rotation is complete, the shoulders are delivered with maternal effort, one at a time to reduce perineal trauma. The anterior shoulder is the first to deliver, after which the head is raised so that the posterior shoulder appears over the perineum. Once the head and shoulders have been delivered, the rest of the body delivers easily.

## Conclusion

The second stage of labour is the most vulnerable period of the pregnancy for the fetus and requires intense surveillance. Complications of the second stage of labour are associated with immediate and long-term maternal as well as fetal morbidities. The attending clinician should be vigilant in detecting aberrations in the labour course at the earliest and take appropriate measures so that the process of labour culminates with a healthy mother and infant.

## References

American College of Obstetricians and Gynecologists. 2003. Dystocia and augmentation of labor. *ACOG Practice Bulletin* 49:1–9.

Archie CL, Biswas MK. 2003. The course and conduct of normal labor and delivery, In: DeCherney AH and Nathan L, eds. *Current Obstetrics and Gynecologic Diagnosis and Treatment*. McGraw-Hill.

Altman MR, Lydon-Rochelle MT. 2006. Prolonged second stage of labor and risk of adverse maternal and perinatal outcomes: a systematic review. *Birth* 33: 315–22.

Basu JK, Buchmann EJ, Basu D. 2009. Role of a second stage partogram in predicting the outcome of normal labour. *Aust NZ J Obstet Gynaecol*. Apr; 49(2): 158–61.

Baydock SA, Flood C, Schultz JA, MacDonald D, Esau D, Jones S, Hiltz CB. 2009. Prevalence and risk factors for urinary and fecal incontinence four months after vaginal delivery. *J Obstet Gynaecol Can*. Jan; 31(1): 36–41.

Brancato RM, Church S, Sione PW. 2008. A meta-analysis of passive descent versus immediate pushing in nulliparous women with epidural analgesia in the second stage of labor. *J. Obstet Gynecol Neonatal Nurs*. Jan–Feb; 37(1):4–12.

Buxton EJ, Redman CW, Obhrai M. 1988. Delayed pushing with lumbar epidural in labor – does it increase the incidence of spontaneous delivery? *J Obstet Gynaecol*. 8:258–61.

Carroli G, Mignini L. 2009. Episiotomy for vaginal birth. *Cochrane Database Syst Rev* Jan 21; (1): CD000081.

Caughey AB. 2009. Is there an upper limit for the management of second stage of labor? *Am J Obstet Gynecol* 201 (4): 337–8.

Cheng Y, Hopkins LM, Caughey AB. 2004. How long is too long?: Does a prolonged second stage of labor in nulliparous women affect maternal and neonatal outcomes? *Am J Obstet Gynecol* 191:933–8.

Cheng Y, Hopkins LM, Laros RK Jr, Caughey AB. 2007. Duration of the second stage of labor in multiparous women: maternal and neonatal outcomes. *Am J Obstet Gynecol*. Jun; 196(6):585.e1-6.

Chiswick ML, James D. 1979. Kielland's forceps. *Br Med J*. Mar 17; 1(6165):747–8.

De Jonge A, Teunissen T, Lagro-Janssen AL. 2004. Supine position compared to other positions during the second stage of labor: a meta-analytic review. *J Psychom Obstet Gynaecol*. 25(1):35–45.

Desai P, Patel P, Gupta A, Virk G, Sinha A. 2006. Epidural analgesia in labor. *J Obstet Gynaecol India* 56(5):417–22.

Dupuis O, Simon A. 2008. Fetal monitoring during the second stage of labor. *J Gynecol Obstet Biol Reprod (Paris)* Feb; 37 Suppl 1:s 93–100.

Enkin M, Keirse MJNC, Neilson J et al. 2000. *A guide to effective care in pregnancy and childbirth* Oxford: Oxford University Press.

Fawole B, Hofmeyr GJ. 2003. Maternal oxygen administration for fetal distress. *Cochrane Database Syst Rev*, Issue 4. Art. No.: CD000136. DOI: 10.1002/14651858.CD000136.

Fitzpatrick M, Behan M, O'Connell PR et al. 2003. Randomised clinical trial to assess anal sphincter function following forceps or vacuum assisted vaginal delivery. *Br J Obstet Gynaecol.* Apr; 110(4):424–9.

Fraser WD, Marcoux S, Krauss I, Douglas J, Goulet C, Boulvain M, et al. 2000. Multicenter, randomized, controlled trial of delayed pushing for nulliparous women in the second stage of labor with continuous epidural analgesia. *Am J Obstet Gynecol*. 182(5):1165–72.

Gei AF, Belfort MF. 1999. Forceps-assisted vaginal delivery. *Obstet Gynecol Clin North Am*. Jun; 26(2):345–70.

Gupta JK, Nikodem VC. 2000. Woman's position during the second stage of labour *Cochrane Database Syst Rev.* Issue 2. Oxford: Update Software.

Fenstein U, E Shelmer, A Levy et al. 2002. Risk factors for arrest of descent during second stage of labor. *Int J Gynecol Obstet*. 77:7–14.

Hansen SL, Clark SL, Foster JC. 2002. Active pushing versus passive fetal descent in the second stage of labor: A randomized trial. *Obstet Gynecol*. 99(2):29–34.

Hansen L. 2009. Second-stage labor care: challenges in spontaneous bearing down. *J Perinat Neonatal Nurs.* Jan–Mar; 23(1):31–9; quiz 40–1.

Healthy beginnings: Guidelines for care during pregnancy and childbirth. 1998. SOGC Clinical Practice Guidelines. *J Soc Obstet Gynaecol Can*; 20:52–8.

Hofmeyr GJ, Kulier R. 1996. Tocolysis for preventing fetal distress in second stage of labour. *Cochrane Database Syst Rev* Issue 1. Art. No.: CD000037. DOI: 10.1002/14651858.CD000037

NICE Clinical Guidelines, No: 55. 2007. *Intrapartum Care: Care of Healthy Women and their Babies during Childbirth*. London: RCOG Press

Johanson RB, Menon V. 1998. Vacuum extraction versus forceps for assisted vaginal delivery. *Cochrane Database Syst Rev*. Issue 4. Art. No.: CD000224. DOI: 10.1002/14651858.CD000224

Johanson RB, Heycock E, Carter J et al. 1999. Maternal and child health after assisted vaginal delivery: five-year follow up of a randomised controlled study comparing forceps and ventouse. *Br J Obstet Gynaecol* Jun; 106(6):544–9.

Janni W, Schiessl B, Peschers U, Huber S et al. 2002. The prognostic impact of a prolonged second stage of labor on maternal and fetal outcome. *Acta Obstet Gynecol Scand*. 81: 214–21.

Kadar N, Cruddas M, Campbell S. 1986. Estimating the probability of spontaneous delivery conditional on time spent in second stage. *Br J Obstet Gynaecol*. 93:568–76.

Lai CY. Cheung HW, His Lao TT, Lao TK, Leung TY. 2009. Is the policy of restrictive episiotomy generalisable? A prospective observational study. *J Matern Fetal Neonatal Med*. Dec; 22(12): 1116–21.

Lu MC, Muthengi E, Wakeel F, Fridman M, Korst LM, Gregory KD. 2009. Prolonged second stage of labor and postpartum hemorrhage. *J Matern Fetal Neonatal Med*. 22(3), 227–32.

Maltau JM, Anderson HT. 1975. Epidural analgesia as an alternative to caesarean section in the treatment of prolonged, exhaustive labor. *Acta Anaesth. Scand*. 19: 349–354.

Merhi ZO, Awonuga AO. 2005. The role of uterine fundal pressure in the management of the second stage of labor: a reappraisal. *Obstet Gynecol Surv*. Sep; 60(9):599–603.

Melchior J, Bernard N. 1991. Second-stage fetal heart rate patterns. In: *Fetal monitoring*. Eds.: Spencer J.A.D. Oxford University Press, 155–158.

Mayberry LJ, Wood S, Strange L, Lee L, Heisler D, Neilsen-Smith K. 2000. *Second stage of labor management: promotion of evidence-based practice and a collaborative approach to patient care*. Washington: AWHONN:1–30.

McKay S, Roberts J. 1990. Obstetrics by Ear: Maternal and caregiver perceptions of the Meaning of Maternal Sounds during second stage of Labor. *Journal of Nurse-Midwifery* 35: 266–273.

Menticoglou SM. 1992. How long should the second stage of labor be allowed to last? *J Soc Obstet Gynaecol Can*. 14(7): 77–9.

Menticoglou SM, Manning F, Harman C, Morrison I. 1995. Perinatal outcome in relation to the second-stage duration. *Am J Obstet Gynecol*. 173(3 Part1): 906–12.

Murphy D. 2001. Failure to progress in the second stage of labor. *Current Opinion in Obstetrics and Gynecology* Dec (Vol 13) Issue 6, 557–61.

Murphy DJ, Liebling RE, Verity L, et al. 2001. Early maternal and neonatal morbidity associated with operative delivery in second stage of labour: a cohort study. *Lancet*. Oct 13; 358 (9289):1203–7.

Myles TD, Santolaya J. 2003. Maternal and neonatal outcomes in patients with a prolonged second stage. *Obstet Gynecol* 102(1):52–8.

Naime Alix AF, Fourquet F, Sigue D, Potin J, Descriaud C, Perrotin F. 2008. How long can we wait at full dilatation. A study of maternal and neonatal morbidity related to the duration of the second stage of labor in nulliparous women. *J Gynecol Obstet Biol reprod (Paris)* May; 37(3):268–75.

Paterson CM, Saunders NS, Wadsworth J. 1992. The characteristics of the second stage of labour in 25,069 singleton deliveries in the North West Thames Health Region. *Br J Obstet Gynaecol*. 99:377–80.

Piquard F, Schaefer A, Hsiung R, Dellenbach P, Haberey P. 1989. Are there two biological parts in the second stage of labor? *Acta Obstet Gynecol Scand*. 68:713–18.

RCOG. 2005. Operative vaginal delivery, Green top guidelines Royal College of Gynaecologists, www.rcog.org.uk.

Roberts J. 2003. A new understanding of the second stage of labor: implications for nursing care. *J Obstet Gynecol Neonatal Nurs*. 32(6):794–801.

Roberts CL, Algert CS, Cameron CA, Torvaldsen S. 2005. A meta-analysis of upright positions in the second stage to reduce instrumental deliveries in women with epidural analgesia. *Acta Obstet Gynecol Scand*. Aug; 84(8):794–8.

Rouse DJ, Weiner SJ, Bloom SL et al 2009. Second stage labor duration in nulliparous women: relationship to maternal and perinatal outcomes. *Am J Obstet Gynecol* Oct. 201(4):337–8.

Saunders NS, Paterson CM, Wadsworth J. 1992. Neonatal and maternal morbidity in relation to the length of the second stage of labour. *Br J Obstet Gynaecol*. 99:381–5.

Schmitz T, Meunier E. 2008. Interventions during labor for reducing instrumental deliveries. *J Gynecol Obstet Biol Reprod (Paris)* Dec; 37 Suppl 8:s179–87.

Schnider SM, Abboud TK, Artal R, Henriksen EH, et al. 1983. Maternal catecholamines decrease during labor after lumbar epidural anesthesia. *Am. J. Obstet. Gynecol*. Sep 1,147:1 13–15.

Simkin P, Ancheta R. 2000. *Labor progress handbook: early interventions to prevent and treat dystocia*. Oxford: Blackwell Science.

Simpson K R; Knox G E. 2001. Fundal pressure during the second stage of labor. *The American Journal of Maternal Child Nursing*; 26(2):64–70; quiz 71.

Simpson KR, James DC. 2005. Effects of immediate versus delayed pushing during second-stage labor on fetal well being. *Nurs Res*. 54(3):149–57.

Sizer AR, Evans J, Bailey SM, Wiener J. 2000. A second-stage partogram. *Obstet Gynecol*, Nov; 96(5 Pt 1):678–83.

Sleep J. 1990. Spontaneous delivery in Alexander J, Levy V, Roch S (eds) *Intrapartum care: a research-based approach*. Hampshire and London: Macmillan Education www.sog.com.

Villar J, Carroli G, Zavaleta N, et al. 2007. Maternal and neonatal individual risks and benefits associated with caesarean delivery: multicentre prospective study. *Br Med J.* Nov 17; 335(7628):1025. Epub 2007 Oct 30.

Wheeler TL II, Richter HE. 2007. Delivery method, anal sphincter tears and fecal incontinence: new information on a persistent problem. *Curr Opin Obstet Gynecol* Oct. 19(5):474–9.

Yildirim G, Beji Nk. 2008. Effects of pushing techniques in birth on mother and fetus: a randomized study. *Birth* Mar; 35(1):31–2.

# CHAPTER 10

# OPERATIVE VAGINAL DELIVERY

*Cruz Winston Justin and Tulika Singh*

## Introduction

The history of the obstetrical forceps is long and interesting. Sanskrit writings from 1500 BC contain evidence of single and paired instruments. Egyptian, Greek, Roman and Persian writings and pictures refer to forceps that were originally used for extraction following fetal demise to save the mother's life. The credit for the invention of the precursor of the modern forceps goes to Peter Chamberlain of England (1600). It was kept a family secret for more than a century. The use of a 'secret' instrument to help deliver the baby when labour went wrong elevated the status of the Chamberlain family to royal obstetricians (Speert 1960). Nearly 400 years on, there are more than 700 varieties of forceps (Gei and Belfort 1999). More recently, refined versions of the obstetric vacuum, initially described by Malmström in 1956, have gained popularity over forceps (Johanson and Menon 2000a). A variety of devices are now available to the modern obstetrician.

The frequency of operative vaginal deliveries is estimated to be 10 per cent of all vaginal deliveries. Currently, most of these are vacuum deliveries, with forceps deliveries comprising less than 3 per cent of total deliveries (Meniru 1996).

## Instrument types

### Ventouse/vacuum extractor

The ventouse consists of a cup which is applied to the fetal head and is connected via a tube to a device which creates vacuum (Figs 10.1 and 10.2). The vacuum allows the operator to provide traction to the fetal head in the axis of the birth canal, thus effecting delivery. They are of two types – the soft cup and the rigid cup. Rigid cups are more likely to achieve vaginal delivery but are also more likely to cause scalp trauma as compared to a soft cup (Johanson and Menon 2000a). Bird innovatively attached the suction tubing to the side of the cup, allowing it to slide into position in the occipito-transverse (OT) and the occipito-posterior (OP) fetal positions. The OP cup is also known as the 'Bird cup'. More recently, a disposable hand-held device (the Kiwi system) has gained popularity. Random-allocation studies show that this device has a comparable safety profile, but is less successful than conventional ventouse in achieving vaginal delivery (Attilakos et al 2005, Groom et al 2006).

## Forceps

All forceps share the same basic design. They are a paired instrument with a handle, shank, lock and blade. The blades usually have a pelvic curve and a cephalic curve (Fig. 10.3). Various versions differ from each other by features like blade length, fenestration, type of lock and the presence or absence of pelvic curve.

Forceps may be broadly divided into those used for non-rotational deliveries (Neville Barnes, Simpsons, Piper's, Wrigley's and Naegle) and those used for rotational deliveries (Kielland's, Tucker-McLane). Rotation forceps like the Kielland's have a less pronounced pelvic curve and a sliding (French) lock to correct asynclitism. In contrast, the Neville-Barnes forceps has a more pronounced pelvic curve and a fixed (English) lock.

## Choice of instrument

For most indications, the vacuum and forceps can be used interchangeably. Because of the lower risk of maternal trauma with vacuum, the RCOG (Royal College of Obstetricians and Gynaecologists, UK) recommends that this be the instrument of first choice (Strachan and Murphy 2005). Obstetricians should be intimately familiar with the details and application of both devices. The forceps and metal cup are associated with a higher chance of successful delivery

> Since the ventouse is associated with less maternal trauma this should be the instrument of first choice.

(Johanson and Menon 2000b). The trade-off is a higher risk of maternal injury with forceps and higher chance of fetal injury with the metal cup (O'Mahony et al 2010). Ultimately, the device used depends on the clinical situation, personal preference and operator skills. The relative merits of vacuum delivery over forceps have been the subject of a Cochrane review and are summarised in Table 10.1.

**Table 10.1** Vacuum versus forceps. Summary of Cochrane review (Johanson and Menon 2000a).

| Vacuum extractor compared with forceps is: | Odds ratio | 95% CI |
| --- | --- | --- |
| More likely to fail at achieving vaginal delivery | 1.7 | 1.3–2.2 |
| More likely to be associated with cephalhematoma | 2.4 | 1.7–3.4 |
| More likely to be associated with retinal hemorrhage | 2.0 | 1.3–3.0 |
| Less likely to be associated with perineal trauma | 0.4 | 0.3–0.5 |
| No more likely to be associated with delivery by cesarean section | 0.6 | 0.3–1.0 |
| No more likely to be associated with low 5-minute Apgar scores | 1.7 | 1.0–2.8 |
| No more likely to be associated with the need for phototherapy | 1.1 | 0.7–1.8 |

## Classification of operative vaginal delivery

A classification adapted by the RCOG is presented in Table 10.2. This classifies the delivery according to station and rotation of the fetal head, which often dictates the type of device to use and potential success of delivery (Strachan and Murphy 2004, ACOG 2000).

Table 10.2  Classification for operative vaginal delivery (Source: Strachan and Murphy, 2005)

| Term | Definition |
|---|---|
| Outlet: | Fetal scalp visible without separating the labia<br>Fetal skull has reached the pelvic floor<br>Sagittal suture is in the antero-posterior diameter or right or left occiput anterior or posterior position (rotation does not exceed 45 degrees)<br>Fetal head is at or on the perineum |
| Low: | Leading point of the skull (not caput) is at station plus 2 cm or more and not on the pelvic floor<br>Two subdivisions: (a) rotation of 45 degrees or less (b) rotation more than 45 degrees |
| Mid: | Fetal head is 1/5 palpable per abdomen<br>Leading point of the skull is above station plus 2 cm but not above the ischial spines<br>Two subdivisions (a) rotation of 45 degrees or less (b) rotation more than 45 degrees |
| High: | Not included in classification |

## Indications

The indications for instrumental delivery are often complex and interdependent, for example, fetal malposition leading to prolonged labour and maternal exhaustion. The clinician will need to develop a clinical sense rather than take the indications in Table 10.3 prescriptively. Broadly speaking however, the indications for instrumental deliveries may be divided into maternal and fetal.

> The indications for instrumental delivery are often complex and interdependent.

### Maternal

A prolonged second stage can lead to maternal and fetal compromise. Prolonged second stage is defined as a second stage lasting more than two hours in a primigravida (three hours with epidural) or more than one hour in a multipara (two hours with epidural) (Strachan and Murphy 2005). Assisted delivery is indicated in this situation, unless delivery is imminent. Maternal exhaustion is a common indication for assistance. In women with maternal medical conditions like cardiac disease, myasthenia gravis, and severe hypertensive disease, it is of benefit to shorten the second stage of labour.

Table 10.3  Indications for operative vaginal delivery

| INDICATIONS |
|---|
| Maternal |
| Prolonged second stage<br>Maternal exhaustion<br>Maternal medical conditions<br>    Myasthenia gravis<br>    Cardiac disease<br>    Severe hypertensive disease<br>    Proliferative retinopathy<br>    Cerebral aneurysm |
| Fetal |
| Fetal malposition<br>Suspected fetal compromise<br>Aftercoming head of breech (forceps only) |

### Fetal

Malposition of the fetal head is a common fetal indication. It results from non-rotation or partial rotation of the fetal head from the OP position. Initial steps in management consist of maternal rehydration and oxytocic use after ruling out disproportion. Assistance is given if spontaneous rotation does not happen within the time frame mentioned above or if maternal or fetal compromise supervenes. Suspected fetal compromise in the form of CTG changes or abnormal pH on a fetal blood sample is an indication for instrumental delivery if suitable. Forceps (outlet) or ventouse (hand-held) can be used to deliver the baby's head at cesarean, especially if difficulty is anticipated. The aftercoming head of breech can be delivered using a long shank forceps like Piper's forceps. The historical use of forceps to deliver a preterm infant (to protect the cranium) has not been supported by studies (Fairweather and Stewart 1983).

## Contraindications

Instrumental delivery is not to be attempted before full dilatation. Doing so, carries the risk of severe and serious cervical lacerations. Non-vertex deliveries are also contraindicated with the exception of face (mento-anterior) and the aftercoming head of breech. In both these instances, forceps (not ventouse) can be used. There is no mechanism for delivery of a fetus with mentoposterior position and an instrumental delivery should not be attempted in this situation. Instrumental delivery should not be carried out when the procedure risks injury to the fetus as in pelvic disproportion, fetal mineralisation disorder or coagulopathy. Forceps or ventouse should not be used when the head is palpable abdominally and has not been engaged. The RCOG recommends that ventouse should not be used when the gestation is below 34 weeks because of higher incidence of fetal injuries. There is not enough evidence regarding safety between the gestation of 34 and 36 weeks. Unfamiliarity of the operator with the instrument obviously precludes safe instrumental delivery. Finally and most important, instrumental delivery is not to be attempted when the operator is unsure of fetal position. Intrapartum ultrasound may be used when clinical examination does not clarify fetal position. Table 10.4 summarises the contraindications.

> Instrumental delivery should not be attempted before full dilatation.

**Table 10.4** Contraindications to operative vaginal delivery

| CONTRAINDICATIONS |
|---|
| Less than full dilation |
| Fetal bleeding disorders |
| Osteogenesis imperfecta |
| Risk of neonatal infection (HIV) |
| Mento-posterior position |
| High station (head not engaged) |
| Non vertex presentation (for ventouse) |
| Prematurity (for ventouse) |
| Unsure fetal position |
| Inexperienced operator |

## Technique Prerequisites

The maternal abdomen should be palpated to confirm engagement of the fetal head. Informed consent should be obtained. This has traditionally been verbal. The RCOG has recently published a consent advice for operative vaginal delivery. The intrapartum period can be a minefield as far as legality of the given advice is concerned. This has prompted many experts to advocate the counselling of all pregnant women regarding operative vaginal delivery because as many as 10 per cent of them may need it. Vaginal examination should be performed to confirm full dilatation of the cervix, assess fetal position, caput, moulding and the colour of liquor. The architecture of the pelvis should be assessed to rule out a contracted pelvis. The landmarks assessed are the sacral hollow, prominence of the ischial spines and shape of the subpubic arch. A good operator will take antepartum factors (like diabetes), intrapartum factors (like secondary arrest) and fetal and maternal factors into consideration before deciding when and how to intervene. The membranes should be absent. The maternal bladder should be emptied. If a urinary catheter is in situ, it should be removed or the bulb deflated. Adequate analgesia should be ensured. This can be in the form of regional (epidural or spinal) or local in the form of perineal infiltration with pudendal block. The instrument to be used should be checked prior to commencement of the procedure. A pediatrician or personnel trained in neonatal resuscitation should be present for all instrumental deliveries, to resuscitate the baby if needed and to examine the baby for birth injuries. Table 10.5 summarises the prerequisites for instrumental delivery.

> A pediatrician or personnel trained in neonatal resuscitation should be present for all instrumental deliveries

**Table 10.5** Pre-requisites for operative vaginal delivery

| PRE-REQUISITES |
| --- |
| Informed consent |
| Engaged head |
| Cervix fully dilated and membranes ruptured |
| Adequate pelvis |
| Vertex presenting |
| Fetal position known |
| Analgesia |
| Bladder empty |
| Aseptic technique |
| Episiotomy if risk of perineal laceration |
| Experienced staff |
| Facilities for cesarean delivery and neonatal resuscitation |
| Willingness to abandon procedure if needed. |

## Ventouse delivery

The woman is placed in lithotomy and analgesia ensured. Crucial to the success of ventouse delivery is the placement of the centre of the cup at the 'flexion point'. This is a point on the saggital suture, 3 cm anterior to the posterior fontanelle. Extreme care should be taken to avoid placement directly over the fontanelle. Correct application promotes flexion and synclitism of the fetal head and promotes delivery. Incorrect or paramedian applications are a common reason for failure and cup detachments ('pop-offs').

> - Placement directly over the fontanelle should be avoided.
> - Incorrect or paramedian applications are a common reason for failure and cup detachments

After the cup is applied, the vacuum is initially set at 0.2 kg/cm$^2$ and a vaginal examination is carried out to confirm that the cup is free of the cervix. Once this is confirmed, the suction is turned up to the operating pressure of 0.6 to 0.8 kg/cm$^2$ (60 to 80 kPa/ 500 to 800 cm H$_2$0). An effective chignon (false caput) is formed in two minutes and it is not necessary to wait for longer before commencing traction. In the past, it was recommended that the vacuum pressure be applied slowly and incrementally, at intervals of two minutes till a pressure of 0.8 kg/cm$^2$ was achieved in approximately 8–10 minutes. This was considered to reduce failure rates by allowing for a firmer application of the cup to the fetal head. However, a randomised control trial of 94 women, comparing stepwise versus rapid pressure application, demonstrated that the rapid technique was associated with a significant reduction in the duration of vacuum extraction by an average of 6 minutes without adversely impacting fetal and maternal outcome (Lim 1997).

The operator then uses the dominant hand to provide traction, while the non-dominant hand steadies the cup with the index and middle fingers on the fetal scalp and the thumb on the cup. Traction is applied perpendicular to the cup, changing direction as the head descends. Angular traction is avoided as it leads to cup detachments and 'cookie-cutter' injures to the fetal scalp. Where the fetal head is in the occiput-transverse or occiput-posterior position, autorotation occurs with traction.

It is vital to avoid rotation traction when using the ventouse. Rocking movements or torque should not be applied to the device; only steady traction in the line of the birth canal should be used (FDA Public Health Advisory 1998). Traction is given with uterine contractions and maternal efforts. Traction should be discontinued when the contraction ends and the mother stops pushing. Descent of the vertex should occur with each application of traction. Once crowning of the fetal head occurs, the suction should be released, the cup removed, and the remainder of the delivery done in the normal fashion.

> Rocking movements or torque should not be applied to the device; only steady traction in the line of the birth canal should be used

The upper limits of safety are not known, but a traction force of 23 kg is accepted as the maximum. Traction force varies with cup size, suction pressure, and the clinical situation. Therefore, it is reasonable and practical to rely on the suction pressure that is displayed on all commercially available devices (Ali and Norwitz 2009).

Unless fetal compromise is suspected, it is important to deliver the fetal head slowly, allowing the perineum to stretch and minimise tears. A modified Ritgen manoeuvre may also be used to minimise perineal trauma.

Attempts at delivery should be halted when there is no descent of the fetal head with 3 pulls. Murphy et al (2001), in an observational study of 393 singleton term pregnancies, found that 82 per cent of successful deliveries were achieved within 1 to 3 pulls, and more than 3 pulls was associated with a 45 per cent risk of neonatal trauma.

> Most successful deliveries are achieved within 1 to 3 pulls, and more than 3 pulls are associated with risk of neonatal trauma.

Ventouse delivery should also be stopped if there is suspicion of fetal injury. Observational studies have shown that nearly all successful vacuum deliveries happen within 15 minutes of commencing the procedure. The risk of fetal injury increases with prolonged operative times. The total vacuum application time should be limited to 20 to 30 minutes (ACOG 2000). Thus, if fetal descent and delivery has not occurred within 20 to 30 minutes and within 3 pulls, the procedure should be abandoned and the baby delivered by cesarean section. This is good clinical practice and is based on common sense, as observational series have shown no long-term differences in neonatal outcome based on these variables (Greenberg 2010).

## Forceps delivery

After placing the woman in the lithotomy position and performing a pelvic examination, the operator checks the forceps blades to check if they are of the same pair and lock easily. After checking the fetal position, by convention, the left blade is applied first. The left blade is in relation to the maternal left. Two or more fingers of the right hand are introduced inside the left posterior portion of the vagina, sliding in between the fetal head and the vaginal wall. The left blade is grasped between the thumb and two fingers of the left hand. The tip of the blade is then gently passed into the vagina between the fetal head and the palmar surface of the right hand and smoothly guided into the sacral hollow. A good clinical tip is to move the handle through a wide arc while slipping the blade behind the fetal head. Care should be taken not to exert unnecessary pressure or to force the blade into the vagina.

Similarly, for the application of the right blade, two or more fingers of the left hand are introduced into the right and posterior part of the vagina, to guard the maternal soft tissues and serve as guides for the right blade, which is held by the operator's right hand. With proper application, the saggital suture of the fetal skull lies in the midline of the blades, the blades are symmetrical, application and locking are smooth. Difficulty with locking signifies asymmetrical application on the fetal head and can cause fetal injuries.

> **Identifying the right and left blades:**
>
> With the patient in the lithotomy position, the blade will be applied with the pelvic curve directed anteriorly and the cephalic curve directed medially.
>
> The forceps can be articulated and held in front of the perineum in the position that the blades will be applied. This makes it easy to identify the left blade from the right.

> **Proper application of forceps:**
> - the saggital suture of the fetal skull lies in the midline of the blades
> - the blades are symmetrical
> - application and locking are smooth.

The operator then ensures there is no maternal tissue between the blades. The operator should be seated in front of the patient, with elbows pressed against the sides of the body. To avoid excessive force during traction, the force should be exerted only through the wrist and forearms. The dominant hand grips the shanks and exerts a downward pull (Pajot's manoeuvre), thus following the J-shaped pelvic curve, or curve of Carus. The non-dominant hand grips the handles and exerts a pull parallel to the floor. As with the ventouse, delivery of the head should be slow and controlled and combined with the Ritgen manoeuvre.

The operator or an assistant can guard the maternal perineum with a large swab to prevent excess trauma to the perineum. Once the fetal head is delivered, the forceps is removed in reverse order of application ('*first one in, last one out*').

## The role of episiotomy

Traditional teaching is to perform an episiotomy routinely with forceps delivery, and selectively when vacuum is used. This is because forceps are thought to take up extra space around the fetal head and their rigid nature is thought to increase the risk of perineal tears. The evidence, however, is limited and further research is needed on this topic. In a small retrospective series, a mediolateral episiotomy was found to be associated with less third and fourth degree perineal tears (Bodner-Adler et al 2003). Another retrospective study showed that using a midline episiotomy for forceps delivery significantly increased the

> If an episiotomy is indicated, mediolateral is preferred to midline episiotomy to avoid third and fourth degree tears

Operative Vaginal Delivery 177

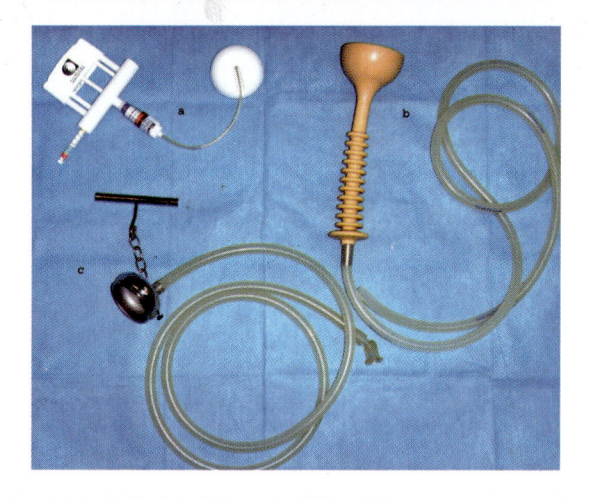

**Figure 10.1** Different types of ventouse. (a) Kiwi® cup with inbuilt hand operated pump, (b) Silastic cup, (c) Bird's OP cup. The latter two need an external vacuum generator shown in Fig. 10.2.

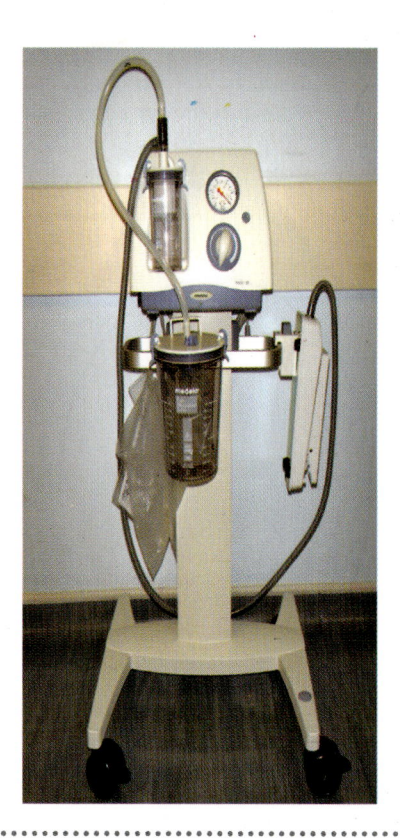

**Figure 10.2** External vacuum generator

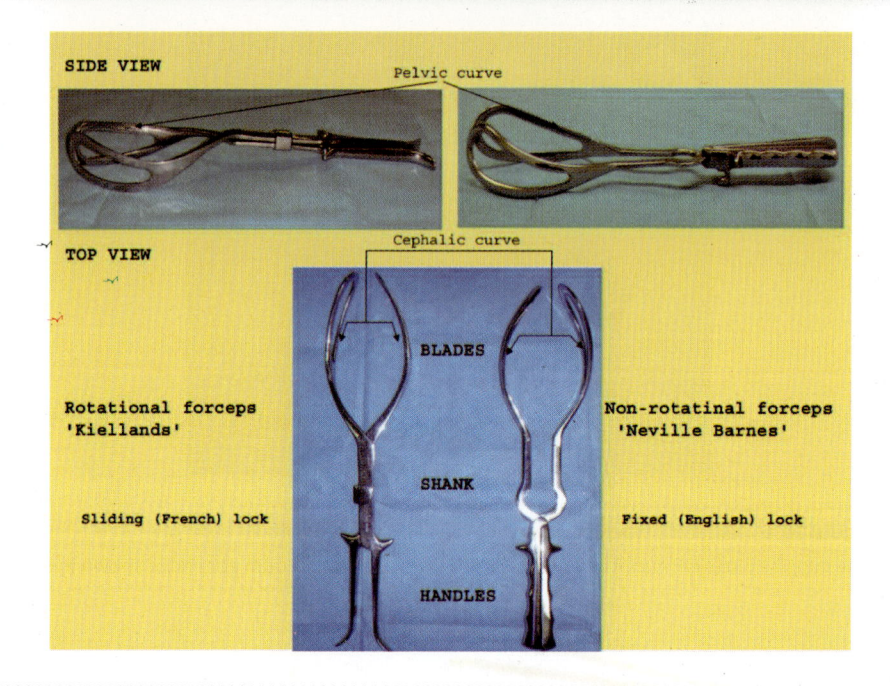

**Figure 10.3** Rotational and non-rotational forceps

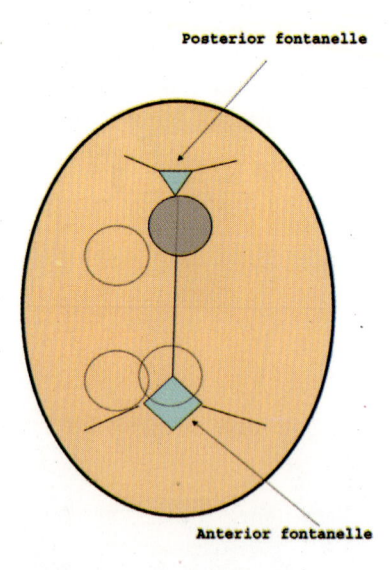

**Figure 10.4** Ventouse cup application. The circle with bold outline shows correct cup placement at the flexion point. The circles with the light outline show incorrect cup placement, which may lead to failure to achieve a delivery.

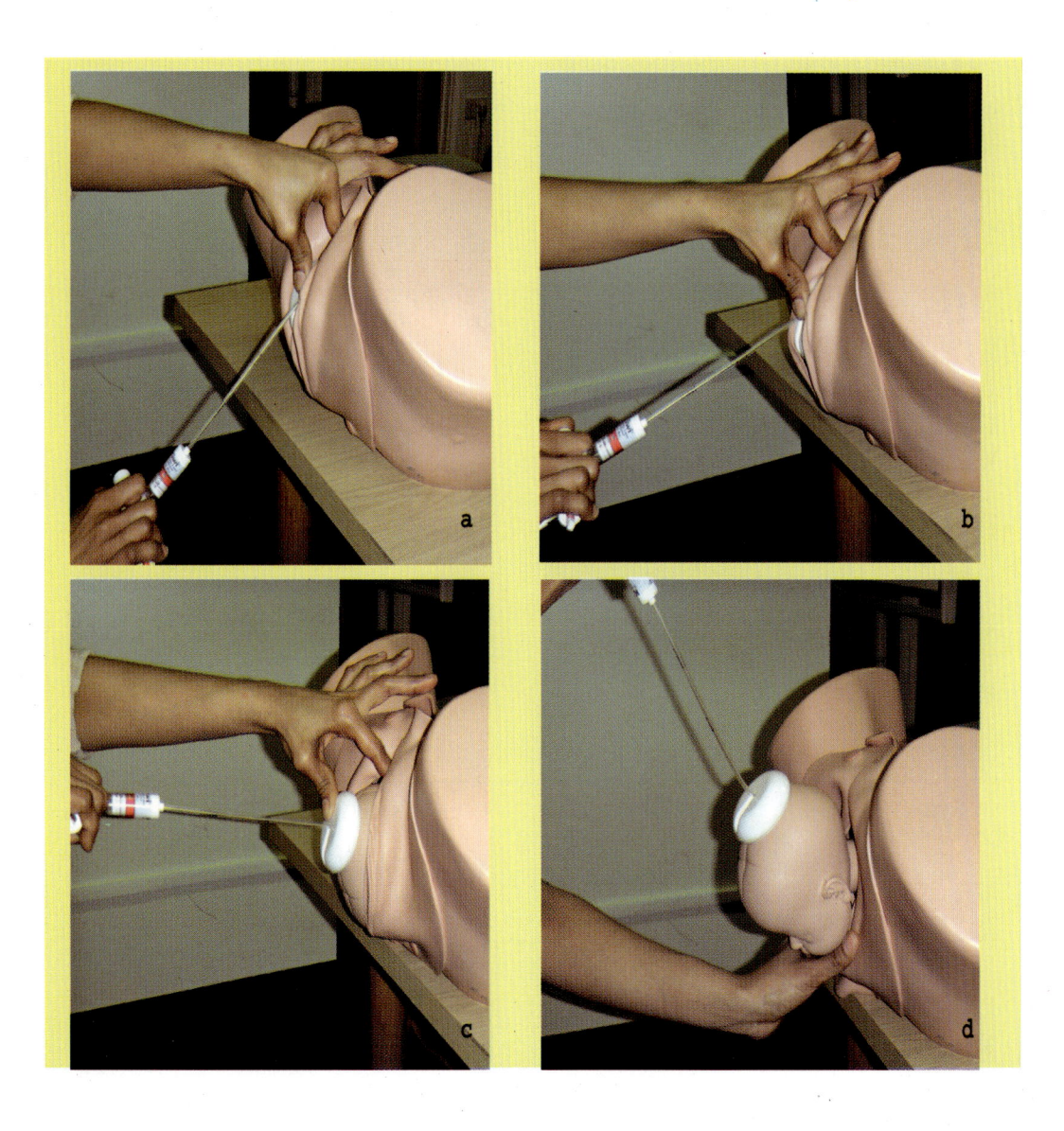

**Figure 10.5** Ventouse delivery: Steps

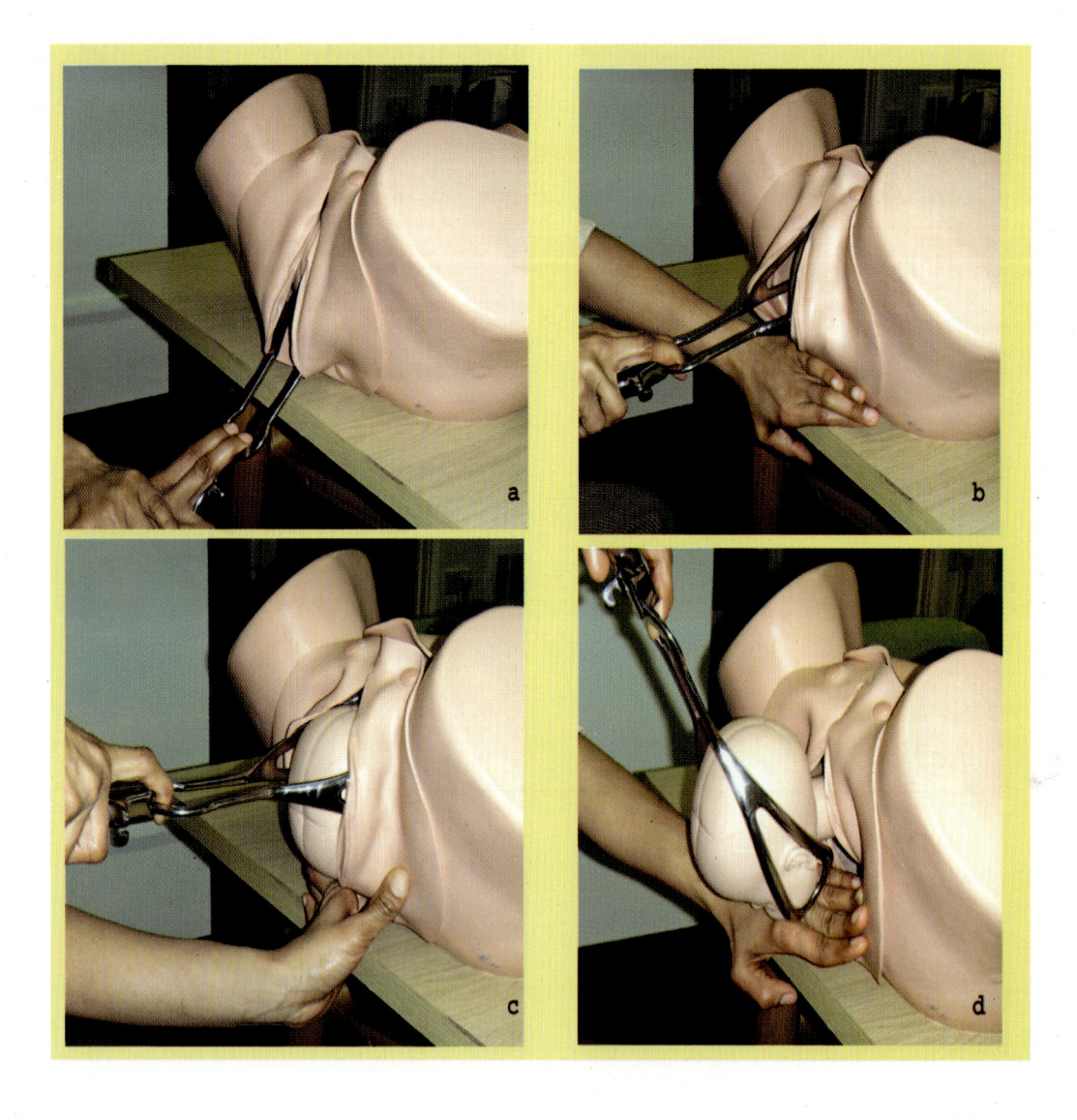

**Figure 10.6** Application of forceps

risk of anal sphincter injury (Kudish et al 2006).

## Rotational instrumental delivery

This can be achieved using either ventouse or rotational forceps like Kielland forceps. The instrument used depends on the choice and expertise of the operator.

Rotational delivery with the Kielland forceps should preferably be carried out by an appropriately trained and experienced operator as its use can be associated with additional risks (Chiswick and James 1979, Chow et al 1987). Alternatively, rotational ventouse or manual rotation followed by traction forceps can be used to achieve delivery in cases of non-OA position of the fetal head (SOGC Clinical practice guideline 2004). In general, vacuum is more likely than forceps to fail when the head is in the mid-cavity (Vacca 1999).

## Sequential use of instruments

The sequential use of instruments leads to an increased risk of trauma to the fetus (Edozien et al 1999). One needs to balance the risks of an emergency cesarean section in the second stage, following failed delivery using vacuum extraction versus forceps application following a failed ventouse extraction. Second stage cesarean sections are known to increase both maternal and perinatal morbidity and mortality (Murphy et al 2001). The RCOG advises that 'the sequential use of instruments should not be attempted by an inexperienced operator without direct supervision and should be avoided wherever possible' (Strachan and Murphy 2005).

> The sequential use of instruments should not be attempted by an inexperienced operator without direct supervision and should be avoided wherever possible

## Trial versus failed instrumental delivery

*Trial of instrumental delivery* refers to an instrumental delivery when vaginal delivery is considered to be difficult or there is a high chance of failure (Lowe 1987). Trial of labour should be carried out in the operating theatre, with facilities for immediate cesarean delivery. Instrumental delivery should be performed in the labour room, only if there is a high chance of successful delivery. Thus, most non-OA, and midcavity instrumental deliveries, where the chance of failure is higher, should be carried out in the operation theatre. *Failed instrumental delivery*, refers to failure to deliver the baby in the labour room, and when the possibility of failure was not considered.

> *Trial of instrumental delivery* is where the chance of failure is expected to be higher. *Failed instrumental* refers to failure to deliver the baby when the possibility of failure was not considered.

Reasons for increased failure rates include maternal body mass index greater than 30, estimated fetal weight > 4000 g or a clinically big baby (Murphy et al 2001). A failed instrumental delivery has great potential to cause panic in both the parturient and staff looking after her. In most obstetric units, failed instrumental would be a risk-management trigger point, whereas failed 'trial' of instrumental is acceptable.

## Post delivery

A good obstetrician will anticipate both *shoulder dystocia* and *uterine atony*, which are common after instrumental births. Prompt implementation of shoulder dystocia drill and use of uterotonics will prevent catastrophic outcomes. The woman should be reassessed for the risk factors of venous thromboembolism and thromboprophylaxis given accordingly (RCOG guideline 37, 2004). A review of the Cochrane database does not reveal much evidence to support routine postnatal antibiotics (Liabsuetrakul et al 2004).

> Shoulder dystocia and uterine atony should be anticipated after instrumental delivery.

> There is not much evidence for routine postnatal antibiotics.

Advice is given to the patient regarding good perineal care. Regular analgesics should be considered in the absence of contraindications. In the postnatal ward, bladder care is vital. It is important to note and record the timing and volume of the first void following delivery (Zaki et al 2004). Regional anesthesia can remove the sensation of bladder filling, leading to overfilling and bladder damage. Leaving an indwelling catheter for all women who have regional anesthesia for instrumental deliveries can prevent this. Pelvic floor physiotherapy has been found to reduce the incidence of urinary incontinence after instrumental delivery (Hay-Smith et al 2008).

## Complications

Complications are common following instrumental delivery and can, on the rare occasion, be serious. However, the risk should be in the context of the alternative, which is cesarean section in the second stage. There is no doubt that the skill of the operator in making a good judgement and skilled choice and use of instruments is pivotal in achieving a safe delivery.

## Fetal morbidity

### Forceps marks

Forceps marks are common, and in most cases, trivial. Rarely, excess pressure and incorrect application can cause serious injury to the fetal soft tissue or cranium.

### Nerve injury

Pressure from the blades can sometimes lead to facial nerve palsy. In most cases, spontaneous resolution occurs (Duval and Daniel 2009). Fetal cervical spine injuries may occur rarely after rotational forceps delivery. Shoulder dystocia is more common in women who undergo instrumental delivery and can be associated with injury to the brachial plexus (Broekhuizen et al 1987).

### Cephalhematoma

A cephalhematoma is a collection of blood under the subperiosteal space. This leads the collection to be confined by the cranial suturelines. They are of little clinical consequence and resolve spontaneously. They can sometimes be associated with neonatal jaundice because of the breakdown of the collected blood. A cephalhematoma is more likely to occur after ventouse as compared to forceps.

### Ocular trauma

Retinal hemorrhage is more common after ventouse application. This does not usually lead to long-term sequelae. Eyelid or eye trauma is an uncommon result of incorrect forceps application. Wrong application of the ventouse to the face can injure facial soft tissue.

### Intracranial hemorrhage

Intracranial hemorrhage is more common in babies delivered after the onset of labour, whatever be the mode of delivery. Rarely, it results from a bleeding tendency of the baby or poor application of the instrument.

### Subgaleal/subaponeurotic hemorrhage

This is a potentially serious injury with a mortality rate of 14 per cent to 20 per cent. It can occur after ventouse, forceps, or more uncommonly after normal birth. Prompt diagnosis and treatment are vital as delays may lead to cardiovascular collapse in the newborn infant (Vacca 2000).

## Maternal morbidity

### Perineal and cervical tears and lacerations

Perineal and cervical lacerations are more common with the use of forceps compared to vacuum, regardless of whether an episiotomy is used or not (Christianson et al 2003). Rotational forceps can lead to spiral tears of the vagina. The role of episiotomy, as mentioned before, is unclear. It is important to allow the head to distend the perineum slowly and perform a controlled delivery. The same precaution should be taken during the delivery of the shoulders. The operator should actively check for perineal and cervical tears by performing both a vaginal and rectal examination and then carefully repair any injuries.

### Urinary and fecal incontinence

Damage to the pelvic floor (levator ani) or the anal sphincter during birth can lead to urinary and fecal incontinence. The damage can be mechanical or because of pudendal denervation. Traumatic vaginal delivery is considered to be the most important risk factor for fecal incontinence in women and may occur not only after recognised third-degree perineal tears, but also after apparently non-traumatic vaginal birth (Sultan and Thakar 2002). The incidence of such damage is increased by intervention with any instrument, rising from an approximate baseline incidence of 10 per cent to 25 per cent following ventouse and 40 per cent following forceps. Studies using endo–anal ultrasonography have shown that persisting sphincter defects are the main cause of fecal incontinence and not, as was previously believed, unrecognised neurological damage. Correct identification and proper repair of anal sphincter injuries along with pelvic floor physiotherapy can prevent long-term problems.

### Psychological trauma

Some women can be psychologically traumatised by an instrumental birth (Astbury et al 1994). It takes a woman and her partner away from the privacy of her birthing room to the often scary and undignified operation theatre. If this is compounded by the need for neonatal resuscitation, the result is often a traumatic birth experience leading to postnatal depression and requests for cesarean birth in subsequent pregnancies. It is important to debrief the new mother before discharge, and in some complicated births, it is important to offer postnatal support and follow up.

## Training issues

A lack of training, reduction in working time and fear of litigation have contributed to an explosion in the rates of cesarean section and reduction in rates of instrumental deliveries in recent times. Extensive media and literature documentation of the rare adverse outcome have made many UK units ban the use of Kielland's rotational forceps (Chiswick and James 1979). It is vital that in the present environment, an intervention that is associated with some fetal and maternal morbidity is carried out either by an expert or a well-supervised trainee. In addition to bedside training, courses like the ALSO (Advanced Life Support in Obstetrics) and MOET (Management of Obstetric Emergencies and Trauma) use mannequins to teach the practical aspects of operative vaginal delivery. The future lies in the use of computer-based simulators which will provide computer-assisted feedback on the acquisition of technical skills. In the meantime, OSATS (Objective Structured Assessment of Technical Skills) will continue to be used in the US, UK and other countries to assess progress in training and certify competence.

## Risk management

Operative vaginal delivery is associated with fetal and maternal morbidity. Complaints and litigation are far too common following an operative birth that goes wrong. Common allegations include poor indication for intervention, improper choice of instrument, excessive use of force, lack of information and poor supervision. Attempts should be made to reduce the rates of instrumental deliveries by interventions like companionship in labour, enhanced mobility, avoidance of regional analgesia, maternal hydration and prudent oxytocic use.

**Table 10.6** Information to be included in a proforma for documentation after operative delivery.

| |
|---|
| Name of person carrying out procedure with designation |
| Consent |
| Abdominal examination finding – fifths palpable |
| Vaginal examination findings – position, station, caput, moulding, liquor |
| Assessment of maternal pelvis adequacy |
| Fetal heart rate |
| Contractions |
| Ease of application of device |
| Degree of traction |
| Number of pulls |
| Number of detachments |
| Duration of procedure |
| Estimated blood loss |
| Swab counts |
| Condition of baby including APGAR |
| Perineal (including rectal) examination |
| Umbilical cord pH |
| Details of repair |
| Post procedure analgesia and thromboprophylaxis |

The training of obstetricians in the art of instrumental vaginal delivery is of crucial importance if we are to reduce the rates of emergency cesarean section in the second stage of labour and achieve a safe and successful vaginal delivery. Practical procedures can be learnt using suitably designed mannequins under directed supervision, but only practice in a 'real' labour ward environment will enable these skills to mature. Further, good record-keeping is important for educational, clinical audit, risk management and medico-legal purposes. Good documentation is vital to any operative delivery and can prove to be invaluable in cases of medico-legal action to build up a defence. Each hospital should have its own protocol/proforma which ensures uniformity and completion of documentation (Agrawal et al 2004). Table 10.6 lists the points to include in a pre-printed proforma.

## Conclusion

The art of operative vaginal birth is an essential skill for every obstetrician. A good instrumental delivery involves adequate case selection, counselling, proper choice of instrument, good execution and aftercare. A skilled operative delivery often means the difference between a good and a bad outcome and birth experience. Although the ventouse remains the more popular device of the two, it remains crucial that practitioners are trained, skilled and comfortable with the use of both vacuum and forceps. Finally, the importance of clear, legible and complete documentation cannot be overemphasised.

## References

Agrawal A, Ghosh S, Lennox CE. 2004. Pre-printed format improves recording of instrumental vaginal delivery. *Clinical Governance: An International Journal*. 9: 91–95.

Ali UA, Norwitz E. 2009. Vacuum-Assisted Vaginal Delivery. *Rev Obstet Gynecol*. Winter; 2(1): 5–17.

American College of Obstetricians and Gynecologists. 2000. Operative Vaginal Delivery: Use of forceps and vacuum extractors for operative vaginal delivery. *ACOG Practice Bulletin* no. 17, June 2000.

Astbury J, Brown S, Lumley J, Small R. 1994. Birth events, birth experiences and social differences in postnatal depression. *Aust J Public Health*. 18(2): 176–84.

Attilakos G, Sibanda T, Winter C, Johnson N, Draycott T. 2005. A randomised controlled trial of a new handheld vacuum extraction device. *Br J Obstet Gynaecol*. Nov; 112 (11):1510–5.

Bodner-Adler B, Bodner K, Kimberger O, Wagenbichler P, Mayerhofer K. 2003 Management of the perineum during forceps delivery. Association of episiotomy with the frequency and severity of perineal trauma in women undergoing forceps delivery. *J Reprod Med*. Apr; 48(4):239–42.

Broekhuizen FF, Washington JM, Johnson F, Hamilton PR. 1987. Vacuum extraction versus forceps delivery: indications and complications, 1979 to 1984. *Obstet Gynecol*. 69(3 Pt 1):338–42.

Chiswick ML, James DK. 1979. Kielland's forceps: association with neonatal morbidity and mortality. *British Medical Journal*. 1:7–8.

Chow SL, Johnson CM, Anderson TD, Hughes JH. 1987. Rotational delivery with Kielland's forceps. *Med J Aust*; 146:616–9.

Christianson LM, Bovbjerg VE, McDavitt EC, Hullfish KL. 2003. Risk factors for perineal injury during delivery. *Am J Obstet Gynecol*. 189(1):255–60.

Duval M, Daniel SJ. 2009. Facial nerve palsy in neonates secondary to forceps use. *Arch Otolaryngol Head Neck Surg*. 135 (7): 634–6.

Edozien LC, Williams JL, Chatterjee IC, Hirsch PJ. 1999. Failed instrumental delivery: how safe is the use of a second instrument? *J Obstet Gynaecol*. 19(5): 460–2.

Fairweather DI, Stewart AI. 1983. How to deliver the under 1500-gram infant. *Reid's Controversy in Obstetrics and Gynaecology* III, 154.

FDA Public Health Advisory. 1998. Need for caution when using vacuum-assisted delivery devices. Center for Devices and Radiological Health., Available at http://www.fda.gov/cdrh/fetal598.html.

Gei AF, Belfort MA. 1999. Forceps-assisted vaginal delivery. *Obstet Gynecol Clin North Am*. 26:345–70.

Greenberg JA. 2010. Procedure for vacuum assisted operative vaginal delivery. UpToDate Web site. http://www.uptodate.com/patients/content/topic.do?topicKey=~cWABY9RJfJlwne.

Groom KM, Jones BA, Miller N, Paterson-Brown S. 2006. A prospective randomised controlled trial of the Kiwi Omnicup versus conventional ventouse cups for vacuum-assisted vaginal delivery. *Br J Obstet Gynaecol*. 113(2):183–9.

Hay-Smith J, Mørkved S, Fairbrother KA, Herbison GP. 2008. Pelvic floor muscle training for prevention and treatment of urinary and faecal incontinence in antenatal and postnatal women. *Cochrane Database Syst Rev*. 8; (4).

Johanson RB, Menon BK. 2000a. Vacuum extraction versus forceps for assisted vaginal delivery.*Cochrane Database Syst Rev*.(2): CD000224.

Johanson R, Menon V. 2000b. Soft versus rigid vacuum extractor cups for assisted vaginal delivery. *Cochrane Database Syst Rev*. (2): CD000446.

Kudish B, Blackwell S, Mcneeley SG, Bujold E, Kruger M, Hendrix SL, Sokol R. 2006. Operative vaginal delivery and midline episiotomy: a bad combination for the perineum. *Am J Obstet Gynecol*. Sep; 195(3): 749–54.

Liabsuetrakul T, Choobun T, Peeyananjarassri K, Islam M. 2004. Antibiotic prophylaxis for operative vaginal delivery. *Cochrane Database Syst Rev*. (2).

Lim FT, Holm JP, Schuitemaker NW, et al. 1997. Stepwise compared with rapid application of vacuum in ventouse extraction procedures. *Br J Obstet Gynaecol*. 104:33–36.

Lowe B.1987. Fear of failure: a place for the trial of instrumental delivery. *Br J Obstet Gynaecol*. 94(1):60–6.

Meniru GI. 1996. An analysis of recent trends in vacuum extraction and forceps delivery in the United Kingdom. *Br J Obstet Gynaecol*. 103(2):168–70.

Murphy DJ, Liebling RE, Verity L, Swingler R, Patel R. 2001. Early maternal and neonatal morbidity associated with operative delivery in second stage of labour: A cohort study. *Lancet*. 358:1203–7.

O'Mahony F, Hofmeyr GJ, Menon V. 2010. Choice of instruments for assisted vaginal delivery. *Cochrane Database Syst Rev*. Nov 10; 11: CD005455.

Royal College of Obstetricians and Gynaecologists. 2004. Thromboprophylaxis During Pregnancy, Labour and after Vaginal Delivery. Guideline No. 37. London: RCOG.

SOGC Clinical Practice Guideline No 148, August 2004. Guidelines for operative vaginal birth. *J Obstet Gynaecol Can*. 26:747–53.

Strachan BM, Murphy DJ. 2004. *Operative vaginal delivery*. Guideline no 26. Royal College of Obstetricians and Gynaecologists, London.

Speert H. 1960. The obstetric forceps. *Clin Obstet Gynecol*. Sep; 3:761–6.

Sultan AH, Thakar R. 2002. Lower genital tract and anal sphincter trauma. *Best Pract Res Clin Obstet Gynaecol*. 16(1):99–115.

Vacca A. 1999. The trouble with vacuum extraction. *Curr Obstet* Gynaecol; 9:41–5.

Vacca A. 2000. Sub-aponeurotic haemorrhage: a rare but life-threatening neonatal complication associated with ventouse delivery. *Br J Obstet Gynaecol*. 107(3):433.

Zaki MM, Pandit M, Jackson S. 2004. National survey for intrapartum and postpartum bladder care: assessing the need for guidelines. *Br J Obstet Gynaecol*. 111:874–6.

# CHAPTER 11

# SHOULDER DYSTOCIA

*VP Paily and K Ambujam*

Despite its low incidence, shoulder dystocia is a worrisome obstetric emergency due to its unpredictability and its potential for fetal and maternal morbidity. Because of the gravity and unexpectedness of the situation, it has long been a major area of obstetric concern. Pecorari (1999) calls it a 'nightmare of modern midwifery.' The most common serious complication following delivery with shoulder dystocia is brachial plexus injury which causes significant lifelong disability. The reported incidence of brachial plexus injury after shoulder dystocia varies widely from 4 per cent to 40 per cent (Doumouchtsis and Arulkumaran 2009).

Gurewitsch (2007) states that clinically relevant and permanent brachial plexus injury is almost universally associated with shoulder dystocia; the injury is caused by the mechanical stresses that occur during shoulder dystocia delivery. However, brachial plexus injuries evident at birth may occur even in the absence of shoulder dystocia and in the absence of traction to the fetal head. One to four per cent of brachial plexus injuries may occur after a cesarean section; a significant proportion occur in utero (Doumouchtsis and Arulkumaran 2009).

A good clinical indicator of shoulder dystocia, is when there is retraction of the delivered fetal head against the maternal perineum ('turtle sign'), immediately after delivery

## Definition

Shoulder dystocia is the failure of delivery of the fetal shoulder(s), whether they are the anterior, posterior, or both fetal shoulders (Pecorari 1999). It has been defined as a delivery that requires additional obstetric manoeuvres following failure of gentle downward traction on the fetal head to effect delivery of the shoulders (Resnik 1980). Spong et al (1995) proposed defining shoulder dystocia as a prolonged head-to-body delivery interval of more than 60 seconds or the need for ancillary obstetric manoeuvres to complete delivery of the shoulders.

> Shoulder dystocia is a delivery that requires additional obstetric manoeuvres following failure of gentle downward traction on the fetal head to effect delivery of the shoulders.

Shoulder dystocia is caused by impaction of the fetal anterior shoulder behind the maternal pubic symphysis. This results from a size discrepancy between the fetal shoulders and the pelvic inlet, either due to macrosomia or due to persistent anteroposterior location of the fetal shoulders as in precipitate labour (Gherman et al 2006). It must be remembered that an arbitrary upper limit of fetal weight is not as important as the morphological distribution of fat, resulting in a larger trunk and chest along with larger shoulders (Kitzmiller et al 1987). Less commonly, it can also result from impaction of the posterior shoulder on the sacral promontory (Gherman 2002).

> Shoulder dystocia is caused by:
> - Impaction of the shoulder behind the maternal pubic symphysis
> - Size discrepancy between the fetal shoulders and the pelvic inlet

## Incidence

There is wide variation in the reported incidence of shoulder dystocia, partly because of clinical variation in diagnosing shoulder dystocia due to lack of a precise definition. This may also be due partially to the anthropometric differences between the populations studied. The reported incidence ranges from 0.6 per cent to 1.4 per cent of vaginal births (ACOG 2002).

## Risk factors

A number of antenatal and intrapartum characteristics have been reported to be associated with shoulder dystocia.

### Antepartum risk factors

*Macrosomia*: Macrosomia at birth is the factor most strongly associated with shoulder dystocia and the incidence of shoulder dystocia is proportional to birth weight (Acker et al 1985). Many of the other risk factors such as maternal obesity, maternal diabetes, prolonged pregnancy and previous large infant predispose to macrosomia, and hence, lead to shoulder dystocia (Gross et al 1987). Although fetal macrosomia and maternal diabetes increase the risk of shoulder dystocia, a considerable proportion of cases occur among women who do not have diabetes and among infants with birth weights less than 4000 g (ACOG 2002). Only 50 per cent to 60 per cent of cases of shoulder dystocia occur in infants weighing >4000 g or in diabetic mothers (Acker et al 1985). Elective cesarean section is not recommended solely on the grounds of suspected macrosomia as the cost and number of cesarean sections to prevent one case of permanent injury from shoulder dystocia is high. Further, most cases of shoulder dystocia will not be prevented by this strategy. Gross and

> Antepartum risk factors
> - Fetal macrosomia
> - Diabetes mellitus
> - Previous history of shoulder dystocia
> - Prolonged pregnancy
> - Male fetal gender
> - High maternal body mass index

> Elective cesarean section is not recommended solely on the grounds of suspected macrosomia as the cost and number of cesarean sections to prevent one case of permanent injury from shoulder dystocia is high.

colleagues (1987) showed that if cesarean deliveries were performed for all patients with fetuses that weighed 4000 g or more, there would be a 27 per cent increase in the total cesarean delivery rate with only a 42 per cent reduction of shoulder dystocia cases.

*Maternal diabetes*: Infants of diabetic mothers have a higher incidence of shoulder dystocia compared to infants of the same birth weight of non-diabetic mothers. Macrosomic infants of diabetic mothers have larger shoulder and extremity circumferences, decreased head-to-shoulder ratio, a significantly higher percentage of body fat, and thicker upper extremity skin folds compared with non-diabetic controls of similar birth weight and length (Gherman et al 2006). Elevated maternal plasma glucose and amino acid concentrations cause fetal pancreatic secretion of insulin. Fetal hyperinsulinemia in turn leads to macrosomia by accelerating fuel utilisation and storage in insulin-sensitive fetal tissues like the abdomen and shoulders. Maternal obesity exaggerates the insulin resistance already present in late pregnancy and has an impact on fetal growth and development. However, the means by which maternal obesity by itself promotes the development of macrosomic babies in non-diabetic pregnancies remains poorly defined (Kalkhoff 1991, Robinson et al 2003).

> Macrosomic infants of diabetic mothers have:
> - larger shoulder and extremity circumferences
> - decreased head-to-shoulder ratio
> - significantly higher percentage of body fat
> - thicker upper extremity skin folds

The American College of Obstetricians and Gynecologists (2002) recommends that a planned cesarean delivery to prevent shoulder dystocia may be considered for suspected fetal macrosomia with estimated fetal weights exceeding 5000 g in women without diabetes and 4500 g in women with diabetes. These upper limits of fetal weight may not be applicable to Indian and South-East Asian populations, where the average maternal and fetal weights may be much less than in the Western population.

> A planned cesarean delivery to prevent shoulder dystocia may be considered for suspected fetal macrosomia with estimated fetal weights exceeding 5000 g in women without diabetes and 4500 g in women with diabetes.

*Previous history of shoulder dystocia*: The risk of having a repeat shoulder dystocia is 1 per cent to 16.7 per cent (Baskett and Allen 1995, Ginsberg and Moisidis 2001, Ouzounian et al 2001). If a nulliparous woman in her index pregnancy had shoulder dystocia, she has an increased risk of shoulder dystocia in the next pregnancy (Ginsberg and Moisidis 2001). Other factors that are statistically significant for recurrent shoulder dystocia include maternal pre-pregnancy weight, maternal weight at delivery, the duration of the second stage of labour, birth weight greater than the index pregnancy, and birth weight more than 4000 g (Gherman et al 2006).

A policy of universal elective cesarean delivery has not been recommended in women with prior shoulder dystocia. The American College of Obstetricians and Gynecologists (2002) states that 'because most subsequent deliveries will not be complicated by shoulder dystocia, the benefit of universal elective cesarean delivery is questionable in patients, who have such a history of shoulder dystocia'. Factors that may aid in the decision-making process for mode of delivery include the estimate of fetal weight compared with the prior pregnancy birth weight (both clinically and by ultrasound), the severity of the prior neonatal injury and maternal diabetes. The records of the previous delivery should be reviewed in the antenatal visit and documented. A decision for trial of labour or an elective cesarean section should be made after discussion with the couple.

**Intrapartum risk factors**

Immediately after delivery, when there is retraction of the delivered fetal head against the maternal perineum (turtle sign), it is a good clinical indicator of shoulder dystocia.

*Prolonged second stage*: Several studies have looked at labour abnormalities and shoulder dystocia. Baskett and Allen (1995) found that 38.6 per cent of cases with shoulder dystocia had a prolonged second stage, in comparison to 11.4 per cent of all deliveries during the same years. It has also been reported that shoulder dystocia occurred with a higher frequency in patients with fetal macrosomia, midpelvic operative delivery, and a prolonged second stage of labour (Benedetti and Gabbe 1978). However, in two large studies, no significant correlation was found between active phase abnormalities (defined as a prolonged second stage of more than 1 hour for multiparas and more than 2 hours for nulliparas or more than 2 hours in length irrespective of parity) and shoulder dystocia (Lurie et al 1995; Mcfarland et al 1995). At the present stage of knowledge, data seems inadequate to suggest that the labour curve is a useful predictor of shoulder dystocia (ACOG 2002).

*Operative vaginal delivery*: Operative vaginal delivery seems to be the only intrapartum risk factor to have a meaningful positive predictive value (Gherman et al 2006). Though both forceps and vacuum extraction are associated with shoulder dystocia, vacuum extraction poses a greater risk for shoulder dystocia than forceps delivery (Bofill et al 1997).

> Vacuum extraction poses a greater risk for shoulder dystocia than forceps delivery.

*Fetal gender*: Male babies may have an increased risk of shoulder dystocia, probably because they are usually bigger than female babies (Spellacy et al 1985). Nassar et al (2003) showed that in a series of fetuses weighing 4500 g or more, 70 per cent were males, whereas only 51 per cent of all newborns were females. Another risk factor for the male fetus could be the wider shoulder girdle compared with that of the female (Dildy and Clark 2000).

## Can shoulder dystocia be predicted antenatally?

Despite the association of these conditions with shoulder dystocia, the majority of cases of shoulder dystocia occur without risk factors. A sizeable number of cases occur among women who do not have diabetes and among infants with birth weights less

> Data seems inadequate to suggest that the labour curve is a useful predictor of shoulder dystocia.

than 4000 g (ACOG 2002). Acker and colleagues (1985) found that the presence of both diabetes and macrosomia accurately predicted only 55 per cent of cases of shoulder dystocia. Further, the antenatal prediction of the main risk factor, macrosomia, is unreliable.

> The presence of both diabetes and macrosomia accurately predicted only 55 per cent of cases of shoulder dystocia.

### Ultrasound in the prediction of macrosomia

Ultrasound is increasingly used to assess fetal weight in cases of suspected macrosomia. However, ultrasonography is not a reliable or accurate predictor of macrosomia (Benacerraf et al 1988; Smith et al 1997).

> Ultrasonography is not a reliable or accurate predictor of macrosomia

Gonen et al (2000) retrospectively analysed a policy that recommended cesarean delivery for macrosomia suspected clinically and confirmed by ultrasound. There was no effect on the incidence of brachial plexus palsy. This resulted from the fact that macrosomia was over-diagnosed in 84 per cent of patients; even the macrosomic infants had a low incidence of brachial plexus injury (3 per cent); and 82 per cent of the infants with brachial plexus injury did not have macrosomia.

## Elective induction or elective cesarean in prevention of shoulder dystocia

### Elective induction

Labour induction in non-diabetic women with suspected macrosomia has not been shown to be effective in decreasing the occurrence of shoulder dystocia or decreasing the rate of cesarean delivery (Kjos et al 1993). Gonen and colleagues (1997) compared labour induction with expectant management in patients with an ultrasound-estimated fetal weight of 4000 g to 4500 g. They found no significant difference in the rate of shoulder dystocia or brachial plexus palsy. On the other hand, induction with an antenatal diagnosis of macrosomia significantly increases the cesarean delivery rate (Leaphart et al 1997). A systematic review of the Cochrane database has concluded that induction of labour for suspected macrosomia in non-diabetic patients does not alter the risk of neonatal morbidity (Irion and Boulvain 2002).

A policy of elective induction of labour versus elective cesarean delivery based on fetal weight does not seem to make a difference in the occurrence of brachial plexus injuries (Conway and Langer 1998).

### Elective cesarean delivery

A policy of planned cesarean delivery is not recommended for suspected macrosomic fetuses (>4000 g) in women who do not have diabetes (ACOG 2002). Such a policy would cause the cesarean delivery rate to increase disproportionately when compared with the reduction in the rate of shoulder dystocia (Langer et al 1991).

> Since fetal weight assessed clinically or by ultrasound is not accurate, a policy of prophylactic cesarean on the basis of suspected macrosomia is bound to increase cesarean rates without consistent reduction in fetal complications.

Gonen et al (2000) predicted that 2345 to 3695 cesarean deliveries would need to be performed to prevent one permanent brachial plexus injury among non-diabetic women.

*Patients with previous history of shoulder dystocia*: The risk of having a repeat shoulder dystocia is 1 per cent to 16.7 per cent (Baskett and Allen 1995, Ginsberg and Mosidis 2001, Ouzounian et al 2001). However, most subsequent deliveries will not be complicated by shoulder dystocia (ACOG 2002). A policy of universal elective cesarean delivery has not been recommended in women with prior shoulder dystocia. The American College of Obstetricians and Gynecologists (2002) states, 'because most subsequent deliveries will not be complicated by shoulder dystocia, the benefit of universal elective cesarean delivery is questionable in patients who have such a history of shoulder dystocia'. Factors that may aid in the decision-making process for mode of delivery include the estimate of fetal weight compared with the prior pregnancy birth weight (both clinically and by ultrasound), the severity of the prior neonatal injury and maternal diabetes. The records of the previous delivery should be reviewed in the antenatal visit and documented. A decision for trial of labour or an elective cesarean section should be made after discussion with the couple.

> The risk of having a repeat shoulder dystocia is 1 per cent to 16.7 per cent. Most subsequent deliveries will not be complicated by shoulder dystocia. A policy of universal elective cesarean delivery has not been recommended in women with prior shoulder dystocia.

## Mechanism of shoulder delivery in spontaneous labour

In spontaneous labour, as the head passes through the pelvic outlet, the shoulders enter the pelvic brim in the oblique diameter. Compression of the shoulder (compaction) helps in reducing the presenting diameter. Once the leading shoulder touches the pelvic floor, it rotates medially. Clinical situations like precipitate labour, hasty instrumental delivery and premature traction on the emerging head, may not allow enough time for the shoulders to rotate and descend. Awaiting the next contraction and its associated spontaneous restitution may be adequate to re-establish normal alignment and progression of labour. Disregarding these facts and pulling prematurely will lead to iatrogenic shoulder dystocia which can also lead to nerve injury.

## Mechanism in shoulder dystocia

In normal labour, as soon as the fetal head emerges, it falls posteriorly, with the face almost touching the maternal anus. The occiput promptly turns towards one of the maternal thighs and the head assumes a transverse position. This movement is called *restitution*. In cases of shoulder dystocia, however, restitution may not occur spontaneously and the delivered head retracts against the maternal perineum ('turtle sign').

> The anterior shoulder may become impacted behind the pubic symphysis if:
> - the bisacromial diameter is large
> - the pelvic brim is more flat than gynecoid
> - the shoulders enter in the antero-posterior diameter of the pelvic brim.

The anterior shoulder may become impacted behind the pubic symphysis if the bisacromial diameter is large, the pelvic brim is more flat than gynecoid, and if the shoulders enter in the antero-posterior diameter of the pelvic brim. Usually, the posterior shoulder will descend below the sacral promontory. On very rare occasions, usually associated with assisted mid-pelvic delivery, both shoulders may be arrested above the pelvic brim. This is known as bilateral shoulder dystocia.

## Complications of shoulder dystocia

### Fetal complications

Gherman et al (1998), in a large retrospective study that evaluated 285 cases of shoulder dystocia, found that the fetal injury rate was 24.9 per cent, including 48 (16.8 per cent) brachial plexus palsies, 27 (9.5 per cent) clavicular fractures and 12 (4.2 per cent) humeral fractures.

*Brachial plexus palsies*: Brachial plexus palsies result from excessive lateral traction and forceful deviation of the fetal head from the axial plane of the fetal body. Unilateral brachial plexus injury is one of the most common fetal complications of shoulder dystocia. The C5–C6 nerve roots are affected in 80 per cent of cases (Erb-Duchenne palsy), leading to paralysis of the deltoid and infraspinatus muscles. The right arm is usually affected (64.6 per cent) because the left occiput anterior presentation leaves the right shoulder impacted against the symphysis pubis (Gherman et al 1998). Fortunately, 88 per cent of brachial plexus injuries will resolve within a year (Chauhan et al 2005).

The incidence of brachial plexus palsy also depends on the number of manoeuvres required to deliver the shoulders, ranging from 7.7 per cent with 1–2 manoeuvres, to 25 per cent with 3 or more manoeuvres (McFarland et al 1996). Nocon et al (1993) found that the number of injuries was the highest (37.9 per cent) with the delivery of the posterior arm.

*Clavicular fracture*: The most common fracture associated with shoulder dystocia is of the clavicle. However, studies have shown that clavicular fractures may occur even without shoulder dystocia. Lam et al (2002) state that 'neonatal clavicular fracture is of little clinical significance, and it does not reflect quality of care'.

*Fetal asphyxia*: Rarely does intractable shoulder dystocia lead to neonatal death and hypoxic ischemic encephalopathy as most shoulder dystocias are resolved within a few minutes (Gherman et al 2006).

Stallings et al (2001) studied the mean umbilical artery pH of shoulder dystocia cases. They found that shoulder dystocia resulted in statistically significant but clinically insignificant reductions in mean umbilical artery blood gas parameters. They did not identify a statistically significant linear relationship between the head-to-body delivery interval and fetal acid–base status.

Ouzounian et al (1998) found that brain injury cases were associated with significantly prolonged head–shoulder intervals. A head–shoulder interval of 7 minutes or more was reasonably reliable in predicting brain injury.

## Maternal complications

Genital tract lacerations are common and associated with the need for a generous episiotomy and the additional manoeuvres required to deliver the shoulders. On rare occasions, uterine rupture may occur in association with vigorous efforts at suprapubic or fundal pressure. Postpartum hemorrhage is more likely due to a combination of uterine atony, prolonged labour, large infant and increased blood loss from lacerations and extensive episiotomy (Benedetti and Gabbe 1978).

## Diagnosis and Management

Shoulder dystocia continues to represent an immense area of clinical interest because it typically occurs without prediction. All patients in labour should be considered at risk for developing shoulder dystocia. Therefore, each delivery unit should have a set of guidelines outlining a sequence of manoeuvres for the management of shoulder dystocia. This should be taught and practised regularly, using a mannequin, by all staff involved in labour management. It is reasonable to propose that shoulder dystocia drills should be as important as cardiopulmonary resuscitation for the mother and neonate.

In normal labour, as soon as the fetal head emerges, it falls posteriorly, with the face almost touching the maternal anus. The occiput promptly turns towards one of the maternal thighs and the head assumes a transverse position. This movement is called *restitution*. In cases of shoulder dystocia, however, restitution may not occur spontaneously and the delivered head retracts tightly against the maternal perineum ('turtle sign'). Gentle traction on the fetal head downwards and backwards fails to deliver the anterior shoulder.

As soon as it is obvious that the normal amount of head traction is unsuccessful, it should be abandoned. Excessive force must not be applied to the fetal head or neck, and fundal pressure must be avoided, because these activities are unlikely to free the impaction and may cause injury to the infant and mother (Baskett and Allen 1995; Gross et al 1987). The commonest cause of brachial plexus injury is excessive traction on the head and neck. Maternal pushing and fundal pressure should also be discouraged.

> Manoeuvres to be avoided once shoulder dystocia is suspected:
> - Application of excessive force to the fetal head or neck
> - Fundal pressure
> - Maternal pushing efforts

### The HELPERR mnemonic

The HELPERR mnemonic from the Advanced Life Support in Obstetrics course (Gobbo and Baxley 2000) is a clinical tool that offers a structured process that deals with shoulder dystocia in a step-wise fashion (Table 11.1). These manoeuvres are designed to do one of three things (Baxley and Gobbo 2004):

❖ utilise the McRoberts' manoeuvre to increase the functional size of the bony pelvis through flattening of the lumbar lordosis and cephalad rotation of the symphysis

- apply suprapubic pressure to decrease the bisacromial diameter (i.e., the breadth of the shoulders) of the fetus
- use internal rotation manoeuvres to change the relationship of the bisacromial diameter within the bony pelvis.

Table 11.1 The HELPERR mnemonic

| | |
|---|---|
| H | Call for help |
| E | Evaluate for episiotomy |
| L | Legs (the McRoberts' manoeuvre) |
| P | Suprapubic pressure |
| E | Enter manoeuvres (internal rotation) |
| R | Remove the posterior arm |
| R | Roll the patient |

## Call for help

Once the problem is suspected or diagnosed, additional personnel should be summoned for help, including a clinician capable of providing anesthesia, and a pediatrician. Nurses and nursing assistants will also be required to carry out various supporting measures. The obstetrician should stay informed of the time that has elapsed since delivery of the head. One means of doing this is by designating a person to call out the time after delivery of the head at fixed intervals, perhaps every 30 seconds.

Shoulder dystocia management is time sensitive. The two competing issues are the amount of time needed to resolve a shoulder dystocia without hypoxic insult and how quickly to progress from one manoeuvre to the next to minimise the risk of peripheral nerve injury. All personnel involved in labour management should be familiar with a logical sequence of manoeuvres to manage shoulder dystocia. Regular hospital drills may be helpful to rehearse this protocol.

## Evaluate for episiotomy

As shoulder dystocia is considered to be a 'bony dystocia,' and is typically not caused by obstructing soft tissue, episiotomy alone will not release the impacted shoulder (ACOG 2002). However, a narrow vaginal fourchette in a primigravida patient may prompt a generous episiotomy or proctoepisiotomy. An episiotomy may also allow the fetal rotational manoeuvres to be performed with ease, and also increase the room for attempted delivery of the posterior arm. Management by episiotomy or proctoepisiotomy has been associated with a nearly seven-fold increase in the rate of severe perineal trauma without reducing the occurrence of neonatal depression or brachial plexus palsy (Gurewitsch et al 2004).

*Decision between vaginal and abdominal routes*: This is the time to rapidly evaluate the situation and decide whether to continue with the vaginal route or to proceed with an abdominal intervention. By manually exploring the area behind the baby's head it may be possible to find out whether or not the posterior shoulder is in the hollow of the sacrum. If the posterior shoulder is not in the hollow of the sacrum, the diagnosis is bilateral shoulder dystocia and the best step would be to restitute the baby's head inside the vagina and perform a cesarean delivery (Zavanelli's manoeuvre).

# Shoulder Dystocia

If the decision is to proceed with the vaginal route, a sequence of steps should be systematically followed.

## McRoberts' manoeuvre

The McRoberts' manoeuvre is the initial step that most obstetricians currently employ for the disimpaction of the shoulder (Gonik et al 1983). This is performed by sharply flexing the maternal thighs onto the abdomen. This results in the straightening of the sacrum relative to the lumbar spine with consequent cephalic rotation of the symphysis pubis, thus disimpacting the shoulder from behind the symphysis (Gherman et al 2000). The McRoberts' manoeuvre is the single most effective intervention for shoulder dystocia. Its success rate is reported as 42 per cent when used alone and 54.2 per cent when combined with suprapubic pressure and/or proctoepisiotomy (Gherman1997).

> The McRoberts' manoeuvre is the single most effective intervention for shoulder dystocia.

## Suprapubic pressure

Suprapubic pressure is typically used along with McRoberts' manoeuvre to improve the success rates. It can be administered by junior doctors or nursing personnel and is given immediately before or in combination with the McRoberts' manoeuvre. External suprapubic pressure is applied firmly in a downward and lateral direction with the heel of the hand (in a cardiopulmonary resuscitation style) to push the anterior shoulder towards the fetal chest. Suprapubic pressure reduces the bisacromial diameter and rotates the anterior shoulder into the oblique diameter. The shoulder is then free to slip underneath the symphysis pubis with the aid of routine traction. (Figure 11.1)

> External suprapubic pressure is applied firmly in a downward and lateral direction with the heel of the hand (in a cardiopulmonary resuscitation style) to push the anterior shoulder towards the fetal chest.

While the assistant(s) give the suprapubic pressure, the operator should give steady traction on the head downwards at an angle of about 45 degrees. It is important to resist the temptation to pull vertically downwards, as that will stretch nerve roots and lead to brachial palsy. If the shoulders do not descend with the above manoeuvres, the operator should decide on the next logical steps.

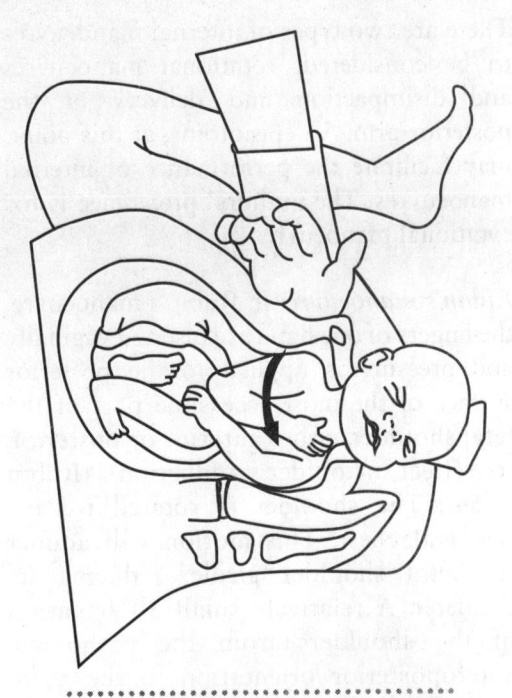

**Figure 11.1** Directed supra-pubic pressure to abdut and rotate anterior shoulder

*Choose between internal manoeuvres and Gaskin's manoeuvre*: Once the McRoberts' manoeuvre and suprapubic pressure have failed to disimpact the shoulders, the clinician has to make a decision between proceeding with internal manoeuvres or rolling the woman to an all-fours position (Gaskin's manoeuvre). Traditionally, internal manipulations are used at this point but the all-fours position may also be successful in certain situations. For a slim, mobile woman not under epidural anesthesia and with a single midwifery attendant, the all-fours position is probably most appropriate. For a less mobile woman under epidural anesthesia and a senior obstetrician in attendance, rotational manoeuvres are more appropriate.

**Internal manoeuvres**

There are two types of internal manoeuvres to be considered: rotational manoeuvres and disimpaction and delivery of the posterior arm. An episiotomy, at this point, may facilitate the performance of internal manoeuvres. The authors' preference is for rotational manoeuvres.

*Rubin's manoeuvre*: In Rubin's manoeuvre, the fingers of one hand are inserted vaginally and pressure is applied to the posterior surface of the most accessible part of the fetal shoulder, either anterior or posterior, to effect shoulder adduction (Rubin 1964). The shoulder is rotated toward the fetal chest. This motion will adduct the fetal shoulder girdle, reducing its diameter. A relatively small 30° rotation of the shoulders from the pathologic anteroposterior orientation to the more physiologic oblique orientation within the pelvis affords approximately 2 cm more room for the passage of the shoulders (Fig 11.2). The McRoberts' manoeuvre can also be applied during this manoeuvre and may facilitate its success.

*Woods' corkscrew manoeuvre*: In this manoeuvre (Fig 11.3), two fingers are placed on the anterior aspect of the posterior shoulder, using the left hand if the infant's back is on the mother's left, and pressure exerted to rotate the baby 180° (Woods 1943).

Thus, the posterior shoulder which is below the level of the pelvic brim is screwed around at that level under the pubic arch and can then be delivered from the anterior position where it will be below the pubic arch. This manoeuvre logically addresses the mechanical relationship between the shoulders and bony pelvis.

When the anterior shoulder is tightly wedged underneath the symphysis pubis, it may be difficult to perform these rotational manoeuvres. It may therefore be necessary to push the fetus upward slightly in order to facilitate the rotation.

*Combined Rubin's and Woods' manoeuvres*: The authors recommend a combination of the two (Rubin's and Woods') manoeuvres to achieve the same goal of rotating the fetus. A liberal episiotomy is essential to allow the index and middle fingers of the two hands to reach the shoulder and accomplish rotation (Fig 11. 4). If the Rubin's or Woods' corkscrew manoeuvres fail, the reverse Woods' corkscrew manoeuvre may be tried. In this manoeuvre, the physician's fingers are placed on the back of the posterior shoulder of the fetus, and the fetus is rotated in the opposite direction as in the Woods' corkscrew or Rubin's manoeuvres (Baxley and Gobbo 2004).

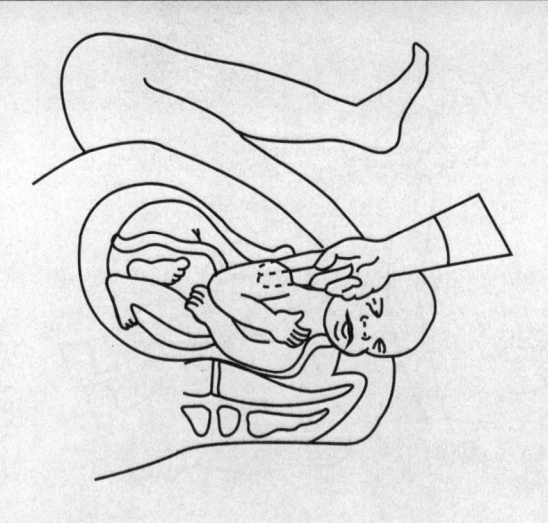

**Figure 11.2** Rubin's manouvere - rotation of anterior shoulder by pressure from behind the scapula - the whole hand may need to inserted inside the vagina

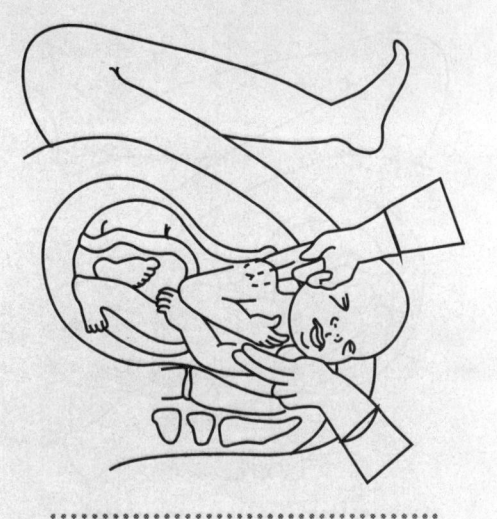

**Figure 11.4** Combined Rubin's and Wood's manouvere

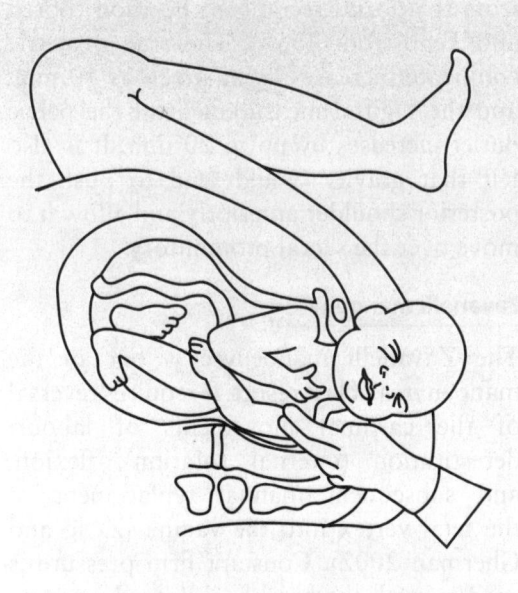

**Figure 11.3** Woods' manouvere – rotation of posterior shoulder by pressure on the anterior aspect – the whole hand inserted inside the vagina may provide greater pressure to rotate

Another possible approach is to use suprapubic pressure to push the anterior shoulder towards the fetal chest and the Woods' manoeuvre to push the posterior shoulder in the opposite direction, both these being complementary.

### Delivery of posterior arm (Barnum manoeuvre)

If rotational manoeuvres fail to disimpact the shoulders, delivery of the posterior arm should be attempted. This is done by passing a hand deep into the vagina underneath the posterior shoulder and following the arm to the elbow. The physician's hand, wrist, and forearm may need to enter the vagina. Pressure on the antecubital fossa will cause the forearm to flex so that it can be grasped and swept over the fetal chest and delivered over the perineum (Fig 11. 5). The upper arm should never be grasped and pulled directly, as this may cause fracture of the humerus.

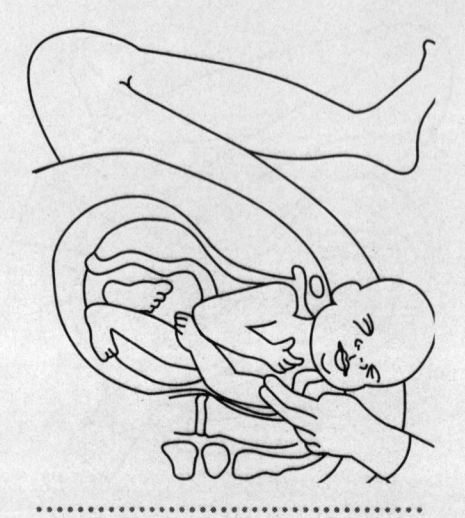

**Figure 11.5** Delivery of posterior arm to reduce the larger bisacromial to smaler axillo-acromial diameter

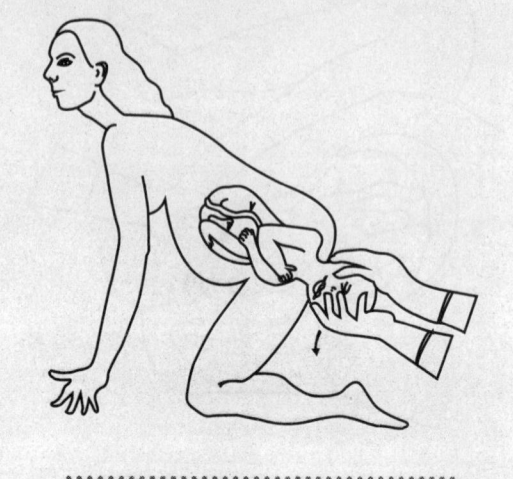

**Figure 11.6** Gaskin's manouvere - delivery on all fours

By replacing the bisacromial diameter with the axilloacromial diameter, posterior arm delivery creates a 20 per cent reduction in shoulder diameter (Poggi et al 2003).

Once the posterior arm is delivered, the delivery of the anterior shoulder will be easy. If it does not come out, rotation of the fetal trunk will help to bring the anterior arm posteriorly and its delivery can be accomplished as described above.

### Roll the patient (Gaskin's manoeuvre)

In the all-fours position (Gaskin's manoeuvre), the labouring woman is assisted onto her hands and knees and downward pressure is applied to the fetal head to deliver the posterior shoulder (Fig 11.6). In Bruner's case series, there were no reports of infants with brachial plexus palsy, and the average time needed to assume the position and complete the delivery was 2 to 3 minutes (Bruner et al 1998). Radiographic studies indicate that pelvic diameters increase when labouring women change from the dorsal recumbent position (Borell and Fendstrom 1957). The true obstetric conjugate increases by as much as 10 mm, and the sagittal measurement of the pelvic outlet increases by up to 20 mm. It is also felt that gravity would tend to push the posterior shoulder anteriorly and allow it to move over the sacral promontory.

### Zavanelli manoeuvre

The Zavanelli manoeuvre is one of the manoeuvres of last resort. It requires reversal of the cardinal movements of labour: derestitution (internal rotation), flexion, and subsequent manual replacement of the fetal vertex into the vagina (Zelig and Gherman 2002). Constant firm pressure is used to push the head back into the vagina and then a cesarean section is performed (Fig 11.7). General anesthesia or tocolytic agents may be administered to facilitate the Zavanelli manoeuvre. It would usually only

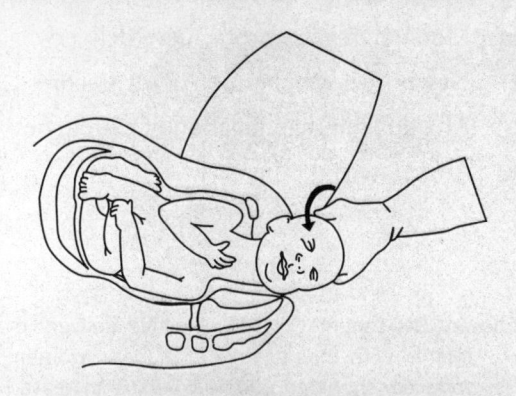

**Figure 11.7** Rotation, flexion and pressure on fetal head to replace it into the vagina before Cesarean section in Zavanelli's manouvere

be applicable in those rare cases of bilateral shoulder dystocia, where the posterior shoulder has not passed the pelvic brim and is therefore not accessible to other vaginal manoeuvres.

Unfortunately, the Zavanelli manoeuvre is often complicated by the clinician's lack of clinical experience with this manoeuvre for performance in emergency conditions, and significant maternal and neonatal complications are inherent in the procedures (Sanberg 1999).

The choice between rotational manoeuvres and the Zavanelli manoeuvre should be made as soon as shoulder dystocia is diagnosed. Pushing back the head after having done the manipulations and traction from below will make it more difficult and the damage to the fetus and the mother would have already occurred. This manoeuvre should never be attempted if a nuchal cord has been clamped and cut (Baxley and Gobbo 2004).

### Other manoeuvres of last resort

Isolated cases of abdominal rescue have been described with failed cephalic replacement. Cesarean section is performed allowing direct manipulation and release of impacted shoulder through the lower segment incision. Vaginal extraction is then accomplished by another physician (O'Shaughnessy 1998).

Deliberate fracture of the clavicle or cleidotomy should only be considered with a dead fetus or one with a lethal anomaly, for fear of trauma to the underlying subclavian vessels.

Symphysiotomy (intentional division of the fibrous cartilage of the symphysis pubis under local anesthesia) has been proposed as a potentially useful procedure, both in the developing and developed world (Crichton and Seedat 1963). However, there is a high incidence of maternal morbidity and poor neonatal outcome.

Of the many techniques proposed to deal with shoulder dystocia, no single manoeuvre has been proved to be superior to another. The simple and atraumatic manoeuvres should be tried first. Fetal manipulations take better advantage of pelvic geometry and require less traction to complete delivery. If one manoeuvre fails to resolve a shoulder dystocia within 30 seconds, another manoeuvre should be performed. When applying traction, it should not be directed too laterally (i.e. maintaining the vertebrae of neck aligned with vertebrae of the fetal trunk as much as possible). Traction should also be applied smoothly without jerky or torsional motion.

After a case of shoulder dystocia, it is important to document clearly on the hospital chart, the type and sequence of manoeuvres used, for clinical audit and potential medicolegal purposes. The following should be documented:

a) Position of fetal head at delivery

b) Which shoulder was the anterior shoulder
c) Time of delivery of the fetal head
d) Staff present at the time of delivery
e) Manoeuvres used to achieve delivery
f) Newborn's weight and APGAR scores
g) Any difficult manipulation of extremities
h) Any maternal injury

## References

Acker DB, Sachs BP, Friedman EA. 1985. Risk factors for shoulder dystocia. *Obstet Gynecol* 66: 762–8.

American College of Obstetricians and Gynecologists. 2002. Shoulder dystocia. ACOG Practice Bulletin No. 40. *Obstet Gynecol* 100:1045

Baskett TF, Allen AC. 1995. Perinatal implications of shoulder dystocia. *Obstet Gynecol* 86:14–7

Baxley EG, Gobbo RW. 2004. Shoulder dystocia. *Am Fam Physician* 1;69(7): 1707–14

Benacerraf BR, Gelman R, Frigoletto FD Jr. 1988. Sonographically estimated fetal weights: accuracy and limitation. *Am J Obstet Gynecol* 159:1118–21.

Benedetti TJ, Gabbe SG. 1978. Shoulder dystocia: a complication of fetal macrosomia and prolonged second stage of labor with midpelvic delivery. *Obstet Gynecol* 52:526–9.

Bofill JA, Rust OA, Devidas M, Roberts WE, Morrison JC, Martin JN Jr. 1997. Shoulder dystocia and operative vaginal delivery. *J Maternal Fetal Med* 6:220–4.

Borell U, Fendstrom I. 1957. A pelvimetric method for the assessment of pelvic mouldability. *Acta Radiol.* 47:365–70.

Bruner JP, Drummond SB, Meenan AL, Gaskin IM. 1998. All-fours maneuver for reducing shoulder dystocia during labour. *J Reprod Med*; 43:439.

Chauhan SP, Rose CH, Gherman RB et al. 2005. Brachial plexus injury: A 23 year experience from a tertiary center. *Am J Obstet Gynecol* 192:1795

Conway DL, Langer O. 1998. Elective delivery of infants with macrosomia in diabetic women: reduced shoulder dystocia versus increased cesarean delivery. *Am J Obstet Gynecol* 178: 922–5.

Crichton D, Seedat EK. 1963. The technique of symphysiotomy. *S Afr Med J.* 37:227–31.

Dildy GA, Clark SL 2000. Shoulder dystocia. Risk identification. *Clin Obstet Gynecol.* 43:265.

Doumouchtsis SK, Arulkumaran S. 2009. Are all brachial plexus injuries caused by shoulder dystocia? *Obstet Gynecol Surv.* 64(9):615–23.

Gherman RB, Goodwin TM, Souter I, Neumann K, Ouzounian JG, Paul Richard. 1997. The McRoberts' maneuver for the alleviation of shoulder dystocia: How successful is it?. *Am J Obstet Gynecol*; 176:656-61.

Gherman RB, Ouzounian JG, Goodwin TM. 1998. Obstetric maneuvers for shoulder dystocia and associated fetal morbidity. *Am J Obstet Gynecol* 178:1126–30.

Gherman RB, Chauhan S, Ouzounian JG, et al. 2006. Shoulder dystocia: the unpreventable obstetric emergency with empiric management guideline. *American Journal of Obstetrics and Gynecology.* 95, 657–72

Gherman RB. 2002. Shoulder dystocia: an evidence-based evaluation of the obstetrical nightmare. *Clin Obstet Gynecol* 45: 345-61 (treatment).

Ginsberg NA, Moisidis C. 2001. How to predict recurrent shoulder dystocia. *Am J Obstet Gynecol* 184:1427–9; 1429–30 (discussion).

Gobbo R, Baxley EG. 2000. Shoulder dystocia. In: *ALSO: advanced life support in obstetrics provider course syllabus.* Leawood, Kansas: American Academy of Family Physicians

Gonen R, Bader D, Ajami M. 2000. Effects of a policy of elective cesarean delivery in cases of suspected fetal macrosomia on the incidence of brachial plexus injury and the rate of cesarean delivery. *Am J Obstet Gynecol* 183:1296–300.

Gonen O, Rosen DJ, Dolfin Z, Tepper R, Markov S, Fejgin MD. 1997. Induction of labor versus expectant management in macrosomia: a randomized study. *Obstet Gynecol* 89:913–7.

Gonik B, Stringer C, Held B: An alternate maneuver for management of shoulder dystocia. *Am J Obstet Gynecol* 145: 882, 1983.

Gross SJ, Shime J, Farine D. 1987. Shoulder dystocia: predictors and outcome. A five-year review. *Am J Obstet Gynecol* 156:334–6.

Gurewitsch Ed, Donithan H, Stallings S, et al. 2004. Episiotomy versus fetal manipulation maneuvers in managing severe shoulder dystocia: a comparison of outcomes. *Am J Obstet Gynecol*. 191: 911–916.

Gurewitsch ED. 2007. Optimizing shoulder dystocia management to prevent birth injury. *Clin Obstet Gynecol*. Sep; 50(3):592–606.

Irion O, Boulvain M. 2002. Induction of labour for suspected fetal macrosomia. *Cochrane Review*. The Cochrane Library, Issue 2.

Kalkhoff RK. 1991. Impact of maternal fuels and nutritional state on fetal growth. *Diabetes*. Dec; 40 Suppl 2:61–5.

Kitzmiller JL, Mall JC, Gin FD, Hendirkcs SK, Newman RB, Scheerer L. 1987. Measurement of fetal shoulder width with computed tomography in diabetic women. *Obstet Gynecol* 70:941–5.27.

Kjos SL, Henry OA, Montoro M, Buchanan TA, Mestman JH. 1993. Insulin-requiring diabetes in pregnancy: a randomized trial of active induction of labor and expectant management. *Am J Obstet Gynecol* 169:611–5.

Lam MH, Wong GY, Lao TT. Reappraisal of neonatal clavicular fracture: relationship between infant size and neonatal morbidity. *Obstet Gynecol*. 2002; 100:115–9.

Langer O, Berkus MD, Huff RW, Samueloff A. 1991. Shoulder dystocia: should the fetus weighing greater than or equal to 4000 grams be delivered by cesarean section? *Am J Obstet Gynecol*. 165:831–7.

Leaphart WL, Meyer MC, Capeless EL. 1997. Labor induction with a prenatal diagnosis of fetal macrosomia. *J Matern Fetal Med* 6:99–102.

Lurie S, Levy R, Ben-Arie A, Hagay Z. 1995. Shoulder dystocia: could it be deduced from the labor partogram? *Am J Perinatology*; 12:61–2.

McFarland M, Hod M, Piper JM, Xenakis EM, Oded L. 1995. Are labor abnormalities more common in shoulder dystocia? *Am J Obstet Gynecol* 173:1211–4.

McFarland MB, Langer O, Piper JM, Berkus MD. 1996. Perinatal outcome and the type and number of maneuvers in shoulder dystocia. *Int. J Gynecol Obstet* 55:219–24.

Nassar AH, Usta IM, Khalil AM et al. 2003. Fetal Macrosomia (>4500 g) perinatal outcome of 231 cases according to the mode of delivery. *J Perinatol*; 23:136

Nocon JJ, McKenzie DK, Thomas LJ, Hansell RS. 1993. Shoulder dystocia: an analysis of risks and obstetric maneuvers. *Am J Obstet Gynecol* 168:1732–9.

O'Shaughnessy MJ. 1998. Hysterotomy facilitation of the vaginal delivery of the posterior arm in a case of severe shoulder dystocia. *Obstet Gynecol*. 924 pt 2:693–5.

Ouzounian JG, Naylor CS, Gherman RB, Kamath M, Johnson M, DeLeon J, et al. 2001. Recurrent shoulder dsytocia: how high is the risk? *Am J Obstet Gynecol* 185:S96.

Ouzounian JG, Korst LM, Ahn MO, et al. 1998. Shoulder dystocia and neonatal brain injury: significance of the head-shoulder interval. *Am J Obstet Gynecol* 178:S76.

Pecorari, D. 1999. A Guest Editorial From Abroad: Meditations on a Nightmare of Modern Midwifery: Shoulder Dystocia. *Obstetrical and Gynecological Survey*: Volume 54 - Issue 6 - pp 353–354.

Poggi SH, Spong CY, Allen RH. 2003. Prioritizing posterior arm delivery during severe shoulder dystocia. *Obstet Gynecol*. 101: 1068–72.

Resnik R. 1980. Management of shoulder girdle dystocia. *Clin Obstet Gynecol*. 23:559–64.

Robinson H, Tkatch S, Mayes DC, et al. 2003. Is maternal obesity a predictor of shoulder dystocia? *Obstet Gynecol*.101:24.

Rubin A. 1964. Management of shoulder dystocia. *JAMA*; 189:835.

Sanberg EC. 1999. The Zavanelli maneuver: 12 years of recorded experience. *Obstet Gynecol* 93: 312–7.

Smith GC, Smith MF, McNay MB, Fleming JE. 1997. The relation between fetal abdominal circumference and birth-weight: findings in 3512 pregnancies. *Br J Obstet Gynaecol*.104:186–90.

Spellacy W, Miller S, Winegar A, Petersen P. 1985. Macrosomia: Maternal characteristics and fetal complications. *Obstet Gynecol* 66: 156–61,

Spong, CY, Beall, M, Rodrigues, D, Ross MG. 1995. An objective definition of shoulder dystocia: prolonged head to body delivery, intervals and /or the use of ancillary obstetric maneuvers. *Obstet Gynecol*. 86:433.

Stallings SP, Edwards RK, Johnson JWC. 2001. Correlation of head- to-body delivery intervals in shoulder dystocia and umbilical artery acidosis. *Am J Obstet Gynecol*; 185:268–74.

Woods CA. 1943. A Principle of physics as applicable to shoulder dystocia. *Am J Obstet Gynecol*. 145:882.

Zelig CM, Gheman RB. 2002. Modified Zavanelli maneuver for the alleviation of shoulder dystocia. *Obstet Gynecol* 100:1112–4.

# CHAPTER 12

# EPISIOTOMY

*Terence Lao*

## Definition

Episiotomy is the surgical excision of the perineum to create additional room during vaginal birth to facilitate delivery of the fetus. There are two types of episiotomy: midline and mediolateral.

## Epidemiology

The prevalence is highly variable from nation to nation, centre to centre, and among different categories of care-givers. There is evidence that the rate has been declining. A study in the US found that it fell from 69.6 per cent in 1983 to 19.4 per cent in 2000. In general, the prevalence was about 40 per cent among vaginal deliveries in the USA (Goldberg et al 2002; Allen and Hanson 2005), while in the UK, the figure varied: it was 15 per cent, 13 per cent, 10 per cent and 22 per cent in England, Scotland, Wales and Ireland, respectively (Williams et al 1998). In Europe, it varied from 8 per cent in Holland to 99 per cent in Eastern Europe. In developing countries, the prevalence tended to be high in the region of 30 per cent to 80 per cent (Carroli and Belizan 2000).

Studies have consistently found that the figures are highest with obstetrician-led delivery in private practice, higher than those in institutions with doctors and midwives under training. The rate is lower with family physicians, and lowest with nurse/midwives.

Ethnicity/race also appeared to influence the rate of episiotomy. One study showed that Caucasian women had episiotomy more frequently than African-American women, while another study demonstrated that women from the Indian subcontinent and South East Asia and the Far East were two to five times more likely than Caucasian women to have an episiotomy.

## Pathology

The surgical incision cuts through the perineal and vaginal skin down to the level of the perineal and vaginal muscles, creating in effect a second degree perineal tear. Performed when necessary and at the appropriate time, an episiotomy may prevent tearing, especially radial tearing, from the fourchette that extends to the perineum and vagina and which may damage the muscles to involve even the anal sphincter and mucosa, due to uncontrolled/excessive stretching by the fetal head or shoulder. Therefore, the rationale for an episiotomy includes the prevention of third and fourth degree perineal tears, facilitating delivery (shortening the second stage of labour in the presence of a non-reassuring fetal heart rate pattern), creating room for the delivery of the aftercoming head in breech delivery, and facilitating delivery of the trunk in shoulder dystocia.

However, there is also much evidence to indicate that episiotomy is actually associated with increased risk of third and fourth degree tears, anal feces/flatus incontinence, rectovaginal fistula, increased blood loss at delivery, postpartum pain, infection, increased length of hospital stay, prolonged period before resumption of sexual intercourse, dyspareunia and sexual dissatisfaction (Fernando and Sultan 2004; Sartore et al 2004). There is also no proven benefit for the newborn.

The restrictive rather than routine use of episiotomy has been shown to reduce clinically important maternal morbidity, at the expense of increased anterior perineal trauma which is of little consequence. Therefore, a restrictive approach not only reduces the prevalence, but also the associated morbidity in the women.

> The restrictive rather than routine use of episiotomy has been shown to reduce clinically important maternal morbidity

The type of episiotomy appears to be an important determinant of third/fourth degree perineal tears (Signorello et al 2000). Mediolateral episiotomy (Fig 12.1) reduces the risk of anal sphincter injury during operative delivery compared with midline episiotomy (Fig 12.2); the latter also increases the risk of fecal and flatus incontinence compared with both an intact perineum as well as a second degree spontaneous tear, an effect that is independent of other factors like duration of second stage, infant birth weight, use of instrumentation and complications of labour (De Leeuw et al 2008). Nevertheless, mediolateral episiotomy does not protect against urinary and anal incontinence or genital prolapse, and was associated with lower pelvic floor muscle strength compared with spontaneous perineal lacerations.

## Etiology

Independent risk factors for episiotomy include the following (Robinson et al 2000):

- nulliparity
- operative delivery (vacuum extraction/forceps delivery)
- fetal macrosomia
- prolonged second stage
- shoulder dystocia
- epidural analgesia

## Prognosis

It has been estimated that 85 per cent of women who have a vaginal delivery have some degree of perineal trauma and that 60 per cent to 70 per cent will require suturing. Left unsutured, most of the lacerations will heal, but there will be poorer wound closure and approximation.

The continuous method of repair was reported to be associated with fewer complaints of pain in the early puerperium, but there was no difference between the use of more rapidly absorbed material

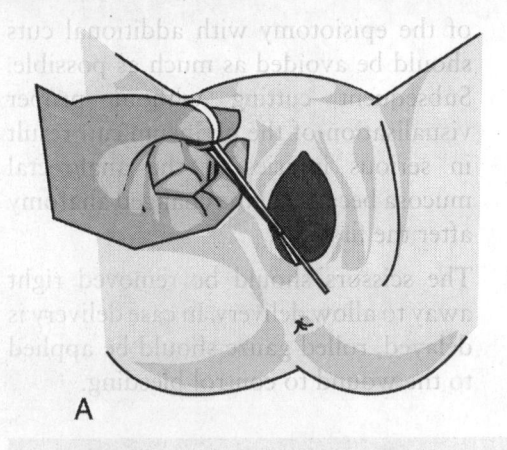

**Figure 12.1** Mediolateral episiotomy
(*Source*: Mudaliar and Menon's *Clinical Obstetrics*, 11th edition. Sarala Gopalan and Vanita Jain eds. Universities Press India Pvt Limited. 2011. Pp 118)

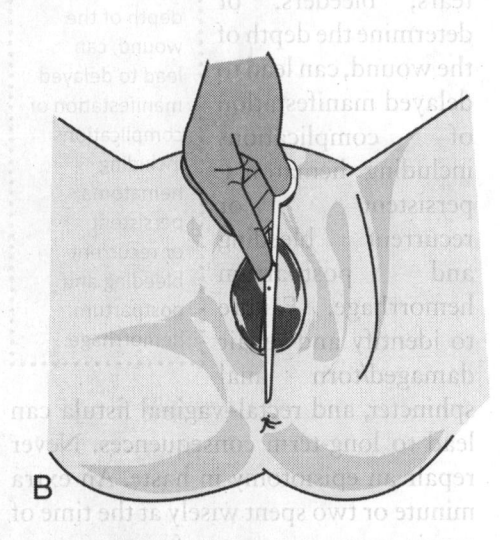

**Figure 12.2** Midline episiotomy
(*Source*: Mudaliar and Menon's *Clinical Obstetrics*, 11th edition. Sarala Gopalan and Vanita Jain eds. Universities Press India Pvt Limited. 2011. Pp 118)

versus the standard material, which is vicryl rapid (Kettle et al 2002). There was also no difference in superficial dyspareunia at 3 months between the continuous versus interrupted method, and the type of material used in the repair. However, suture removal was required more often with the standard suture material.

## Clinical approach

Episiotomy should be restricted to situations in which its use is indicated by clinical judgment on an individual basis, rather than as a routine procedure for certain categories of women or mode of delivery. In fact, even 'absolute' indications described in the literature have been challenged.

### Indications for episiotomy

- delay in delivery/prolonged second stage (often attributed to a rigid perineum)
- imminent perineal tear
- instrumental delivery
- breech delivery
- preterm delivery (to prevent the 'champagne cork' effect on the fetal head)
- fetal distress
- shoulder dystocia
- fetal macrosomia

## Performing an episiotomy

1. Consent must be obtained before the second stage of labour, preferably before the onset of labour.
2. If indicated, an episiotomy should be performed at the second stage when the perineum is stretched, or after application of the instrument for operative delivery.

3. Local analgesia must be infiltrated into the perineum of the intended site, or top up should be given if epidural analgesia is used.

4. If instrumental delivery is decided after an episiotomy has been made, the cut surface must be protected with the hand, while the instrument is introduced into the vagina and applied to the fetal head.

5. Mediolateral episiotomy is recommended. The cut is best made with a pair of strong and sharp curved scissors to ensure clean and straight edges. The scissors blades are opened and applied to the posterior part of the fourchette, one blade resting on the perineal skin, while the other rests on the vaginal mucosa. The tip of the scissors must curve away from the anus. The blade should be inserted into the vagina and guided by the index and middle fingers, which are inserted between the fetal head (or presenting part) and vaginal mucosa. These fingers are used to pull up the perineum to create room between the perineum and fetal head for the passage of the blade.

6. Before cutting, make sure no other tissue is trapped between the blades and vaginal muscoa. The cut is best made at the height of a contraction when the stretching is maximum, starting in the midline along the less vascular area of the aponeurosis rather than the bodies of the muscles, and the incision should be curving away from the anus (at least 1 cm from the anal verge), so that any extension will not involve the anal sphincter.

7. The length of the cut should have been determined before hand; enlargement of the episiotomy with additional cuts should be avoided as much as possible. Subsequent cutting without proper visualisation of the perineum can result in serious injuries of the anal/rectal mucosa because of the changed anatomy after the first cut.

8. The scissors should be removed right away to allow delivery. In case delivery is delayed, rolled gauze should be applied to the wound to control bleeding.

## Repairing an episiotomy

1. Assessment of the episiotomy wound should be made under adequate lighting. This is the most important part of the repair. Failing to detect additional tears, bleeders, or determine the depth of the wound, can lead to delayed manifestation of complications including hematoma, persistent or recurrent bleeding and postpartum hemorrhage. Failure to identify and repair damaged/torn anal sphincter, and rectal–vaginal fistula can lead to long-term consequences. Never repair an episiotomy in haste. An extra minute or two spent wisely at the time of repair can prevent many future regrets.

   > Failure to detect additional tears, bleeders, or determine the depth of the wound, can lead to delayed manifestation of complications including hematoma, persistent or recurrent bleeding and postpartum hemorrhage.

2. Inspect the length, depth and extension of the wound under direct vision. Look for active bleeders. To facilitate this, the surgeon should be seated comfortably and the height of the bed should be

adjusted so that the vaginal orifice is at eye level and illuminated with adequate lighting; the direction of light should be adjusted to eliminate any shadows. Clean the vagina with rolled gauze and determine the source and amount of bleeding. If more than the usual bleeding is coming from above the episiotomy, other causes of bleeding such as vaginal vault tears, cervical laceration, retained placental tissue etc should be excluded before repairing the episiotomy.

3. Apply pressure and/or artery forceps to the bleeders to control the bleeding until a good view of the size, extent and any extension can be seen. Identify the apex and look for bleeders and submucosal extension of the episiotomy upwards or laterally towards the bladder or lateral fornix. In case of a deep wound/ additional second degree laceration, palpate with fingers for any defects at the base of the wound. Look out for third and fourth degree perineal lacerations. In case of doubt, a combined vaginal and rectal digital examination is warranted.

> In case of doubt, a combined vaginal and rectal digital examination is warranted to rule out third and fourth degree perineal lacerations

4. Inject local anesthetic agent (1 per cent lignocaine) to painful sites unless there is already adequate analgesia from prior injection of local anesthetic agent or epidural analgesia.

5. In case of generalised oozing and significant tissue edema, try compression with rolled gauze soaked in ice-cold normal saline for several minutes to stop the oozing. If this is ineffective, add 1 ml of adrenaline (1:1000) to 5 ml of sterile KY Jelly in a galipot and mix thoroughly. Then smear the mixture to the new gauze roll and press this against the bleeding areas for 3–5 minutes. Unless there are big arterial bleeders, this method will help to stop the oozing and reduce the edema.

6. When the surgeon is satisfied with the inspection, a long rolled gauze or a vaginal pad can be inserted high in the vagina to prevent blood from the uterus obscuring the view. Then the repair process can begin.

## Methods of repair

In the absence of any extensions, additional lacerations, or third and fourth degree lacerations, the episiotomy can be repaired by either the interrupted or continuous method (Fig 12.3). Any additional second degree lacerations connected to the episiotomy should be repaired first with a running stitch using size '2/0' or '3/0' absorbable material, starting from the apex of the trauma to a point about 0.5 cm from the main episiotomy wound. Tie the knot outside the mucosa. The tension should be adjusted to achieve approximation of the edges and hemostasis, but without the stitch 'pulling down' or biting into the vaginal mucosa, or pulling the ipsilateral edge of the episiotomy away from the contralateral edge. The aim is to restore the vagina to its original configuration before repair.

### Interrupted suturing

1. Insert the first stitch above the apex of the vaginal wound. In case of a shallow or short 'tunnel' extending beyond the apex in the mucosa, the needle can be

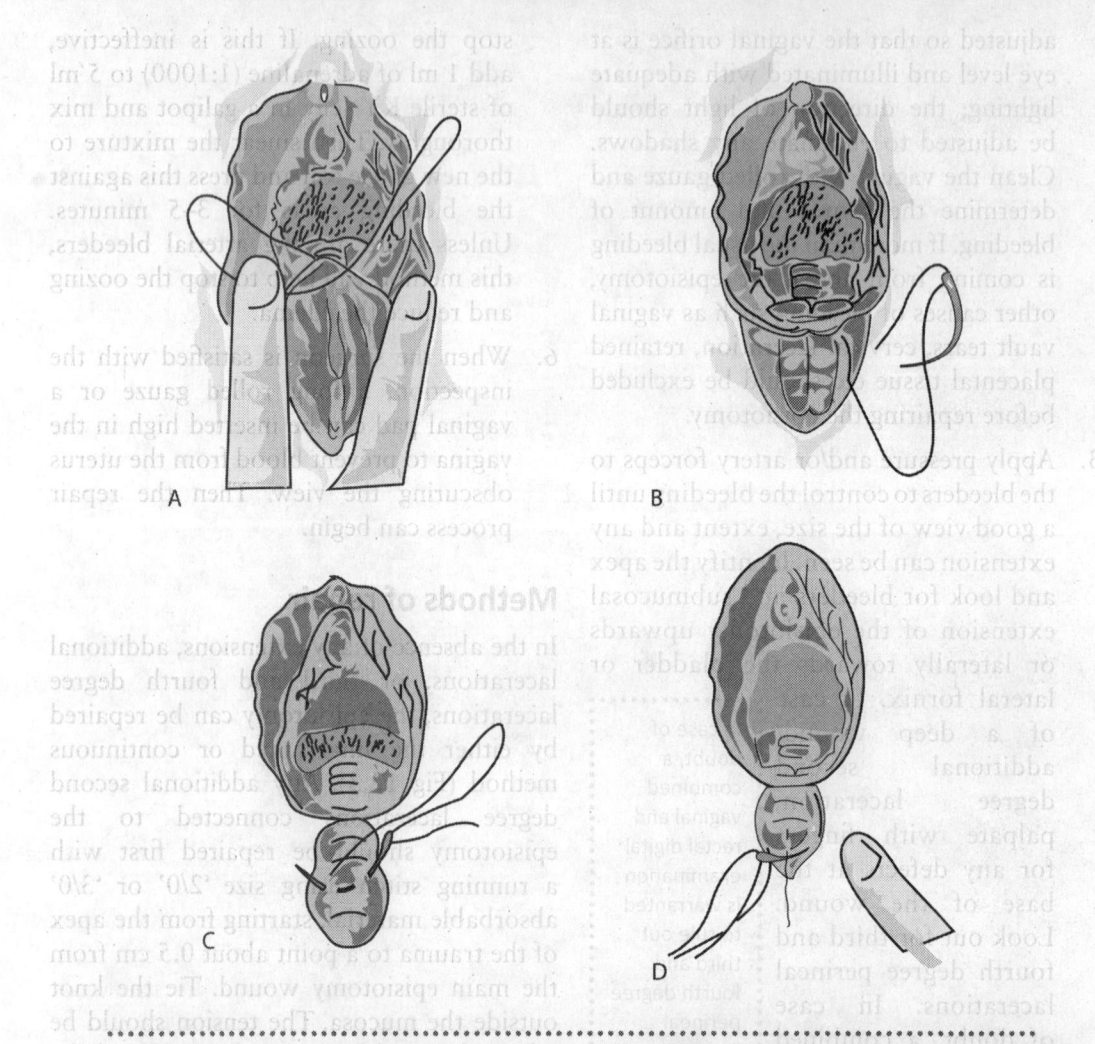

**Figure 12.3** Repair of a midline episiotomy: A. Continuous locked 00 or 000 absorbable sutures closes the vaginal epithelium from the apex to the hymeneal ring; B. Interrupted sutures are used to close the deep perineal fascia and underlying levator ani muscles; C. Continuous suture is used to close the superficial fascia; D. Subcuticular stitch is applied to the skin (*Source*: Mudaliar and Menon's *Clinical Obstetrics*, 11th edition. Sarala Gopalan and Vanita Jain eds. Universities Press India Pvt Ltd. 2011. Pp 123)

inserted just deep enough to include the side walls and the floor of the 'tunnel', either under direct vision by tracking the needle as it is being inserted, or by using a finger to trace the path of the needle following its insertion. For a left-sided mediolateral episiotomy being repaired by a right-handed surgeon, the needle-holder can be used as a retractor. The surgeon grasps the needle-holder with the wrist in supination so that the needle tip is pointing upwards. The needle-holder is inserted into the vagina along the posterior wall, which is retracted away from the needle-holder with the fingers of the left hand. For a right-sided mediolateral episiotomy repaired by a right-handed surgeon, the approach is similar, except that the left hand is used to retract away the right vaginal sidewall, while the needle-holder is used to retract away the posterior vaginal wall. Tying the knot on the posterior instead of the lateral wall has two advantages. It is much easier to tighten the knot and apply proper tension with the finger by pushing the throws against the posterior wall rather than upwards and sideways against the lateral wall, and the suture is less easy to cut through the thicker and more mobile posterior wall than the lateral wall even if the tension is excessive.

2. Close the vaginal wound with a continuous running stitch. In apposing the cut edges, ensure proper alignment by paying attention to the direction and angle of the episiotomy, which may curve or point more laterally or medially in different patients. The distance between each needle insertion and exit points on the two edges should be approximately 1 cm, but care must be exercised to avoid 'plucking' on any side, or unequal edges will become apparent when the stitch reaches the level of the fourchette and the repair has to be redone. It is not necessary to pass the needle too deeply or beneath the floor of the wound after the first two stitches since this may result in the stitch going into the rectum, or the fourchette being pulled towards the anus when the perineum is repaired. Ensure that the depth of the needle insertion is uniform, so that the result of the repair resembles that of a blanket (blanket stitch). To avoid excessive tension and to achieve adequate hemostasis, an inter-locking stitch may be preferable, but in case of a small uncomplicated episiotomy, this is not always necessary.

3. At the level of the posterior fourchette, a loop knot is tied, preferably above the level of the hymenal remnants, so that the knot will not cause any discomfort when the patient sits down. The changing colours between the vaginal mucosa and the perineal skin at this point also facilitate the positioning of the knot.

4. The perineal muscles are then closed with two to four interrupted sutures using the same material. The stitches are placed about 1 cm apart. The depth of needle insertion should be sufficient to obliterate any dead space but without overlapping with the vaginal muscles. The tension is adjusted to be sufficiently in approximation and hemostasis, without the stitches biting into the muscles. The purpose is to avoid turning the vagina and perineum into one piece of solid non-compliant scar tissue.

5. The skin edges are approximated with three to five interrupted transcutaneous non-absorbable (mersilk is preferred) size '0' or '2/0' stitches placed roughly 1.0 cm apart. The depth of the needle insertion should be above the layer of the approximated perineal muscles so that when the perineal muscles contract, the skin edges and the stitches are not pulled. If the skin edges extend towards the anus, the interrupted stitches should be placed as close as possible to the anus, because of the change in the curvature

of the skin and the skin movements associated with bowel motion. This will avoid the edges gaping open later. The knots should be tied on the lateral side, as this causes less discomfort while sitting. The use of non-absorbable suture has two advantages. First, this will avoid too much suture material being left inside the skin, with the potential of causing pain, discomfort, small abscesses, granulomas, and excessive fibrosis and scarring later. Second, once the stitches, and hence the knots, are removed, there is immediate relief. The stitches should be removed on the fifth day postpartum.

**Continuous suturing**

1. The vaginal wound is repaired as described above. An interlocking or a non-locking technique may be used. For a non-locking stitch, tie a large loop knot (with the loop at least 3 cm) at the level of the fourchette. The loop is divided 0.5 cm from the knot and the longer loose end is held with artery forceps for the tying of the terminal knot after the complete repair. This knot will help avoid the inadvertent pulling and shortening of the vaginal part of the episiotomy, and hence, distorting the vaginal canal when the suture is tightened as the perineal muscles are apposed. If a knot is not tied, then after locking, a 2 cm loop of the suture should be left behind and held with artery forceps for later use.

2. The needle is re-inserted after the knot is tied through the vaginal tissue on the medial side and exited beneath the perineal skin just above the muscle layer. The muscle layer is then approximated with a loose continuous stitch just tight enough to close all dead space and bring the edges of the skin together to a distance of about 1 cm apart. To facilitate this, the needle insertion should be placed closer to the subcutaneous tissue and the stitches should take the form of flatter loops than those used in the interrupted method. The aim of this is to allow adequate skin approximation without too much tension in the subcutaneous stitch. Once the stitch reaches the apex of the skin incision, the stitch is locked again after the rest of the loose suture is pulled out from the muscle after the needle.

3. There are two methods of skin closure. In the first method, the needle can be used to approximate the skin by vertical sutures placed at right angles to and just beneath the epidermis of the skin wound with the needle inserted in between the sutures in the muscle layer, passing from the lateral to the medial side and overlapping slightly with the muscle layer. In the second method, the needle is placed parallel to the skin wound and inserted through the subcutaneous tissue without leaving any tracts visible on the skin; taking small 0.5 cm bites alternatively on the lateral and then the medial side in a zigzag manner. In either method, the stitch is brought from the apex of the skin incision towards the fourchette. Finally, at the last stitch, the needle is passed back into the vagina exiting on the lateral side. The stitch is pulled just tight enough to ensure the complete approximation of the skin edges without plucking of the apex or anywhere along its course. The loose end of the vaginal loop is then tied to the terminal knot just inside the level of the hymen.

### Vaginal drain

In case the episiotomy is deep (≥ 1 cm below the floor of the vaginal wound) or long (≥ 1 cm beyond the apex or side wall of the vaginal wound), extra care should be used to close the vaginal wound. Depending on the location of the 'tunnel', it may not be wise or safe to close the dead space with the stitch for fear of damage to surrounding organs and structures. In such cases, after thorough examination and exclusion of injury to neighbouring organs, a corrugated drain tailored with scissors to just fit the width of the tunnel and with the end rounded should be left to drain this tunnel. The drain should be placed along the floor of the vaginal wound and should exit through the skin wound. The rest of the drain should be cut away leaving about 1 cm to protrude from the skin surface. The episiotomy should be repaired with the interrupted method. There is usually no need to anchor the drain with a stitch. Vaginal packing is usually unnecessary, but in case of doubt, rolled gauze can be used to pack the vagina. The drain can be removed 12–24 hours later if hemostasis is achieved.

Note: The continuous non-locking technique is associated with a significant reduction in perineal pain and need for suture removal (Kettle et al 2008). The interrupted method is recommended for any complicated episiotomy, including very edematous tissue, additional or multiple second degree lacerations, following evacuation of hematomas, and in patients with bleeding tendency. Interrupted repair may allow drainage of collected blood, whereas continuous repair may lead to trapping of blood inside the episiotomy and a delay in diagnosis. The more rapidly absorbed suture material should be used where available. In any case, avoid leaving too much suture material inside the wound and avoid leaving knots beneath the mucosa/skin layer. After the repair, perform a gentle vaginal examination to check for missed lacerations, inappropriate apposition of anatomy and tension. Remove the pad and make sure all gauze swabs are removed. Look for any continuous or recurrent bleeding. Then perform a rectal examination to make sure no sutures have passed through the rectal mucosa and that the anal sphincter is intact. Any sutures through the rectum must be removed and replaced.

> A rectal examination is recommended to make sure no sutures have passed through the rectal mucosa and that the anal sphincter is intact. Any sutures through the rectum must be removed and replaced.

### Suture material

Absorbable suture, such as polyglactin or the recently available Vicryl rapide®, mounted on an atraumatic needle should always be used, except for the skin in case of interrupted repair. For the usual episiotomy, size '0' or '2/0' suture is sufficient. Size '2/0' or '3/0' suture is usually indicated for first and second degree vaginal lacerations. For the interrupted stitches for the skin, mersilk is preferable as the material is softer and the knot causes less discomfort when the patient is sitting.

## Post-repair management

- ❖ Adequate analgesia is important. Non-steroidal anti-inflammatory drugs given orally or as rectal suppositories are most helpful.
- ❖ Pain and edema due to lacerations and from the repaired episiotomy can

lead to urine retention. An in-dwelling Foley catheter for 24 hours may be required. Even if the patient can pass urine afterwards, look for evidence of a distended bladder after micturition or perform an ultrasound scan to check residual urine. If there is a palpable bladder or the estimated volume is ≥150 ml, insert the Foley catheter for 24 hours.

❖ The episiotomy, its repair, and any associated perineal tears must be clearly documented in the delivery record. If non-absorbable sutures are used for the skin, the time of their removal must be clearly entered in the postpartum orders.

## References

Allen RE, Hanson RW Jr. 2005. Episiotomy in low-risk vaginal deliveries. *J Am Board Fam Pract*; 18: 8–12.

Carroli G, Belizan J. 2000. Episiotomy for vaginal birth. *Cochrane Database Syst Rev.*(2):CD000081.

De Leeuw JW, de Wit C, Kuijken JPJA, Bruinse HW. 2008. Mediolateral episiotomy reduces the risk for anal sphincter injury during operative vaginal delivery. *BJOG* 115: 104–108.

Goldberg J, Holtz D, Hyslop T, Tolosa JE. 2002. Has the use of routine episiotomy decreased? Examination of episiotomy rates from 1983 to 2000. *Obstet Gynecol* 99: 395–400.

Fernando RJ, Sultan AH. 2004. Risk factors and management of obstetric perineal injury. *Current Obstetrics and Gynaecology*; 14 320–326.

Kettle C, Hills RK, Jones P, Darby L, Gray R, Johanson R. 2002. Continuous versus interrupted perineal repair with standard or rapidly absorbed sutures after spontaneous vaginal birth: a randomized controlled trial. *Lancet* 359: 2217–2223.

Kettle C, Hills RK, Ismail KMK. 2007. Continuous versus interrupted sutures for repair of episiotomy or second degree tears. *Cochrane Database of Systematic Reviews* Issue 3. Art.No.:CD000947. DOI.10.1002/14651858 CD000947.pub2.

Robinson JN, Norwitz ER, Cohen AP, Lieberman E. 2000. Predictors of episiotomy use at first spontaneous vaginal delivery. *Obstet Gynecol* 96: 214–218.

Sartore A, De Seta F, Maso G, Pregazzi R, Grimaldi E, Guaschino S. 2004. The effects of mediolateral episiotomy on pelvic floor function after vaginal delivery. *Obstet Gynecol* 103: 669–673.

Signorello LB, Harlow BL, Chekos AK, Repke JT. 2000. Midline episiotomy and anal incontinence: retrospective cohort study. *BMJ* 320: 86–90.

Williams FLR, Florey C du V, Mires GJ, Ogston SA. 1998. Episiotomy and perineal tears in low-risk UK primigravidae. *J Publ Health Med* 20: 422–427.

## Useful websites

www.patient.co.uk

## Patient information and contacts

www.rcog.org.hk

# CHAPTER 13

# BREECH DELIVERY

*Lakshmi Seshadri*

Breech presentation is the most common malpresentation and occurs in about 3 per cent to 4 per cent of all pregnancies at term (Cruickshank and White 1973). It is associated with a higher perinatal mortality and morbidity than vertex presentation at all gestational ages (Brenner et al 1974). In order to improve outcomes for the mother and for the baby and to define optimal management strategy, several clinical trials have been conducted in the last two decades.

## Incidence

The incidence of breech presentations decreases as pregnancy advances. It is seen in about 25 per cent of pregnancies at less than 28 weeks, but decreases to 7 per cent at 32 weeks and 3 per cent to 4 per cent at term (Collea 1980; Hickok et al 1992).

## Risk Factors

Fetal and maternal factors that increase the risk of breech presentation are listed in Table 13.1.

### Fetal factors

*Prematurity* is the most common cause of breech presentation, because the higher volume of liquor makes it easier for the fetus to keep changing its lie and presentation. The large head in *hydrocephalus* finds it easier to occupy the broad fundus of the uterus. *Anencephaly* is associated with polyhydramnios and the increase in liquor predisposes to abnormal presentations. *Congenital anomalies* are present in 18 per cent of preterm breech and 4 per cent to 8 per cent of term breech infants (Brenner et al 1974; Green et al 1982). *Chromosomal abnormalities* such as Trisomy 13, 18 and 21 are also seen more often in fetuses presenting by breech (Braun et al 1975), but whether there is a causal relationship between these anomalies and breech presentation is unclear. Neuromuscular abnormalities in the fetus, such as *myotonic dystrophy* reduce the ability of the fetus to turn within the uterus. In *Potter syndrome*, the associated oligohydramnios may prevent the fetus from turning from a breech presentation.

### Maternal factors

Of the maternal factors, the most common are *uterine abnormalities*. The presence of a uterine septum makes it difficult for the fetus to turn. *Cornuofundal location of placenta* reduces the space available at the uterine fundus and the breech tends to settle in the lower pole. Tumours in the lower uterine segment and placenta previa displace the presenting part upwards and cause abnormal presentations. Breech presentation is more common in multiparous women and in women with previous breech presentation.

**Table 13.1 Risk factors for breech presentation**

Relative/absolute increased liquor
    Prematurity
    Polyhydramnios
Fetal anomalies
    Neural tube defects
        Hydrocephalus
        Anencephaly
    Neuromuscular disorders
        Myotonic dystrophy
        Trisomy 13, 18, 21
        Potter syndrome
Uterine anomalies
    Septate uterus
    Bicornuate uterus
Abnormal placentation
    Placenta previa
    Cornuofundal insertion
Multifetal pregnancies
Tumours in the lower uterine segment
    Myoma
    Ovarian tumours
Multiparity
Previous breech presentation

## Classification

There are three types of breech presentations (Table 13.2) (Fig 13.1):

1. *Frank breech* (60 per cent to 70 per cent): The fetus is flexed at the hips and extended at the knees. This is the most common type of breech presentation. The compact frank breech fits snugly in the lower uterine segment; therefore, cord prolapse is less common than in other types of breech. Labour progresses more easily. The extended legs splint the body, making external version difficult. Diagnosis of frank breech presentation may be missed on abdominal examination, since the breech is compact and difficult to distinguish from a deeply engaged head. The head is also less ballotable, being flanked by the legs and can be mistaken for the buttocks.

2. *Complete breech* (5 per cent to 10 per cent): The fetus is flexed at the hips and knees. This is the least common type of breech presentation. The irregular complete breech does not effectively dilate the cervix. The risk of cord prolapse, head entrapment and cesarean section are increased.

**Table 13.2 Types of breech presentation**

**Frank breech**
    Flexed at hips and extended at knees
    Occurs in 60 per cent to 70 per cent
    Lower risk of cord prolapse
    Better progress of labour
**Complete breech**
    Flexed hips and knees
    Occurs in 10 per cent to 12 per cent
    Increased risk of
        Cord prolapse
        Cesarean section
**Incomplete breech (Footling)**
    Extended hips and /or knees
    Foot below the breech in footling
    Occurs in 20 per cent to 25 per cent
    Highest risk of
        Cord prolapse
        Head entrapment
        Cesarean section

Frank or extended    Complete    Footling

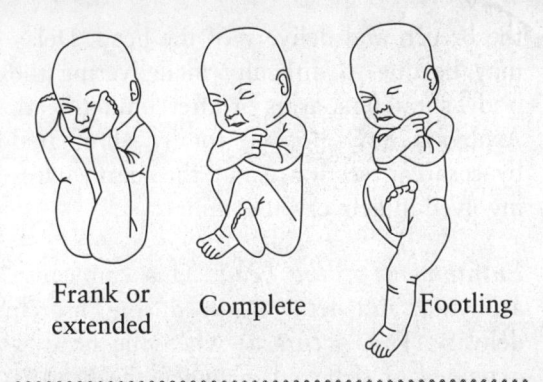

**Figure 13.1** Types of breech

3. *Incomplete breech* (20 per cent to 25 per cent): One or both hips are extended and a foot or knee is below the breech. In footling breech, one or both feet lie below the breech. Risk of cord prolapse and head entrapment is higher than in complete breech. Therefore, footling breech is considered an indication for cesarean section.

## Maternal complications

Maternal morbidity is increased in breech presentation and delivery. The causes are listed in Table 13.3. Complications depend on the mode of delivery. Vaginal breech delivery involves vaginal, and occasionally, intrauterine manipulations. These can cause vaginal/cervical lacerations, extension of episiotomy or perineal tears. Intrauterine manipulations can result in uterine rupture. Cesarean section, for any indication, is associated with mortality and morbidity due to increased blood loss, longer hospitalisation, anesthetic complications, sepsis and thromboembolic phenomena.

**Table 13.3    Causes of maternal morbidity**

Operative vaginal delivery/intrauterine manipulations
    Vaginal/cervical lacerations
    Extension of episiotomy/perineal tears
    Postpartum hemorrhage
    Infection
    Rupture uterus
Cesarean section
    Morbidity
    Mortality

## Perinatal morbidity and mortality

Perinatal morbidity and mortality are higher in breech presentation and delivery (Morgan and Kane 1964; Brenner et al 1974; Schutte et al 1985). In the past few decades, owing to an increase in cesarean section for breech presentation, the perinatal mortality rate has decreased, but has not been eliminated (Albrechtsen et al 1997; Herbst 2005). The increased risk to the fetus is due to inherent problems in the fetus presenting as breech and also from complications of breech delivery.

> The increased risk to the fetus is due to inherent problems in the fetus presenting as breech and also from complications of breech delivery.

### Inherent problems in the fetus presenting as breech

These have already been listed in Table 13.1 and include prematurity, congenital anomalies and chromosomal anomalies, and neuromuscular disorders. Mortality/morbidity due to this cannot be reduced by mode of delivery.

## Complications of breech presentation/delivery

The incidence of complications is higher in vaginal breech delivery compared to vaginal delivery of a fetus presenting by vertex. The causes are listed in Table 13.4.

### Table 13.4 Complications of breech delivery

Cord accidents
- Cord prolapse
- Short cord
- Cord entanglement

Birth asphyxia
Entrapment of aftercoming head
Birth trauma

***Cord accidents***: Cord prolapse is increased 5- to 20-fold in breech presentation (Collea 1980) and is an important cause of asphyxia and mortality. Cord prolapse is most common in footling breech (18 per cent), less in complete breech (5 per cent) and is the least in frank breech (0.5 per cent). A short cord is a known association with breech presentation and may undergo traction during delivery. The cord can get entangled and coiled around the legs, especially in footling presentation.

> Cord prolapse is increased 5- to 20-fold in breech presentation and is most common in footling breech.

***Birth asphyxia***: Birth asphyxia is three to four times higher in vaginal breech delivery (Brenner et al 1974; Green et al 1982). It is related to the time interval between delivery of the breech and delivery of the head. Delay may be due to difficulty in delivering the body, shoulders, arms or aftercoming head. Asphyxia may not be totally eliminated by cesarean section, since the manoeuvres involved in delivery are similar.

> Birth asphyxia is three to four times higher in vaginal breech delivery and is related to the time interval between delivery of the breech and delivery of the head.

***Entrapment of the head***: This can cause asphyxia and fetal death during breech delivery. This occurs a) when the head is extended or deflexed, b) when the head is larger than the body as in prematurity and c) when the delivery of the breech occurs through a cervix which is not fully dilated.

***Birth injuries***: Birth injuries are 13 times higher in vaginal breech delivery (Collea 1980). The types of injuries encountered are listed in Table 13.5. Fracture of the femur occurs when delivering extended legs or during breech extraction; fracture of the humerus occurs in nuchal arms and extended arms. Epiphyseal separations occur with undue traction. Abdominal viscera may be damaged if the fetus is grasped around the abdomen rather than by a femoro-pelvic grip. Brachial plexus injuries are usually due to traction on the neck while delivering the arms or the aftercoming head. Cervical spinal cord injuries occur during the delivery of the aftercoming head when the head is hyperextended, when undue traction is applied on the neck or when delivery of the head is attempted prematurely. Fracture of the skull bones can occur during delivery of the head. If the delivery of the head is not controlled, sudden decompression as it delivers, can cause tentorial tears and intracranial hemorrhage.

> Birth injuries are 13 times higher in vaginal breech delivery.

**Table 13.5 Fetal birth injuries in breech delivery**

Fracture of long bones
   Humerus
   Femur
Separation of epiphyses of femur, humerus
Brachial plexus injury
Depressed fracture of skull
Tentorial tears/intracranial hemorrhage
Spinal cord injuries
Injury to external genitalia
Injury to abdominal viscera

## Prematurity – the preterm breech

Mortality and morbidity are increased in preterm fetuses presenting by breech. Mortality in preterm breech deliveries beyond 32 weeks and weighing more than 1500 g is low, irrespective of the mode of delivery. However, for fetuses weighing between 1000 and 1500 gm, mortality is high if delivered vaginally (Goldenberg and Nelson 1977; Ulstein 1980; Robertson et al 1996). Cesarean section is therefore recommended, when the estimated fetal weight is in this range. Mortality in preterm breech is not entirely due to the mode of delivery, but also due to the higher incidence of congenital anomalies and growth restriction. The preterm fetus is prone to intraventricular and periventricular damage, which may result from hemorrhage or hypoxic insult. This cannot be entirely eliminated by cesarean section (Tejani et al 1984; Robertson et al 1996).

> Mortality and morbidity are increased in preterm fetuses presenting by breech. Mortality is high for fetuses weighing between 1000 and 1500 gm, delivered vaginally.

Vaginal breech delivery, however, can increase the risk of mortality (Table 13.6). The preterm head is larger than the body; therefore, entrapment of the head is common. The small body slips out through a partially dilated cervix. The occipital bone of the preterm fetus is easily damaged during vaginal breech delivery (occipital diastasis). The bone moves forward and damages the cerebellum and/or the spinal cord. Bruising of the fetal body during delivery and the resultant hemoglobinemia and myoglobinemia can lead to acute renal failure, hyperbilirubinemia and shock lung syndrome. Fracture of long bones, damage to abdominal viscera, spinal cord injury and brachial plexus injury occur more easily in the preterm baby.

Birth injuries occur during cesarean section as well. The lower segment is not well formed, the incision may be too small and the delivery of the head may be difficult. Manoeuvres during delivery of the fetus through the small incision can result in birth injuries similar to those encountered during vaginal delivery. If the lower segment is not well formed, the head may get stuck at the small circumference of the isthmus just above the lower segment incision. The incision may have to be extended as J or U or inverted T, to deliver the head. The use of short acting acute tocolysis to relax the uterus may be useful.

> Birth injuries occur during cesarean section as well since the lower segment is not well formed, the incision may be too small and the delivery of the head may be difficult.

**Table 13.6 Mortality and morbidity in preterm breech**

*Mortality unrelated to mode of delivery*
   Congenital anomalies
   Neuromuscular disorders
   Intrauterine growth restriction
   Intraventricular and periventricular damage
   Injuries due to antepartum hypoxia
*Mortality related to mode of delivery*
   Entrapment of aftercoming head
   Occipital diastasis
      Cerebellar injury
      Spinal cord injury
   Hemoglobinemia/myoglobinemia
      Acute renal failure
      Hyperbilirubinemia
      Shock lung
Visceral injuries
Fracture of long bones

## Mechanism of labour in breech presentation

The engaging diameter is the bitrochanteric diameter which is 9.5 cm. The fetal sacrum is the denominator. There are six positions: right sacro-anterior, posterior and lateral and left sacro-anterior, posterior and lateral (Fig 13.2) Mechanism of labour is described in three stages:
a. Delivery of the breech
b. Delivery of the shoulders
c. Delivery of the head

> The engaging diameter in a breech is the bitrochanteric diameter (9.5 cm).

### Delivery of the breech

The right sacro-anterior is the most common position. The bitrochanteric diameter of the breech engages in the right oblique diameter of the pelvis (Table 13.7). With uterine contractions, compaction of the fetus and descent occurs. When the breech touches the pelvic floor, the anterior buttock rotates through 45° and the bitrochanteric diameter lies in the anteroposterior diameter of the pelvis. The anterior breech hitches under the pubic symphysis, the posterior breech sweeps the perineum and the breech is born by lateroflexion. The anterior buttock slips under the pubic symphysis.

**Table 13.7 Mechanism of delivery of breech**

Engaging diameter- bitrochanteric (9.5 cm)
Denominator – sacrum
Positions
      Left sacro-anterior
      Left sacro-posterior
      Right sacro-anterior
      Right sacro-posterior
Cardinal movements
   Engagement
   Descent with compaction
   Internal rotation of anterior buttock
   Delivery by lateroflexion

### Delivery of shoulders

The bisacromial diameter of the shoulder engages in the same (right) oblique diameter of the pelvis. The anterior shoulder rotates through 45° and hitches under the pubic symphysis. The posterior shoulder sweeps the perineum and the shoulder is born. The shoulders then undergo restitution (Table 13.8).

### Delivery of the head

The suboccipito frontal diameter of the head engages in the opposite (left) oblique diameter. Internal rotation of the head through 45° results in the occiput hitching under the pubic symphysis. The face sweeps the perineum and

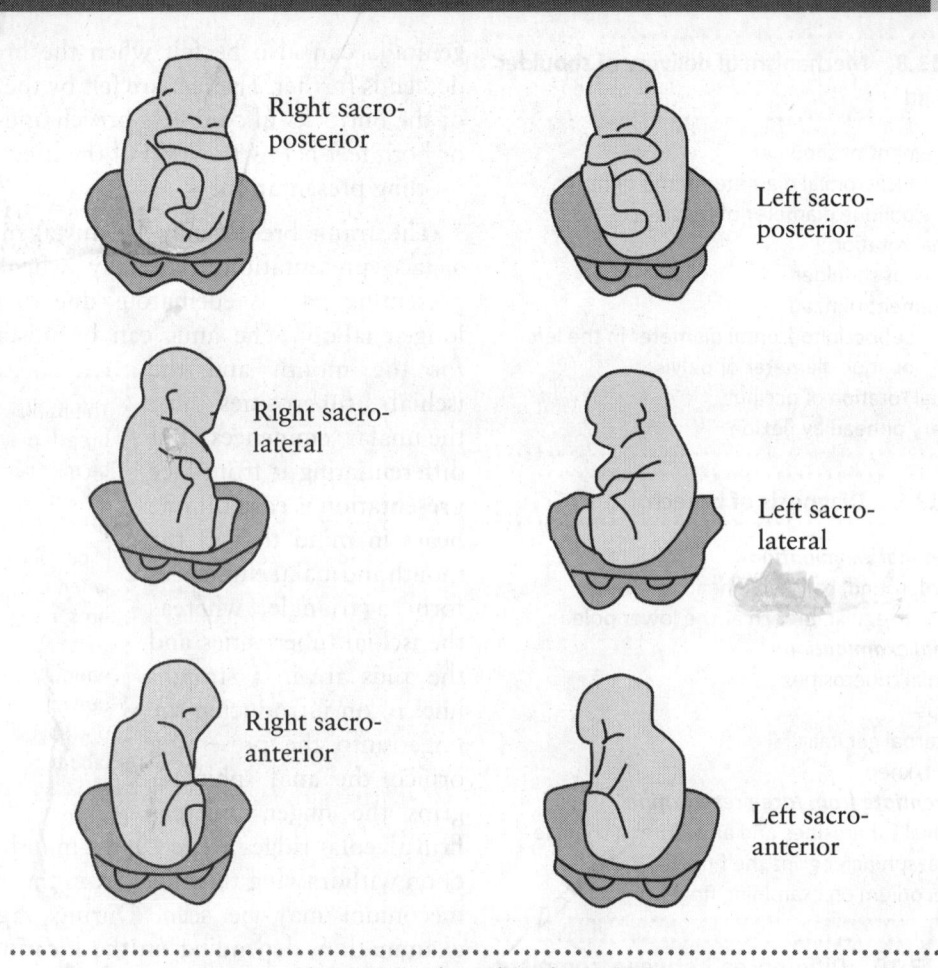

**Figure 13.2** The six breech positions

- Right sacro-posterior
- Left sacro-posterior
- Right sacro-lateral
- Left sacro-lateral
- Right sacro-anterior
- Left sacro-anterior

is born by flexion and then the occiput slips from under the symphysis pubis.

## Antenatal management of breech presentation

### Diagnosis

Diagnosis of breech presentation is by abdominal and vaginal examination (Table 13.9).

### Abdominal examination

Abdominal examination reveals the hard, ballotable head occupying the fundus, with the back to one side and limbs on the other. The firm, broad, irregular and not so ballotable breech is felt on pelvic grip. On auscultation, the fetal heart sounds are heard best above the umbilicus. There are some characteristic findings in complete breech presentation which aid in differentiating it from extended breech (Table 13.10)

#### Table 13.8 Mechanism of delivery of shoulder and head

Engagement of shoulder
    Bisacromial diameter in the right oblique diameter of pelvis
Internal rotation
Delivery of shoulder
Engagement of head
    Suboccipito frontal diameter in the left oblique diameter of pelvis
Internal rotation of occiput
Delivery of head by flexion

#### Table 13.9 Diagnosis of breech

*Abdominal examination*
    Hard, round, ballotable head at fundus
    Firm, irregular, breech at the lower pole
*Vaginal examination*
    Ischial tuberosities
    Anus
    External genitalia
    Feet/knee
*Differentiate from face presentation*
    Ischial tuberosities and anus form a triangle
    Anal sphincter grips the finger
    Meconium on examining finger

#### Table 13.10 Differences between complete and extended breech

| Complete breech | Extended breech |
| --- | --- |
| Common in multigravida | Common in primigravida |
| Head is freely mobile | Head is less mobile |
| Breech is soft, broad | Breech is compact |
| Breech is usually mobile | Breech may be engaged |
| ECV- higher success rate | ECV-lower success rate |

### Vaginal examination

The sacrum, anus and ischial tuberosities are felt on vaginal examination. The external genitalia can also be felt when the breech descends further. The feet are felt by the side of the buttocks in complete breech and one or both feet below the level of the breech in footling presentation.

The frank breech may be mistaken for a face presentation, especially when the presenting part is edematous due to prolonged labour. The anus can be mistaken for the mouth and the ischial tuberosities for the malar eminences. But differentiating it from face presentation is easier if one bears in mind that a) the mouth and malar eminences form a triangle, whereas the ischial tuberosities and the anus are in a straight line; b) on introducing the finger into the presenting orifice, the anal sphincter grips the finger, whereas firm alveolar ridges are felt in the mouth and c) on withdrawing the finger from the anus, meconium may be seen. During vaginal examination, depending on the location of the fetal sacrum, positions are designated as left sacro-anterior (LSA), left sacro-posterior (LSP), right sacro-anterior (RSA) and right sacro-posterior (RSP) or sacro-transverse (LST/RST).

> The frank breech may be mistaken for a face presentation, especially when the presenting part is edematous due to prolonged labour.

### Ultrasonography

This should be done where possible in all women diagnosed to have breech presentation. It must be performed before external version is undertaken and before decision regarding mode of delivery is made. Information that can be obtained from ultrasonography is listed in Table 13.11.

### Table 13.11 Ultrasonography in breech presentation

- Type of breech
- Estimated fetal weight
- Hyperextension/flexion of fetal head
- Liquor volume
- Location of placenta
- Gestational age (± 3 weeks at late gestation)
- Fetal anomalies
- Uterine anomalies

Other investigations like computerised tomography and radiopelvimetry are not recommended as a routine.

## External cephalic version

Since breech presentation is associated with risks to the mother and fetus and a high risk of cesarean section, converting it into cephalic presentation, if possible, is logical. This is accomplished by external cephalic version (ECV); this is the manipulation of the fetus through the mother's abdomen to convert a breech presentation, oblique or transverse lie into a cephalic presentation. ECV reduces the incidence of non-cephalic presentations (RR 0.42), and thereby, reduces the rate of cesarean section (RR 0.52) according to a Cochrane review (Hofmeyr 2000).

> Entrapment of the head usually occurs in preterm breech or with premature bearing down efforts.

Before 36 weeks, spontaneous version to cephalic presentation can occur. Performing ECV before 36 weeks has a higher success rate, but also a higher chance of spontaneous reversion to breech presentation. After 36 weeks, spontaneous version rate is less than 8 per cent and reversion to breech after version is less likely (<5 per cent) (Collaris and Oei 2004). Therefore, external version to cephalic presentation is recommended only if breech presentation persists beyond 36 weeks. In multiparous women, it may be performed at 37 weeks.

Even after successful ECV, risks of obstetric intervention and cesarean section are higher in women with breech presentation than in women who had a cephalic presentation to begin with (Chan et al 2004).

### Factors influencing success of ECV

These are listed in Table 13.12. The success rate of external cephalic version is about 60 per cent in multiparous women and 40 per cent in primigravidae. Success rate is higher when there is more liquor, in non-whites, when the fetus is smaller and in complete breech. A Cochrane systematic review has shown that use of tocolytics increases the success rate (Hofmeyr 2004).

### Table 13.12 Factors influencing success of ECV

- Parity
- Type of breech
- Liquor volume
- Engagement of the breech
- Fetal size
- Use of tocolysis
- Placental position
- Maternal ethnicity

### Risks of ECV

Complications occur in a small number of women following ECV. Fetal bradycardia may occur in a few (8 per cent), but this

> ECV is an indication for the administration of anti-D immunoglobulin since fetomaternal hemorrhage may occur.

is transient. Few cases of placental abruption and rupture uterus have been reported. Fetomaternal hemorrhage occurs in 3 per cent and anti-D immunoglobulin should be administered if the mother is Rh-negative. There is a slight (0.5 per cent) increase in immediate emergency cesarean section rate (Ben-Arie et al 1995), but no increase in perinatal mortality.

### Contraindications

The absolute and relative contraindications are listed in Table 13.13. The procedure may be difficult in obese women, primigravidae and when the placenta is located anteriorly but these are not contraindications to ECV.

Table 13.13   Contraindications to ECV

**Absolute contraindications**
Multifetal pregnancy
Antepartum hemorrhage
Major uterine anomalies
Placenta previa
Severe proteinuric hypertension
Oligohydramnios
Rupture of membranes
When elective cesarean section is planned
**Relative contraindications**
Previous cesarean section
Intrauterine growth restriction
Major fetal anomaly
Non reassuring features in cardiotocography
Fetal macrosomia

### Procedure

ECV should be performed according to strict guidelines. Facilities for cardiotocography, ultrasonography and immediate cesarean section, if required, should be available. Tocolysis is administered prior to ECV. Randomised trials using epidural analgesia have shown higher success rate and less pain in women who have been given epidural analgesia prior to ECV (MacArthur et al 2004). However, sedation and epidural analgesia are not recommended by some, since they may reduce maternal perception of pain, which is an important indicator of undue force. Further studies are needed before definite recommendations for sedation or epidural analgesia can be made.

- Ultrasonography and cardiotocography should be performed before ECV.
- The patient should be placed in a slight head down position to promote disengagement of the breech. Lateral tilt is recommended to avoid supine hypertension.
- The procedure should be performed under ultrasound guidance. Fetal heart should be monitored intermittently throughout the procedure.
- Tocolytic should be administered. Terbutaline 0.25 mg subcutaneously or ritodrine 0.2 mg/minute intravenously may be given
- The breech should be disengaged from the pelvis
- The fetal head is manipulated towards the pelvis. Forward roll is preferred but if this does not succeed, backward flip should be tried. (Fig 13.3)
- Vibroacoustic stimulation is used by some to promote fetal movement and aid the procedure.
- After completion of version, the fetal head should be held in position for a few minutes.
- Cardiotocography should be performed after the procedure
- Version can be repeated if the presentation reverts to breech. This can be performed in early labour as well.

# Breech Delivery

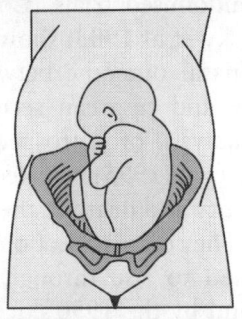

Fetus is in complete breech position

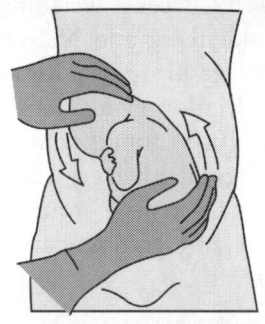

Disengaging breech from the pelvis

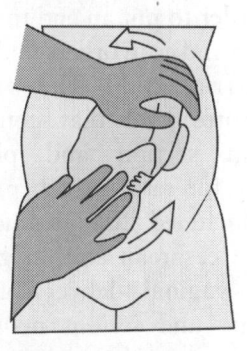

Fetal head being manipulated towards the pelvis

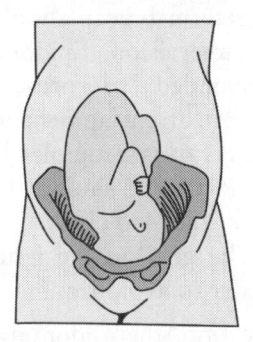

After completion of version, fetal head should be held in position for a few minutes

**Figure 13.3** External cephalic version

## Mode of delivery

### Preterm breech

Mode of delivery of the preterm breech has been controversial. The majority of obstetricians deliver them by cesarean section, but evidence in favour of this mode of delivery is lacking.

* Diagnosis of preterm labour should be established first.
* If the preterm fetus is presenting by breech, ultrasound evaluation must be performed to rule out congenital anomalies and to estimate the fetal weight.
* Earlier studies have reported unacceptably high mortality and morbidity with vaginal delivery for preterm fetuses

> Routine cesarean section is not recommended for the preterm breech.

between 26 and 32 weeks weighing 1000–1500 g (Goldenberg and Nelson 1977; Duenhoelter et al 1979). More recent studies by Malloy et al (1991) and Kayem et al (2008) found similar outcome with vaginal delivery and cesarean section. Currently, routine cesarean section is not recommended for the preterm breech.

### Delivery of preterm breech – special considerations

Vaginal delivery of preterm breech should be performed under supervision. Epidural analgesia is recommended to prevent premature bearing down. If entrapment of the head occurs and the cervix is incompletely dilated, Duhrssens's incisions should be made on the cervix at the 4 o'clock and 8 o'clock positions. The grip on the fetus should be gentle in order to avoid trauma.

During cesarean section, the abdominal incision should be large enough. The uterine incision should be adequate to deliver the head. If the lower segment is not formed, a 'J' shaped incision or low vertical incision from the lower to upper segment may be used.

## Term breech

Mode of delivery of the term breech is a topic of debate in current day obstetrics. Vaginal breech delivery is associated with higher risk of perinatal mortality and morbidity compared to delivery of fetus in vertex presentation. Wright in 1959 suggested that cesarean section for all term breech presentations would reduce the perinatal mortality drastically. But the practice of vaginal breech delivery continued till the mid 1970's. Observational studies and two randomised trials (Collea et al 1980; Gimovsky et al 1983) showed no difference in perinatal outcome between the vaginal delivery and cesarean section groups, but meta-analysis of retrospective studies by Gifford et al (1995) revealed a higher risk of fetal injury and death in the vaginal delivery group. The cesarean section rates for breech continued to rise through the subsequent years and by the 1990's, it was 60 per cent in Norway, 69 per cent in the UK and 80 per cent in USA (Vidaeff 2006).

In order to put an end to this uncertainty, Hannah and co-workers undertook the Term Breech Trial (2000). This was a randomised multicentre trial that compared planned cesarean section and planned vaginal delivery for term breech presentation. The study included 2088 women, 1041 in the planned cesarean section group and 1042 in the vaginal delivery group. Perinatal mortality and serious neonatal morbidity were significantly higher in the vaginal delivery group (5 per cent vs. 1.6 per cent, RR 0.33, 95 per cent CI 0.19–0.56, p<0.0001). The risk reduction with cesarean section was more in countries with low perinatal mortality rate. There was no difference in maternal outcome. They concluded that planned cesarean section should be recommended for all singleton term breech deliveries.

There are several criticisms of the Term Breech Trial. The number of patients recruited, rate of vaginal delivery and level of expertise in vaginal delivery were not uniform among the centres; deaths not due to vaginal delivery

> The Term Breech Trial found that perinatal mortality and serious neonatal morbidity were significantly higher in the vaginal delivery group.

were also included in the intention to treat analysis; the results were not generalisable since the risk reduction was not as good in developing countries with a high perinatal mortality rate. Nevertheless, the cesarean section rate increased dramatically in all countries after the publication of the results of the Term Breech Trial. Other studies from Sweden (Herbst and Thorngren-Jerneck 2001) and the Netherlands (Rietberg et al 2005) also found cesarean section to be safer.

Subsequently, results of small retrospective studies and a prospective observational multicentric study in France and Belgium (Goffinet et al 2006) were published. They used strict selection criteria for vaginal delivery and found no difference in neonatal outcome between the two groups. Follow up of the Term Breech Trial recruits at two years (Whyte et al 2003) showed no difference in neurodevelopmental abnormalities or death or maternal outcome.

The American College of Obstetricians and Gynecologists (ACOG) in 2006 has recommended that 'decision regarding mode of delivery should depend on the experience of the obstetrician' and 'planned vaginal delivery of a term singleton breech fetus may be reasonable under hospital specific protocol guidelines'. Informed consent must be obtained before making the decision.

**Vaginal breech delivery**

Stringent criteria must be used for selection of patients for vaginal delivery (Table 13.14). Assessment of the pelvic capacity by clinical examination, though subjective, is useful. CT pelvimetry is safer than radiopelvimetry, but is not recommended as a routine.

Contraindications for vaginal delivery are (Todd and Steer 1963; Beischer 1966):
a. antero-posterior diameter of <11 cm
b. transverse diameter of <12 cm at the inlet
c. interspinous diameter of <9 cm

A primigravida with breech presentation is not considered a contraindication for vaginal delivery. Estimated fetal weight of up to 3800 g may be considered safe for vaginal delivery in some populations, but not in others. When the maternal anthropometric measurements and the average birth weight are lower in a population, babies weighing more than 3400–3500 g may have to be delivered by cesarean section.

**Table 13.14 Criteria for selection of patients for vaginal breech delivery**

Uncomplicated breech
Extended or complete breech
Fetal weight >2000 grams < 3500 grams
No hyperextension of head
Presence of skilled obstetrician
Adequate pelvis on clinical/X-ray/CT pelvimetry

Quite often, women are admitted in labour with breech presentation. Prognosis for successful vaginal delivery in these situations can be assessed by using scoring systems. Several are available, but the one devised by Zatuchni and Andros (1967) is the most popular (Table 13.15). A score of 3 or less is an indication for cesarean section, since the perinatal mortality rate is high. Women with higher scores can be allowed vaginal delivery.

**Cesarean section for term breech**

Cesarean section is the preferred mode of delivery when there are associated maternal complications like severe preeclampsia,

## Table 13.15 Zatuchini–Andros prognostic scoring (1967)

|  | 0 | 1 | 2 |
|---|---|---|---|
| Parity | Primigravida | Multi-gravida |  |
| Gestational age | 39 weeks or more | 38 weeks | 37 weeks |
| Estimated fetal weight | >8lb (3630 gm) | 7–8 lb (3176–3629 gm) | <7 lb (3175 gm) |
| Previous breech delivery > 2500 g | none | 1 | 2 or more |
| Cervical dilatation at admission | 2 cm or less | 3 cm | 4 cm or more |
| Station of breech at admission | -3 or higher | -2 | -1 or lower |

abruption, placenta previa or contracted pelvis. Other indications are listed in Table 13.16.

## Table 13.16 Indications for cesarean section

Large baby > 3500 g
Footling or incomplete breech presentation
Hyperextension of fetal head
Inadequate pelvis
Associated maternal complications
Placenta previa

## Vaginal breech delivery

Vaginal delivery of a breech may fall under one of the following:
a. Assisted breech delivery
b. Breech extraction
c. Spontaneous breech delivery

General guidelines for a vaginal breech delivery are as follows:

- Informed consent should be obtained. The risks of vaginal delivery, cesarean section and the chances of successful vaginal delivery should be discussed.
- Facilities for immediate cesarean section should be available.
- The chances of successful vaginal delivery are higher with spontaneous labour. There is controversy regarding induction of labour and increase in perinatal mortality was found in the oxytocin induction group in the term Breech Trial (Hannah et al 2000). Most authors, therefore, do not recommend induction of labour.
- Membranes should not be ruptured early. Vaginal examination should be performed to exclude cord prolapse when membranes rupture spontaneously.
- Electronic fetal monitoring is recommended.
- Epidural analgesia is useful since it prevents premature bearing down effort, but the second stage may be prolonged.
- Oxytocin augmentation should be used with caution. Poor progress in labour may be a sign of disproportion and careful assessment is required. If required, oxytocin should be used under supervision for a limited period of time.
- Partogram must be maintained.
- Passage of meconium in the first stage may be indicative of possible fetal hypoxia, but in the second stage, it is physiological.

❖ An intravenous line should be in place for addition of oxytocin if required, in the second and third stage of labour.

## Assisted breech delivery

Assisted breech delivery is one where the fetus is delivered spontaneously, with manoeuvres to assist delivery of the arms and aftercoming head. The following personnel and equipment should be available:

1. A skilled obstetrician
2. An able assistant
3. A neonatologist
4. Facilities for lithotomy position
5. Forceps for delivering the aftercoming head

### Procedure

1. In the second stage, the patient should be placed in the lithotomy position, with the buttocks just over the edge of the couch, when the fetal anus is seen at the introitus between contractions (i.e. the breech 'climbs up' the perineum).
2. With the next contraction, an episiotomy may be performed in a nullipara, but this may not be needed in a multipara. More space at the introitus and inside the vagina helps with manipulations to deliver the shoulders and the aftercoming head.
3. The fetus should be allowed to deliver spontaneously until the nape of the neck. The feet may be gently hooked out if required.
4. If the legs are extended, the obstetrician should introduce the hand along the fetal thigh, slightly abduct it and apply gentle pressure in the popliteal fossa to flex the limb and deliver (Pinard's manoeuvre). (Fig 13.4).
5. The lower half of the fetus is wrapped in a sterile towel to avoid cutaneous stimulation. This also makes it easier to hold the baby.

   The fetus should be held by placing the thumbs on the sacrum and the index fingers on the iliac crests – known as the femoro-pelvic grip. (Fig 13.5)
6. The back of the fetus should face the obstetrician throughout the procedure.
7. If the cord is coming along with the baby, the loop of cord is pulled down and kept to one side to prevent compression and traction.
8. The duration between delivery of the fetus up to the umbilicus and delivery of the mouth is crucial to avoid asphyxia. This usually takes 2–3 minutes, but really should not exceed 5 minutes.

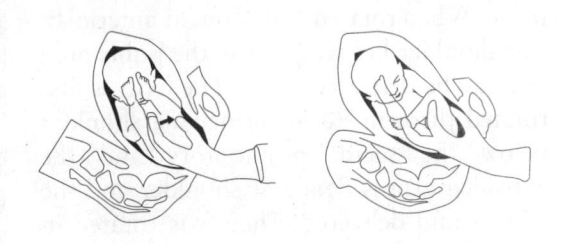

**Figure 13.4** Pinard's maneouvre

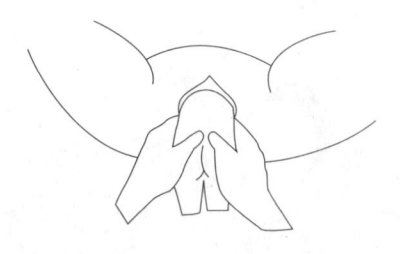

**Figure 13.5** The dorsum of the baby should face upwards

### Delivery of the shoulders and arms

With the next few contractions, the mother should be encouranged to push and this will ensure the birth of the body of the baby. When the inferior angle of the scapula is visible, the arms may be flexed and in front of the body; the anterior arm may be helped out by sweeping the obstetrician's hand over the fetal back and then anteriorly to abduct, flex and bring it down over the chest (Fig 13.6). The other arm of the fetus is swept down by this manoeuvre.

### Extended arms

The arms may be extended at the shoulder and elbow. Two techniques are used in this situation.

*Lovset's manoeuvre*: The principle behind this technique is that the posterior shoulder is always lower due to the inclination of the pelvis. When rotated and brought anteriorly, this shoulder lies well below the pubic arch and can be delivered easily. The fetus is first rotated through 90° to bring one shoulder below the sacral promontory and the extended arm is flexed at shoulder and the elbows and delivered. Then it is rotated in the clockwise or anti-clockwise direction through 180° to bring the posterior arm anteriorly under the pubic symphysis. The hands usually slip out or can be helped out gently (Fig 13.7). The posterior arm can be delivered as it is or the fetus can be rotated again through 180° in the opposite direction to bring this shoulder anteriorly and the delivery is accomplished.

*Bringing down the posterior arm*: This technique is more difficult and may require general anesthesia. The right hand must be used to deliver the right arm of the fetus and the left hand to deliver the left arm. If the back of the fetus is towards the mother's right side, the fetus is grasped by the legs using the obstetrician's right hand and pulled towards the mother's left groin (Fig 13.8). The left hand is introduced into the sacral hollow, along the arm, to the elbow. The arm is swept over the face and chest and delivered. The fetus is then rotated till the back faces the mother's left, pulled sharply towards the right groin with the left hand, and the arm is delivered by the right hand.

### Nuchal arms

When the arm is extended at the shoulder but flexed at the elbow, it assumes a nuchal position with the forearm behind the occiput. The fetus should be rotated in the direction in which the nuchal arm points and then rotated back to its normal position. This releases the nuchal arm and the breech delivery can be continued as described (Fig 13.9).

### Delivery of the aftercoming head

No attempt should be made to deliver the head until the head has descended into the pelvis and the nape of the neck is visible. Undue traction and haste at this time can

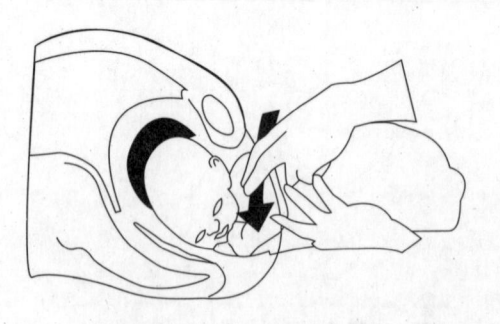

**Figure 13.6** Delivery of the arm

Breech Delivery 231

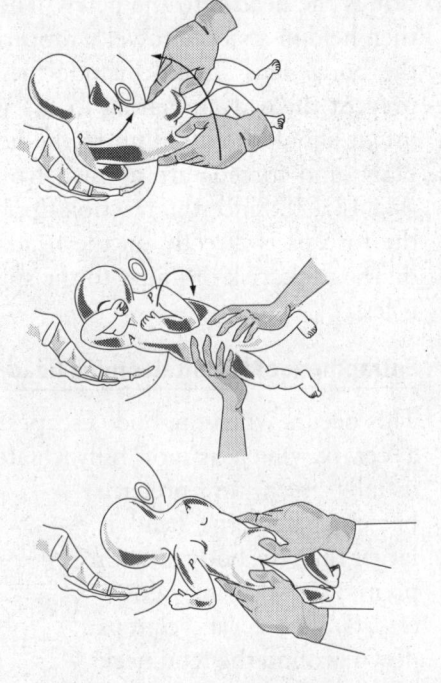

a) The fetus is held by the pelvis on the sacrum and anterior iliac spines and rotated in the clockwise direction

b) This brings the extended posterior shoulders below the symphysis pubis which can be delivered.

c) The baby is rotated in the anti-clockwise direction to bring the opposite shoulder below the symphysis pubis.

**Figure 13.7** Lovset's manoeuvre

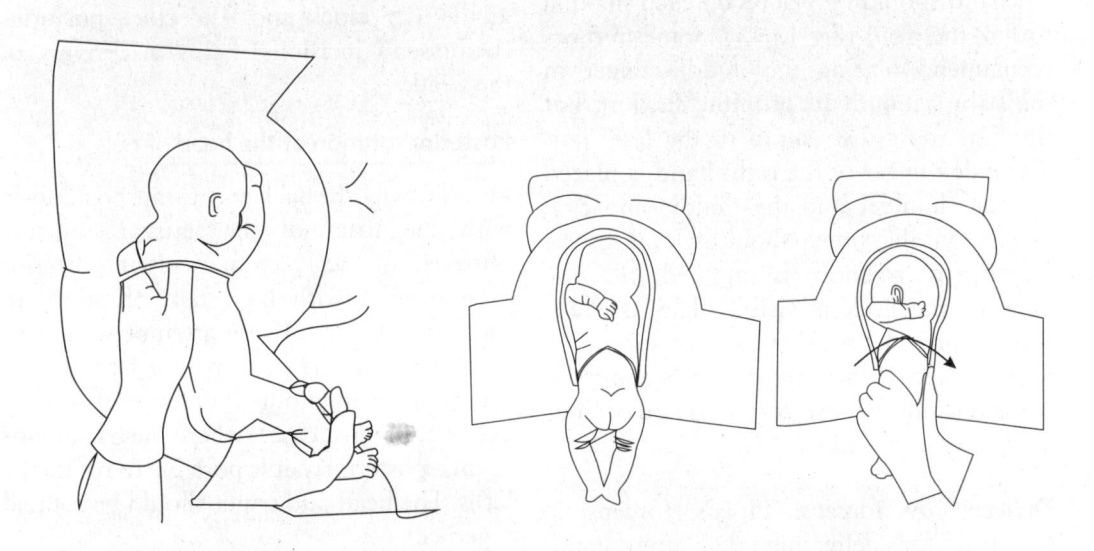

**Figure 13.8** Delivery of posterior arms

**Figure 13.9** Release of nuchal arm

lead to extension of the head. Delivery of the head may be performed by the Burns-Marshall technique, the Mauriceau-Smellie-Veit technique or by forceps.

***Burns-Marshall technique***: Once the shoulders and arms are delivered, the baby is allowed to hang vertically, partially supported by the obstetrician till the nape of the neck (which is identified by the hairline), is visible under the pubic arch. The assistant should apply suprapubic pressure to flex the head. The baby is then swung in an arc over the mother's abdomen, holding it with the index and middle fingers between the heels and the thumb and ring finger on the lateral aspect of the feet (Fig 13.10). The delivery of the head should be controlled by the assistant providing perineal support.

***Mauriceau-Smellie-Veit technique***: After delivery of the arms, the fetal body should be held astride on the obstetrician's left forearm. The index and middle finger of the left hand should be placed on each maxilla to flex the head (Fig 13.11). Some authors recommend placing the middle finger in the baby's mouth to promote flexion, but this can cause dislocation of the fetal jaw. The index finger of the right hand is placed on one shoulder and the middle and ring fingers on the other shoulder and gentle downward traction is applied till the nape of the neck is visible. The assistant should provide suprapubic pressure. The fetus is lifted towards the mother's abdomen while the mouth, nose, forehead and occiput are born.

***Delivery by forceps***: Piper's forceps is designed for delivering the aftercoming head, but any low forceps can be used. Suprapubic pressure and gentle traction brings the head into the pelvis. The fetus is then held in a sterile towel wrapped around the body. This should include the arms to prevent them from getting in the way. The infant should be lifted up to the horizontal plane and forceps are applied from below (Fig 13.12). Since the traction applied with the forceps is directly on the head and not on the neck, risk of injury to the spinal cord is less.

### Entrapment of the aftercoming head

This occurs when the body escapes through a cervix which is not fully dilated. It is usually seen in preterm breech, where the head is larger than the body or with premature bearing down efforts. The cervix clamps down around the fetal neck after the body is delivered. An attempt may be made to push the cervix up but if this fails, incising the cervix at the 4 o' clock and 8 o' clock positions (Duhrssen's incisions) helps in delivery of the head.

> Entrapment of the head usually occurs in preterm breech or with premature bearing down efforts.

### Posterior rotation of the head

Occasionally, the back may rotate posteriorly with the front of the fetus facing the obstetrician. Delivery as occiput posterior is associated with high risk of injury to the cervical spine. Every attempt should be made to keep the back of the fetus facing upwards throughout the assisted breech delivery. In most cases, where the back tends to turn posteriorly, it is possible to rotate the fetus. The head and trunk should be rotated together.

If rotation fails, the delivery of the head poses problems. The head has to be delivered

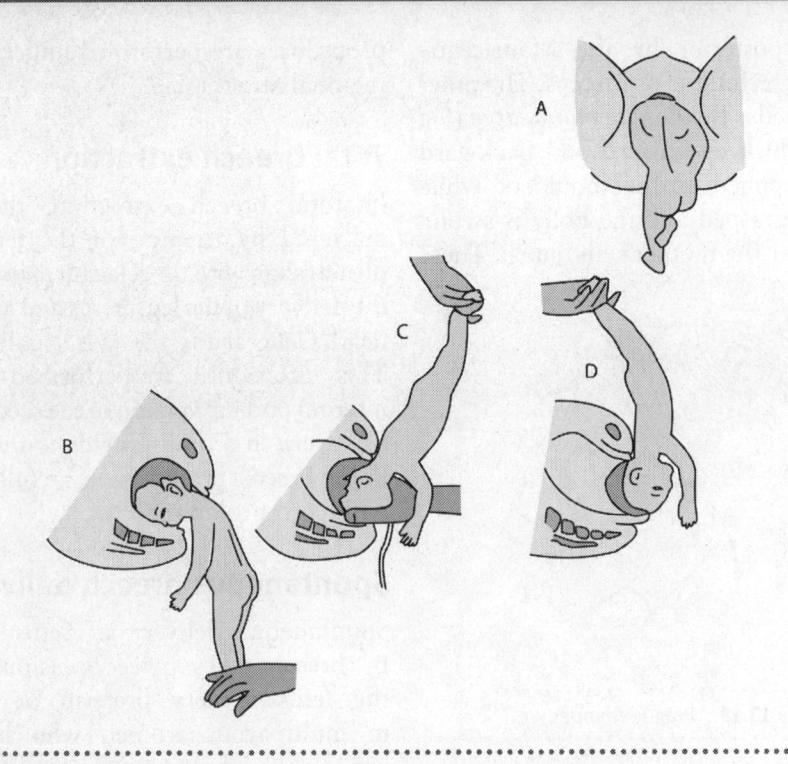

**Figure 13.10** The Burns-Marshall technique

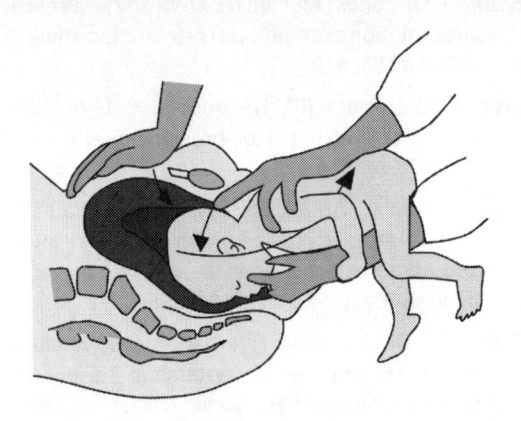

**Figure 13.11** Mauriceau-Smellie-Veit's technique

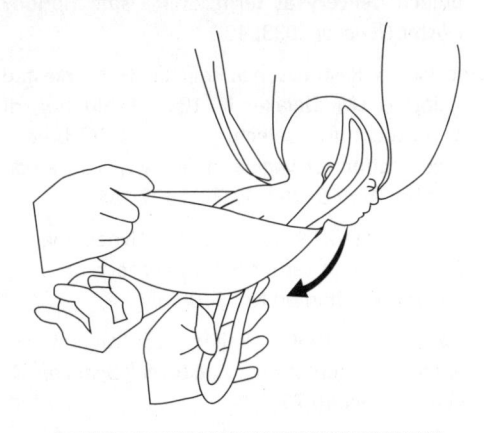

**Figure 13.12** Delivery of head using forceps

as occiput posterior by the Mauriceau–Smellie–Veit technique or forceps. The other technique used is the *Prague manoeuvre* (Fig 13.13) in which downward and backward traction is applied on the shoulders, while the feet are grasped and the body is swung in an arc over the mother's abdomen. These procedures are performed under general or regional anesthesia.

## Total breech extraction

In total breech extraction, the fetus is delivered by traction of the fetus by the obstetrician with the relevant manoeuvres for the delivery of the legs, arms and aftercoming head. General anesthesia is usually required. This procedure is performed following internal podalic version in the second of twin or, rarely, in a multigravida with transverse lie or breech presentation at full dilatation with cord prolapse.

## Spontaneous breech delivery

Spontaneous delivery of fetus presenting by breech takes place occasionally, when the fetus is very preterm or dead and in multiparous women who have rapid progress or labour.

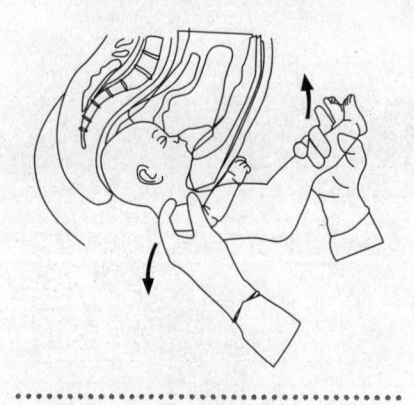

**Figure 13.13** Prague manoeuvre

## References

Alarab M, Regan C, O'Connell MP, Keane DP, O'Herlihy C, Foley ME. 2004. Singleton vaginal breech delivery at term: still a safe option? *Obstet Gynecol* 1033: 407

Albrechtsen S, Rasmussen S, Reigstad H, Markestad T, Irgens LM, Dalaker K. 1997. Evaluation of a protocol for selecting fetuses in breech presentation for vaginal delivery or caesarean section. *Am J Obstet Gynecol* 177: 586

American College of Obstetricians and Gynecologists. 2006. Mode of term singleton breech delivery. Committee Opinion No. 340, July

Beischer NA. 1966. Pelvic contraction in breech presentation. *J Obstet Gynecol Br Commonwealth* 73: 421

Ben-Arie A, Kogan S, Schachter M, Hagay ZJ, Insler V. 1995. The impact of external cephalic version on the rate of vaginal and caesarean breech deliveries: a 3-year cumulative experience. *Eur J Obstet Gynecol Reprod Biol* 63: 125

Braun FHT, Jones KL, Smith DW. 1975. Breech presentation as an indicator of fetal abnormality. *J Pediatr* 86: 419

Brenner WE, Bruce RD, Hendricks CH. 1974. The character and perils of breech presentation. *Am J Obstet Gynecol* 118: 700

Chan LY, Tang JL, Tsoi KF, Fok WY, Chan LW, Lau TK. 2004. Intrapartum cesarean delivery after successful external cephalic version: a meta-analysis. *Obstet Gynecol* 104: 155

Collaris RJ, Oei SG. 2004. External cephalic version: A safe procedure? A systematic review of version-related risks. *Acta Obstet Gynecol Scand* 83: 511

Collea JV. 1980. Current management of breech presentation. *Clin Obstet Gynecol* 23: 525

Collea JV, Chein C, Quilliga, EJ. 1980. The randomized management of term frank breech presentation–A study of 208 cases. *Am J Obstet Gynecol* 137:235

Cruickshank DP, White CA. 1973. Obstetric malpresentation : twenty years experience. *Am J Obstet Gynecol*. 116: 1097

Duenhoelter JH, Wells CE, Reisch JS, Santos-Ramos R, Jimenez JM. 1979. A paired controlled study of vaginal and abdominal delivery of the low birth weight breech fetus. *Obstet Gynecol* 54:310

Gifford DS, Morton SC, Fiske M, Kahn K. 1995. A meta-analysis of infant outcomes after breech delivery. *Obstet Gynecol*. 85: 1047

Gimovsky ML, Wallace RL, Schifrin BS, Paul RH. 1983. Randomized management of the nonfrank breech presentation at term: a preliminary report. *Am J Obstet Gynecol*. 146: 34

Goffinet F, Carayol M, Foidart JM, Alexander S, Uzan S, Subtil D, Bréart G. 2006. PREMODA Study Group. *Am J Obstet Gynecol*. 194: 1002

Goldenberg RL, Nelson JG. 1977. The premature breech. *Am J Obstet Gynecol* 127: 240,

Green JE, McLean F. Smitt LP, Usher R. 1982. Has an increased caesarean section rate for term breech delivery reduced the incidence of birth asphyxia, trauma and death? *Am J Obstet Gynecol* 142: 643

Hannah ME, Hannah WJ, Hewson SA, Hodnett ED, Saigal S,Willan AR, *et al*. 2000. Planned caesarean section versus planned vaginal birth for breech presentation at term: a randomized multicentre trial. *Lancet Term Breech Trial Collaborative Group*. 356: 1375

Herbst A. 2005. Term breech delivery in Sweden: Mortality relative of fetal presentation and planned mode of delivery. *Acta Obstet Gynecol Scand* 84 (6) : 593

Herbst A, Thorngren-Jerneck K. 2001. Mode of delivery in breech presentation at term: increased neonatal morbidity with vaginal delivery. *Acta Obstet Gynecol Scand*. 80: 731

Hickok DE, Gordon DC, Milberg JA, Williams MA, Daling JR. 1992. The frequency of breech presentation by gestational age at birth: A large population-based study. Am *J Obstet Gynecol* 166:851

Hofmeyr GJ. 2000. External cephalic version facilitation for breech presentation at term. *Cochrane Database Syst Rev*. 2: CD000184 (update : 23001; 4 : CD 000184)

Hofmeyr GJ. 2004. Interventions to help external cephalic version for breech presentation at term. *Cochrane Database Syst Rev* (1): CD000184.

Kayem G, Baumann R, Goffinet F, et al. 2008. Early preterm breech delivery: Is a policy of planned vaginal delivery associated with increased risk of neonatal death? *Am J Obstet Gynecol* 198 (3): 289. e1

Malloy MH, Onstad L, Wright E. 1991. National Institute of Child Health and Human Development Neonatal Research Network: The effect of cesarean delivery on birth outcome in very-low-birthweight infants. *Obstet Gynecol* 77:498

Macarthur AJ, Gagnon S, Tureanu LM, Downey KN. 2004. Anesthesia facilitation of external cephalic version: a meta-analysis. *Am J Obstet Gynecol*. 191:1219

Morgan ES, Kane SH. 1964. An analysis of 16,327 breech births. *JAMA*. 187: 262

Rietberg CC, Elferink-Stinkens PM, Visser GH. 2005. The effect of the Term Breech Trial on medical intervention behaviour and neonatal outcome in The Netherlands: an analysis of 35,453 term breech infants. *BJOG*. 112: 205

Robertson PA, Foran CM, Croughane-Minihane MS, Kilpatrick SJ. 1996. Head entrapment and neonatal outcome by mode of delivery in breech deliveries from 28 to 36 weeks of gestation. *Am J Obstet Gynecol* 174 : 1742

Schutte MF, van Hemel OJ, Van de Berg C, Van de Pol A. 1985. Perinatal mortality in breech presentations as compared to vertex presentations in singleton pregnancies:

An analysis based upon 57,819 computer registered pregnancies in the Netherlands. *Eur J Obstet Gynecol Reprod Biol* 19:391

Tejani N, Rebold B, Tuck S, Ditroia D, Sutro W, Verma U. 1984. Obstetric factors in the causation of early periventricular – intraventricular haemorrhage. *Obstet Gynecol.* 64: 510

Todd WD, Steer CM. 1963. Term breech: Review of 1006 term breech deliveries. *Obstet Gynecol* 22: 583

Ulstein M. 1980. Breech delivery, *Ann Chir Gynecol Fenn* 69: 70.

Vidaeff AC. 2006. Breech delivery before and after Term Breech Trial. *Clin Obstet Gynecol* 49: 198

Whyte H, Hannah M, Saigal S. 2003. Term Breech Trial Collabourative Group. Outcomes of children at 2 years of age in the Term Breech Trial. *Am J Obstet Gynecol.* 189: S57

Zatuchni GI, Andros GJ. 1967. Prognostic index for vaginal delivery in breech presentation at term: Prospective study. *Am J Obstet Gynecol.* 98(6): 854–7.

# CHAPTER 14

# STRATEGIES TO REDUCE THE RATE OF CESAREAN SECTION

*Michael Stephen Robson*

Before discussing strategies to reduce the rate of cesarean section, the most important issue to consider is why the need for such reduction? The cesarean section rate can be reduced, but only if it can be medically justified, accepted by women and society, and safely implemented.

Cesarean section rates cannot be considered on their own. Maternal and perinatal morbidity, maternal and staff satisfaction, financial cost, complaints and medico-legal cases pertaining to cesarean sections must also be analysed. The appropriate cesarean section rate will be derived from all these factors.

Finally, cesarean section rates are not homogeneous in nature and have to be analysed in a standard way to determine whether they are actually appropriate or not. Cesarean section audit, including relevant outcomes, should always be implemented before contemplating a strategy to reduce a cesarean section rate; such a reduction must be part of a long-term strategy. In practice, merely implementing good quality audit and ensuring simple organisational changes will result in an appropriate cesarean section rate. Whether or not this means a reduction in the cesarean section rate will depend on what it was to start with.

## Cesarean section rates – how much do we know, and how much do we need to know?

## The need for information

Although there is much disagreement on what an appropriate cesarean section rate is, it is agreed that it has become an issue that needs investigation and discussion. In most countries in the world, there is very poor routine data collection on all aspects of childbirth, but especially about cesarean sections, considering the interest and strong reaction cesarean section rates provoke. A cesarean section is considered by some as the most significant intervention in childbirth. The rate is increasing in most countries. The cost of a cesarean section is significant and it will increase with subsequent deliveries. The cost of not doing a cesarean section may also be significant. The justification for a cesarean section is difficult to prove, not only in economic terms, but also in terms of maternal satisfaction and fetal and maternal morbidity and mortality. By any of these criteria, more detailed information about cesarean sections must now be considered as necessary, and therefore, should be collected and returned centrally on a statutory, regular basis rather than by sporadic, small, audits using different definitions.

## Information collection on cesarean sections – general principles

There are five principles that need attention in order to ensure successful, good quality, routine, information collection. The information has to be relevant, carefully defined, accurately collected, timely and available. Information collection also calls for adequate resources and careful organisation.

The number of cesarean sections performed can easily be arrived at, but their indications will be more difficult to standardise. An attempt must be made to ensure one main indication, rather than a list of indications. This has to be carried out using an agreed, standard hierarchical system.

The importance of accurate collection of data on cesarean sections and their indications will need to be continually emphasised. There has to be a balance between quantity and quality of data collection. It is more important to have an accurate, standardised, minimum data set than a lot of data, poorly collected. Within the data set there will be a requirement for information on maternal satisfaction, morbidity and mortality. These outcomes also have to be carefully defined. Data on long-term maternal and fetal morbidity and mortality will be more difficult to collect accurately, but would, ideally, still be necessary. This would only be possible to carry out successfully with the implementation of a national database.

## Cesarean section rate – how could we reduce it?

## Classification of cesarean sections

At present, there is no accepted classification system for cesarean sections (Knight and Sullivan 2010; Bragg et al 2010). There have been many descriptive studies, but no standard classification system that has been used to make changes in specific prospective groups of women. Cesarean section rates have been analysed by comparing overall rates, by indication for cesarean section, by sub-groups of women, and by primary and repeat cesarean section rates; all of which have their disadvantages (Torloni et al 2011).

## The 10-group classification of cesarean sections

The 10-group classification makes it possible to compare cesarean section rates over time in one unit and between different units, and is shown in Table 14.1. This would, if implemented on a *continuous* basis, allow the possibility of critically assessing perinatal care thereby leading to change, if thought necessary. The obstetric concepts, with their parameters, used to classify the women in the 10-group classification are: the category of the pregnancy, the previous obstetric record of the woman, the course of labour and delivery and the gestational age of the pregnancy. From these concepts and their parameters, the 10-groups were formed.

The concepts and their parameters are all prospective, mutually exclusive, totally

**Table 14.1** The 10-Group Classification

| Groups | Number of CS over total number of women in each group | Relative size of groups % | CS rate in each group % | Contribution made by each group to the overall CS rate % |
|---|---|---|---|---|
| | *Overall Caesarean Section (CS) Rate (%) 2023/9756 (20.7%) The National Maternity Hospital Ireland* | | | |
| 1. Nulliparous, single cephalic, ≥ 37 weeks, in spontaneous labour | 202/2685 | 27.5 (2685/9756) | 7.5 (202/2685) | 2.1 (202/9756) |
| 2. Nulliparous, single cephalic, ≥ 37 weeks, induced or CS before labour | 508/1472 | 15.1 (1472/9756) | 34.5 (508/1472) | 5.2 (508/9756) |
| 3. Multiparous (excluding prev. CS), single cephalic, ≥ 37 weeks, in spontaneous labour | 35/2801 | 28.7 (2801/9756) | 1.3 (35/2801) | 0.4 (35/9756) |
| 4. Multiparous (excluding prev. CS), single cephalic, ≥ 37 weeks, induced or CS before labour | 112/908 | 9.3 (908/9756) | 12.3 (112/908) | 1.1 (112/9756) |
| 5. Previous CS, single cephalic, ≥ 37 weeks | 560/926 | 9.5 (926/9756) | 60.5 (560/926) | 5.7 (560/9756) |
| 6. All nulliparous breeches | 194/204 | 2.1 (204/9756) | 95.1 (194/204) | 2.0 (194/9756) |
| 7. All multiparous breeches (including prev. CS) | 106/130 | 1.3 (130/8756) | 81.5 (106/130) | 1.1 (106/9756) |
| 8. All multiple pregnancies (including prev. CS) | 135/204 | 2.1 (204/9756) | 66.2 (135/204) | 1.4 (135/9756) |
| 9. All abnormal lies (including prev. CS) | 28/28 | 0.3 (28/9756) | 100 (28/28) | 0.3 (28/9756) |
| 10. All single cephalic, ≤ 36 weeks (including prev. CS) | 143/398 | 4.1 (398/9756) | 35.9 (143/398) | 1.4 (143/9756) |

inclusive, simple and easy to understand and organise and are shown in Table 14.2. They are particularly clinically relevant to midwives and obstetricians, because the information they depend on is required whenever an assessment is made of a pregnant woman, who is either in labour or about to deliver. A pregnancy can only be single cephalic, single breech, multiple or a transverse or oblique lie (category of pregnancy). A woman can only be nulliparous, multiparous without a previous scar or multiparous with at least one previous scar (Previous obstetric record). A woman can only deliver by either going into spontaneous labour, have labour induced or be delivered by cesarean section before labour (Course of

**Table 14.2** Obstetric concepts and their parameters

| Obstetric concept | Parameter |
|---|---|
| Category of pregnancy | Single cephalic pregnancy |
| | Single breech pregnancy |
| | Single oblique or transverse lie |
| | Multiple pregnancy |
| Previous obstetric record | Nulliparous |
| | Multiparous (without a uterine scar) |
| | Multiparous (with a uterine scar) |
| Course of labour and delivery | Spontaneous labour |
| | Induced labour |
| | Caesarean section before labour (Elective or emergency) |
| Gestation | Gestational age in completed weeks at time of delivery |

pregnancy). Lastly, a pregnancy's gestational age is unique, provided an accepted method for calculating it is agreed upon. All the four obstetric concepts and their parameters fit the principles required for a classification system. Their definitions are mostly self-explanatory, but there are two parameters where there may be slight differences in interpretation. The definition of the parameters of spontaneous labour and induction within the obstetrical concept of course of labour and delivery will always be controversial. Likewise, the calculation of gestational age may also differ between different units, but the simplicity of term or pre-term is attractive and feasible in most cases. The advantages, though, of using these particular concepts and their parameters in practice outweigh their disadvantages; if the same definitions are consistently applied, the analysis and sub-analysis of the groups will identify any significant variations in practice.

Each of the 10-groups can and should be further subdivided when indicated. The indications for cesarean section should be specifically defined within each group of women because the definition and the management will vary in each group and will have different risk–benefit ratios.

Therefore, assuming that there is a belief that a cesarean section rate was too high, and also assuming that all the other information required is available, including outcome and maternal satisfaction, then the 10-groups can be used to assess any cesarean section rate, and in particular, compare with other lower or higher cesarean section rates either within the same delivery unit from previous years, or with other delivery units elsewhere. It would be possible to see in which groups of women, the differences in the incidence of cesarean sections occur. It will not immediately explain why there is a difference in the rates of cesarean sections, and further analysis would be required, but it will provide a useful overview to start from. From this, it will be possible to target different groups of women and change the management according to available evidence.

In terms of cesarean section rates, the most important areas of management to assess are ensuring fetal well-being and efficient uterine action in labour, together with auditing the indications for induction and pre-labour cesarean sections. Indications for cesarean sections in labour should be classified into fetal or dystocia.

## The use of the 10-group classification to analyse cesarean section rates

The simplest way to demonstrate how the 10-group classification could be used to assess and then possibly instigate changes in management that may alter the cesarean section rate, is to explain and then use Table 14.1 with the data supplied, to go through each of the groups showing how each of the columns are useful in interpreting the available information.

The most important point is that all the women from the obstetric population being studied are represented in Table 14.1. There are no exceptions.

At the top of the table, the numerator indicates the total number of cesarean sections carried out, and the denominator, the total number of women in the obstetric population. This gives the overall cesarean section rate.

The first column from the left hand side of the table describes each of the 10-groups of women.

The numerator in each group in the second column indicates the number of cesarean sections in each group and the denominator indicates the number of women in each of the groups. The first check that should be made when assessing the 10-groups is that these numbers add up to the totals at the top of the table.

In the third column, the relative size of each of the 10-groups has been calculated by taking the denominator of each group, and dividing it by the total denominator of the obstetric population and expressing this as a percentage.

The fourth column shows the cesarean section rate within each group. This is calculated by dividing the numerator in each group by the denominator in each group and is also expressed as a percentage.

Lastly, the fifth column shows the absolute percentage contributions made by each group to the overall cesarean section rate. This is calculated by dividing the numerator of each group, the number of cesarean sections, by the total denominator of the obstetric population. The contribution made by each group to the overall cesarean section rate is not only dependent on the cesarean section rate within the group, but also on the size of the group.

Using the figures provided in Table 14.1, it is immediately possible to see from columns 2 (overall numbers) and 5 (percentages), which group contributes most to the cesarean section rate. In the example shown and in most general obstetric populations, it is Group 5. This group consists of women with at least one previous cesarean section and a single cephalic pregnancy at 37 weeks gestation or greater. Columns 3 and 4 from that group are then used to compare with either previous data from the same unit, or data from other units to see whether any differences in the contribution to the overall cesarean section rate from this group is due to a difference in the size of the group or to a difference in the cesarean section rate within the group, or possibly a combination of the two. Group 5 is a heterogeneous group of women. It contains women with one or more previous scars and also some women who have previously delivered vaginally. Therefore, to interpret the cesarean section rate in this group more accurately, more information is required. More detailed analysis of the cesarean section rate in this group would consist of assessing what proportion of the cesarean sections were carried out in spontaneous labour, induced labour, or by pre-labour cesarean section. Depending on those results, further assessment would depend again on which sub-group contributed to the most cesarean sections. The cesarean section rate within spontaneous labour would need to be assessed, as would the cesarean sections from Group 5 resulting from women who were either induced or who had a cesarean section before labour. It is at this stage that the standardised indications for either inductions or cesarean sections before labour have to be known and justified. Other outcome information would also be required at this stage to determine the balance of risks to mother and baby, of either inducing labour or delivering by cesarean section as against waiting for the onset of spontaneous labour. Awaiting spontaneous labour should, at least in theory, result in a lower cesarean section rate, but this would also have to be proven. The size of group 5 generally reflects previous cesarean sections in nulliparous women and the simplest way of reducing the size is by avoiding the first cesarean section; in particular, in nulliparous, single cephalic pregnancies at greater or equal to 37 weeks gestation in spontaneous labour. A cesarean section rate of 50 per cent to 70 per cent in Group 5 is a reasonable target. The aim should be a short spontaneous labour. Although the largest contributor to the cesarean section rate, Group 5, should be treated with respect because of the unpredictable nature of uterine rupture.

Group 2 in Table 14.1 is the next largest contributing group to the overall cesarean section rate. Columns 3 and 4 are again used to compare with other data in order to assess whether it is the size of the group that differs or whether it is the cesarean section rate within the group that differs. Group 2 consists of nulliparous women, with a single cephalic pregnancy at greater than or equal to 37 weeks gestation, who either had labour induced or were delivered by pre-labour cesarean section. To analyse the group further, it has to be first divided into: those women who had labour induced and those who were delivered by pre-labour cesarean section. The reason why they are initially included in the same group is because in both sub-groups of women, delivery was indicated before waiting for the onset of spontaneous labour. Whether induction of labour was attempted as against pre-labour cesarean section would depend on different individual or institutional practice. As in Group 5, at this stage, other information would be required to determine the balance of risks to mother and baby of either inducing labour or delivering by cesarean section as against waiting for the onset of spontaneous labour. Waiting for spontaneous labour would again, in theory at least, result in a lower cesarean section rate, but this would need to be confirmed in practice. The standardised indications for either inductions or cesarean sections before labour also need to be known and justified. The contribution of Group 2 to the overall cesarean section rate depends more on the size of the group, in particular, the pre-labour cesarean section group rather than the cesarean section rate in the inductions. Therefore, more emphasis should be placed on the necessity and indications for inductions as opposed to the methods of induction. In Table 14.1, Groups 2 and 5 are responsible for almost half the total number of cesarean sections.

Groups 1 and 3 are significant, in the sense that they are usually the two largest groups in most obstetric populations and consist of single cephalic pregnancies, in spontaneous labour at 37 weeks or greater gestation. They would be considered as normal, low-risk pregnancies. Group 1 includes only nulliparous women. Group 3 includes only multiparous women with no previous scar. These two groups are usually looked after by midwives, and have never been audited as separate groups. The cesarean section rate in Group 3 rarely deviates outside 1 per cent to 3 per cent, if the information has been accurately collected. It is the most consistent figure in the 10-group classification, and this is probably because all the women in this group tend to deliver without needing any significant obstetric intervention. Indeed, the cesarean section rate in this group is so consistent that, if it is found to be greater than 3 per cent, that figure is more likely to be due to inaccurate data collection than any other reason. The most common reason why this may occur is because some women who have had one or more previous uterine scars are wrongly included in this group. Alternatively, these are women who although thought to be in spontaneous labour, on review of the notes, were actually found to be clinically, cases of labour induction.

Group 1 is probably the most important group in the entire obstetric population, the gold standard of any labour ward. Like Group 3, it is rarely audited as a separate group, yet it is one of the groups that not only varies most in methods of management, but also in terms of outcome, in particular the cesarean section rate (Brennan et al 2009). The cesarean section rate in Group 1 will depend not only on the type of management used, but also to a certain extent on the relative size of Group 2. This, in most obstetric populations, will depend on the delivery unit's policy on induction in general and post-dates in particular. Cesarean section rates increase with gestation from 37 weeks and upwards in nulliparous women, with single cephalic pregnancies in spontaneous labour. Therefore, if post-date pregnancies are induced before the onset of spontaneous labour, their incidence in Group 1 will decrease and that should contribute to a lower cesarean section rate in Group 1. The cesarean section rate target for Group 1 should be 5 per cent to 10 per cent and is achievable with appropriate management ensuring fetal well-being at the same time as efficient uterine action. This figure will also depend on the age and body mass index profile within the group.

Group 4 is similar to Group 2, but consists of multiparous women (without a previous scar), with a single cephalic pregnancy, who either had labour induced or were delivered by cesarean section before labour. A similar analysis to that of Group 2 should take place. The contribution of this group to the overall cesarean section depends mainly on the incidence of pre-labour cesarean section. In Group 4, this will be mainly due to maternal request as there are not many medical reasons for pre-labour cesarean section. Again, audit will be required to confirm this. The incidence of cesarean section in inductions in Group 4 is relatively low, at about 5 per cent as opposed to inductions in Group 2, which will vary between 25 per cent and 30 per cent, depending on the relative size and profile of Group 2.

Groups 6 and 7 consist of all breech presentations, whatever the gestation. A significant number of breeches are delivered by cesarean section and although that rate may vary, it is never going to be very low. Therefore, the contribution to the overall cesarean section rate will be more dependent on the incidence of breeches than anything else. The incidence of breeches depends on two main variables: the success of external cephalic version and the incidence of preterm delivery. Interestingly, there is also an increased incidence of breeches in nulliparous women. The cesarean section rate in these two groups are now close to 100 per cent, but because the groups are no bigger usually than 3 per cent to 4 per cent (of the total number of deliveries), together they will never make a large contribution to the overall cesarean section rate; there is a maximum contribution, after which it can be no higher. These groups are not the ones to target when trying to reduce the overall cesarean section rate.

Group 8 covers all multiple pregnancies. Relatively speaking, this group usually makes a small contribution to the overall cesarean section rate, but it seems to be increasing, partly due to an increase in the size of the group, and also to an increase in the cesarean section rate within the group. The size of the group will vary, mainly according to the different types of infertility treatment. The cesarean section rate within the group may be affected by the decrease in availability of the clinical skills required to deliver twins, in particular the delivery of the second twin by breech. It may also be affected by the earlier diagnosis of monochorionicity and growth discrepancy in all twin pregnancies which are picked up in specialised twin clinics leading to an increase in pre-labour cesarean section or induction of labour, but reduction in perinatal mortality. Group 8 also needs to be analysed based on previous obstetric record and course of the pregnancy. However, like Groups 6 and 7, it will never make a large contribution to the overall cesarean section rate, and therefore, it is not the group to be targeted to reduce the overall cesarean section rate.

Group 9 is the smallest of the groups, but is nonetheless important. Its consistent but small size is important for confirming accurate data collection. Its size should be no more than 0.6 per cent and the cesarean section rate in the group should always be 100 per cent. It consists of all the deliveries by cesarean section that take place for transverse or oblique lies. Further analysis, if the size of the group is larger, would include gestational age and whether the cesarean sections were in labour or pre-labour. Some women may be delivered earlier than necessary at their own request rather than opting for a more conservative approach allowing time for the baby to revert to a longitudinal lie and the onset of spontaneous labour. This group makes an insignificant contribution to the overall cesarean section rate, unless it is abnormally large in size.

Group 10 is often cited as the reason why many delivery units, especially tertiary referral centres, have a high cesarean section rate. This is rarely the reason for a high overall cesarean section rate. It consists of a group of women where there is probably most consistency in clinical management, in terms of the decision-making by obstetricians to deliver by cesarean section, because the options are limited. The contribution made by this group to the overall cesarean section rate is usually, therefore, more dependent on the size of the group, the incidence of pre-term labour and pre-term obstetrical complications. This group, too, needs to be analysed, not only according to the previous obstetric record, but also by course of labour and delivery (Table 14.2). A high incidence of pre-term spontaneous labour usually lowers the cesarean section rate in this group and a high cesarean section rate in this group, more than 30 per cent, usually signifies a high incidence of fetal and maternal medical conditions such as intrauterine growth restriction and preeclampsia. The size of the group may vary significantly, but the average is around 5 per cent.

As more data becomes available from different units (McCarthy et al 2007, Betran et al 2009, Howell et al 2009, Allen et al 2010, Scarella et al 2011) and over time from the same unit (Brennan et al 2011) in this standardised format, the 10-group classification will become more useful. Interestingly, similar overall cesarean section rates from different units may have completely different contributions from the different groups. Likewise, the overall cesarean section rate in a unit may remain the same, but the contribution to the overall cesarean section rate from each of the groups may change.

## Reducing the cesarean section rate

The methods that are required to do this successfully depend on the implementation of the labour ward audit cycle (Figure 14.1). It depends on auditing labour ward events and outcome, classifying them, assessing them, and then subsequently, modifying the management. The principles of labour ward audit have been described elsewhere (Robson 1997). Active participation in collecting the information should be part of the responsibility of all the professionals working on the labour ward. After classification of the crude data, the information has to be disseminated among the professionals involved in labour and delivery. Assessment of management at some stage involves setting targets of care that are thought to be desirable. One of those targets will be an appropriate cesarean section rate, but this cannot be considered, as it often is, in isolation from other targets such as fetal and maternal morbidity and mortality. Available resources and expertise also need to be taken into account when setting targets. The most significant target to consider today is maternal satisfaction, and this target may unfortunately often be contradictory to other targets set, making it both difficult and confusing for health professionals. Maternal satisfaction is best assessed by providing debriefing forms to all women who deliver in the unit.

In order to set targets, and indeed, to assess management as well as modify management, regular multidisciplinary meetings are required. There are different ways in which these can be held, but it is the author's view that daily morning meetings lasting approximately half an hour are the best way. These need to be attended, supported and led by senior midwifery and medical staff. This should include a discussion of relevant events in the previous 24 hours in the delivery suite. The success of these meetings depends on the existence of a good information system and adequate preparation for each meeting. The return for this commitment by all the

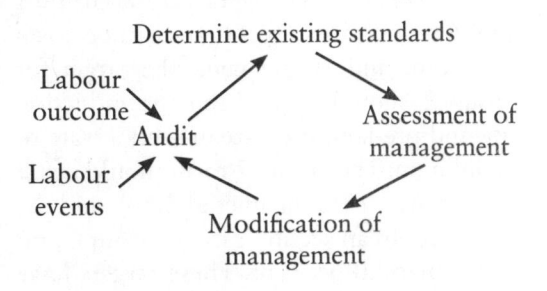

**Figure 14.1** The Labour Ward Audit Cycle

staff is good teamwork and communication in the department. Written guidelines in the management of labour and delivery may be helpful as an adjunct, but should not replace the daily morning meetings and continuous education. The cesarean section rate is an important target within the framework described, but should never be the only target and, therefore, never considered in isolation.

The methodology of using the labour ward audit cycle has been described previously (Robson et al 1996). In that study, the cesarean section rate was reduced by using the audit cycle to identify and instigate changes in the management of labour in a specific group of woman (Group 1). The groups of women that need to be targeted in any population have to be identified by carrying out audit using the 10-groups.

It is the author's opinion that the groups that will be identified most often are Groups 1, 2 and 5. The single cepalic nulliparous woman at greater or equal to 37 weeks gestation (Groups 1 and 2 together) is the most important group in maternity care. Its contribution to both maternal and fetal perinatal outcome in any maternity unit is considerable. It is also the driving force behind the increase in cesarean section rates (Brennan et al 2011). The target for Group 1 should be a cesarean section rate of between 5 per cent and 10 per cent; the target for Group 2 should be to keep the induction rate and pre-labour cesarean section rate to a minimum. The Group 2 ratio should be no lower than 2:1 (Brennan et al 2009) and the overall cesarean section rate in Group 2, no higher than 30 per cent. These targets have to be considered in relation to all the other outcomes. The cesarean section rate for Groups 1 and 2 together (all single cephalic nulliparous women greater than or equal to 37 weeks gestation) should 15 per cent to 17 per cent. This takes into account, relative sizes of groups as well as the cesarean section rate within the groups.

Group 5 should be managed with care, as there is a significant and unpredictable risk to trying to reduce the cesarean section rate too radically here, namely uterine rupture. The aim should be to encourage all women to aim for a short spontaneous labour, avoid induction, and if oxytocin is to be used, then it should be used only for a limited time and with strict rules.

It is the author's view that Groups 6, 7, 8, 9 and 10 should not be targeted in trying to reduce the cesarean section rate. The relative risk reward is too high. As for the remaining two groups, Group 3 is unlikely to contribute significantly to the overall cesarean section rate and Group 4 may or may not be significant in their contribution, but this will have to be confirmed by audit.

With continuous critical review as described and frequent comparison with other delivery units, the cesarean section rate in each individual unit will find its appropriate level. Whether that will mean a reduction in the overall cesarean section rate will depend on how high the rate was before.

The aim in future should not be to worry whether the cesarean section rate is too high or too low, but rather what it is, why and whether it can be considered to be appropriate, taking into consideration all the relevant outcome factors. This assessment should take place on a continuous basis in all delivery units using a similar kind of system.

## Conclusion

Any strategy to reduce the cesarean section rate requires good information both on cesarean section rates and outcomes. Good classification systems will allow a strategy to target certain groups of women where the risk–reward ratio will be most favourable (Torloni et al 2011). Comparing results and management with other units will result in arriving at the most appropriate care to suit each individual population of women.

Successful implementation requires regular multidisciplinary meetings involving as many of the staff as is practically possible in assessing and subsequently changing management.

## References

Allen VM, Baskett TF, and O'Connellon CM. 2010. Contribution of select maternal groups to temporal trends in rates of caesarean section. *J Obstet Gynaecol Can* vol. 32 (7) pp. 633–41

Betrán A, Gulmezoglu A, Robson M, Merialdi M, Souza J, D Wojdyla D, Widmer M, Carroli G, Torloni M, Langer A, Narváez A, Velasco A, Faúndes A, Acosta A, Valladares E, Romero M, Zavaleta N, Reynoso S and Bataglia V. 2009. WHO Global Survey on Maternal and Perinatal Health in Latin America: classifying caesarean sections. *Reprod Health* vol. 6 (1) pp. 18

Bragg F, Cromwell DA, Edozien LC, Gurol-Urganci I, Mahmood T, Templeton A and Van Der Meulen JH. 2010. Variation in rates of caesarean section among English NHS trusts after accounting for maternal and clinical risk: cross sectional study. *BMJ*. Vol. 341 (Oct06 1) pp. c5065–c5065

Brennan D, Murphy M, Robson M and O Herlihy C. 2011. The Singleton, Cephalic, Nulliparous Woman After 36 Weeks of Gestation. *Obstetrics and Gynecology* vol. 117 (2, Part 1) pp. 273-279

Brennan D, Robson M, Murphy M and O'Herlihy C. 2009. Comparative analysis of international cesarean delivery rates using 10-group classification identifies significant variation in spontaneous labor. *Am J Obstet Gynecol* vol. 201 (3) pp. 308.e1–8

Howell S, Johnston T and Macleod SL. 2009. Trends and determinants of caesarean sections births in Queensland, 1997-2006. *The Australian & New Zealand Journal of Obstetrics and Gynaecology* vol. 49 (6) pp. 606–11

Knight M and Sullivan EA. 2010. Variation in cesarean delivery rates. *BMJ* vol. 341 pp. c5255

McCarthy FP, Rigg L, Cady L and Cullinane F. 2007. A new way of looking at Caesarean section births. *The Australian & New Zealand Journal of Obstetrics and Gynaecology* vol. 47 (4) pp. 316–20

Robson M. 1997. *Labour Ward Audit. Management of Labor and Delivery*. Ed R Creasy. Blackwell Science pp. 559—70. pp. 1–12

Robson M, Scudamore IW and Walsh SM. 1996.Using the medical audit cycle to reduce cesarean section rates. *Am J Obstet Gynecol* vol. 174 (1 Pt 1) pp. 199–205

Robson M. 2001. Classification of caesarean sections. *Fetal and Maternal Medicine Review*. 12:1 23–39

Scarella A, Chamy V, Sepúlveda M, Belizán J. 2011. Medical audit using the Ten Group Classification System and its impact on the cesarean section rate. *Eur J Obstet Gynecol Reprod Biol*. 154 (2): 136–40.

Torloni MR, Betran AP, Souza JP, Widmer M, Allen T, Gulmezoglu M and Merialdi M. 2011. *Classifications for cesarean section: a systematic review*. PLoS ONE vol. 6 (1) pp. e14566.

CHAPTER 15

# CESAREAN SECTION: PROCEDURE AND TECHNIQUE

*Gita Arjun, S Rajasri, Soumya Balakrishnan and Vinotha Thomas*

A cesarean delivery is defined as the birth of a fetus via both a laparotomy (an incision in the abdominal wall) and a hysterotomy (incision in the uterus). At least 1 in 5 women delivers by cesarean section, so it is important for an obstetrician to know the indications, techniques and complications of a cesarean section.

Cesarean sections are life-saving procedures that are firmly ensconced in obstetric practice. With the immense advances in anesthetic services and improved surgical techniques, the morbidity and mortality of this procedure has come down considerably. This has, albeit wrongly, emboldened obstetricians to perform more and more cesarean sections. The universal upswing in cesarean rates has hit both developing and developed countries. Unfortunately, given economic constraints, developing countries are hardly equipped to handle the repercussions of such an unprecedented increase in surgical interventions.

## Rising rates of cesarean sections

Over the last 20 years, there has been a disturbing increase in the rate of cesarean sections around the world, including India. It used to be a matter of pride to have low cesarean section rates, especially in teaching hospitals. A collaborative study done by the Indian Council of Medical Research in the 1980s showed a cesarean section rate of 13.8 per cent in teaching hospitals in India (ICMR 1990). This rate has risen significantly. A study to examine the escalating rates of cesarean sections in teaching hospitals in India compared the rates between 1993–1994 and 1998–1999. The data was from 30 medical colleges/teaching hospitals (Kambo et al 2002). The overall rate of cesarean section increased from 21.8 per cent in 1993–1994 to 25.4 per cent in 1998–1999. What was alarming was that 42.4 per cent were primigravidas and 31 per cent were from rural areas. Because of the rise in primary cesarean sections, there is a proportionate rise in repeat sections. Between 1990 and 1992, the repeat cesarean section rate was between 30 per cent to 45 per cent in teaching hospitals in Madurai and Chennai, India (Rao et al 1994).

In a study over a two-year period in an urban area of India, the total cesarean section rates even in the public and charitable sectors were 20 per cent and 38 per cent respectively. In the private sector, the rate was an astonishing 47 per cent (Sreevidya and Sathiyasekaran 2003). A similar study from an affluent part of Chennai, India, showed that almost 1 out of 2 women (45 per cent) had a cesarean section (Pai et al 1999).

> In the private sector, the cesarean section rate was an astonishing 47 per cent. (Sreevidya and Sathiyasekaran 2003).

A study from the United Kingdom (Bragg et al 2010), showed that among 620,604 singleton births, 147,726 (23.8 per cent) were delivered by cesarean section. Women were more likely to have a cesarean section if they had had one previously (70.8 per cent) or had a baby with breech presentation (89.8 per cent).

A survey of cesarean rates in Latin America showed that the median rate of cesarean delivery was 33 per cent, with the highest rates of cesarean delivery noted in private hospitals (51 per cent) (Villar et al 2006).

In the United States, the overall cesarean section rate was 32 per cent in 2007 (Hamilton et al 2009).

It is difficult to pinpoint the exact cause for the rising rates of cesarean sections. Contributing factors may include reluctance on the part of the obstetrician to attempt a vaginal delivery after a previous cesarean section or in a breech presentation, patient perception that a cesarean is safer for the fetus leading to cesareans-on-demand and social-cultural influences (e.g. choosing an auspicious time).

It is also not easy to fix an optimal cesarean section rate. In the United States, a 15 per cent cesarean section rate is seen as the goal to achieve (USDHHS 2000). The World Health Organization (WHO) too recommends 15 per cent as the optimal cesarean section rate. It is interesting to note that even a decade ago, only three countries had rates lower than 15 per cent (Walker et al 2002). India has not established guidelines for acceptable cesarean section rates.

## Do increasing rates of cesarean decrease perinatal mortality?

High-risk patients do not show a large variation in cesarean rates, regardless of where they deliver. The largest variation occurs in the low-risk patient, specifically the nulliparous patient with term singleton fetuses with vertex presentation without other complications. It has been shown that in this group, perinatal morbidity and mortality rates are not improved by the performance of a cesarean section (O'Driscoll and Foley 1987). In another study, perinatal mortality increased despite doubling of the cesarean section rate (Mukherjee et al 1993). These findings suggested that the increase in cesarean sections did not decrease perinatal deaths. A study from a hospital in Mumbai showed that the cesarean section rate increased from 1.9 per cent to 16 per cent in 40 years, but without any improvement in overall perinatal outcome beyond a cesarean section rate of 10 per cent (Mehta et al 2001).

> The increase in cesarean sections does not decrease perinatal deaths in low-risk patients

In fact, an unindicated cesarean section may do more harm than good. In a low risk, uncomplicated pregnancy, cesarean section has an eight-fold higher mortality than vaginal delivery (Pettiti 1985), 8–12 times higher morbidity (Boehm and Graves 1994) and a higher incidence of complications in subsequent pregnancies.

## Indications for cesarean section

A cesarean section may be done in a labouring woman (*emergency* cesarean section) or in a woman who has not gone into labour (*elective* cesarean section). Uniformly, across nations, the commonest indications for 85 per cent of cesareans performed are:

* dystocia
* fetal distress
* previous cesarean delivery
* breech presentation

Cesarean sections may be done for several reasons. The indications usually fall into four categories (NICE Guidelines, 2004):

1. Immediate threat to the life of the woman or fetus
2. Maternal or fetal compromise which is not immediately life threatening
3. No maternal or fetal compromise, but needs early delivery
4. Delivery timed to suit woman or staff

## Elective cesarean section

An elective cesarean section is a planned cesarean for reasons that arise in the antepartum period. Repeat cesarean sections are a leading indication for cesarean sections. It is therefore important to be absolutely certain about the indication for a primary section since doing a cesarean section considerably increases the risk for a subsequent cesarean.

Some evidence-based indications for elective cesareans are:

1. A twin pregnancy with first twin breech (Hogle et al 2003)
2. Maternal HIV (International Perinatal HIV Group 1999)
3. Primary genital herpes with visible lesions at time of labour or ruptured membranes (ACOG 2007)
4. Grade 3 and 4 placenta previa
5. A term singleton breech, if external cephalic version is contraindicated or has failed, is considered an indication for an elective cesarean section (Hannah et al 2000). However, each obstetric unit needs to work out its policy for allowing a vaginal delivery in selected cases of breech presentation.

An elective cesarean need not be offered for the following indications:

1. Twin pregnancy, if first twin is cephalic at term (Hogle et al, 2003)
2. Preterm birth
3. A 'small for gestational age' baby (ACOG 2002)
4. Hepatitis B virus
5. Hepatitis C virus
6. *Recurrent* genital herpes at term with no visible lesions (ACOG 2007)

## Cesarean section on demand

Patient demand has complicated this already complex issue. In the United Kingdom, patient demand was the third commonest indication for elective cesarean section in 1992 (Atiba et al 1993)). Fear of the pain of labour, and avoiding injury to the perineum, which may lead to sexual dysfunction, are some of the reasons quoted. In India, as in many Asian countries, there is great emphasis placed on the astrological calendar.

The demand for the baby to be born at an auspicious time has placed great pressure on obstetricians and when they acquiesce to this demand, the rate will naturally go up (Kabra et al 1994).

Bewley and Cockburn (2002a, 2002b) in their commentary on patient 'request' cesareans, state that demand cesareans cannot be supported, either on ethical or medical grounds.

> Demand cesareans cannot be supported, either on ethical or medical grounds.

## Emergency or intrapartum cesarean section

### Dystocia

A labour abnormality is the commonest cited cause for an intrapartum cesarean section. Dystocia is defined as the slow, abnormal progression of labour. Freidman (1978) introduced terms for labour abnormalities. These were more precise than terms used earlier, and explained which part of labour had failed. He established terms like 'secondary arrest of dilatation' and 'arrest of descent' to describe the specific failure in the process of labour.

> Dystocia is defined as the slow, abnormal progression of labour.

Cesarean sections are also done for more imprecise terms like 'cephalo-pelvic disproportion' or 'failure to progress'.

Attempts have been made to predict dystocia but have met with mixed success. Abnormal labour or dystocia in the first or second stage of labour can be associated with one or more abnormalities of the cervix, uterus, maternal pelvis, or fetus. Some of the factors that may contribute to longer active labours include advanced maternal age, nulliparity, maternal anxiety, multiple gestation, and intrauterine infections. In analysing factors influencing prolongation of the second stage, Piper et al (1991) found that epidural analgesia, prolonged first stage of labour, nulliparity, large fetuses, and high station at complete cervical dilation were associated with a longer second stage.

> Longer active phase of labour may be caused by:
> - Advanced maternal age
> - Nulliparity
> - Maternal anxiety

Risk factors for difficult delivery among nulliparous women in the second stage of labour include short stature (less than 150 cm), age greater than 35 years, gestational age greater than 41 weeks, interval between epidural induction and full cervical dilation of greater than 6 hours, fetal station above +2 cm at full cervical dilatation, or occiput posterior fetal position (Fraser et al 2002).

### Fetal distress

The term fetal distress is imprecise, but is the indication for many cesarean sections. Contrary to expectation, electronic fetal monitoring increased the rate of cesarean section by as much as 40 per cent (Thacker et al 2001), but did not bring down the risk of cerebral palsy and perinatal death (Scheller and Nelson 1994).

In the presence of a fetal heart rate tracing which shows significant changes (absent baseline variability, recurrent variable decelerations, recurrent late decelerations, or bradycardia), the optimal time frame to effect delivery has not been established (ACOG 2010). However, good clinical practice suggests that for optimal outcome, the labour team should be able proceed with a cesarean section within 30 minutes of making the decision.

An immediate cesarean section may be the only option when faced with an acute or catastrophic worsening of the fetal condition.

## Technique of Cesarean Delivery

Being the most common surgical procedure in obstetrics, the steps of a cesarean section have been standardised over the years. Berghella and colleagues have reviewed the steps based on current evidence (2011).

### Pre-operative care

It is preferable to stop oral intake for at least 8 hours prior to an elective cesarean section. Women who have been in labour should ideally have been on clear liquids. In these women or those who need to undergo an emergency cesarean soon after a meal, prevention of acid aspiration syndrome is of prime concern. Regional anesthesia is preferred in these women. Most units use non-particulate antacids and ranitidine intravenously to increase gastric pH. If general anesthesia is being used, cricoid pressure should be maintained till the cuff of the endotracheal tube has been inflated.

If there is hair which will interfere with the operative area, it is shaved on the day of surgery. Shaving on the night before surgery increases the risk of wound infection. In elective cesareans, bathing with chlorhexidine has been shown to decrease surgical site infection.

It is good clinical practice to document fetal heart tones prior to surgery.

An indwelling bladder catheter is placed and is usually removed 24 hours after surgery.

### Skin cleansing techniques

There has been only one randomised trial for skin cleansing techniques for cesarean deliveries. Extrapolating from surgeries on non-pregnant patients, the use of a povidone-iodine solution is considered reasonable.

## Opening the Abdomen

### Skin incision

The commonly used skin incisions for a cesarean delivery include vertical (midline and paramedian) incisions and transverse incisions (Pfannenstiel, Joel-Cohen, Maylard and Cherney). The type of incision is usually dictated by the clinical situation and the preferences of the operator.

Though vertical incisions generally allow faster abdominal entry, are associated with less bleeding and nerve injury, and can be easily extended cephalad if more space is required for access, they do not improve neonatal outcomes. Vertical midline incisions are associated with a greater risk of postoperative wound dehiscence and development of incisional hernia. The scar is cosmetically less pleasing.

A midline incision is the preferred vertical incision. Paramedian incisions are not usually recommended.

Currently, a low transverse skin incision is most commonly used for a cesarean delivery. A transverse incision is associated with less postoperative pain, greater wound strength, and better cosmetic results than the vertical midline incisions (Berghella et al 2005). Compared to the Pfannenstiel incision, the Joel-Cohen incision is associated with less fever, pain and analgesic requirements, less blood loss, shorter duration of surgery and hospital stay (Mathai and Hofmeyer 2007).

**Length of skin incision**

Difficulty in delivery of the fetus is minimal with skin incisions measuring at least 15 cm in length (Ayers and Morley 1987). This is the length of a standard Allis clamp – 'the Allis clamp test' (Finan et al 1991). Shorter incisions may lead to difficulty in exposure of the peritoneal cavity and delivery of the baby's head.

**Types of transverse incisions**

*Pfannenstiel incision*: The Pfannenstiel incision results in good exposure to the central pelvis, but has limited access to the lateral pelvis and upper abdomen. This is because the fascia is cut transversely, but the rectus muscles are just pulled laterally, thus limiting exposure.

*Technique*

The skin incision is located two fingerbreadths above the pubic symphysis. The incision is a low transverse incision that curves gently upward, placed in a natural fold of skin (the 'smile' incision). The subcutaneous tissue is incised sharply with a scalpel. The fascia is then nicked on either side of the midline. The fascial incision is extended transversely with curved Mayo scissors. The upper and then the lower fascial edges are grasped with Allis clamps, and elevated. Under continuous tension, the fascia is then separated from the underlying rectus muscles by blunt and sharp dissection. Once the upper and lower fascia have been dissected free, and any perforating vessel sutured or electrocoagulated, the underlying rectus abdominus muscles are separated with finger dissection. Sharp dissection may be necessary to separate adherent muscles. The peritoneum is then nicked open in the midline. The opening in the peritoneum is then widened sharply with fine scissors, exposing intraperitoneal contents.

*Joel-Cohen incision*: Joel-Cohen (1977) described a transverse skin incision, which has been adapted and is considered a good incision for cesarean sections. This modified incision is placed about 3 cm below the line joining the anterior superior iliac spines. The skin incision is higher than the traditional Pfannenstiel incision and is not curved. In the Joel-Cohen incision, sharp dissection is minimised. The rectus muscles are separated by finger traction. The fascia may be incised in the midline and both the fascia and subcutaneous tissue are rapidly divided by blunt finger dissection (Joel-Cohen 1977). The fascia may also be opened by pushing laterally with slightly opened scissor tips (Holmgren et al 1999).

When exposure is limited and additional space is required, the Maylard or Cherney modification may be used.

*Maylard incision*: Maylard proposed a transverse muscle-splitting incision. This incision usually refers to a sub-umbilical transverse incision. It allows greater access to the abdomen.

*Technique*

The Maylard incision length is usually longer than the Pfannenstiel incision. After incising the fascia transversely, sharp dissection or electrocautery is used to transversely cut the rectus muscle, approximately 2 cm above the insertion into the pubic bone. The underlying artery may be entered, but it can be clamped and cauterised immediately. The peritoneum is opened and cut laterally.

*Cherney incision*: Cherney described a transverse muscle-cutting incision that allows excellent surgical exposure to the space of Retzius and the pelvic sidewall. It has been adapted for cesarean section.

*Technique*
The skin and fascia are cut in a manner similar to a Maylard incision. The lower fascia is reflected, exposing the tendinous attachment of the rectus abdominus muscle bodies to the fascia of the pubis. Using electrocautery, the rectus tendons are cut from the pubic bone. The rectus muscles are retracted and the peritoneum opened.

## Opening the peritoneum

Once a small incision is made in the peritoneum, the incision can be extended with sharp or blunt dissection. Some authors favour using the fingers to bluntly open the peritoneum to minimise the risk of inadvertent injury to the bowels or other organs that may be adherent to the underlying surface (Holmgren et al 1999, Wallin and Fall 1999, Berghella 2011). Blunt versus sharp entry into the peritoneum has not been compared in a randomised trial.

## Raising the bladder flap

Once the peritoneal cavity is entered and the lower part of the uterus exposed, it is important to know that the uterus is often dextrorotated, with the left round ligament lying more anterior and nearer the midline than the right round ligament. This dextrorotation can be quickly corrected by inserting a hand between the uterus and the right pelvic sidewall and lifting the uterus gently upwards and to the left.

The uterovesical fold of peritoneum is grasped with toothed forceps, just above the upper margin of the bladder. A small nick is made in the midline with fine scissors. The blades of the scissors are then inserted under the loose fold of peritoneum and intermittently opened and closed to separate the peritoneum from the underlying tissue. This strip is then cut sharply to both sides, taking care to cut so that the incision forms a curve, with the lateral ends curving upwards. The lower edge of the peritoneal flap is then grasped with a toothed forceps or artery clamp and the bladder is separated gently by blunt dissection. In the presence of a previous cesarean scar, sharp dissection may be required.

There is only one small study which has evaluated the need for raising the bladder flap (Hohlagschwandtner et al 2001). It found a reduction in operating time and incision-to-delivery interval, reduced blood loss, and need for analgesics if a bladder flap was not raised. However, the long-term consequences of this intervention were not evaluated. Raising the bladder flap may be particularly useful in cases where adhesions may not allow access to the lower uterine segment. In these cases, pushing the bladder out of harm's way may decrease the risk of inadvertent bladder injury.

## Uterine incision

It is important to be aware of the placental position, particularly if the ultrasound has indicated an anterior low-lying placenta or anterior placenta previa. This may prepare the surgeon to avoid lacerating the placenta and also to plan the delivery of the fetus.

The uterine incision may be transverse or vertical. There are no randomised trials that have compared the two techniques. The uterine incision must be large enough to allow atraumatic delivery of the fetal head and trunk without either tearing into or having to cut the uterine vessels at the lateral margins of the uterus.

> It is important to be aware of the placental position at the time of making the uterine incision, especially if an ultrasound scan has indicated a low-lying placenta or placenta previa.

The type of incision depends upon several factors, including the position and size of the fetus, location of the placenta, presence of leiomyomas, and development of the lower uterine segment.

## Transverse incision

The transverse lower uterine segment incision is recommended for most cesarean deliveries (Monroe-Kerr or Kerr incision). The advantages of the transverse incision include less blood loss, less need for bladder dissection, easier reapproximation, and a lower risk of rupture in subsequent pregnancies (Berghella et al 2005)

> The advantages of the transverse incision include:
> - less blood loss
> - less need for bladder dissection
> - easier re-approximation
> - lower risk of rupture in subsequent pregnancies

The transverse incision has the disadvantage of extending laterally, causing laceration of major blood vessels. A 'J' or inverted 'T' extension is often required if a larger incision is needed. In the long-term, the 'J' or 'T' incision may have problems because the 'J' extension goes into the lateral fundus and the angles of the inverted 'T' incision are poorly vascularised, both of which potentially result in a weaker uterine scar.

*Technique of transverse uterine incision*: The uterus is entered through the lower uterine segment, 1 cm below the upper margin of the peritoneal reflection. In women who have been in labour and may have undergone significant cervical effacement and dilatation, it is prudent to place the incision relatively higher. This will not only prevent lateral extension into the uterine vessels, but will also avoid opening into the vagina.

A small incision is made in the midline with the scalpel. Care must be taken not to nick the baby's skin. This is more common when the lower uterine segment is thinned out. This may also occur in breech presentations where the differentiation between maternal muscle and fetal skin of the breech may become difficult. If possible, membranes are left intact until complete extension of the incision.

When entry into the uterine cavity is achieved, the hysterotomy incision can be extended using blunt expansion with the surgeon's fingers. Blunt expansion is fast and has less risk of inadvertent trauma to the fetus. It may also reduce blood loss and extension of the incision. Two trials have found that sharp dissection with bandage scissors was associated with greater blood loss (Magann et al 2002, Sekhavat et al 2010). There have been case reports of fetal parts being cut while extending the uterine incision with scissors.

### Vertical incision

The two types of vertical incisions are the low vertical (Kronig, De Lee, or Cornell) and the 'classical' vertical. The low vertical is performed in the lower, noncontractile uterine segment and may be as strong as the low transverse incision. Comparing the low vertical and the low transverse incisions, Shipp and colleagues (1999) suggested that there is no increased risk of a low vertical uterine incision when compared to a low transverse incision. The major disadvantage of the low vertical incision is the possibility of extension upwards into the uterine fundus or downwards into the bladder, cervix or vagina.

> The main disadvantage of the low vertical incision is the possibility of extension upwards into the uterine fundus or downwards into the bladder, cervix or vagina.

The low vertical incision has not found much favour in practice because the separation between lower and upper uterine segments is not easily identifiable clinically.

A vertical incision that extends into the upper uterine segment/fundus is termed a 'classical' incision. This incision is not performed in modern obstetrics because of the higher frequency of catastrophic uterine rupture (4 to 9 per cent) compared with low transverse (0.2 to 1.5 per cent) incisions. The rupture may occur spontaneously even before the woman goes into labour. It is also associated with a higher rate of maternal morbidity (Patterson et al 2002). The only indication for a classical cesarean incision may be a need for a quick delivery where the patient will also be undergoing tubal ligation.

> A classical cesarean is not performed in modern obstetrics because of the higher frequency of catastrophic uterine rupture compared with low transverse incisions.

### Delivering the fetus

After the uterine incision is made, the obstetrician inserts a hand into the uterine cavity, and quickly assesses the presentation (if not known earlier). When the fetus is in a cephalic presentation, the hand is used to scoop the head up and bring it to the level of the uterine incision. The head is then extracted through the uterine incison. To facilitate the delivery of the head through the uterine incision, transabdominal fundal pressure is usually applied by the surgical assistant. The shoulders are then delivered by gentle traction and the rest of the body will readily follow. The mouth and nostrils of the infant are immediately aspirated with a bulb syringe.

Once the infant's cord is clamped and cut, it is handed over to an appropriately trained clinician who will take over the care of the infant.

### Instrumental delivery at cesarean

Instrumentation has been associated with maternal (particularly with forceps) or fetal (particularly with vacuum) morbidity in vaginal deliveries. Extrapolating from this, therefore, manual delivery of the fetal head during cesarean delivery should be favoured whenever possible, until further data is available (Berghella et al 2005). At this time, there are no controlled studies comparing

> Manual delivery of the fetal head during cesarean delivery should be favoured whenever possible.

manual with instrumental delivery of the fetal head at cesarean delivery.

### Delivering the deeply impacted head

A complication of cesarean delivery following prolonged labour can be a deeply impacted fetal head. The head may be wedged deep in the pelvis and can be hard to disengage and deliver. The fingers of one hand are insinuated between the fetal head and the cervix and vagina and the fingers are wiggled gently. This releases the suction with which the fetal head is stuck in the pelvis. There is a sucking sound as the air rushes into the space between the head and the pelvis, and then the head can be extracted. However, with prolonged labour, the tissues may be very edematous and friable and this could lead to extension of the incision laterally into the broad ligament and uterine vessels.

If this procedure fails, upward pressure applied by the assistant's hand in the vagina can push the head back through the vagina and out of the pelvis.

### The Patwardhan technique for deeply impacted head at cesarean

When the head is impacted deep in the pelvis in cases of occipito-transverse or occipito-anterior positions of the vertex, the fetal shoulder is usually found at the level of the uterine incision. As soon as the uterine incision is made, the anterior shoulder tends to 'pop' out. If it does not, it is gently extracted through the incision. Next, the posterior shoulder is also delivered out of the incision line. The surgeon now hooks the fingers through both the fetal axillae and with gentle traction, brings the fetal body out of the uterus. This is aided by fundal pressure by the assistant. When the back is posterior after delivering the anterior shoulder, a hand is introduced into the uterus and a foot is sought. By traction on the foot coupled with fundal pressure, the breech is delivered followed by the trunk. The head is delivered by traction on the legs (Patwardhan and Motashaw 1957).

In a retrospective study of 100 patients, Khosla and associates (2003), found that hemorrhage due to extension of incision requiring blood transfusion occurred in 24 per cent of patients in whom the head was delivered first, as compared to none where the Patwardhan technique was used.

A deeply impacted head could also be delivered by extending the uterine incision into an inverted 'T' or a 'J' shape to deliver the fetus, as a large incision may be required.

### Delivering the placenta

Spontaneous delivery of the placenta is encouraged with gentle traction on the cord and use of oxytocin to enhance uterine expulsive forces. Though many surgeons remove the placenta manually, waiting for the spontaneous expulsion of the placenta is recommended. A systematic review of the Cochrane database (Anorlu et al 2008) showed that manual extraction results in more postoperative endometritis, greater blood loss and lower postpartum hematocrit.

After placental extraction, it is important to ensure that the entire placenta, along with the membranes, has been removed. The uterine cavity is explored with the hand or the uterine cavity is wiped with one hand holding a sponge. The fundus of the uterus is stabilised with the other hand.

## Prevention of uterine hemorrhage

The uterus is massaged immediately after the delivery of the placenta, to promote uterine contraction. The commonest uterotonic used is oxytocin. This is usually given at a dose of 10–20 units in 500 ml of normal saline. The next three bottles of postoperative intravenous solutions also contain the same dosage and the fluid is run in at 125 ml/hour. Oxytocin has fewer side effects than ergot alkaloids, especially in hypertensive women.

> Oxytocin given at a dose of 10–20 units in 500 ml of normal saline is recommended as an uterotonic after a cesarean section.

## Closure of the uterine wound

Closure of the uterine incision may be aided by exteriorisation of the uterus. Prior to suturing the uterine incision, temporary removal of the uterus from the abdominal cavity (exteriorisation of the uterus) to facilitate repair of the uterine incision may be a good technique. It is particularly valuable when exposure of the incision is difficult or there is need for hemostasis due to excessive bleeding. The adnexae can also be visualised easily and this allows easy identification of any incidental adnexal pathology, like an ovarian neoplasm. Exteriorisatoion allows easy access to the tubes for tubal ligation.

In a systematic review of the Cochrane database, Jacobs-Jokhan and Hofmeyr (2004) did not find enough evidence to either recommend or refute this technique. In a recently published randomised study, Coutinho and colleagues (2008) found no significant difference between extra-abdominal and intra-abdominal repair of the uterine incision at cesarean delivery, but found that the number of sutures required was lower and surgical time was shorter with extra-abdominal repair. Another advantage of exteriorisation is that it allows rapid recognition of a non-contracted, flabby uterus which can benefit from uterine massage. The adnexae can be easily accessed and inspected when the uterus is exteriorised.

If the cesarean has been done under regional anesthesia, the patient may experience discomfort and vomiting when the uterus is exteriorised.

### Technique for closure of the uterine wound

Traditionally, the uterine incision is closed by a two-layer repair. The first layer is closed with a locking suture which ensures hemostasis. This is followed by an imbricating layer.

In 1988, Lal and Tsomo, and in 1992, Hauth and associates, advocated the use of a single-layer repair. These studies showed that there is considerable saving of operating time if a single-layer closure is used, with no increase in blood loss or occurrence of endometritis. A systematic review of the Cochrane database, (Enkin and Wilkinson 2005) showed no advantages or disadvantages for routine use of single-layer closure compared to two-layer closure, except perhaps a shorter operation time.

> The risk of uterine rupture in pregnancies after single-layer closure increased two- to four-fold compared with pregnancies after a double-layer closure.

However, the choice of single- or double-layer closure of the uterine incision has an impact on the occurrence of uterine rupture in subsequent pregnancies. Two studies

(Bujold et al 2002, 2010) reported that the risk of uterine rupture in pregnancies after single-layer closure was increased two-to four-fold compared with pregnancies after a double-layer closure.

Taking these factors into consideration, a two-layer uterine closure is recommended for women who are not undergoing a tubal sterilisation. These women have the potential for uterine rupture if they undergo a trial of labour after cesarean (TOLAC) in a subsequent pregnancy. This seems to be a good option in developing countries where women may not have, or maintain, their medical records. Given the available data, a one-layer technique is acceptable in women who undergo tubal sterilisation with the cesarean delivery. A double (or even triple) layer closure may be necessary when the myometrium is thick, such as with a classical cesarean, low vertical incisions or a 'T' extension.

> A single-layer closure can be used in women undergoing tubal sterilisation.

## Abdominal irrigation

Other than suctioning out excessive amniotic fluid and blood which may have collected in the peritoneal cavity, there is no necessity for intra-abdominal irrigation (Harrigill et al 2003).

## Inspection of adnexae

It is a good idea to inspect the ovaries and tubes at this time. This ensures that a cyst or mass is not missed. Dede et al (2007) suggest that an ovarian cyst or mass identified incidentally at the time of cesarean section should be removed. Excision of the mass is preferred, without which, malignancy could be missed. If malignancy is suspected and facilities for frozen section are available, then oophorectomy is done if frozen section confirms the presence of malignancy. A staging laparotomy will have to be done at a later date.

> Examining the adnexae during a cesarean section is good clinical practice.

## Closure of peritoneum

There is currently no evidence to justify the time taken and cost of peritoneal closure (Berghella 2005). In a systematic review of the Cochrane database, Bamigboye and Hofmeyr (2003) concluded that 'leaving the peritoneum unsutured is not likely to be hazardous in the short term and may in fact, be of benefit'. In a review, Tulandi and Al-Jaroudi (2003) encouraged clinicians not to close both parietal and visceral peritoneum. The fear of adhesion formation due to non-closure is not supported by most randomised studies. In fact, non-closure of visceral and parietal peritoneum results in significantly fewer adhesions at subsequent surgery (Komoto et al 2006; Malomo et al 2006).

> There is currently no evidence to justify the time taken and cost of peritoneal closure.

## Rectus muscles

There is no necessity to reapproximate the rectus muscles. When the fascial edges are approximated, the muscles will come together naturally. Suturing the muscles will only lead to increased post-operative pain (Berghella et al 2005)

## Fascial closure

This is probably the most important step in the closure of the abdomen. A properly done fascial closure is essential in preventing the occurrence of incisional hernia. Prior to suturing the fascial edges, it is important to inspect the subfascial plane for bleeders and to achieve meticulous hemostasis.

The suture material used for fascial closure can be a delayed absorbable suture like polydiaxonone or polyglactin. A permanent suture like 1-0 nylon or polypropylene has also been recommended. In developing countries, nylon is a cost-effective permanent suture which has less incidence of suture sinus formation than polypropylene. The recommendation for fascial closure is a continuous non-locking technique, with the sutures placed 1 cm from the edge of the fascia and placed 1 cm apart.

> The fascia can be closed with a delayed absorbable suture (polydiaxonone/polyglactin) or a permanent suture (1-0 nylon) or polypropylene.

## Closure of the subcutaneous tissue

Routine subcutaneous tissue closure in women with a depth <2 cm cannot be recommended. A Cochrane review of methods of abdominal wall closure at cesarean was unable to make any recommendations based on a small number of studies. If adhesive paper strips are being used to close the skin, a few sutures may be placed in the subcutaneous tissue to reduce the tendency of the skin to gape.

Placing a drain in the subcutaneous tissue is unnecessary and may lead to infection (Hellums et al 2007).

## Closure of skin

The skin can be closed with vertical mattress sutures; 3-0/ 4-0 silk or fine nylon can be used. Better cosmesis and patient satisfaction can be achieved with subcuticular sutures using delayed-absorbable suture.

Adhesive paper strips are the least painful and have excellent cosmetic results. The skin edges are cleaned with saline and dried. An adhesive skin preparation like tincture benzoin can be used on the edges to help the strips stick better. Care should be taken not to let the tincture benzoin touch the raw surface of the wound. The edges are held together with forceps and the adhesive strips are applied by placing them on one edge and then pulling gently across to the other skin edge.

## Wound dressing

A light protective gauze dressing is recommended. One or two narrow strips of tape can hold the dressing in place. An occlusive dressing is not necessary. The dressing can be removed after 24 to 48 hours.

## Prophylactic antibiotics for cesarean delivery

Prophylactic antibiotics have been shown to have excellent benefit in women undergoing both elective and emergency cesarean section. A systematic review of the Cochrane database showed a decrease of 60 per cent to 75 per cent in the rates of endometritis in women who had received prophylactic antibiotics for a

> Prophylactic antibiotics have been shown to have excellent benefit in women undergoing both elective and emergency cesarean section.

cesarean delivery (Smaill and Hofmeyr 2005). The decrease in wound infection was approximately 25 per cent in elective cesareans and approximately 65 per cent in women who had been in labour.

Both ampicillin and first generation cephalosporins like cefazolin, have similar efficacy in reducing postoperative endometritis (Hopkins and Smaill 2005). However, ampicillin is no longer recommended due to emerging drug resistance. In reviewing 51 trials, Hopkins and Smaill (2005) concluded that 'there does not appear to be added benefit in utilising a more broadspectrum agent or a multiple dose regimen'. Later-generation, more expensive broadspectrum agents do not improve efficacy further. The optimal timing of administration (immediately after the cord is clamped versus pre-operative) has not been determined. In a randomised trial, Sullivan and colleagues (2007) provided evidence that pre-incision administration of antibiotics is superior to administration after cord clamping, in preventing endometritis and total infectious morbidity.

The recommended dosage is 2 g of cefazolin as a single intravenous bolus at the time of induction of anesthesia.

> There does not appear to be added benefit in utilising a more broad-spectrum agent or a multiple dose regimen as prophylaxis for cesarean section.

> Prophylactic antibiotic for cesarean section: 2 g of cefazolin as a single intravenous bolus at the time of induction of anesthesia.

## Incidental surgery during cesarean section

The two common incidental findings at cesarean section are adnexal masses and fibroids.

It is mandatory to inspect the adnexa after closing the uterine incision. If an ovarian mass is found during cesarean, and the mass is suspected of being a neoplasm, excision may be required. The decision to proceed with an oophorectomy may be made if facilities for frozen section are available and confirm the presence of malignancy. In most developing countries, facilities for frozen section may not be readily available. In that case, the mass may be excised in toto and if proven to be malignant, oophorectomy may be done at a later date, along with a staging laparotomy.

> It is mandatory to inspect the adnexae after closing the uterine incision at cesarean section.

Myomectomy in the pregnant uterus has the potential for severe blood loss. Myomectomy is generally contraindicated for this reason, although Burton and colleagues (1989) in a small series have described successful excision in selected cases. On the other hand, pedunculated myomas can usually be removed safely during a cesarean section.

## Postoperative care

Intravenous fluids are continued after cesarean till the patient is able to tolerate and retain oral feeding. Typically, lactated Ringer solution or a similar crystalloid solution containing 5% dextrose is used. The usual amount administered is 500 ml every 4 hours. Urine output is recorded.

Pain relief is provided by narcotic analgesics like meperidine (Pethidine) 75–100 mg every 6 hours, according to requirement. Buprenorphine is also a good choice for postoperative pain and can be given in the dosage of 0.3–0.6 mg intramuscularly every 6–8 hours (Vadivelu and Anwar 2010).

A systematic review of the Cochrane database regarding early feeding after cesarean section showed that early oral fluids or food were associated with reduced time to first food intake, reduced time to return of bowel sounds, reduced postoperative hospital stay following surgery under regional analgesia and a trend to reduced abdominal distension. No significant differences were identified with respect to nausea, vomiting, time to bowel action/passing flatus, paralytic ileus and number of analgesic doses (Mangesi and Hofmeyr 2002). Other studies also recommend resumption of feeding (clear liquids or solids according to the patient's preference) within 8 hours of surgery (Kovavisarach and Atthakorn 2005, Bar et al 2008).

> Early intake of oral fluids or food is associated with
> - reduced time to first food intake
> - reduced time to return of bowel sounds
> - reduced postoperative hospital stay

## References

American College of Obstetricians and Gynecologists. 2010. Management of intrapartum fetal heart rate tracings. Practice Bulletin No. 116. *Obstet Gynecol*. 116:1232–40.

American College of Obstetricians and Gynecologists. 2007. Management of herpes in pregnancy. Practice Bulletin No.82

American College of Obstetricians and Gynecologists. 2002. Perinatal care at the threshold of viability. Practice Bulletin No.38,

Anorlu, RI, Maholwana, B, Hofmeyr, GJ. 2008. Methods of delivering the placenta at cesarean section. *Cochrane Database Syst Rev*. CD004737.

Atiba EO, Adeghe AJ, Murphy PJ, Felmingham JE, Scott GI. 1993. Patients' expectations and cesarean section rates. *Lancet* 341:246

Ayers JWT, Morley GW. 1987. Surgical incision for cesarean section. *Obstet Gynecol* 70:706–8.

Bamigboye AA, Hofmeyr GJ. 2003. Closure versus non-closure of the peritoneum at cesarean section. *Cochrane Database Syst Rev* 1.

Bar, G., Sheiner, E., Lezertovitz, A., Lazer, T. and Hallak, M. 2008. Early maternal feeding following cesarean delivery: a prospective randomised study. *Acta Obstetricia et Gynecologica Scandinavica*, 87: 68–71. doi: 10.1080/00016340701778849

Berghella, V, Baxter, JK, Chauhan, SP. 2005. Evidence-based surgery for cesarean delivery. *Am J Obstet Gynecol* 193:1607.

Berghella, V. 2011. Cesarean delivery Technique In: *UpToDate*, Lockwood CJ (Ed), UpToDate, Waltham, MA. URL: http://www.uptodate.com

Bewley S, Cockburn J. 2002a. The unethics of 'request' cesarean section [commentary]. *Br J Obstet Gynaecol* 109:593,

Bewley S, Cockburn J. 2002b. The unfacts of 'request' cesarean section [commentary]. *Br J Obstet Gynaecol* 109:597

Bhasker Rao, K. 1994. Global aspects of a rising cesarean section rate. Global Health Today: Perspectives on current research and clinical practice. The proceedings of the XIV world congress of obstetrics and gynecology, Montreal, Eds. D R Popkins, L J Peddle

Boehm FH, Graves CR. Caesarean birth. In: Rivlin ME, Martin RW, eds. *Manual of Clinical Problems in Obstetrics and Gynecology*. Boston: Little Brown, 1994:158–162.

Bragg F, Cromwell DA, Edozien LC et al. 2010. Variation in rates of cesarean section among English NHS trusts after accounting for maternal and clinical risk: cross sectional study. *BMJ* 341: c5065

Bujold, E, Bujold, C, Hamilton, EF, et al. 2002. The impact of a single-layer or double-layer closure on uterine rupture. *Am J Obstet Gynecol* 186:1326.

Bujold, E, Goyet, M, Marcoux, S, et al. 2010. The role of uterine closure in the risk of uterine rupture. *Obstet Gynecol* 116:43.

Burton, CA, Grimes, DA, March, CM. 1989. Surgical management of leiomyomata during pregnancy. *Obstet Gynecol* 74:707.

Collaborative study on high risk pregnancies and maternal mortality. 1990. ICMR task force study. New Delhi: ICMR

Coutinho, IC, Ramos de Amorim, MM, Katz, L, Bandeira de Ferraz, AA. 2008. Uterine exteriorization compared with in situ repair at cesarean delivery: a randomized controlled trial. *Obstet Gynecol* 111:639.

Dede, M, Yenen, MC, Yilmaz, A, et al. 2007. Treatment of incidental adnexal masses at cesarean section: a retrospective study. *Int J Gynecol Cancer* 17: 339.

Enkin MW, Wilkinson C. 2003. Single versus two layer suturing for closing the uterine incision at Caesarean section (Cochrane Review). *The Cochrane Library*, Issue 1, 2003.

Finan MA, Mastrogiannis DS, Spellacy WN. 1991. The Allis test for easy cesarean delivery. *American Journal of Obstetrics and Gynecology* 64:772–5.

Friedman EA. 1978. *Labour: Clinical Evaluation and Management*, 2nd ed. New York, Appleton-Century-Crofts

Fraser WD, Cayer M, Soeder BM, Turcot L, Marcoux S. 2002. PEOPLE (Pushing Early or Pushing Late with Epidural) Study Group. Risk factors for difficult delivery in nulliparas with epidural analgesia in second stage of labor. *Obstet Gynecol* 99: 409–18.

Hamilton BE, Martin JA, Ventura SJ. 2009.Births: Preliminary data for 2007. National vital statistics reports; vol 57 no 12. Hyattsville, MD. National Center for Health Statistics, Released March 18

Hannah ME, Hannah WJ, Hewson SA, Hodnett ED, Saigal S, Willan AR 2000. Planned cesarean section versus planned vaginal birth for breech presentation at term: a randomized multicentre trial. Term Breech Trial Collaborative Group. *Lancet*, 356:1375-1383.

Harrigill, KM, Miller, HS, Haynes, DE. 2003. The effect of intraabdominal irrigation at cesarean delivery on maternal morbidity: a randomized trial. *Obstet Gynecol* 101:80.

Hauth JC, Owen J, Davis RO. 1992. Transverse uterine incision closure: one versus two layers. *Am J Obstet Gynecol* 167: 1108–11.

Hellums, EK, Lin, MG, Ramsey, PS. 2007. Prophylactic subcutaneous drainage for prevention of wound complications after cesarean delivery— a metaanalysis. *Am J Obstet Gynecol* 197:229.

Hogle KL, Hutton EK, McBrien KA, Barrett JF, Hannah ME. 2003. Cesarean delivery for twins: a systematic review and meta-analysis. *Am J Obstet Gynecol* 188:220–7

Hohlagschwandtner, M, Ruecklinger, E, Husslein, P, Joura, EA. 2001. Is the formation of a bladder flap at cesarean necessary? A randomized trial. *Obstet Gynecol* 98:1089.

Holmgren G, Sjoholm L, Stark M. 1999. The Misgav-Ladach method for cesarean section: method description. *Acta Obstetricia et Gynecologica Scandinavica* 78:615–21.

Hopkins L, Smaill F. 2006. Antibiotic prophylaxis regimens and drugs for cesarean section. *Cochrane Database Syst Rev* 1.

International Perinatal HIV Group. 1999. The mode of delivery and the risk of vertical transmission of human immunodeficiency virus type 1: A meta-analysis of 15 prospective cohort studies. *N Engl J Med* 340: 977

Jacobs-Jokhan, D, Hofmeyr, G. 2004. Extra-abdominal versus intra-abdominal repair of the uterine incision at cesarean section. *Cochrane Database Syst Rev.* :CD000085.

Joel-Cohen S. 1977. *Abdominal and vaginal hysterectomy.* 2nd Edition. Philadelphia: JB Lippincott,18–23.

Kabra SG, Narayanan R, Chaturvedi M, Anand P, Mathur G. 1994. What is happening to cesarean section rates? *Lancet* 343(8890): 179– 180.

Kambo I, Bedi N, Dhillon BS., Saxena NC. 2002. A critical appraisal of cesarean section rates at teaching hospitals in India. *International Journal of Gynecology and Obstetrics* 79 151–158

Khosla AH, Dahiya K, Sangwan K. 2003. Cesarean section in a wedged head. *Indian J Med Sci* 57:187–91

Komoto, Y, Shimoya, K, Shimizu, T et al. 2006. Prospective study of non-closure or closure of the peritoneum at cesarean delivery in 124 women: Impact of prior peritoneal closure at primary cesarean on the interval time between first cesarean section and the next pregnancy and significant adhesion at second cesarean. *J Obstet Gynaecol Res* 32:396.

Kovavisarach E, Atthakorn M. 2005. Early versus delayed oral feeding after cesarean delivery. *International Journal of Gynecology and Obstetrics* Volume 90, Issue 1 , Pages 31–34, July

Lal K, Tsomo P. 1988. Comparative study of single layer and conventional closure of uterine incision in cesarean section. *Int J Gynecol Obstet* 27:349–52.

Magann EF, Chauhan SP, Bufkin L, Field K, Roberts WE, Martin JN. 2002. Intra-operative haemorrhage by blunt versus sharp expansion of the uterine incision at cesarean delivery: a randomised clinical trial. *BJOG*; 109:448-52.

Malomo, OO, Kuti, O, Orji, EO, et al. 2006. A randomised controlled study of non-closure of peritoneum at cesarean section in a Nigerian population. *J Obstet Gynaecol* 26:429. 52.

Mangesi L, Hofmeyr GJ. 2002. Early compared with delayed oral fluids and food after cesarean section. *Cochrane Database of Systematic Reviews* Issue 3. Art. No.: CD003516. DOI: 10.1002/14651858.CD003516

Mathai M, Hofmeyr GJ. 2007. Abdominal surgical incisions for cesarean section. *Cochrane Database of Systematic Reviews* Issue 1. Art. No.: CD004453. DOI: 10.1002/14651858.CD004453.pub2.

Mehta A, Apers L, Verstraelen H, and Temmerman M. 2001. Trends in Caesarean Section Rates at a Maternity Hospital in Mumbai, India. *J Health Popul Nutr.* Dec

Mukherjee J, Bhattacharya PK, Lahiri TK, Samaddar JC, Mehta R. 1993. Perinatal mortality in cesarean section: a disturbing picture of unfulfilled expectations. *J Indian Med Assoc.* Aug; 91(8):202–3.

National Collaborating Centre for Women's and Children's Health. 2004. Caesarean section. Clinical Guideline 13. London: RCOG Press.

O'Driscoll K, Foley, M. 1987. Caesarean section and perinatal outcome. *Am J Obstet Gynecol* 158:449–52.

Pai M, Sundaram P , Radhakrishnan KK, Thomas K, Muliyil JP. 1999. A high rate of Cesarean sections in an affluent section of Chennai. Is it a cause of concern? *Natl Med J India* 12:56–58

Patterson, LS, O'Connell, CM, Baskett, TF. 2002. Maternal and perinatal morbidity associated with classic and inverted T cesarean incisions. *Obstet Gynecol* 100:633.13.

Patwardhan BB, Motashaw ND. 1957. *J Obstet Gynaec Ind*; 8:1.

Petitti DB. 1985. Maternal mortality and morbidity in cesarean section. *Clin Obstet Gynecol* 28(4):763–769 (December).

Piper JM, Bolling DR, Newton ER. 1991. The second stage of labor: factors influencing duration. *Am J Obstet Gynecol* 165:976–9.

Scheller JM, Nelson KB. 1994. Does cesarean delivery prevent cerebral palsy or other neurological problems of childhood? *Obstet Gynecol* 83:624

Sekhavat L, Dehghani Firouzabadi R, Mojiri P. 2010. Effect of expansion technique of uterine incision on maternal blood loss in cesarean section. *Arch Gynecol Obstet*. 282(5):475-9.

Shipp, TD, Zelop, CM, Repke, JT, et al. 1999. Intrapartum uterine rupture and dehiscence in patients with prior lower uterine segment vertical and transverse incisions. *Obstet Gynecol* 94:735.

Smaill F, Hofmeyr GJ. 2005. Antibiotic prophylaxis for cesarean section. *Cochrane Database Syst Rev.* Issue 3

Sreevidya S, Sathiyasekaran BWC. 2003. High cesarean rates in Madras (India): a population-based cross-sectional study. *BJOG* 110: 106–111.

Sullivan SA, Smith T, Chang E, Hulsey T, Vandorsten JP, Soper D. 2007. Administration of cefazolin prior to skin incision is superior to cefazolin at cord clamping in preventing postcesarean infectious morbidity: a randomized, controlled trial. *Am J Obstet Gynecol* 196:455.e1–5.

Thacker SB, Stroup D, Chang M. 2001. Continuous electronic heart rate monitoring for fetal assessment during labor. *Cochrane Database Syst Rev.* (2):CD000063.

Tulandi T, Al-Jaroudi D. 2003. Nonclosure of peritoneum: a reappraisal. *Am J Obstet Gynecol* 189:609–12.

Vadivelu N, Anwar M. 2010. Buprenorphine in postoperative pain management. *Anesthesiology Clin* 28 601–609 doi:10.1016/j.anclin.2010.08.01

Villar J, Valladares E, Wojdyla D et al. 2006. Caesarean delivery rates and pregnancy outcomes: the 2005 WHO global survey on maternal and perinatal health in Latin America. *Lancet*, Volume 367, Issue 9525, Pages 1819–29, June

Walker R, Turnbull D, Wilkinson C. 2002. Strategies to Address Global Cesarean Section Rates: A Review of the Evidence. *BIRTH* 29:1 March

Wallin, G, Fall, O. 1999. Modified Joel-Cohen technique for cesarean delivery. *Br J Obstet Gynaecol* 106:221.

US Department of Health and Human Services, Public Health Service. 1991. *Healthy people 2000: National health promotion and disease prevention objectives.* Washington, DC: DHHS,

# CHAPTER 16

# VAGINAL BIRTH AFTER CESAREAN DELIVERY

*Pranathi Reddy*

There is widespread public and professional concern about the increasing proportion of births by cesarean section. This increase is the result of several changes in the practice environment, including the introduction of electronic fetal monitoring and the decrease in the use of vaginal breech deliveries and forceps deliveries (Clark and Hankins 2003; Lee et al 2003; Goetzinger and Macones 2008). Even in developing countries like India, there has been an alarming increase in cesarean rates (ICMR Task Force 1990; Sreevidya and Sathiyasekaran 2003; Pai et al 1999). Increasing rates of primary cesarean section have led to an increased proportion of the obstetric population with a history of prior cesarean delivery. This in turn increases the risk of a repeat cesarean. The experience of a prior cesarean appears to have become a major indication for a repeat cesarean for a large proportion of mothers, even if there is no other reported medical indication. Many factors influence the increasing rates of repeat cesarean section, including the capacity of a hospital to support vaginal birth after cesarean (VBAC) delivery, differences in physician practice patterns and patient preferences (Zweifler et al 2006). The increase in cesarean delivery rate has been partly perpetuated by the dictum 'once a cesarean always a cesarean' (Cragin 1916).

However, large cohort studies have established the fact that a large number of women may have a successful and safe vaginal birth after cesarean with reported figures of 70 per cent to 80 per cent (Flamm et al 1990). The National Institutes of Health Consensus Development Conference Statement on VBAC states, 'Given the available evidence, trial of labor is a reasonable option for many pregnant women with one prior low transverse uterine incision' (NIH 2010). The American College of Obstetricians and Gynecologists concurs and states, 'Most women with one previous cesarean delivery with a low-transverse incision are candidates for and should be counseled about VBAC and offered Trial of Labour after Cesarean (TOLAC) (ACOG 2010)'.

> A large number of women may have a successful and safe vaginal birth after cesarean (VBAC) with reported figures of 70 per cent to 80 per cent.

Pregnant women with a previous cesarean section can deliver in one of the following ways:

- Trial of labour after previous cesarean delivery ending in vaginal birth
- Trial of labour after previous cesarean delivery ending in emergency cesarean section
- Planned elective repeat cesarean section (ERCS).

Evidence for infrequent but significant and serious risks following VBAC does exist and must be kept in mind when attempting TOLAC. VBAC may not be as safe as originally thought (Landon et al 2004; Smith et al 2002). A trial of labour after previous cesarean delivery should be offered judiciously and with extensive counselling offered to the patient. It should also be undertaken only at facilities capable of emergency deliveries and short decision-to-cesarean times. Uterine rupture and other complications may be unpredictable, and therefore, TOLAC should be undertaken in facilities with staff immediately available to provide emergency care (ACOG 2010).

> TOLAC should be undertaken in facilities with staff immediately available to provide emergency care.

## Maternal risks of TOLAC

### Risk of uterine rupture

One of the major determinants of severe adverse outcome associated with VBAC is whether uterine rupture occurs. The incidence of this is generally estimated to be in the region of 0.5 per cent to 1.0 per cent. However, there is no dependable way to predict who will have a uterine rupture.

Considering all gestational ages, uterine rupture occurs in approximately 325 per 1,00,000 women undergoing trial of labour. The risk of uterine rupture for women who undergo trial of labour at term is 778 per 100,000. The risk of uterine rupture for women who undergo elective repeat cesarean delivery is 26 per 100,000 when all gestational ages are evaluated and 22 per 100,000 for women who are at term at the time they give birth (NIH 2010).

The reported incidence of uterine rupture varies, in part because some studies have grouped true, catastrophic uterine rupture together with asymptomatic scar dehiscence. Additionally, early case series did not stratify rupture rates by the type of prior cesarean incision (i.e., low transverse versus classical) (Leung et al 1993). When uterine rupture occurs there is a significant risk of bladder injury, transfusion and infection. There may be the need for hysterectomy (approximately 25 per cent). Maternal death from uterine rupture in planned VBAC occurs in less than 1/100,000 cases in the developed world; this estimate is based on information from case reports (Farmer et al 1991, Wen et al 2004). This rate may be much higher in developing countries.

> Maternal death from uterine rupture in planned VBAC occurs in less than 1/100,000 cases in the developed countries. The rate may be much higher in developing countries.

### Risks associated with failed TOLAC

The major determinant of morbidity associated with a decision for TOLAC is whether the attempt is successful. In a study from Nigeria, failed VBAC was associated with higher incidence of chorioamnionitis, postpartum hemorrhage, blood transfusion, uterine rupture, hysterectomy, and composite major neonatal morbidities. The risk factors which predicted failure were younger age, lack of previous vaginal delivery, induction of labour and fetal weight >4,000 g (Obori et al 2010).

## Risks of TOLAC to fetus/neonate

It is a fact that women undergoing VBAC face a slightly higher risk of perinatal death than women undergoing cesarean delivery. TOLAC carries a 2–3/10,000 additional risk of birth-related perinatal death when compared with elective repeat cesarean section (ERCS). However, the absolute risk of such birth-related perinatal loss is comparable to the risk for women having their first birth (Lyerly et al 2007). Smith and colleagues (2002), in a study of more than 300,000 singleton births, showed that the risk of perinatal death associated with TOLAC was comparable to that of nulliparas in labour.

Although rates of delivery-related perinatal death are the same between VBAC and primary vaginal delivery, this equation changes once uterine rupture has occurred. The rate of hypoxic–ischemic encephalopathy can increase significantly with uterine rupture. However, it is

> The risk of perinatal death associated with TOLAC is comparable to that of nulliparas in labour.

> Uterine rupture, though rare, increases perinatal morbidity and mortality.

important to remember that this complication is also extremely rare.

In a study comparing 17,898 women undergoing VBAC with 15,801 women undergoing ERCS, Landon and colleagues (2005) found that the probability of hypoxic–ischemic encephalopathy (HIE) was 0.00046 in infants whose mothers underwent TOLAC at term. HIE occurred in none of those infants whose mothers underwent elective repeated cesarean delivery.

**Table 16.1** Neonatal Risks

| Neonatal Risks | ERCS (%) | TOLAC (%) | Comment |
|---|---|---|---|
| Antepartum Still birth | | | |
| 37 to 38 weeks | 0.08 | 0.38 | |
| 39 weeks or greater | 0.01 | 0.16 | |
| HIE | 0–013 | 0.08 | Secondary analysis |
| Neonatal death | 0.05 | 0.08 | Not significant |
| Perinatal death | 0.01 | 0.13 | Increase seen due to intrapartum hypoxia |
| Neonatal admission | 6.0 | 6.6 | Not significant |
| Respiratory morbidity | 1–5 | 0.1–1.8 | |
| Transient tachypnea | 6.2 | 3.5 | |
| Hyperbilirubinemia | 5.8 | 2.2 | |

If uterine rupture occurs, risk of HIE 6.2% (95% CI, 1.8–10.6%), risk of neonatal death 1.8% (95% CI, 0–4.2%)

(Adapted from ACOG Practice Bulletin no. 115, August 2010)

## Advantages of achieving VBAC

Women who achieve VBAC avoid major abdominal surgery, resulting in lower rates of hemorrhage, infection, and a shorter recovery period compared with elective repeat cesarean delivery (Flamm et al 1990). Additionally, for those considering larger families, VBAC may help avoid potential future maternal consequences of multiple cesarean deliveries such as hysterectomy, bowel or bladder injury, transfusion and infection (Ananth et al 1997; Landon 2004), and abnormal placentation such as placenta previa and placenta accreta (Silver et al 2006; Varner et al 2007). Neither elective repeat cesarean delivery nor TOLAC, are without maternal or neonatal risk.

These findings underline the importance of developing methods to predict the likelihood of success of a VBAC in relation to maternal characteristics. Several investigators have attempted to create scoring systems to assist in the prediction of VBAC, but most have had limited success (Macones et al 2001; Srinivas et al 2007)

## Selecting Women for TOLAC

Good candidates for planned TOLAC are those women in whom the balance of risks (as low as possible) and chances of success (as high as possible) are acceptable to the patient and doctor. The balance of risks and benefits appropriate for one patient may seem unacceptable for another.

## Contraindications to TOLAC

Women with a prior history of a classical cesarean section are recommended to give birth by ERCS. There is limited evidence on whether maternal or neonatal outcomes are significantly influenced by the number of prior cesarean births or type of prior uterine scar.

Nonetheless, due to higher absolute risks of uterine rupture or unknown risks, planned TOLAC is contraindicated (Landon et al 2005; Guise et al 2005; Macones et al 2005) in women with:

- Previous uterine rupture; risk of recurrent rupture is unknown
- Previous high vertical classical cesarean section where the uterine incision has involved the whole length of the uterine corpus (200–900/10,000 risk of uterine rupture)
- Three or more previous cesarean deliveries (reliable estimate of risks of rupture unknown), or
- Where the woman herself refuses

Women with a previous uterine incision, other than an uncomplicated low transverse cesarean section incision, who wish to consider vaginal birth should be assessed by a senior consultant with full access to the details of the previous surgery.

## Factors influencing success of VBAC

### Factors which increase success of VBAC

(Gyamfi et al 2004; Macones et al 2005, Smith et al 2005)

- Previous vaginal birth, particularly previous VBAC, is the single best predictor for successful VBAC. It is associated with an approximately 87 per cent to 90 per cent success rate for planned VBAC. The rate of rupture increases with each successive labour, but a prior vaginal delivery also increases the chance of a successful VBAC attempt.

- Having at least 24 months between the date of the last cesarean birth and the due date for this pregnancy increases the chance of a successful VBAC and decreases the risks of uterine rupture.
- Spontaneous onset of labour
- Gestation below 40 weeks at onset of labour further contributes to a greater chance of having a VBAC.

**Factors contributing to unsuccessful VBAC**

(Goodall et al 2005, Gyamfi et al 2004, Juhasz et al 2005, Bujold et al 2004)

- Induced labour
- No previous vaginal birth
- Body mass index greater than 30
- Previous cesarean section for dystocia
- Gestation beyond 41 weeks
- Birth weight greater than 4000
- No epidural anesthesia
- Previous preterm cesarean birth
- Cervical dilatation at admission less than 4 cm
- Less than 2 years from previous cesarean birth
- Advanced maternal age
- Non-white ethnicity
- Short stature
- A male infant.

Where relevant to the woman's circumstances, this information should be shared during the antenatal counselling process to enable the woman to make the best informed choice.

## Special considerations for management of antenatal period in a woman with a previous cesarean section

Counselling regarding mode of delivery should ideally start at the time of the sentinel cesarean. Women should be offered information regarding the need for the first cesarean and the implications it may have for future pregnancies and deliveries.

Identify, at the first antenatal visit, all women who have had a previous cesarean section or have a uterine scar. A senior consultant should assess them.

Factors to note at the booking visit include:

- Number and type of previous uterine scar/s
- Indication/s for prior cesarean section. Are the notes available?
- Were there any puerperal complications?
- Gestation at time of prior cesarean section
- Anticipated family size: this is important as the longer term risks related to further repeat cesarean section scars must be taken into consideration (placenta previa, placenta accreta, blood loss/transfusion, hysterectomy and mortality)
- History of a successful vaginal delivery and whether this was before or after the uterine scar. The rupture rate rises with each successive labour, but a prior vaginal delivery also increases the chance of a successful VBAC attempt.
- What is the inter-conception interval?

❖ Are there any other associated medical problems?

## Antenatal counselling

Counselling of the women about choices with regard to mode of delivery should begin at the booking visit itself. Women should also be informed that this assessment would be an ongoing process and the ultimate decision would depend on the course of the current pregnancy.

Women with a prior history of one uncomplicated lower-segment transverse cesarean section, in an otherwise uncomplicated pregnancy at term, with no contraindication to vaginal birth, should be able to discuss the option of planned VBAC and the alternative of an elective repeat cesarean section.

The antenatal counselling of women with a prior cesarean birth should be documented in the notes. A patient information leaflet should be provided with the consultation.

A final decision for mode of birth should be agreed between the woman and her obstetrician before the expected/planned delivery date, ideally by 36 weeks of gestation (Flamm et al 1990).

A plan for the event of labour starting prior to the scheduled date should also be documented.

Women considering their options for birth after a single previous cesarean should be informed that, overall, the chances of successful planned VBAC are between 72 per cent and 76 per cent (Smith et al 2002; Landon et al 2004; Wen et al 2004).

Placenta previa/accreta should be excluded with ultrasonography. Identifying and treating anemia early on is important in these women.

If a decision is made for TOLAC, the woman should be advised:

1. To present to the obstetric unit early in labour or if there is spontaneous rupture of membranes (SROM)
2. That the decision made in the antenatal clinic is not binding
3. To have a clear understanding with the obstetric team which states the boundaries of safe practice to which they have agreed and indicate the circumstances under which they would request that a repeat cesarean section be carried out
4. The decision should be clearly documented in the antenatal records

## Intrapartum Management

### The setting in which TOLAC should be attempted

Women who have had a previous cesarean section should be offered care during labour in a unit where:

1. There is immediate access to cesarean section (within 30 minutes of the indication arising)
2. There are on-site blood transfusion services or blood can be obtained within a reasonable amount of time.
3. Facilities for continuous fetal heart monitoring are available, preferably electronic fetal heart monitoring
4. Specialist obstetricians, anesthetists and pediatricians are available round the clock

It is known that at least 20 per cent to 30 per cent of all women attempting VBAC are likely to need a repeat emergency cesarean section, and in some cases this may be very urgent. In hospitals which do not have an on-site theatre and anesthetic staff throughout a 24-hour period, it is essential that staff can be called in at very short notice to enable a theatre to be opened quickly.

## Continuous fetal monitoring

Continuous electronic fetal monitoring is recommended following the onset of uterine contractions for the duration of TOLAC.

An abnormal cardiotocograph (CTG) is the most consistent finding in uterine rupture and is present in 55 per cent to 87 per cent of these events (Guise et al 2004). Continuous electronic fetal monitoring is generally used for women during planned VBAC, and thus, the estimates of risk of both lethal and non-lethal perinatal asphyxia associated with VBAC are in this context (RCOG, Evidence based Clinical Guideline Number 8, 2001). The relative and absolute risks of severe adverse events in the absence of continuous electronic fetal monitoring are unknown.

## Partograms for progress of labour

Partographic progress of labour enhances safety. A partogram, in addition to monitoring progress of labour, enables effective monitoring of maternal parameters like blood pressure and pulse rate. Tachycardia can be an early indication of scar dehiscence. Monitoring the intensity, duration and frequency of uterine contractions is best accomplished manually. The routine use of intrauterine pressure catheters in the early detection of uterine scar rupture is not recommended. The duration of labour should be closely monitored with special reference to alert and action lines on partogram. Prolongation of labour is an important sign of dystocia.

There is no available evidence to guide clinical practice in terms of length of either first or second stages of labour. However, it is recommended that in cases of prolonged first or second stage, the threshold for resorting to repeat cesarean section should be lower than in women with an intact uterus.

## Analgesia

Epidural analgesia for labour may be used as part of TOLAC, and adequate pain relief may encourage more women to choose TOLAC (Sakala et al 1990; Flamm et al 1998). There is no high quality evidence to suggest that epidural analgesia is a causal risk factor for an unsuccessful TOLAC (Sakala et al 1990; Landon et al 2005).

In addition, effective regional analgesia should not be expected to mask signs and symptoms of uterine rupture, particularly because the most common sign of rupture is fetal heart tracing abnormalities.

## Early diagnosis of uterine scar rupture

Early diagnosis of uterine scar rupture followed by expeditious laparotomy and resuscitation is essential to reduce associated morbidity and mortality in mother and infant.

There is no single pathognomonic clinical feature that is indicative of uterine rupture, but the presence of any of the following peripartum signs and symptoms should raise the concern of the possibility of this event (Turner 2002)

- Abnormal CTG tracing
- Severe abdominal pain, especially if persisting between contractions
- Chest pain or shoulder tip pain
- Sudden onset of shortness of breath
- Acute onset scar tenderness
- Abnormal vaginal bleeding or hematuria
- Cessation of previously efficient uterine activity
- Maternal tachycardia, hypotension or shock
- Loss of station of the presenting part.

The diagnosis of uterine rupture is ultimately confirmed at emergency cesarean section or postpartum laparotomy.

## Delivery

The length of the second stage should not exceed 2 hours: one hour to allow for passive descent, but no more than one hour of active pushing (or 30 minutes if the woman has had a prior vaginal delivery). Assisted delivery, in the presence of a prior uterine scar, should ideally only be performed by an experienced consultant. This should be in the operating theatre with provision for immediate cesarean section.

Manual uterine exploration after VBAC and subsequent repair of asymptomatic scar dehiscence has not been shown to improve outcomes. Excessive vaginal bleeding or signs of hypovolemia are potential signs of uterine rupture and should prompt complete evaluation of the genital tract (Cahill et al 2005; Varner et al 2007).

## Role of induction and augmentation of labour

Women with a previous cesarean should be informed of the two- to three-fold increased risk of uterine rupture and around 1.5-fold increased risk of cesarean section in induced and/or augmented labours compared with spontaneous labour. Women should be informed that there is a higher risk of uterine rupture with induction of labour with prostaglandins.

The additional risks in augmented TOLAC mean that:

- Although augmentation is not contraindicated it should only be preceded by careful obstetric assessment, maternal counselling and be a consultant-led decision
- Oxytocin augmentation should be titrated such that it should not exceed the maximum rate of contractions of four in 10 minutes; the ideal contraction frequency would be three to four in 10 minutes
- Careful serial cervical assessments, preferably by the same person, are necessary to show adequate cervicometric progress, thereby allowing augmentation to continue.
- The intervals for serial vaginal examination and the selected parameters of progress that would necessitate discontinuing TOLAC should be consultant-led decisions.

## TOLAC in special circumstances

**Preterm labour:** Women who are preterm and considering the options for birth after a previous cesarean should be informed that planned preterm VBAC has similar success rates to planned term VBAC, but with a lower risk of uterine rupture. Therefore, following appropriate counselling and in a carefully selected population, planned VBAC may be offered as an option to women undergoing preterm birth with a history of prior cesarean birth.

**Multiple gestation:** Women with one previous cesarean delivery with a low transverse incision, who are otherwise appropriate candidates for twin vaginal delivery, may be considered candidates for TOLAC. In two analyses of large populations, women with twin gestations had a similar chance of achieving VBAC as women with singleton gestations and did not incur any greater risk of uterine rupture or maternal or perinatal morbidity (Cahill et al 2005; Varner et al 2007).

## References

American College of Obstetricians and Gynecologists. 2010. Vaginal birth after previous cesarean delivery. Practice Bulletin No. 115. *Obstet Gynecol* 116:450–63

Ananth CV, Smulian JC, Vintzileos AM. 1997. The association of placenta previa with history of cesarean delivery and abortion: a meta-analysis. *Am J Obstet Gynecol* 177:1071–8. (Meta-analysis)

Bujold E, Hammoud AO, Hendler I, Berman S, Blackwell SC, Duperron L, et al. 2004. Trial of labor in patients with a previous cesarean section: does maternal age influence the outcome? *Am J Obstet Gynecol*

Cahill A, Stamilio DM, Pare E, Peipert JP, Stevens EJ, Nelson DB et al. 2005. Vaginal birth after cesarean (VBAC) attempt in twin pregnancies: is it safe? *Am J Obstet Gynecol* 193

Clark SL, Hankins GD. 2003. Temporal and demographic trends in cerebral palsy--fact and fiction. *Am J Obstet Gynecol* 188:628–33

Cragin EB. 1916. Conservatism in obstetrics. *N Y Med J* 104:1–3.

Lee HC, El-Sayed YY, Gould JB. 2008. Population trends in cesarean delivery for breech presentation in the United States, 1997–2003. *Am J Obstet Gynecol* 199:59

Farmer RM, Kirschbaum T, Potter D, Strong TH, Medearis AL. 1991. Uterine rupture during trial of labor after previous cesarean section. *Am J Obstet Gynecol* 165:996–1001.

Flamm BL, Lim OW, Jones C, Fallon D, Newman LA, Mantis JK. 1988. Vaginal birth after cesarean section: results of a multicenter study. *Am J Obstet Gynecol* 158: 1079–84.

Flamm BL, Newman LA, Thomas SJ, Fallon D, Yoshida MM. 1990. Vaginal birth after cesarean delivery: results of a 5-year multicenter collaborative study. *Obstet Gynecol* 76:750–4.

Goetzinger KR, Macones GA. 2008. Operative vaginal delivery: current trends in obstetrics. *Women's Health* 4:281–90.

Goodall PT, Ahn JT, Chapa JB, Hibbard JU. 2005. Obesity as a risk factor for failed trial of labor in patients with previous cesarean delivery. *Am J Obstet Gynecol* 192:1423–6.

Guise JM, McDonagh MS, Osterweil P, Nygren P, Chan BK, Helfand M. 2004. Systematic review of the incidence and consequences of uterine rupture in women with previous caesarean section. *BMJ* 329:19–25.

Guise JM, Hashima J, Osterweil P. 2005. Evidence–based vaginal birth after Caesarean section. *Best Prac Res Clin Obstet Gynaecol* 19:117–30.

Gyamfi C, Juhasz G, Gyamfi P, Stone JL. 2004. Increased success of trial of labor after previous vaginal birth after cesarean. *Obstet Gynecol* 104:715–19.

Indian Council of Medical Research. 1990. *Collaborative study on high risk pregnancies and maternal mortality (ICMR task force study)*. New Delhi: ICMR

Juhasz G, Gyamfi C, Gyamfi P, Tocce K, Stone JL. 2005. Effect of body mass index and excessive weight gain on success of vaginal birth after cesarean delivery. *Obstet Gynecol* 106:741–6.

Landon MB, Hauth JC, Leveno KJ, Spong CY, Leindecker S, Varner MW, et al. 2004. Maternal and perinatal outcomes associated with a trial of labour after prior cesarean delivery. National Institute of Child Health and Human Development, Maternal-Fetal Medicine Units Network. *N Engl J Med* 351:2581–9.

Landon MB, Leindecker S, Spong CY, Hauth JC, Bloom S, Varner MW, et al. 2005. The MFMU Cesarean Registry: factors affecting the success of trial of labor after previous cesarean delivery. *Am J Obstet Gynecol* 193:1016–23

Leung AS, Leung EK, Paul RH. 1993. Uterine rupture after previous cesarean delivery: maternal and fetal consequences. *Am J Obstet Gynecol* 169:945–50.

Lyerly, A. D., Mitchell, L. M., Armstrong, E. M., Harris, L. H., Kukla, R., Kuppermann, M., et al. (2007). Risks, values, and decision making surrounding pregnancy. *Obstetrics and Gynecology, 109*(4), 979–984.

Macones GA, Hausman N, Edelstein R, Stamilio DM, Marder SJ. 2001. Predicting outcomes of trials of labor in women attempting vaginal birth after cesarean delivery: a comparison of multivariate methods with neural networks. *Am J Obstet Gynecol* 184:409–13.

Macones GA, Cahill A, Pare E, Stamilio DM, Ratcliffe S, Stevens E, et al. 2005. Obstetric outcomes in women with two prior cesarean deliveries: is vaginal birth after cesarean delivery a viable option? *Am J Obstet Gynecol* 192:1223–8.

National Institutes of Health. NIH. 2010. Consensus Development Conference: vaginal birth after cesarean: new insights. Consensus Development Conference statement. Bethesda (MD): NIH. Available at: http://consensus.nih.gov/2010/images/vbac/vbac_statement.pdf.

Obori V, Adewunmi A, Ande A et al. 2010. Morbidity associated with failed vaginal birth after cesarean section. *Acta Obstetricia et Gynecologica Scandinavica* Volume 89, Issue 9, 1229–32

Pai M, Sundaram P, Radhakrishnan KK, Thomas K, Muliyil JP. 1999. A high rate of caesarean sections in an affluent section of Chennai: is it cause for concern? *Natl Med J India* 12: 156–158.

Royal College of Obstetricians and Gynaecologists. 2001. The Use of Electronic Fetal Monitoring. The use and interpretation of cardiotocography in intrapartum fetal surveillance. Evidence based Clinical Guideline Number 8. London: RCOG Press

Sakala EP, Kaye S, Murray RD, Munson LJ. 1990. Epidural analgesia. Effect on the likelihood of a successful trial of labor after cesarean section. *J Reprod Med* 35: 886–90.

Silver RM, Landon MB, Rouse DJ, Leveno KJ, Spong CY, Thom EA, et al. 2006. Maternal morbidity associated with multiple repeat cesarean deliveries. National Institute of Child Health and Human Development Maternal-Fetal Medicine Units Network. *Obstet Gynecol* 107:1226–32.

Smith GC, Pell JP, Cameron AD, Dobbie R. 2002. Risk of perinatal death associated with labor after previous cesarean delivery in uncomplicated term pregnancies. *JAMA* 287:2684–90.

Smith GC, White IR, Pell JP, Dobbie R. 2005. Predicting cesarean section and uterine rupture among women attempting vaginal birth after prior cesarean section. *PLoS Med* 2: 871–8.

Sreevidya S, Sathiyasekaran BWC. 2003. High caesarean rates in Madras (India): a population-based cross-sectional study. *BJOG* Feb;110 (22):106–11.

Srinivas SK, Stamilio DM, Stevens EJ, Odibo AO, Peipert JF, Macones GA. 2007. Predicting failure of a vaginal birth attempt after cesarean delivery. *Obstet Gynecol*. 109: 800–5.

Turner MJ. 2002. Uterine rupture. *Best Prac Res Clin Obstet Gynaecol* 16: 69–79.

Varner MW, Thom E, Spong CY, Landon MB, Leveno KJ, Rouse DJ, et al. 2007. Trial of labor after one previous cesarean delivery for multifetal gestation. National Institute of Child Health and Human Development (NICHD) Maternal-Fetal Medicine Units Network (MFMU). *Obstet Gynecol* 110: 814–9.

Wen SW, Rusen ID, Walker M, Liston R, Kramer MS, Baskett T, et al. 2004. Comparison of maternal mortality and morbidity between trial of labor and elective cesarean section among women with previous cesarean delivery. *Am J Obstet Gynecol* 191: 1263–9.

Zweifler, J., Garza, A., Hughes, S., et al. 2006. Vaginal birth after cesarean in California before and after a change in guidelines. *Ann Fam Med*, 4(3), 228–234.

# CHAPTER 17

# ANTEPARTUM HEMORRHAGE

*Amarnath Bhide*

Antepartum hemorrhage (APH) defined as bleeding from the genital tract in the second half of pregnancy, remains a major cause of perinatal mortality and maternal morbidity even in the developed world. In approximately half of all women presenting with APH, a diagnosis of placental abruption or placenta praevia will be made; no firm diagnosis will be made in the other half even after investigations. In cases presenting with APH, the evaluation consists of history of symptoms and clinical signs. Once the mother is stabilised, a speculum examination and an ultrasound scan is useful to derive a diagnosis.

Causes of antepartum hemorrhage are:
- Abruptio placentae
- Placenta previa
- APH of indeterminate origin
- Vasa previa
- Bleeding from the lower genital tract

## Placental abruption

Placental abruption is the premature separation of a normally situated placenta from the uterine wall, resulting in hemorrhage before the delivery of the fetus. It occurs in approximately one in 80 deliveries and remains a significant source of perinatal mortality and morbidity.

### Incidence

Recent large epidemiological studies report an incidence ranging from 5.9 to 6.5 per 1000 singleton births and 12.2 per 1000 twin births. Perinatal mortality is reported to be 119 per 1000 births complicated by abruption (Ananth et al 1999). The risk of abruption recurring in a subsequent pregnancy is increased as much as 10-fold.

### Pathology and etiology

The precise cause of abruption is unknown. Abruption arises from hemorrhage into the deciduas basalis of the placenta, which results in the formation of hematoma and an increase in hydrostatic pressure leading to separation of the adjacent placenta. The resultant hematoma may be small and self-limited or may continue to dissect through the decidual layer. However, the bleeding may be in whole or in part concealed, if the hematoma does not reach the margin of the placenta and cervix for the blood loss to be revealed. Therefore, the correlation between the amount of revealed hemorrhage and the degree of actual blood loss is poor. The bleeding may infiltrate the myometrium resulting in the so-called 'Couvelaire' uterus.

> Infiltration of the myometrium by blood results in a 'Couvelaire' uterus.

A causal relationship between hypertension and abruption is controversial. Most explanations implicate vascular or placental abnormalities, including increased fragility of vessels, vascular malformations, or abnormalities in placentation. The absence of transformation from muscular arterioles to low-resistance, dilated vessels as in normal pregnancy and the lack of trophoblastic invasion of uterine vessels is thought to result in decreased placental blood flow and abnormal endothelial responses to vaso-active substances. These abnormal placental vessels may predispose to ischemia and rupture of involved vessels, thus causing placental abruption.

Placental abruption is associated with gestational hypertensive disease, advanced maternal age, increasing parity, the presence of multiple gestations, polyhydramnios, chorioamnionitis, prolonged rupture of membranes, trauma, and possibly, thrombophilias. Potential preventable risk factors include maternal use of recreational drugs, such as cocaine, and maternal smoking. Unexplained

> Placental abruption is associated with:
> - gestational hypertension
> - advanced maternal age
> - increasing parity
> - multiple gestation
> - polyhydramnios
> - chorioamnionitis
> - prolonged rupture of membranes
> - trauma

elevation of maternal serum alpha-fetoprotein (MSAFP) levels in the second trimester is associated with pregnancy complications such as placental abruption.

## Clinical presentation

The diagnosis of placental abruption is clinical, based on characteristic signs and symptoms. This is then confirmed by evaluation of the placenta after delivery. It presents classically with vaginal bleeding, abdominal pain, uterine contractions and tenderness. On clinical examination, the uterus is irritable, with increased baseline tone. There may be evidence of fetal distress. In severe cases, the mother may show signs and symptoms of hypovolemia. Fetal cardiac activity may be absent, and there is a serious risk of development of coagulopathy in the mother due to consumption of the clotting factors. The clinical signs of blood loss are more pronounced than the amount of visible vaginal bleeding. Ultrasound is an insensitive and unreliable tool for detecting or excluding placental abruption, as negative sonographic findings are common with clinically significant abruptions. The diagnosis may be confirmed postpartum on gross examination of the placenta, which reveals a clot and/or depression in the maternal surface, known as a 'delle'.

> Ultrasound is an insensitive and unreliable tool for detecting or excluding placental abruption.

In less severe cases, the diagnosis of placental abruption may not be obvious, particularly if the hemorrhage is largely concealed and it may be misdiagnosed as idiopathic preterm labour. The majority of fetal morbidity is thought to be due to prematurity. Low birth-weight, fetal growth restriction, neonatal anemia and hyper-bilirubinemia are significantly more common. Premature separation of the placenta also leads to fetal hypoxia. In cases presenting with the fetus still alive, fetal heart rate abnormalities are common.

Placental abruption cannot be eliminated as a potential diagnosis in the absence of vaginal bleeding, as hemorrhage may be retro-placental and completely concealed. Placental abruption is concealed in 20 per cent to 35 per cent and revealed in 65 per cent to 80 per cent of cases. In severe abruption, complications include hemorrhage requiring transfusion, disseminated intravascular coagulopathy (DIC), infection and rarely, maternal death. Couvelaire uterus may occur and occasionally may require hysterectomy. The incidence of stillbirth is related to the size of the abruption and the uterine irritability that causes polysystole and sustained uterine contractions. Separation exceeding 50 per cent of the placenta causes a marked elevation in stillbirth rate.

> Bleeding in placental abruption is revealed in 65 per cent to 80 per cent of cases and concealed in 20 per cent to 35 per cent.

> Separation exceeding 50 per cent of the placenta increases the risk of stillbirth.

## Management

Once placental abruption has been suspected, action should be swift and decisive because the prognosis for mother and fetus is worsened by delay. Treatment consists of initial resuscitation and stabilisation of the mother and recognition and management of complications. It is individualised based on the extent of the abruption, maternal and fetal reaction to this insult, and gestational age of the fetus. Maternal resuscitation and treatment of hypovolemic shock are a subject of a review in its own right, and will not be discussed further. For the purpose of management, Sher and Statland (1985) divided placental abruption into three degrees of severity. These are:

**Mild (Grade 1):** This is not recognised clinically before delivery and is usually diagnosed by the presence of a retro-placental clot. This is a retrospective diagnosis.

**Moderate (Grade 2):** This is an intermediate grade in which the classical clinical signs of abruption are present, but the fetus is still alive. The frequency of fetal heart rate abnormalities is high.

**Severe (Grade 3):** This is the severe grade in which the fetus is dead and coagulopathy may be present. The volume of blood loss is appreciable in this condition. If the mother presents with Grade 3 abruption, immediate arrangements to cross-match at least four units should be made. Blood transfusion should begin early, since abruption large enough to lead to fetal demise is associated with significant blood loss.

There are three practical options for management:

- ❖ Expectant: in the hope that the pregnancy will continue
- ❖ Immediate cesarean section
- ❖ Rupture the membranes and aim at vaginal delivery

In mild placental abruption, the bleeding may stop and the symptoms gradually resolve with satisfactory fetal monitoring, and the patient can often be discharged after a few days and managed as an outpatient. The management of moderate or severe placental abruption is resuscitation, delivery of the fetus and observation for, and correction of any coagulation defect that arises. This requires management in the labour ward with intensive monitoring of both mother and fetus. A trial of labour and vaginal delivery is recommended whenever tolerated by the maternal–fetal pair. Labour is usually rapid and progress should be monitored with continuous fetal heart rate monitoring. Delivery should be expedited in the form of an emergency cesarean section if fetal distress is evident.

Major abruption should be regarded as an emergency, requiring multidisciplinary input from the obstetrician, anesthetist and hematologist. A fulminant maternal DIC can ensue within hours of a complete abruption and delivery should be arranged, as it is the only means with which to halt the DIC. Replacement of blood and its components should begin before surgery. Abruption also places the mother at a high risk of severe postpartum hemorrhage. This is due to a combination of uterine atony and coagulation failure. Invasive monitoring with arterial lines and central venous access may be necessary, and patients are best treated in the high-dependency unit. Urine output should be closely monitored, as renal failure is a potential complication. In the triennium, 2003–2005, two maternal deaths were reported to be attributable to placental abruption in the UK.

Multiple studies have shown expectant management, with or without tocolytics, to be safe and effective in a select population of patients with preterm placental abruption provided that the fetal heart rate tracing is normal (Combs et al 1991). In some observational studies, tocolysis allowed a median delay of delivery of several days without increasing neonatal or maternal morbidity, including the need for transfusion or delivery by cesarean section (Towers et al 1990). However, in the absence of randomised controlled trials, the benefits of tocolysis remain uncertain.

> The high risk of severe postpartum hemorrhage with abruption is due to a combination of uterine atony and coagulation failure.

> The probability of a recurrence of abruption increases in future pregnancies and therefore it is reasonable to deliver electively after fetal maturity is reached in the subsequent pregnancy.

The probability of a recurrence of abruption increases in future pregnancies following a history of placental abruption. There are no reliable predictors of the timing in pregnancy at which this may happen, and there are no known interventions to reduce recurrence. The practice of elective delivery after fetal maturity is reached in the subsequent pregnancy, is reasonable.

## Placenta previa

Placenta previa is defined as a placenta that lies wholly or partly within the lower uterine segment. The prevalence of clinically-evident placenta previa at term is estimated to be approximately 4 or 5 per 1000 pregnancies (RCOG Green top guideline No. 27, 2005).

## Classification

Classification of placenta previa is important in making management decisions, because the incidence of morbidity and mortality in the fetus and mother increases as the grade increases. Classically, placenta previa is divided into four types or grades (Figure 17.1 and Table 17.1).

Types I and II are regarded as minor, and types III and IV as major degrees of placenta previa. Care must be taken not to confuse these grades with grades of placental maturity. The classification is difficult to use in practice, because the definition of lower uterine segment is more conceptual than anatomical. In any case, with the availability

**Table 17.1** Types of placenta previa

| Type | Description |
| --- | --- |
| 1 | Placenta is in the lower uterine segment but the lower edge does not reach the internal os (stops short by 3 cm) |
| 2 | Lower edge of the placenta reaches internal os but does not cover it |
| 3 | Placenta covers the internal os asymmetrically |
| 4 | Placenta covers the os symmetrically |

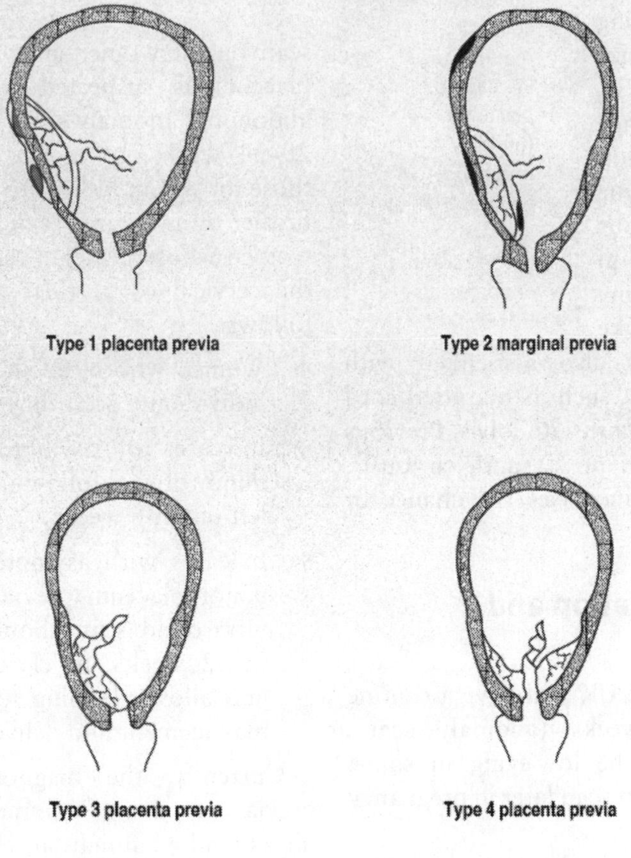

Type 1 placenta previa

Type 2 marginal previa

Type 3 placenta previa

Type 4 placenta previa

**Figure 17.1** Different types of placenta previa

of ultrasound, this classification has become obsolete. Currently, the condition is most commonly diagnosed on ultrasound examination. Ultrasound remains the method of choice because it is safe, relatively cheap and readily available.

## Etiology and associated factors

Placenta previa is caused by implantation of the blastocyst low in the uterine cavity. Factors associated with the development of placenta previa include increasing maternal parity, advancing maternal age, increasing placental size (multiple pregnancy), endometrial damage (previous dilatation and curettage), uterine scars like previous Cesarean section or myomectomy and pathology like endometritis. It is also associated with placental pathology, such as marginal cord insertions and succenturiate lobes. Previous history of placental previa and, curiously, cigarette smoking increases the chance of placenta previa.

> Placenta previa is associated with:
> - increasing maternal parity
> - advancing maternal age
> - increasing placental size (multiple pregnancy)
> - endometrial damage
> - uterine scars
> - endometritis

## Clinical presentation and diagnosis

Most women in the UK will have a routine scan at 21–23 weeks (anomaly scan). The placenta will be low-lying in some, necessitating a repeat scan later in pregnancy (See Figure 17.2).

A reasonable antenatal imaging policy is to perform a trans-vaginal ultrasound

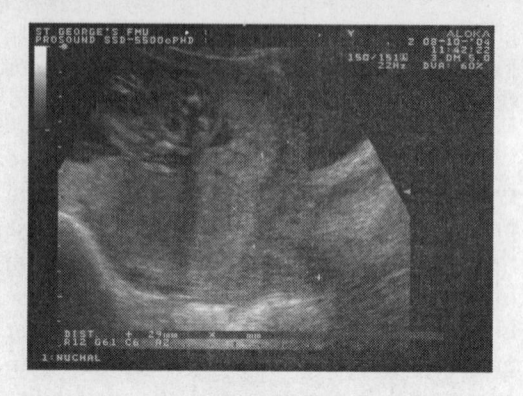

**Figure 17.2** Abdominal ultrasound scan showing posterior placenta previa. The cervical canal is marked by callipers.

scan on all women in whom a low-lying placenta is suspected from their trans-abdominal anomaly scan, at approximately 20–24 weeks, to reduce the numbers of those for whom follow-up will be needed. A further trans-vaginal scan is required for all women whose placenta reaches or overlaps the cervical os at their anomaly scan as follows:

❖ Women who bleed should be managed individually according to their needs.

❖ In cases of asymptomatic suspected minor previa, follow-up imaging can be left until 36 weeks.

❖ In cases with asymptomatic suspected major placenta previa, a trans-vaginal ultrasound scan should be performed at 32 weeks, to clarify the diagnosis and allow planning for third-trimester management and delivery.

Currently, the diagnosis of placenta previa is most commonly made on ultrasound examination. Up to 26 per cent of placentas are found to be low lying on ultrasound examination in the early second trimester. Several studies have demonstrated that unless the placental edge is at least reaching the internal cervical os at mid-pregnancy, placenta previa at term will not be encountered (Becker et al 2001; Bhide and Thilaganathan 2004). Trans-vaginal ultrasound is safe in the presence of placenta previa, and is more accurate than trans-abdominal ultrasound in locating the placental edge. Ultrasound has been used to observe and document the phenomenon of placental migration from the lower uterine segment. It is thought that this process is not a true migration of placental tissue but, rather, a degeneration of the peripheral placental tissue that receives a suboptimal vascular supply and has slow placental growth in better perfused uterine areas at the same time, so-called placental trophotropism. None of the cases presented with placenta previa at term, unless the placental edge overlapped the internal os at least by 1 cm at the mid-trimester scan. There was a minimal placental migration rate of 0.1 mm/week in this group. In contrast, cases where the placenta eventually migrated away from the internal os showed a mean rate of migration of 4.1 mm/week. Placental edge overlapping the internal os at the mid-trimester scan, and a thick placental edge (where the angle between the placental edge and the uterine wall is less than 135°) are known to be associated with reduced likelihood of placental migration. Placental migration is less likely with posterior placentae and with previous cesarean section (Predanic et al 2005). If the placental edge is overlapping the internal os or is within 2 cm on trans-vaginal scan at 38 weeks, elective cesarean section is a reasonable option (Figure 17.3).

> Unless the placental edge is at least reaching the internal cervical os at mid-pregnancy, placenta previa at term will not be encountered.

In women where the placenta failed to migrate, increased rates of interventional cesarean delivery, manual placental removal and a higher prevalence of placenta accreta were encountered.

Women classically present with painless vaginal bleeding. The bleeds tend to occur due to the formation of the lower uterine segment. Fetal malpresentation or unstable lie is found in at least a third of cases, and many women with placenta previa do not bleed until the onset of labour.

## Management

The management of placenta previa depends upon clinical presentation, gestational age, severity of bleeding and degree of previa. Currently, the diagnosis of placenta previa is made using ultrasound. Most cases presenting with APH would already be known to have a low-lying placenta. Those cases, in which the placenta was low-lying at the time of routine anomaly scan should

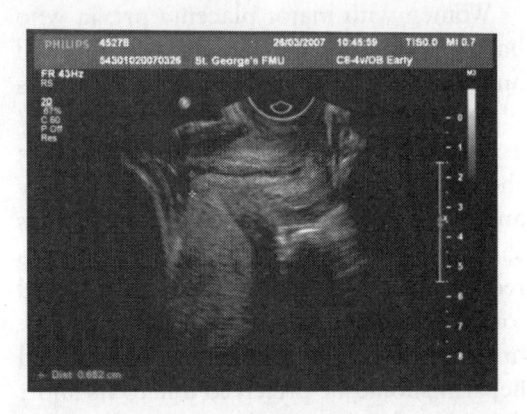

Figure 17.3 Trans-vaginal ultrasound scan showing a posterior low placenta. The distance of the placental edge from the internal os is 6.5 mm.

receive a repeat ultrasound scan at 36 weeks to check placental location. Some of these cases will present with antepartum bleeding. Initial hemorrhages, referred to as 'warning hemorrhages' are often small and tend to stop spontaneously. Delivery may be needed for severe, intractable or recurrent bleeding. Fetal morbidity is associated with iatrogenic prematurity. In the report of confidential enquiries into maternal mortality in the UK ('Why mothers die 2000–2002'), there were 14 maternal deaths due to hemorrhage. Three out of these 14 deaths were due to placenta previa.

> If the placenta was low-lying at the time of routine anomaly scan, a repeat ultrasound scan should be done at 36 weeks to check placental location.

Antenatal imaging by colour flow Doppler ultrasonography should be performed in women with placenta previa who are at increased risk of placenta accreta. Where this is not possible locally, such women should be managed as if they have placenta accreta until proven otherwise.

Women with major placenta previa who have previously bled should be admitted and managed as inpatients from 34 weeks of gestation. The risk of thrombo-embolism associated with prolonged hospitalisation should be kept in mind. Gentle mobility and the use of elastic compression stockings should be encouraged. Anticoagulation to reduce the risk of clots should be reserved for those women at a particularly high risk of thrombosis, and regular un-fractionated heparin should be preferred due to its short duration of action.

Those with major placenta previa who remain asymptomatic, having never bled, require careful counselling before contemplating outpatient care. Any home-based care requires close proximity to the hospital, the constant presence of a companion and full informed consent from the woman. They should be advised to contact the hospital early in the event of abdominal pain or vaginal bleeding. Prior to the delivery, a discussion about the delivery plan, risks of severe hemorrhage, need for blood transfusion and the possibility of surgical intervention, including removal of the uterus, should take place.

Traditionally, cesarean section has been the recommended mode of delivery for major placenta previa (types III and IV), whereas for minor previa (types I and II), an attempt at vaginal delivery was deemed appropriate. Until recently, no evidence-based protocol was available for management of delivery guided by the findings of the ultrasound scan. We reported that when the placental edge was within 1 cm of the internal cervical os within 2 weeks of delivery, all patients required a cesarean delivery due to bleeding. We proposed that cases with placental edge to internal os distance of less than 2 cm be referred to as major placenta previa and an elective cesarean section should be recommended. In contrast, if the placental edge to internal cervical os distance is 2–3.5 cm at the last ultrasound scan within 2 weeks of delivery, the likelihood of achieving a vaginal delivery is at least 60 per cent. It is recommended that these cases be still referred to as low-lying placenta, because the risk of postpartum hemorrhage remains high in this group. An attempt at vaginal delivery is appropriate. RCOG Guidelines recommend that any women going to the operation theatre with known major placenta previa should be attended by an experienced obstetrician and anesthetist, with consultant presence available, especially if these women have previous uterine scars, an anterior placenta or are suspected to be associated with placenta accreta (RCOG Green top guideline No. 27, 2005). Four units of cross-matched blood should be kept ready, even if the mother has never experienced vaginal bleeding. Delivery of women with placenta previa should not be planned in units where blood transfusion facilities are unavailable. The choice of anesthetic technique for cesarean sections is usually made jointly by the anesthetist, the obstetrician and the pregnant women. The timing of surgery should be deferred till 38 weeks, if possible, in order to reduce neonatal morbidity.

## Placenta accreta

Although placenta accreta is very rare (0.004%) in women with a normally situated placenta, it occurred in 9.3 per cent of women with placenta previa according to data from Southern California (Comstock 2005). Ultrasound features of placenta accreta in second and third trimesters include visualisation of irregular vascular sinuses (see Figures 17.4a and 17.4b) with turbulent flow (Comstock 2005), abnormalities of the bladder wall on ultrasound inspection and possibly myometrial thickness of less than 1 mm. Absence of the sonolucent space between the myometrium and the placenta is not a reliable sign. Colour flow-mapping is a useful test for the diagnosis. Magnetic resonance imaging is not yet a completely sensitive and specific test for the diagnosis and is not warranted routinely.

> Placenta accreta occurs more commonly in women with placenta previa.

When a probability of placenta accreta is raised, multidisciplinary input involving the patient and her family, the anesthetist, obstetrician and the sonographer should be arranged. The risks from placenta accreta include massive hemorrhage, risk of hysterectomy, infection and even maternal death.

> The risks from placenta accreta include:
> • massive hemorrhage
> • risk of hysterectomy
> • infection
> • maternal death

Advance planning should be made for management of delivery. The options are

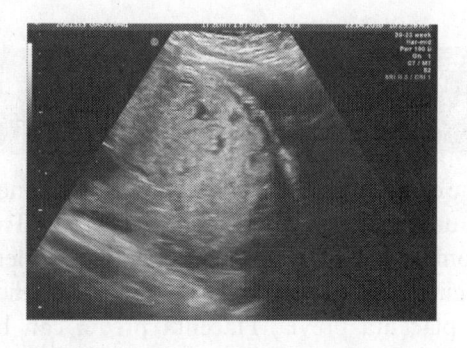

**Figure 17.4a** Trans-abdominal ultrasound of an anterior low placenta, later shown to be accreta. Note the irregular echo-lucent areas (vascular sinuses)

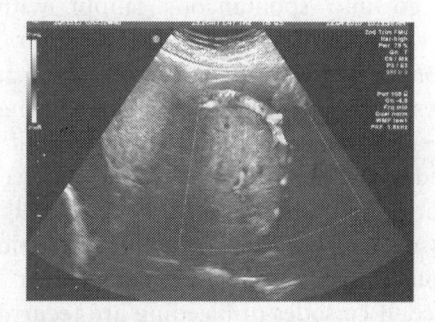

**Figure 17.4b** Colour flow-mapping in a case of placenta accrete showing vascular spaces.

subsequent hysterectomy after delivery or leaving the placenta in-situ in order to reduce surgical complications and blood loss. Conservative management of placenta accreta can be successful and can preserve fertility. Uterine artery embolisation, ligation of anterior division of the internal iliac artery, and Methotrexate treatment, in order to accelerate the process of absorption of the adherent placenta which had been left in-situ, have all been tried with variable success. Following a decision of leaving the placenta in situ, delayed hemorrhage requiring hysterectomy has also been reported.

## Bleeding of indeterminate origin

The exact cause of bleeding in late pregnancy is unknown in about half of cases. The woman typically presents with painless vaginal bleeding without ultrasound evidence of placenta previa. Placenta previa can be excluded by an ultrasound scan, but the diagnosis of placental abruption is based on clinical signs and symptoms, and is difficult to confirm in mild cases. Approximately 15 per cent of women with unexplained APH will go into spontaneous labour within two weeks of the initial hemorrhage. In the majority of cases, the bleeding is mild and settles spontaneously. Further management will either be expectant, or delivery will be expedited. If pregnancy is beyond 37 weeks gestation and the bleeding is recurrent or is associated with fetal growth restriction, labour induction is the management of choice. If episodes of bleeding are recurrent and significant, there may be a need for immediate delivery even if the gestation is below 37 weeks. If a policy of expectant management is adopted, fetal well-being should be monitored. Once the bleeding has settled and the woman has been observed as an inpatient for 24–48 h, it may be considered safe to allow her to be managed as an outpatient. If the gestational age is below 34–36 weeks, antenatal steroids should be administered in view of the risk of preterm delivery. In a small proportion of cases, where placenta previa and placental abruption have been excluded, a cause may still be found. They include 'show', cervicitis, trauma, vulval varicosities, genital tract tumours, hematuria, genital infections and vasa previa. Many of these conditions are evident on the initial speculum examination.

## Vasa previa

Vasa previa is the presence of unsupported fetal vessels below the fetal presenting part, where the cord insertion is velamentous (Figure 17.5).

It is rare, but the consequences are catastrophic, if not prenatally diagnosed. Vasa previa has an incidence of approximately one per 6000 deliveries. Classically, vaginal bleeding follows amniotomy with subsequent severe fetal heart rate decelerations or bradycardia, which may be suggestive of vasa previa. The diagnosis of this condition before these events is difficult, but the experienced observer may be able to feel vessels on digital examination below the presenting part. A speculum examination

> Vaginal bleeding following amniotomy, with subsequent severe fetal heart rate decelerations or bradycardia, may be suggestive of vasa previa

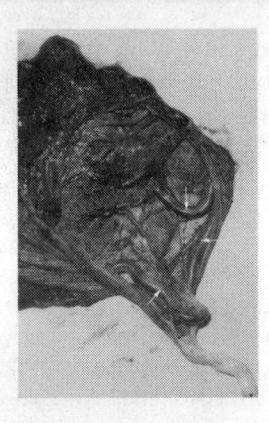

**Figure 17.5** Velamentous insertion of the cord. Note the unsupported fetal vessels in the membranes. If present over the internal os, these constitute vasa previa.

may also reveal the vessels on inspection. An Apt test on the blood can be performed to demonstrate the presence of fetal blood. Immediate cesarean delivery is needed if fetal blood is confirmed to be present in the vaginal bleeding. Oyelese et al (2004) demonstrated the importance of prenatal diagnosis. In the group where prenatal diagnosis of vasa previa had been made, 97 per cent infants survived, as opposed to only 44 per cent where the diagnosis had not been made before birth. Echogenic parallel or circular lines near the cervix representing the umbilical cord, seen by grey-scale ultrasound, should raise the possibility of vasa previa. The diagnosis of vasa previa can be confirmed by Doppler and transvaginal ultrasound studies if aberrant vessels over the internal cervical os are suspected. Several reports have linked vasa previa to in-vitro fertilisation.

The diagnosis should be kept in mind in cases of in-vitro fertilisation pregnancies with low placenta, and cases where the placenta had been low-lying at the mid-trimester scan, but has receded from the internal os on repeat assessment. Delivery by elective cesarean section after fetal pulmonary maturity is established and preferably at term prior to the onset of labour should be recommended, unless obstetric complications supervene.

**Practice points:**

- The exact cause of bleeding in late pregnancy is unknown in about half of cases.
- The diagnosis of placenta abruption is clinical, based on characteristic signs and symptoms. Ultrasound has a limited role in the diagnosis.
- Once placental abruption has been suspected, action should be swift and decisive, because the prognosis for mother and fetus is worsened by delay.
- Major abruption should be regarded as an emergency, requiring multidisciplinary input from the obstetrician, anesthetist and hematologist.
- Currently, the diagnosis of placenta previa is most commonly made following the mid-trimester ultrasound scan demonstrating low-lying placenta.
- Ultrasound remains the method of choice in suspected placenta previa, because it is safe, relatively cheap and readily available. It is also useful for planning the mode of delivery.
- Ultrasound features of placenta accreta in second and third trimesters include visualisation of irregular vascular sinuses with turbulent flow and abnormalities of the bladder wall on ultrasound inspection.
- Prenatal diagnosis of vasa previa has a major impact on improving fetal

survival. The diagnosis should be kept in mind in IVF pregnancies with low placenta, and cases where the placenta had been low-lying at the mid-trimester scan, but has receded from the internal os on repeat assessment.

## References

Ananth CV, Berkowitz GS, Savitz DA, et al. 1999. Placental abruption and adverse perinatal outcomes. *JAMA* 282: 1646–51.

Becker R, Vonk R, Mende B, et al. 2001. The relevance of placental location at 20–23 gestational weeks for prediction of placenta praevia at delivery: evaluation of 8650 cases. *Ultrasound Obstet Gynecol* 17:496–501.

Bhide A, Thilaganathan B. 2004. Recent advances in the management of placenta praevia. *Curr Opin Obstet Gynecol* 16: 447–51.

Combs CA, Nyberg DA, Mack LA, et al. 1991. Expectant management after sonographic diagnosis of placental abruption. *Am J Perinatol* 9:170–4.

Comstock CH. 2005. Antenatal diagnosis of placenta accreta: a review. *Ultrasound Obstet Gynecol* 26:89–96.

Oyelese Y, Catanzarite V, Prefumo F, et al. 2004. Vasa praevia: the impact of prenatal diagnosis on outcomes. *Obstet Gynecol* 103:937–42.

Royal College of Obstetrician's and Gynaecologists. 2005. Green Top Guideline No. 27. *Placenta Praevia and Placenta Praevia Accreta: Diagnosis and management.* Royal College of Obstetricians and Gynecologists. Revised October

National Institute for Clinical Excellence (NICE). 2001. *The Confidential Enquiries into Maternal Deaths in the United Kingdom: Why Mothers Die 1997–1999.* London: Department of Health.

Predanic M, Perni S, Chasen S, Baergen R, Chervenak F. 2005. A sonographic assessment of different patterns of placenta praevia 'migration' in the third trimester of pregnancy. *J Ultrasound Med* 24:773–80.

Sher G, Statland BE. 1985. Abruptio placentae with coagulopathy: a rational basis for management. *Clin Obstet Gynaecol* 28:15–23.

Towers CV, Pircon RA, Heppard M. 1990. Is tocolysis safe in the management of third trimester bleeding? *Am J Obstet Gynecol* 180:1572–8.

# CHAPTER 18

# THE THIRD STAGE OF LABOUR

*Melina Georgiou and Leonie K Penna*

The third stage of labour is the period from the delivery of the baby until the delivery of the placenta. Following the excitement of the birth of the baby, delivery of the placenta is often viewed as dull and unimportant. However, management of this stage can directly influence important maternal outcomes such as blood loss, the need for manual removal of the placenta and the incidence of postpartum hemorrhage.

Worldwide, there are an estimated 500,000–600,000 deaths of mothers in childbirth annually (WHO 1990; Adamson 1996). In the developing world, the majority of these deaths result from complications of the third stage. In the developed world, death rates have fallen dramatically over the last 50 years. This is due to a number of improvements in care during pregnancy and childbirth, including the provision of antenatal care, improvement in women's nutritional status, oxytocics to prevent and treat postpartum hemorrhage and the wider availability of blood transfusion services and effective antibiotics.

The best management of the third stage would be one that effectively minimises serious problems such as blood loss and retained placenta, while interfering as little as possible with the physiological mechanisms of placental delivery and bonding between mother and baby, and has few side effects.

## Physiological mechanisms

Recognition of the physiological events taking place during normal labour is important in the correct management of obstetric complications. At term, the normal volume of blood flow through the placenta is 500–800 ml per minute. At placental separation, this has to be arrested within seconds, otherwise serious hemorrhage will occur. There are three interrelated physiological mechanisms for this:

> Bleeding after placental separation is arrested by the following mechanisms:
> - retraction of the oblique uterine muscle fibres causing compression of torn blood vessels
> - uterine contraction bringing the uterine walls into apposition
> - increased activation of the coagulation and fibrinolytic systems around the placental site

❖ Retraction of the oblique uterine muscle fibres in the upper uterine wall. This acts as a ligature to the torn blood vessels, which intertwine through the muscle. In cases of placenta previa, where the placenta is located in the lower segment where oblique muscle fibres are absent, this mechanism is absent, and therefore, there is greater risk of postpartum hemorrhage.

❖ Following separation, the strong uterine contraction brings the uterine walls into apposition so that further pressure is exerted on the placental site.

❖ There is evidence to suggest that there is transitory increased activation of the coagulation and fibrinolytic systems around the placental site, so clot formation in the torn vessels is intensified. Following separation, the placental site is rapidly covered by a fibrin mesh utilising 5–10 per cent of the circulating fibrinogen.

Following delivery of the infant, there is an immediate lowering of the uterine fundus due to so-called 'retraction'. This is probably facilitated by the typical arrangement of the uterine musculature (circular) fibres. The retraction reduces the area of the uterine surface to which the relatively incompressible placenta is attached, therefore, separation occurs. Once separation occurs, the uterus contracts strongly, forcing the placenta and membranes into the lower segment of the uterus.

## Expectant Management of the Third Stage

Expectant management of the third stage is also described as conservative management or as a physiological third stage. It involves waiting for signs of separation and allowing the placenta to deliver spontaneously or aided by gravity or nipple stimulation (manually or by breastfeeding).

This line of practice is the usual one in a domiciliary setting and in the developing world. Despite the overall definition of expectant management, it means different things to different people. In the Netherlands, expectant management means waiting for signs of placental separation, after which the placenta is delivered, either by maternal effort alone or by maternal effort aided by fundal pressure. In some parts of Africa, it means controlled cord traction without the use of an oxytocic drug. In the UK, it usually describes a 'hands-off' approach, with no intervention of any kind other than putting the baby to the breast to aid separation and encouraging maternal effort to deliver the placenta as soon as separation is obvious. This difference in definitions results in lack of standardisation in studies comparing expectant and active management and makes careful interpretation of these studies on the third stage difficult.

## Active Management of the Third Stage

Active management implies a 'cascade of interventions' aimed at prevention of complications of the third stage, such as postpartum hemorrhage and retained placenta. The management

Active management of the third stage involves:
- prophylactic administration of a parenteral oxytocic drug
- early clamping of the umbilical cord
- controlled cord traction

includes prophylactic administration of a parenteral oxytocic drug, early clamping of the umbilical cord and controlled cord traction. The package of active management is standard practice in the UK, Australia and many other countries.

## Use of Oxytocics and other Uterotonics

It has been shown that the prophylactic use of oxytocic drugs as part of routine management of the third stage reduces the risk of postpartum hemorrhage by about 40 per cent (De Groot 1996; Prendiville et al 1988).

Standard management is to administer oxytocin with the delivery of the anterior shoulder in a vaginal delivery of a singleton cephalic presentation, and as the head delivers in a vaginal breech delivery. The overall aim is not to administer oxytocin before delivery is inevitable as a tonic uterine contraction (in the event that there is delay in delivery of the shoulders or the aftercoming head), as it would worsen neonatal prognosis by increasing the hypoxic insult. In twin gestations, oxytocin should not be given until delivery of the second baby. In a cesarean section, oxytocin is usually given as the cord is clamped, but administration after delivery of the head would be unlikely to result in problems, as the incidence of true shoulder dystocia in a cesarean section is low. Instrumental vaginal delivery is associated with a higher incidence of postpartum hemorrhage and an oxytocic drug should be given in all cases.

### Oxytocics

Oxytocics were initially introduced in the treatment of postpartum hemorrhage and their role in this context is undisputed. However, there is more controversy regarding prophylactic use in order to try to prevent hemorrhage. The theoretical objective of prophylactic use is to ensure adequate uterine contraction following delivery of the infant, thus, reducing the amount of blood loss. This is achieved by early and complete placental separation and occlusion of the vessels and capillaries on the placental site.

There are three main groups of oxytocic drugs: the ergot alkaloids (ergometrine), oxytocin, and prostaglandins (such as misoprostol or $PGF_{2\alpha}$). The choice of oxytocic will depend on factors such as drug effectiveness, route of administration, pharmacokinetic properties, cost, adverse effects and stability for storage.

*Ergot alkaloids*: Ergot alkaloids such as ergometrine act by enhancing the muscle tone of the uterus, by causing fast rhythmic contractions of the myometrium, an effect described as tetany. This promotes separation of the placenta and, in addition, the myometrial blood vessels are compressed resulting in a restriction of the loss of blood. The tetany continues for several hours. A mean terminal half-life of 120 minutes has been reported for ergotamine, although this varies between individuals (De Groot 1996).

Ergot alkaloids can be administered orally, intravenously or intramuscularly. Methyl ergometrine is the only oxytocic available in tablets. The feasibility of oral ergometrine as prophylaxis for postpartum hemorrhage has been studied; if effective, it could be

> Oral ergometrine is not effective in the prevention of postpartum hemorrhage.

used by traditional birth attendants who may be unable to administer injections. Unfortunately, the oral route does not appear to be a reliable route of administration. Studies have showed that oral ergometrine is not effective in the prevention of postpartum hemorrhage (De Groot 1996). In addition, instability during transport and storage in hot climates is a major problem. Oral ergometrine is very unstable when stored unrefrigerated as it was found to be affected by the higher relative humidity levels in developing countries. The parenteral form of ergometrine (for intravenous or intramuscular use) must also be refrigerated, either in hospital or in the fridge of the pregnant woman having a planned home birth (De Groot 1995).

The recommended safe and effective dose of ergometrine is 0.2 to 0.5 m intravenously or intramuscularly. This can be repeated following prophylaxis, as a treatment for bleeding on one occasion to a maximum total dose of 1mg.

> The recommended safe and effective dose of ergometrine is 0.2 to 0.5 mg intravenously or intramuscularly.

The main side effects of ergot alkaloids are nausea, vomiting and hypertension. The latter side effect is such that ergometrine is contraindicated in any woman suffering from preexisting hypertension or cardiac disease in pregnancy, where another oxytocic should be given instead. The nausea and vomiting are sufficiently troublesome, hence, concurrent administration of an antiemetic should be considered if the drug is given intravenously.

> Ergometrine is contraindicated in any woman suffering from preexisting hypertension or cardiac disease in pregnancy.

*Oxytocin*: Oxytocin is a naturally occurring uterotonic, which Du Vigneaud first reported in 1953. During pregnancy, the human myometrium contains oxytocin receptors, which increase as gestational age increases. During labour, the number of oxytocin receptors in both the myometrium and the decidua are high. The effect of an oxytocin injection is to increase the frequency and amplitude of contractions. It has a short half life of 3–5 minutes, and therefore, if a sustained effect is required, an intravenous infusion is necessary.

Oxytocin can be administered intravenously or intramuscularly, but not orally, as it is ineffective by that route. While intravenous administration provides immediate drug availability, pharmacokinetic data show that even with the intramuscular route, oxytocin is circulating in the blood within 2–3 minutes of administration (Gülmezoglu et al 2002).

Chemically, oxytocin is closely related to an antidiuretic hormone and, thus, may lead to fluid retention and water intoxication. These are unusual side effects and would not be expected with the relatively low doses used for prophylaxis of postpartum hemorrhage. However, caution is required in women who have received large doses of oxytocin for labour augmentation, especially when given with large volume electrolyte-free intravenous fluids or where another risk factor for fluid retention, such as preeclampsia, exists (Brucker 2001).

Intravenous bolus injections of 10 units of oxytocin have been shown to cause transient but profound hypotension due to peripheral vasodilatation in some women (Secher et al 1998). In normotensive women, this is followed by an increase in cardiac output, but in women with preexisting hypotension (such as in cases of postpartum hemorrhage), or with a known cardiac abnormality, cardiac arrest and maternal death has been reported (NICE 2001). The dose is 5 units as an intravenous bolus, 10 units intramuscularly or 20 units in 500 ml saline as an infusion.

- Oxytocin can be administered intravenously or intramuscularly, but not orally.
- The dose is 5 units as an intravenous bolus, 10 units intramuscularly or 20 units in 500 ml saline as an infusion.

Oxytocin is cheap, has significantly fewer side effects when compared to ergometrine and is the most stable injectable oxytocic drug, although refrigeration is still recommended for storage.

*Syntometrine®*: Syntometrine® combines five units of a synthetic oxytocin, Syntocinon®, and 500 mg of ergometrine. This combination is administered intramuscularly. As the oxytocin acts within 2–3 minutes and the ergometrine within 6–7 minutes, their combination results in a rapid uterine contraction enhanced by a stronger, more sustained contraction lasting several hours.

A number of trials have compared oxytocin to ergot alkaloids for the prevention of postpartum hemorrhage and have found no evidence of a difference in the incidence of hemorrhage with either drug. The use of oxytocin is associated with a trend toward less postpartum hemorrhage, and is less likely, than the ergots, to lead to a delay in placental delivery or to a rise in blood pressure. However, none of these differences reached statistical significance (Enkin et al 1995).

McDonald reviewed six studies in a meta-analysis for the Cochrane database comparing the effects of the use of oxytocin and Syntometrine®. The analysis showed that there was a significant reduction in the risk of postpartum hemorrhage, for 500–1000 ml of Syntometrine® when compared to 5 units of oxytocin (McDonald et al 2002). The advantage of Syntometrine® was smaller, but still significant when compared to those receiving 10 units of oxytocin (McDonald 2002). There was no difference seen between the groups for larger postpartum hemorrhage (1000 ml or more). No significant differences were seen for the need of blood transfusion or manual removal of the placenta. Based on recent studies, both the WHO and RCOG has recommended oxytocin for the routine prophylactic management of PPH (WHO 2007, RCOG Green top Guidelines 2009).

These results have to be taken in the context of the place of administration of drugs for prophylaxis against postpartum hemorrhage. In developing countries, where risks of undiagnosed preeclampsia and eclampsia are already high, and the availability of trained health professionals is low, the risks of hypertension as a side effect of an ergot-containing preparation may outweigh the small decrease in the amount of blood loss, making intramuscular oxytocin the preferred choice for third stage management (Elbourne et al 2002).

In developing countries intramuscular oxytocin may be the preferred choice for third stage management.

*Prostaglandins*: Prostaglandins have strong uterotonic properties, which are independent of gestational age. They encompass one branch of a large family of agents that are based on 20 carbon polyunsaturated fatty acids. After administration, prostaglandins cause a strong myometrial contraction by inducing calcium release from the myometrial cell, resulting in increased uterine tone. In addition to this direct effect on the myometrium, prostaglandins also increase oxytocin levels.

Prostaglandin preparations are available in oral, parenteral or local absorption form. Parenteral prostaglandins include $PGF_2\alpha$ and $PGE_2\alpha$ and in the tablet form of misoprostol (PGF1 analogue) which can be given orally or used locally. $PGF_2\alpha$ causes vasodilatation, increasing heart rate, systemic arterial blood pressure and cardiac output. Vomiting, abdominal pain and diarrhea are more common with intramuscular prostaglandins than with oral prostaglandins.

Parenteral $PGF_2\alpha$ (marketed as carboprost) is mainly used in the management of the third stage when intractable postpartum hemorrhage occurs and other measures fail. Experience of parenteral $PGF_2\alpha$ for routine use in the third stage is very limited. Available data suggest that intramuscular prostaglandins are more effective than injectable oxytocin and ergometrine in reducing the blood loss in the third stage of labour. However, concerns regarding safety, side effects and cost have limited the use of prostaglandins for routine prophylaxis in the third stage in low-risk women (Gülmezoglu 2002).

Misoprostol is inexpensive and can be administered orally, rectally or vaginally. It is stable at ambient temperatures. There is considerable experience with misoprostol use for peptic ulcer disease, and to a lesser degree, as a uterotonic in obstetrics and gynecology, although the latter use is unlicensed. Pharmacokinetic data on oral misoprostol has demonstrated that peak plasma levels occur 20–30 minutes after oral administration (Gülmezoglu 2002). Its main side effects are nausea, vomiting, diarrhea, shivering and elevated body temperature.

Oral misoprostol is more effective than placebo, but less effective than injectable oxytocin (Hofmeyr and Gulmezoglu 2008). Misoprostol 800 to 1000 micrograms has been found to be a good second line uterotonic when the PPH is refractory to oxytocin (Hofmeyr et al 2005).

Although the side effects were mainly nausea, vomiting, diarrhea, shivering and pyrexia, and have been described as not severe, they cause discomfort, may require the administration of antibiotics for suspected postpartum infections and also delay blood transfusions. The observed high rate of these side effects makes use of higher doses of misoprostol to improve its efficacy, undesirable among healthy women. It is therefore suggested that misoprostol should not replace oxytocin or ergometrine in the routine management of the third stage as it is less effective (Gülmezoglu 2002). After detailed analysis, FIGO and ICM (2006) have recommended the use of 600 micrograms of misoprostol orally for prophylaxis in low resource settings, where injectable oxytocins are not available.

- Misoprostol should not replace oxytocin or ergometrine in the routine management of the third stage as it is less effective
- 600 micrograms of oral misoprostol can be used in low resource settings, where injectable oxytocins are not available.

## Clamping of the Cord

Active management of the third stage of labour usually entails the clamping and dividing of the umbilical cord relatively early, before beginning controlled cord traction. The duration of the third stage is reduced by cord clamping (Enkin et al 1995). However, the time of the clamping in relationship to delivery does not appear to influence the rate of postpartum hemorrhage, although the numbers in available studies are small (Enkin 1995). Overall, the efficacy of this intervention can be questioned; however, as it is an integral step in the active management in most units, it is difficult to evaluate it as an individual intervention.

Early cord clamping reduces the amount of blood returning to the fetus; therefore, it results in lower hemoglobin values and hematocrits in the newborn. By 6 weeks after birth, these effects are only minimal and by 6 months, they are undetectable. This issue may be of importance when the baby is premature or asphyxiated, where early clamping is often carried out to allow early resuscitation of the baby by the pediatricians. A delay of clamping of as little as 30 seconds while holding the baby below the level of the placenta, may, therefore, be an advantage (Mercer 2001; Rabe and Reynolds 2002).

> A delay of clamping of as little as 30 seconds while holding the baby below the level of the placenta may be an advantage.

Early cord clamping results in lower neonatal bilirubin levels as a result of a lower hematocrit. The effect on the incidence of neonatal jaundice is unclear, however, and no detectable differences were noted in trials that reported on this (Mercer 2001).

As a larger proportion of blood remains in the placenta following early cord clamping, the likelihood of fetomaternal transfusion increases. Venous pressure is further increased as uterine retraction continues and may be sufficiently high to the rupture of surface placental vessels, thus facilitating transfer of fetal cells in the maternal circulation. This may be a critical factor when the mother's blood group is rhesus negative. Allowing time for fetal transfusion or free bleeding from the placental end of the cord in these women reduces the risk of feto-maternal transfusion and would be expected to reduce the incidence of rhesus isoimmunisation.

## Controlled Cord Traction

Following clinical signs of placental separation, delivery of the placenta is facilitated by controlled cord traction. Evidence of placental separation includes the fundus becoming more globular (rising), a small gush of blood loss per vagina and lengthening of the umbilical cord with uterine contractions.

The border of one hand is placed on the mother's abdomen below the level of the uterine fundus, suprapubically, and the other hand grasps the umbilical cord and applies steady traction posteriorly and downward, while the uterus is being held upward to prevent uterine inversion. Once the placenta and its membranes are delivered, the uterus can then be massaged to stimulate contractions, expel any small blood clots and prevent any further bleeding.

There have been two controlled trials in which controlled cord traction was compared to less active approaches, although one of the studies did include fundal pressure (Enkin et al 1995). They showed that controlled cord traction was associated with a lower mean blood loss and a shorter third stage. They did not, however, provide conclusive data about its effect on the incidence of postpartum hemorrhage or retained placenta. In one of the studies, there was a 3 per cent incidence of umbilical cord rupture.

## Active Versus Expectant Management in the Third Stage of Labour

Prendiville summarised the five major trials exploring active versus expectant management in the Cochrane database of systematic reviews, aiming to determine which line of management is most likely to prevent postpartum hemorrhage.

Routine active management was shown to be superior to expectant management in that there was a statistically significant reduction in the incidence of moderate hemorrhage of 500–1000 ml, severe hemorrhage of over 1000 ml, postpartum maternal hemoglobin of less than 9 g/dl, postnatal blood transfusion, the need for therapeutic oxytocics and the third stage lasting more than 20 minutes. Women were more satisfied with the third stage if they had active management. These findings were confirmed in general populations and also in women considered to be at low risk of third stage complications (Prendiville et al 2002).

However, active management also resulted in a statistically significant increase in the incidence of maternal diastolic blood pressure greater than 100 mmHg and maternal vomiting, nausea and headache postdelivery. There was some inconsistency in the results with regard to the need for manual removal of placenta and the incidence of secondary postpartum hemorrhage. In the Dublin trial, these complications were more common in the active management group (Begley 1990), but in the Bristol trial they were more common in the expectant management group (Prendiville et al 1988). The latest trial found no difference in the two groups (Rogers et al 1998). The overall meta-analysis showed that there was a tendency for the active management group to have higher incidence of these complications, but this did not reach statistical significance. The oxytocic used in the Dublin trial was intravenous ergometrine, whereas in the other trials they used intramuscular Syntometrine® and this may account for the observed difference in complications. There was no statistically significant difference in neonatal outcome or breastfeeding rates, and no difference in long-term maternal outcome.

> Active management of the third stage significantly reduces:
> - moderate hemorrhage (500–1000 ml)
> - severe hemorrhage (> 1000 ml)
> - postpartum maternal hemoglobin of < 9 g/dl
> - postnatal blood transfusion
> - the need for therapeutic oxytocics
> - the third stage lasting > 20 minutes

## Examination of the Placenta and the Membranes

The placenta should be examined soon after delivery so that if there is a doubt about its completeness, further action can be taken immediately, if necessary. The placenta should be laid on a flat surface. The maternal surface should be examined for any evidence of missing cotyledons. The completeness of the membranes is difficult

> The placenta should be laid on a flat surface and the maternal surface should be examined for any evidence of missing cotyledons.

to assess, but a careful examination will give some indication and retained membranes will usually be passed spontaneously. If it is certain that placental tissue is missing, then a vaginal examination is indicated, as fragments may be present there and if these are absent, exploration of the uterus should be considered. Expectant management may be undertaken in women who have not had excessive bleeding at delivery, are not actively bleeding, have a well-contracted uterus and who are being managed within an environment where observation can be provided.

The placental fetal surface should be inspected for any blood vessels that radiate beyond the placental edge into the membranes, with no corresponding placental tissue. These denote a possible succenturiate lobe, which may have been retained. The position of insertion of the cord is noted. This is usually central, but in a few cases it can be at the very edge of the placenta (battledore insertion of the cord). This is unimportant, unless the attachment is fragile. If the cord is inserted into the membranes at some distance from the edge of the placenta, it is called velamentous insertion of the cord. The umbilical vessels then run through the membranes from the cord to the placenta. If the placenta is normally situated, no harm will result to the fetus, but the cord is likely to become detached upon applying traction during active management of the third stage of labour. If the placenta is low lying, the vessels may pass across the cervical os. The term applied to these vessels is vasa previa. If these vessels tear, either at spontaneous rupture of membranes or at artificial rupture of membranes, it will lead to rapid exsanguination of the fetus.

Examination of the vessels of the cord should reveal one umbilical vein and two umbilical arteries. The absence of one artery may be associated with congenital abnormality, particularly of the renal and cardiovascular systems. The presence of a two-vessel cord may have been noted on an antenatal ultrasound scan. With the appropriate checks of renal and cardiac anatomy performed, all postnatal diagnoses should be communicated to a pediatrician so that postnatal checks can be organised. The cord length averages 50 cm and is still recorded in many units, although this information is of no value. In addition, the placental weight may be recorded. However, as outlined above, the weight will vary depending on the time of cord clamping. Delayed clamping produces a placenta weighing about a sixth of the baby's birth weight and early clamping results in the placenta weighing about a fifth of the baby's weight.

> Examination of the vessels of the cord should reveal one umbilical vein and two umbilical arteries. The absence of one artery may be associated with congenital abnormality of the renal and cardiovascular systems

Information derived from examination of the placenta may also provide good retrospective evidence of an intrauterine problem. Recent placental infarctions appear bright red, old infarctions form grey patches, whereas localised calcification can be seen as flattened white plaques, which feel gritty to touch. In twins, chorionicity can be established as well as vascular anastomoses. The need for formal histopathology of the placenta should be considered in all cases.

Depending on local resources, the measurement of paired umbilical artery and vein pH is recommended in all women and is mandatory in all cases of perinatal asphyxia, deliveries for suspected fetal distress and emergency operative delivery.

> Examination of the placenta can reveal:
> - recent placental infarctions (bright red)
> - old infarctions (grey patches)
> - localised calcification (flattened white plaques)
> - chorionicity and vascular anastomoses in twins

## Complications of the Third Stage

### Postpartum Hemorrhage

Primary postpartum hemorrhage denotes a blood loss of more than 500 ml in the first 24 hours postpartum. The care of a woman with postpartum hemorrhage depends on a rapid but careful assessment of the cause and prompt arrest of the bleeding. In the management of postpartum hemorrhage, drugs given for prophylaxis in the third stage should be remembered when prescribing further oxytocics.

### Retained Placenta

This diagnosis is made when the placenta remains undelivered after a specified period, usually 30 minutes to one hour following delivery of the baby. In rare cases, non-delivery of the placenta indicates a morbid adherence of the placenta with an absence of a plane of cleavage. Bleeding will only occur if there is partial separation.

> The diagnosis of retained placenta is made when the placenta remains undelivered after a period of 30 minutes to one hour following delivery of the baby.

Risk factors for a retained placenta include previous history of retained placenta, preterm delivery, multiparity, induced labour and small placenta (Adelusi et al 1997; Titiz et al 2001). Most cases of retained placenta are due to one of two problems:

1. The placenta has failed to separate, although a normal plane of cleavage exists. If this is complete there may be little bleeding, but if partial separation has occurred, heavy bleeding may occur. The uterus is often poorly contracted and an infusion of oxytocin may help to bring about placental separation and delivery.

2. The placenta has separated as normal, but has been trapped in the cervix prior to being expelled. The uterus will usually be well contracted and there will be little bleeding. However, the presence of 'retained products' in the uterus may result in uterine relaxation and hemorrhage. Oxytocin infusion may reduce the risk of bleeding, but will not help delivery of the placenta.

The conventional treatment for a retained placenta is to commence an oxytocin infusion and follow this by manual removal of the retained placenta under regional or general anesthesia. As there is a significant risk of hemorrhage, blood products should be available for the rapid treatment of hemorrhage.

The procedure is done with aseptic technique. The fundus of the uterus is grasped and stabilised with one hand, while the other hand is inserted in the vagina and then through the cervix. The palm of the hand is then introduced between the uterine wall and the placenta, using the fingers in a side-to-side motion. Once the whole of the placenta is separated, the entire placenta is grasped and removed. It is important to re-explore the (hopefully) empty uterus to ensure that no retained placental tissue or clots remain. When the uterine cavity is confirmed empty, an oxytocin infusion is commenced. Under no circumstances should instruments be used to remove the placenta, as this will increase the risk of causing uterine perforation. If the placenta cannot be removed digitally, the possibility of morbid adherence should be considered and the management will depend on the degree of bleeding. Prophylactic antibiotic (broadspectrum such as ampicillin and metronidazole) cover should be administered to reduce the risk of endometritis.

Waiting for 60 minutes before resorting to manual removal will reduce the number who will require manual removal. In the absence of bleeding, this is a more effective approach than embarking on manual removal too early.

Early evidence suggested that an injection of oxytocin into the umbilical vein of the attached placenta reduces the need for manual removal. However, when required, manual removal following oxytocin may be more difficult than usual because of a firmly contracted uterus (Carroli and Bergel 2002). The same procedure with saline suggested reduced need for manual removal (Carroli and Bergel 2002). The 'RELEASE' trial, a randomised controlled study, has shown that this technique is not effective (Weeks et al 2010). It is possible that intraumbilical vein injection of prostaglandins may be an effective method for management of a retained placenta and further research in this area has been recommended (Carroli and Bergel 2002). Another alternative that is being studied is the use of larger volumes and different oxytocics (Rogers et al 2007).

Eight hundred micrograms of misoprostol rectally have been proposed as an effective alternative to the treatment of a retained placenta (Li et al 2001). Side effects include nausea, vomiting, shivering, diarrhea and pelvic cramping pain.

## Placenta Accreta

Placenta accreta is an abnormal adherence, either in whole or in part, of the placenta to the underlying uterine wall. Placenta increta occurs when the placenta invades deeply into the myometrium and placenta percreta implies penetration to the uterine serosa.

- Placenta accreta: abnormal adherence to the underlying uterine wall
- Placenta increta: deep invasion into the myometrium
- Placenta percreta: penetration to the uterine serosa.

They arise because implantation of the ovum occurred in an area of the uterus in which the endometrium was deficient or damaged, possibly due to previous scarring (from previous curettage, infection, uterine scar) or congenital anomaly. About 50 per cent of placenta accretas occur in cases of placenta previa. This is believed to be due to the inadequacy of the decidua in the lower segment.

Placenta accreta is diagnosed when difficulty is encountered during delivery of the placenta at manual removal or during cesarean section. Effective treatment, if there is significant hemorrhage, will require hysterectomy, but more conservative treatment like oxytocin, oversewing the implantation site or surgical placental excision may be successful in carefully selected women who are hemodynamically stable and desire more children (Riggs et al 2000).

Ultrasound may aid the diagnosis of placenta accreta in clinically suspected cases, especially when the placenta overlies a previous uterine scar. The ultrasound characteristics of placenta accreta include the loss of decidual hyperechoic zones, marked thinning of the placental-site wall, invasion of the placenta in the myometrium and in cases of low anterior placenta percreta, the disruption of hypoechoic uterine serosa–bladder interface (Panoskaltsis et al 2000; Herman 2000). Colour Doppler can be used to demonstrate persistent blood flow between the basal placenta and the myometrium and to highlight the extent of myometrial invasion. Magnetic resonance imaging (MRI) also provides information regarding the extent of placental invasion, especially in cases of posterior high placentation. In a prospective study of 19 women at risk of placenta accreta, the sensitivity and specificity of ultrasound was 86 per cent and 92 per cent, respectively, for the diagnosis. The sensitivity increased to 100 per cent by the addition of MRI. In cases with a posterior placental site (previa or not), MRI appeared to provide a more confident diagnosis (Levine et al 1997).

> The ultrasound characteristics of placenta accreta include:
> - loss of decidual hyperechoic zones
> - thinning of the placental-site wall
> - invasion of the placenta in the myometrium
> - disruption of hypoechoic uterine serosa–bladder in cases of low anterior placenta percreta

There have been several reports of conservative management of placenta accreta with methotrexate (Panoskaltis et al 2000; Mussalli et al 2000; Legro et al 1994; Arulkumaran et al 1986). The benefits are the avoidance of major surgery, such as cesarean, hysterectomy with the consequent morbidity, as well as preservation of future fertility. The treatment uses intravenous, intramuscular or oral methotrexate and folinic acid, but there was no agreement on a standardised protocol of methotrexate administration. All women require close follow-up with regular hematological investigations to avoid an immunosuppressive toxic reaction and ultrasound scan to look at placental regression. This method has been described, both for placenta accreta diagnosed at cesarean section (when the uterus is closed leaving the placenta in situ) and at manual removal when the cord should be ligated as high as possible with an absorbable suture (Mussalli et al 2000). Antibiotic therapy is recommended and the woman and her carers must be aware of the risk of secondary postpartum hemorrhage during conservative treatment. A second surgical procedure may be required to remove the placenta after the initial methotrexate treatment (Mussalli et al 2000).

## Uterine Inversion

This is a rare but serious complication. It may occur as a result of excessive cord traction in the presence of a relaxed uterus, over-vigorous fundal pressure, or exceptionally high intraabdominal pressure as result of coughing or vomiting. It can present with pain, hemorrhage or shock. Prompt recognition and treatment is the key to a good outcome. Options for treatment include manual or hydrostatic replacement or laparotomy and 'repair from above'. Use of a tocolytic may assist in reduction of the uterus (Baskett and Arulkumaran 2002).

## Conclusion

Active management of the third stage of labour with prophylactic oxytocic drugs and cord traction has reduced the incidence of serious complications following delivery. Some complications such as retained placenta and uterine inversion may increase as a result of active management. Careful implementation of active management policy is necessary to ensure that the risk of these complications is low, and hence, acceptable in the context of prevention of postpartum hemorrhage.

## References

Adelusi B, Soltan MH, Chowdhury N, Kangave D. 1997. Risk of retained placenta:multivariate approach. *Acta Obstet Gynecol Scand* 76(5):414–18.

Arulkumaran S, Ng CSA, Ingermarsson I, Ratnam SS. 1986. Medical treatment of placenta accreta with methotrexate. *Acta Obstet Gynecol Scand* 65:285–86.

Adamson P, 1996. A failure of imagination. In *Progress of Nations*, 2–9. UNICEF.

Baskett T, Arulkumaran S. 2002. Postpartum haemorrhage In *Intrapartum care*, 145–60. London: RCOG Press.

Begley CM. 1990. A comparison of 'active' and 'physiological' management of the third stage of labour. *Midwifery* 6:3–17.

Brucker MC. 2001. Management of the third stage of labor: An evidence-based approach. *J Midwifery Wom Health* 46(6):381–92.

Carroli G, Bergel E. 2002. Umbilical vein injection for management of retained placenta (Cochrane Review). In *The Cochrane Library*, Issue 3, Oxford: Update Software.

De Groot AN. 1995. Prevention of postpartum haemorrhage. *Bailliere's Clin Obstet Gynaecol* 9(3):619–31.

De Groot AN. 1996. The role of oral (methyl) ergometrine in the prevention of postpartum haemorrhage. *Eur J Obstet Gynecol Reprod Biol* 69(1):31–36.

National Institiute for Clinical Excellence (NICE). 2001. *The Confidential Enquiries into Maternal Deaths in the United Kingdom: Why Mothers Die 1997–1999*. London: Department of Health.

Elbourne DR, Prendiville WJ, Carroli G, Wood J, McDonald S. 2002. Prophylactic use of oxytocin in the third stage of labour (Cochrane Review). In *The Cochrane Library*, Issue 3. Oxford: Update Software.

Enkin M, Keirse MJNC, Renfew M, Neilson J. 1995. *A guide to effective care in pregnancy and childbirth*. 2nd ed. Oxford: Oxford University Press.

Gülmezoglu AM, Forna F, Villar J, Hofmeyr GJ. 2002. Prostaglandins for prevention of postpartum haemorrhage (Cochrane Review). In *The Cochrane Library*, Issue 3, Oxford: Update Software.

Herman A. 2000. Complicated third stage of labor: Time to switch to the scanner. *Ultrasound Obstet Gynaecol* 15:89–95.

Hofmeyr GJ, Gulmezoglu AM. 2008, Misoprostol for the prevention and treatment of postpartum haemorrhage. *Best Pract Res Clin Obstet Gynecol* 22:1025–1041

Hofmeyr GJ, Walraven G, Gulmezoglu AM, Maholwana B, Alfirevic Z, Villar J. 2005.: Misoprostol to treat postpartum haemorrhage: a systematic review. *Br J Obstet Gynecol.* 112:547–553

ICM and FIGO 2006. Joint statement: active management of third stage of labour in low resource settings – www.figo.org

Legro RS, Price FV, Hill LM, Caritis SN. 1994. Nonsurgical management of placenta percreta: A case report. *Obstet Gynaecol.* 83(5 Pt 2):847–49.

Levine D, Hulka CA, Ludmir J, Li W, Edelman PR. 1997. Placenta accreta: Evaluation with color Doppler US, power Doppler US, MR imaging. *Radiol* 205:773–76.

Li Y T, Yin CS, Chen FM. 2001. Rectal administration of misoprostol for the management of retained placenta – A preliminary report. *Chin Med J* 64(12):721–24.

McDonald S, Prendiville WJ, Elbourne D. 2002. Prophylactic syntometrine versus oxytocin for delivery of the placenta (Cochrane Review). In *The Cochrane Library*, Issue 3. Oxford: Update Software

Mercer JS. 2001. Current best evidence: a review of the literature on umbilical cord clamping. *J Midwifery Women's Health* 46(6):402–14.

Mussalli GM, Shah J, Berck DJ, Elimian A, Tejani N, FA Manning. 2000. Placenta accreta and methotrexate therapy: Three case reports. *J Perinat* 20(5):331–34.

Panoskaltsis TA, Ascarelli A, De Souza N, Sims CD, Edmonds KD. 2000. Placenta increta: evaluation of radiological investigations and therapeutic options of conservative management. *Br J Obstet Gynaecol* 107:802–806.

Prendiville WJ, Elbourne D, McDonald S. 2002. Active versus expectant management in the third stage of labour (Cochrane Review). In *The Cochrane Library*, Issue 3, Oxford: Update Software.

Prendiville WJ, Harding JE, Elbourne DR, Stirrat GM. 1988. The Bristol third stage trial: Active vs physiological management of the third stage of labour. *BMJ* 297:1295–1300.

Rabe H, Reynolds G. 2002. Delayed cord clamping in preterm infants (Protocol for a Cochrane Review) In *The Cochrane Library*, Issue 3. Oxford: Update Software.

Riggs JC, Jahshan A, Schiavello HJ. 2000. Alternative conservative management of placenta accreta. A case report. *J Reprod Med.* 45(7):595–98.

Rogers J, Wood J, McCandlish R, Ayers S, Truesdale A, Elbourne D. 1998. Active vs expectant management of the third stage of labour: the Hinchingbrooke randomised controlled trial. *Lancet* 351:693–99.

Rogers MS, Yuen PM, Wong S. 2007. Avoiding manual removal of the placenta: evaluation of intra-umbilical injection of uterotonics using the Pipingas technique for management of adherent placenta. *Acta Obstet Gynecol Scand* 86:48–51.

Royal College of Obstetricians and Gynaecologists. 2009. Green-Top Guidelines 52 – Prevention and management of postpartum haemorrhage www.rcog.org.uk

Secher NJ, Arnsbo P, Wallin L. 1998. Haemodynamic effects of oxytocin (syntocinon) and methyl ergometrine (methergin) on the systemic and pulmonary circulations of pregnant anaesthetized women. *Acta Obstet Gynecol* 105:353–36.

Titiz H, Wallace A, Voaklander DC. 2001. Manual removal of the placenta: A case control study. *Aust NZ J Obstet Gynaecol* 41(1):41–44.

Weeks AD, Alia G, Vernon G et al. 2010. Umbilical vein oxytocin for the treatment of retained placenta (RELEASE Study): a double-blind, randomised controlled trial. *Lancet* 375;141–147.

WHO. 1990. *WHO Report of technical working group – The prevention and management of postpartum haemorrhage.* Geneva: World Health Organization. www.who.int

WHO. 2007. *Recommendations for the prevention of postpartum haemorrhage.* www.who.int

# CHAPTER 19

# MANAGEMENT OF POSTPARTUM HEMORRHAGE

*Gita Arjun, S Rajasri, Soumya Balakrishnan and Vinotha Thomas*

The risk of maternal death from childbirth represents one of the greatest inequities in global health. According to a report by the World Health Organization (WHO), women in developing countries are more than 40 times more likely than women in developed countries to die in childbirth. This translates to 1 in 61 women in developing countries versus 1 in 2800 women in developed countries (WHO 2000). Even within developing countries, the risk of maternal death differs for women who have access to basic essential obstetrical care compared to those who do not. Poverty contributes significantly to the risk, and poorer nations, therefore, have an increased rate of maternal death.

Obstetric hemorrhage is the world's leading cause of maternal mortality, causing 24 per cent of maternal deaths annually (an estimated 127,000). Postpartum hemorrhage (PPH) is the most common type of obstetric hemorrhage and accounts for the majority of the 14 million cases of obstetric hemorrhage that occur each year (WHO 2004).

> Obstetric hemorrhage is the world's leading cause of maternal mortality and postpartum hemorrhage accounts for the majority of deaths.

In developed countries, PPH has become largely preventable and manageable. However, in developing countries, mortality from PPH continues to remain high. While data are limited, studies have shown that PPH causes up to 60 per cent of all maternal deaths in developing countries.

Women who survive severe postpartum hemorrhage experience significant morbidity, including problems caused by blood products, intensive care admission, further surgical interventions, infection and prolonged hospitalisation (Zelop 2011).

## Definition

Traditional teaching defines primary postpartum hemorrhage as the loss of 500 ml or more of blood from the genital tract within 24 hours of the birth of a baby, with severe PPH occurring with a blood loss of 1000 ml or more (Mousa and Alfirevic 2007). However, an average of 1000 ml of blood is lost at cesarean section. Moreover, estimates of blood loss at delivery are quite often inaccurate, with significant underreporting being the rule.

Chesley (1972) estimated that over the course of pregnancy, the plasma volume increases by approximately 40 per cent and the red cell mass increases by approximately 25 per cent. This should usually compensate for the blood loss that will occur at delivery. Unfortunately, in developing countries, pre-existing anemia may make the woman more susceptible to hemodynamic changes with even the usual amount of blood loss.

Clinically, postpartum hemorrhage can be defined as any amount of blood loss that results in hemodynamic instability. The American College of Obstetricians and Gynecologists defines PPH as blood loss which decreases the hematocrit by 10 per cent or necessitates transfusion (ACOG 2006)

> PPH is best defined as blood loss that results in hemodynamic instability and necessitates transfusion.

PPH is classified as *primary PPH*, which occurs within the first 24 hours postpartum, and *secondary PPH* which occurs between 24 hours and up to six weeks postpartum (Kominiarek and Kilpatrick 2007).

## Causes of Postpartum Hemorrhage

*Primary postpartum hemorrhage* is commonly due to abnormalities of one or more of the following processes (Anderson and Etches 2008):

*Tone*:
- a non-contracting, atonic uterus is the commonest cause

*Tissue*:
- retained products of conception
- adherent placenta

*Trauma*:
- genital tract lacerations and hematomas
- uterine rupture (rare)
- uterine inversion (rare)

*Thrombin*:
- coagulation defects/abnormalities (rare)

Investigators have tried to identify risk factors for the occurrence of primary PPH. However, primary PPH may occur unpredictably in women who have no apparent risk factor.

Risk factors for primary PPH include first pregnancy, maternal obesity, a large baby, twin pregnancy, prolonged or augmented labour, and antepartum hemorrhage (Mousa and Alfirevic 2007). High multiparity does not appear to be a risk factor, either in high- or low-income countries, even after control for maternal age (Drife 1997; Stones et al 1993).

> Risk factors for primary PPH:
> - first pregnancy
> - maternal obesity
> - a large baby
> - twin pregnancy
> - prolonged or augmented labour
> - antepartum hemorrhage

Although the majority of postpartum hemorrhage is due to uterine atony, the rising incidence of cesarean delivery is leading to an increase in PPH due to retained placenta, secondary to abnormally adherent placenta (Silver et al 2006).

*Secondary postpartum hemorrhage* is commonly due to the following causes (Alexander et al 2002):

### Abnormalities of placentation

- Subinvolution of the placental site
- Retained products of conception

- Placenta accreta
- Infection
- Endometritis, myometritis, parametritis
- Infection/dehiscence of cesarean scar

## Initial Evaluation of PPH

An atonic uterus is the commonest cause of PPH. To confirm the presence of uterine atony, the bladder should be emptied and a bimanual pelvic examination should be performed. The uterus will be soft and feels 'boggy'. Compression or massage of the uterus can reduce the bleeding, help in expulsion of blood clots, and allow time for other procedures to be initiated.

In spite of these measures, if bleeding persists, other etiologies, besides atony, must be considered. Even in the presence of uterine atony, other contributing factors may play a role in PPH.

The placenta should be inspected again for missing bits. The uterine cavity must be carefully assessed to rule out retained placental bits or membranes.

The patient must be positioned for proper visualisation of the cervix and vagina. Good lighting and proper instruments must be utilised to carefully assess the lower genital tract.

An obstetric unit should establish a protocol which should be followed by everybody in such a situation. A speculum may be used for better visualisation. Using a folded gauze in a sponge-holding forceps to push up the cervix, the vaginal walls should be carefully inspected, all the way up to the fornices. The cervix should be held with two sponge-holding forceps and the entire circumference visualised to rule out tears. Sometimes the patient may need to be moved to a well-equipped operating room and adequate anesthesia may be necessary for the identification and proper repair of lacerations.

- Every obstetric unit should establish a protocol for the evaluation and management of PPH
- A drill should be held regularly to prepare the staff to deal with PPH

## Atonic Postpartum Hemorrhage

Atonic PPH is the most common cause of PPH and the leading cause of maternal death. Myometrial contraction is responsible for placental separation and constriction of the blood vessels that supply the placental bed. In uterine atony, the myometrium remains flabby, and hence, the blood vessels are not obliterated. This results in bleeding.

### Risk factors

Although there are known risk factors that may lead to atonic PPH (Table 19.1), PPH is not always a predictable event. Women at high risk should be identified, so that appropriate measures can be taken during labour. However, only 40 per cent of women with PPH with vaginal birth have an identifiable risk factor (Combs et al 1991). Similarly, Rouse and colleagues (2006) found that half the women who had atonic PPH after a primary cesarean section had no risk factors.

**Table 19.1  Risk factors for atonic PPH**

**Antepartum risk factors**
Over-distended uterus (hydramnios, twins, macrosomia)
Previous PPH
Placenta previa
Asian ethnicity
Obesity (BMI >35)
Anemia (<9g/dl)
Uterine abnormalities/ fibroids

**Intrapartum risk factors**
Prolonged labour
Prolonged use of oxytocin
Precipitate labour
Retained placental tissue
Halogenated anesthetics

## Prevention

Prevention of PPH includes antenatal risk assessment and their management e.g. correction of anemia. Prendiville and colleagues (2000), in a systematic review of the Cochrane database found that active management of the third stage of labour resulted in lower maternal blood loss and with reduced risks of PPH and prolonged third stage.

The WHO held a Technical Consultation on the Prevention of Postpartum Hemorrhage (Mathai and Gulmezoglu 2007) and recommended that:

❖ Active management of the third stage of labour should include administration of a uterotonic soon after the birth of the baby, delayed cord clamping and delivery of the placenta by controlled cord traction, followed by uterine massage.

❖ Skilled attendants should offer active management of the third stage of labour, as potential risk such as uterine inversion, might result from inappropriate cord traction.

❖ Oxytocin (10 IU IM) should be offered for prevention of PPH in preference to ergometrine/methylergometrine or oral, sublingual, and rectal misoprostol. If oxytocin is not available, ergometrine/methylergometrine can be used for women without hypertension or heart disease.

❖ Injectable prostaglandins (carboprost/sulprostone) should not be used for prevention of PPH in preference to oxytocin.

❖ In the absence of active management of the third stage of labour, a uterotonic drug (oxytocin or misoprostol) should be offered.

The active management of the third stage of labour results in fewer maternal deaths, fewer admissions to an intensive care unit, less blood loss, less use of blood transfusion, less use of additional uterotonics, less postpartum anemia, earlier establishment of breastfeeding and less anemia in infancy.

## Management

The two important steps to be implemented immediately are to call for help, and simultaneously, start the steps of resuscitation. Monitoring of the patient should be done concomitantly with investigation of cause and measures to arrest the bleeding.

- Call for help
- Initiate steps of resuscitation immediately

Extra personnel must be roped in for help and the anesthetist, hematologist and blood bank staff should be alerted.

At all times, the patient must be reassured and all procedures being carried out should be explained to her. As a patient goes into shock, her anxieties increase exponentially and these must be addressed constantly. A member of the team (if it is possible to spare him/her) should be assigned to specifically keep the patient calm and to explain all that is going on with her.

> The patient should be reassured at all times and the procedures being carried out should be explained to her.

## Resuscitation

The urgency and measures undertaken to resuscitate the patient depends on the amount of blood loss and the presence or absence of shock. When the blood loss is between 500–1000 ml, and there are no clinical signs of shock, PPH is considered to be *minor*. When the blood loss is more than 1000 ml and the patient is continuing to bleed or when there are clinical signs of shock, it is considered to be *major* PPH. Clinical signs of shock include tachycardia, hypotension, tachypnea, oliguria or delayed peripheral capillary filling.

> Minor PPH: Blood loss of 500–1000 ml
> Major PPH: Blood loss > 1000 ml with clinical signs of shock

The following guidelines are recommended by the RCOG Greentop Guidelines Number 52 (2009).

### Resuscitation measures in minor PPH:

- Establish intravenous access with a large bore (16–18 gauge) cannula.
- Initiate infusion with crystalloid solution (0.9% normal saline or lactated Ringer's solution)

### Resuscitation measures in major PPH:

Restoration of both blood volume and oxygen-carrying capacity are vital in this situation.

- Compromise of airway and breathing must be assessed and corrected
- Blood pressure and pulse rate must be monitored continuously
- Oxygen may be administered by mask at 10–15 liters/minute
- Establish intravenous access with a large bore (16–18 gauge) cannula. Another line must be started on the opposite arm.
- The head end of the table may be flat – do not prop up the head
- The patient may be kept warm with blankets
- Transfuse blood as soon as possible. Blood is preferably warmed before transfusing. If special equipment is not available to do this, the blood bag may be placed in a warm water bath to raise its temperature
- Until blood is available, infuse up to 3.5 litres of crystalloids and/or colloid as rapidly as required. Isotonic crystalloids should be used in preference to colloids which are more expensive and may cause adverse effects
- Replacement with coagulation factors and platelets may be necessary

Table 19.2 lists blood components, indications for transfusions and hematological effects.

Table 19.2  Blood component therapy (ACOG 2006)

| Product | Volume (ml) | Contents | Effect (per unit) | Indication |
|---|---|---|---|---|
| Packed red cells | 240 | RBC, WBC, plasma | Increases HcT By 3%, Hb by 1g/dl | Anemia |
| Platelets | 50 | Platelets, RBC, WBC and plasma | Increases platelet count 5,000–10,000/mm³ per unit | If platelet count <50 × 10⁹/L |
| Fresh frozen plasma | 250 | Fibrinogen, anti thrombin III, factors V and VIII | Increases fibrinogen by 10 mg/dl | 4 units for every 6 units of red cells/ or aPTT PT >1.5x normal |
| Cryo-precipitate | 40 | Fibrinogen, factors VIII and XIII, von Willebrand factor | Increases fibrinogen by 10 mg/dl | If fibrinogen <1g/L |

The therapeutic goals of management of massive blood loss are to maintain:

* Hemoglobin > 8g/dl
* Platelet count > 75x10⁹/l
* Prothrombin < 1.5 x mean control
* Activated prothrombin time < 1.5x mean control
* Fibrinogen > 1g/L

## Investigation and Monitoring

### Minor PPH

* Pulse and blood pressure recording every 15 minutes
* Complete blood count
* Coagulation screen including fibrinogen

*Clot observation test* provides a simple measure of fibrinogen: 5 ml of the patient's blood is placed into a clean, test tube and observed frequently. Normally, blood will clot within 8–10 minutes and the clot will remain intact even when shaken. If fibrinogen is less than 150 mg/dl, the blood in the tube will not clot, or if it does, it will undergo partial or complete dissolution in 30–60 minutes

### Major PPH

* Continuous pulse, blood pressure recording and respiratory rate
* Cross-match blood (4 units minimum)
* Full blood count, coagulation screen including fibrinogen, baseline renal and liver function tests
* Monitor temperature
* Foley catheter to monitor urine output
* Consider arterial line monitoring
* Documentation of fluid balance, blood, blood products and procedures

Fluid replacement and the use of blood and blood products should be strictly monitored and the amount given should be dictated by the clinician leading the resuscitation measures. The full blood count will include estimation of hematocrit and platelet count. The clotting screen should include prothrombin time, thrombin time, partial thromboplastin time and fibrinogen assay.

## Arresting the Bleeding

Mechanical and pharmacological measures should be instituted in turn, until the bleeding stops. If pharmacological measures fail, surgical measures should be initiated sooner rather than later. Uterine tamponade is considered as first line surgical intervention. If this fails to stop bleeding, conservative surgical interventions may be attempted, depending on clinical circumstances and available expertise.

## Mechanical measures

Massaging the fundus, bimanual uterine compression and emptying the bladder to stimulate uterine contraction form the first line management of PPH. Bimanual uterine compression is a simple, and usually effective, method to control bleeding from uterine atony. A hand on the abdomen massages the posterior aspect of the uterus while the fist of the other hand is in the vagina pushing against the anterior aspect of the uterus (Fig 19.1).

## Pharmacological measures

In the management of PPH, oxytocin should always be offered as the first line of treatment and should be preferred over ergometrine alone, oxytocin–ergometrine combination, and prostaglandins. If the bleeding does not respond to oxytocin, ergometrine or oxytocin–ergometrine combination should be offered as second line treatment. If bleeding continues despite these measures, injectable prostaglandin should be offered as the third line of treatment. In the absence of injectable uterotonics, 1000 mcg of rectal misoprostol may be considered, because of its ease of administration and its low cost (Table 19.3).

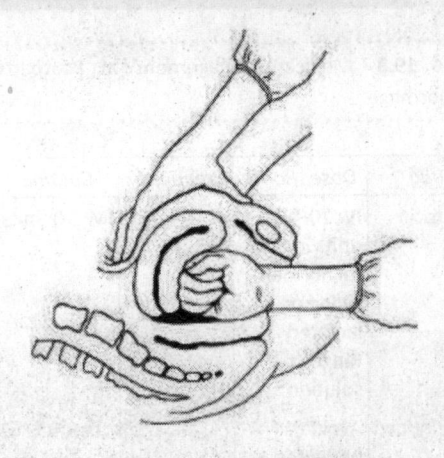

**Figure 19.1** Bimanual compression

## Tamponade techniques

Tamponade of the uterus can be tried when uterotonics fail to control bleeding. If prompt response is not seen, preparations should be made for exploratory laparotomy. Though uterine packing with gauze had fallen from favour due to the fear of concealed hemorrhage, it seems to be making a limited comeback. It is particularly useful in controlling hemorrhage from uterine atony and placental site bleeding caused by placenta previa or placenta accreta (Maier 1993;

> Uterine tamponade is particularly useful in controlling hemorrhage from uterine atony and placental site bleeding caused by placenta previa or placenta accreta

**Table 19.3** Medical Management of Postpartum Hemorrhage

| Drug* | Dose/Route | Frequency | Comment |
|---|---|---|---|
| Oxytocin | IV: 10–40 units in 500 ml normal saline or lactated Ringer's solution | | IM: 10 units |
| Continuous | Avoid undiluted rapid IV infusion, which causes hypotension. | | |
| Methyl-ergonovine | IM: 0.2 mg | Every 2–4 h | Avoid if patient is hypertensive or has cardiac disease. |
| 15-methyl PGF$_2\alpha$ | IM: 0.25 mg | Every 15–90 min, 8 doses maximum | Avoid in asthmatic patients; relative contraindication if hepatic, renal, and cardiac disease. Diarrhea, fever, tachycardia can occur. |
| Misoprostol (PGE$_1$) | 800–1,000 mcg rectally | | |

Abbreviations: IV, intravenously; IM, intramuscularly; PG, prostaglandin.
*All agents can cause nausea and vomiting.

Adapted from: Dildy GA, Clark SL. 1993. Postpartum hemorrhage. Contemp Ob/Gyn. 38(8):21–9.

Hsu et al 2003)). Uterovaginal packing may be used to gain time to stabilise the patient while arranging for a surgical procedure. A 4-inch gauze is layered tightly from side to side in the uterine cavity.

Foley catheters have been advocated for creating a tamponade in atonic PPH. 24 F Foley catheters with a 30 ml bulb can be stocked in the labour room for such emergencies. The tip is guided into the uterine cavity and inflated with 60–80 ml of saline. Additional Foley catheters can be inserted, if necessary, until bleeding stops. However, this method has not found favour with many obstetricians, since the Foley balloon is too small to be effective in the flabby, atonic uterine cavity.

Coundous and colleagues (2003) have described the 'tamponade test' to decide on surgical intervention for massive PPH. A Sengstaken-Blakemore esophageal catheter is inserted into the uterus and inflated. If bleeding continues despite insertion with a Sengstaken-Blakemore esophageal catheter, it is considered an indication for surgical intervention. The Bakri balloon catheter has also been described for tamponade in atonic PPH. The Bakri tamponade-balloon is made of silicone and has a ductile shape which allows it to conform to the uterine anatomy (Bakri 2001).

## Surgical techniques for uterine atony

### Uterine artery and internal iliac artery ligation

When all the above techniques have failed, surgical intervention may be life saving. It is important not to postpone surgical intervention till the patient is morbidly ill.

# Management of Postpartum Hemorrhage

The O'Leary technique involves devascularising the post-cesarean section uterus with bilateral mass ligation of the ascending branches of the uterine arteries and veins (O'Leary 1995). Though uterine artery ligation and internal iliac artery ligation have been described, the procedures are technically difficult and time consuming in an already sick patient. The failure rate is also high and hysterectomy may have to be resorted to. Joshi and colleagues (2007) reported hysterectomy in a third of the patients who had internal iliac artery ligation for atonic PPH.

> Uterine artery ligation and internal iliac artery ligation are technically difficult and time consuming in an already sick patient. The failure rate is also high and hysterectomy may have to be resorted to.

## Uterine compression sutures

### B-Lynch suture and modifications

The B-Lynch suture, also known as the 'brace suture', was described by B-Lynch and co-workers in 1997, as an alternative surgical method for controlling PPH due to uterine atony. At the end of the procedure, the sutures have the appearance of suspenders or braces, hence the name. The sutures compress the anterior and posterior atonic walls of the uterus, achieving hemostasis. This technique is simple and safe, life saving and preserves fertility. It is a revolutionary surgical intervention.

> The B-Lynch compression suture is simple and safe, life saving and preserves fertility.

### Materials:

* 70 mm round body needle or straight needle
* No.2 chromic catgut

Technique (Fig 19.2)

1. The patient, under general anesthesia, is catheterised and placed in the lithotomy position, to allow objective assessment vaginally of the control of bleeding.
2. The abdomen is opened by a low transverse incision if the patient has had a vaginal delivery, and if following a cesarean section, the same incision is reopened.
3. The uterovesical fold of the peritoneum is incised transversely and the bladder pushed down gently.
4. A lower segment incision is made or sutures of a recent cesarean section are removed and the uterine cavity is examined and swabbed out.

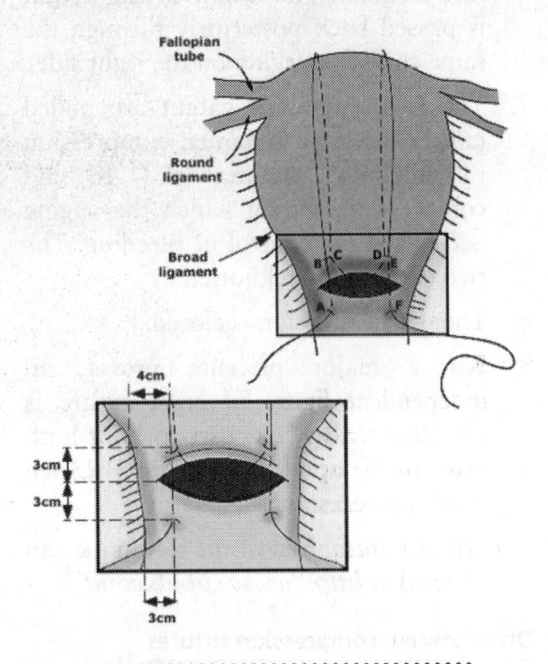

**Figure 19.2** The B-Lynch uterine compression suture technique

5. The uterus is exteriorized and rechecked to identify any bleeding points. A bimanual compression is first tried to assess the potential chance of success of the technique.
6. The uterus is punctured 3 cm from the right lower edge of the uterine incision and 3 cm from the right lateral border. The catgut is rethreaded through the uterine cavity to emerge at the upper incision margin, 3 cm above and 4 cm from the lateral border, and is passed over to compress the uterine fundus approximately 3–4 cm from the right cornual border. The catgut is fed posteriorly and vertically to enter the posterior wall of the uterine cavity at the same level as the upper anterior entry point. The suture is pulled under moderate tension by bimanual compression exerted by the first assistant. The length of the catgut is passed back posteriorly through the same surface marking on the right side.
7. The two lengths of catgut are pulled taut, assisted by bimanual compression to minimise trauma and to aid compression, during which the vagina is checked for control of bleeding. The two ends are then knotted.
8. The uterine incision is closed.
9. For a major placenta previa, an independent figure of eight suture is placed anteriorly or posteriorly or both prior to the application of the B-Lynch suture, if necessary.

Further information of the technique can be obtained at *http://www.cbl.uk.com/*

### Other uterine compression sutures

There have been multiple modifications and simplifications of this technique. Kayem and colleagues (2011) performed a population-based study in the United Kingdom that evaluated the effectiveness of uterine compression suture placement used to manage postpartum hemorrhage. The commonest suture used (37 per cent) was the B-Lynch technique.

Several other modifications of uterine compression sutures have been described (Cho et al 2000; Malibary 2000; Hayman et al 2002; Bhal et al 2005; Nelson and Birch 2006). Failure to preserve the uterus, suture erosion, and partial and total uterine necrosis have been reported after uterine compression sutures (Grotegut et al 2004; Joshi and Shrivastava 2004). Cho's square suture has been associated with pyometria, synechia and Asherman's syndrome (Ochoa et al 2002; Wu and Yeh 2005).

## Uterine artery embolisation

A hemodynamically stable patient with persistent bleeding, especially if the rate of loss is not excessive, is a suitable candidate for arterial embolisation. Reported primary success rate (i.e. rate of success of the first embolisation) for this uterine atony ranges from 73 per cent to 100 per cent (Chaleur et al 2008). Radiographic identification and percutaneous trans-catheter arterial embolisation of uterine artery with gel foam, coils, or glue can be done in institutions where facilities exist. Balloon occlusion is also a technique used in such circumstances. Embolisation can be used for bleeding that continues after hysterectomy or can be used as an alternative to hysterectomy to preserve fertility (Saloman et al 2003). The technique requires significant resources in terms of cost of treatment, facilities and training.

## Hysterectomy

Hysterectomy is reserved for the situation where all other measures available have been tried and failed, where bleeding continues with a severely shocked patient and in cases of coagulopathy, where no replacement blood products are available. In most instances, a subtotal hysterectomy, which is quicker, simpler, safer and associated with less blood loss, is adequate.

Kayem et al (2011) showed that vaginal delivery and a delay between delivery and uterine suture placement of 2 to 6 hours were significantly associated with an increased risk of hysterectomy. It is understandable that the clinician may be reluctant to proceed with laparotomy after vaginal delivery. However, a prolonged delay may predispose patients to unrecognised blood loss, thereby further increasing the risk of compression suture failure. If mechanical tamponade techniques are not successful within a reasonable time period, the clinician should proceed with laparotomy and uterine compression suture placement. Delay in making this decision may result in a hysterectomy.

## PPH due to retained placenta and placenta accreta

Retained placenta affects 0.6 per cent to 3.3 per cent of normal deliveries. There is no consensus as to the length of the third stage beyond which a placenta should be called retained. The risk of hemorrhage rises after 30 minutes have elapsed and the possibility of spontaneous delivery rate after 60 minutes is non-existent.

Intraumbilical vein injection of oxytocin with saline may be offered for the management of retained placenta. If in spite of controlled cord traction, administration of uterotonics and intraumbilical vein injection of oxytocin and saline, the placenta is not delivered, manual extraction of the placenta should be offered as the definitive treatment.

Placenta accreta and uterine atony are the two most common reasons for postpartum hysterectomy (Combs et al 1991; Mousa and Alfirevic 2007). Risk factors for placenta accreta include placenta previa, with or without previous uterine surgery, prior myomectomy, prior cesarean delivery, Asherman's syndrome, submucous leiomyomata, and maternal age older than 35 years (Mousa and Alfirevic 2007). Ultrasonography may be helpful in establishing the diagnosis in the antepartum period. Colour Doppler technology may be an additional adjunctive tool for suspected accreta. Despite advances in imaging techniques, no diagnostic technique affords the clinician complete assurance of the presence or absence of placenta accreta.

> Risk factors for placenta accreta:
> - placenta previa
> - prior cesarean delivery
> - prior myomectomy
> - Asherman's syndrome
> - submucous leiomyomata
> - maternal age older than 35 years

If the diagnosis or a strong suspicion is formed before delivery, a number of measures should be taken:

❖ The patient should be counselled about the likelihood of hysterectomy and blood transfusion.

❖ Blood products and clotting factors should be available.

❖ The appropriate location and timing for delivery should be considered to allow access to adequate surgical personnel and equipment.

❖ A pre-operative anesthesia assessment should be obtained.

The extent (area, depth) of the abnormal attachment will determine the surgical intervention: curettage, wedge resection, medical management or hysterectomy. Uterine conserving options may work in small focal accretas, but abdominal hysterectomy is usually the definitive treatment.

## PPH due to uterine inversion

Uterine inversion is usually due to mismanagement of the third stage, either due to excessive cord traction on a fundally implanted placenta that has not been separated or secondary to fundal pressure given to aid placenta separation. The accompanying shock was traditionally thought to be disproportionate to the blood loss and was considered to be partly neurogenic due to traction on the uterine supports. However, it has been shown that blood loss is usually massive and underestimated.

On bimanual examination, the finding of a firm mass, below or near the cervix, coupled with absence of identification of the uterine corpus on abdominal examination suggests inversion. If the inversion occurs before placental separation, no further attempt should be made to detach or remove the placenta as this will lead to additional hemorrhage.

Replacement of the uterine corpus involves placing the palm of the hand against the fundus (now inverted and lowermost at or through the cervix), as if holding a tennis ball, with the fingertips exerting upward pressure circumferentially. To restore normal anatomy, relaxation of the uterus may be necessary. Terbutaline, magnesium sulfate, halogenated general anesthetics and nitroglycerin have been used for uterine relaxation (You and Zahn 2006).

The hydrostatic method described by O' Sullivan involves replacing the inverted uterus in the vagina and rapid infusion of 2 liters of warm saline into the vagina, with one hand sealing the vagina. This leads to ballooning of the vaginal fornices, exerting an even hydrostatic pressure which forces open the constricting cervix, usually reducing the inverted uterus. An oxytocin infusion is commenced only after the uterus has been restored to its normal configuration.

Manual replacement, with or without uterine relaxants, is usually successful. In the unusual circumstance in which it is not, laparotomy is required. Two procedures have been reported to return the uterine corpus to the abdominal cavity. The Huntington procedure involves progressive upward traction on the inverted corpus using Babcock or Allis forceps. The Haultain procedure involves incising the cervical ring posteriorly, allowing for digital repositioning of the inverted corpus, with subsequent repair of the incision.

## PPH due to injuries to the genital tract

Obstetric injuries to the genital tract can be divided into lacerations and hematomas. The lacerations are subdivided into vulval, vaginal and cervical tears and uterine rupture. Hematomas are classified depending on the site of occurrence as infralevator (below the levator ani muscle) or supralevator (above the levator ani muscle). Hematomas can also be classified as vulvar, vulvovaginal and paravaginal or retroperitoneal.

Vaginal tears are commonly seen in the lower 2/3 of the vagina, on the posterolateral walls. The upper 1/3 of the vagina is less commonly involved, but if it occurs, it may be associated with tears in the cervix, broad ligament, or even the lower uterine segment, necessitating a laparotomy.

> Optimal repair of genital tract lacerations requires:
> - correct positioning of the patient
> - satisfactory analgesia/anesthesia
> - adequate lighting and exposure
> - appropriate assistance
> - special vaginal retractors
> - long needle holders.

Cervical tears can lead to torrential bleeding. Right-angled retractors and sponge holders are used to visualise the tears. Those tears, which are larger than 2 cm and bleeding, are closed with continuous locking 00 polyglactin sutures.

Small hematomas can be treated conservatively, but expanding ones with hemodynamic instability require surgical intervention. Hematomas should be opened, bleeding points should be secured and the dead space should be approximated with figure-of-eight sutures. Supralevator hematomas may require a laparotomy and a partial or complete rupture in the uterine wall should be looked for.

## PPH due to defects in coagulation

Clotting abnormalities should be suspected on the basis of patient or family history, or clinical circumstances. HELLP syndrome, abruptio placentae, prolonged intrauterine fetal demise, sepsis and amniotic fluid embolism are associated with clotting abnormalities. Significant hemorrhage from any cause can lead to consumption of coagulation factors. When coagulopathy is suspected, appropriate testing should be ordered, with blood products infused as indicated.

In the presence of persistent, uncontrollable bleeding, it has been recommended that up to 1 litre of fresh frozen plasma (FFP) and 10 units of cryoprecipitate (two packs) may be given empirically, while awaiting the results of coagulation studies and a hematologist's consult (Walker et al 1994). It would be appropriate to order these blood components as soon as a need for them is anticipated, because it usually takes time to procure them.

> Clotting abnormalities can occur with:
> - HELLP syndrome
> - abruptio placentae
> - prolonged intrauterine fetal demise
> - sepsis
> - amniotic fluid embolism.

### Role of Factor VII A therapy

Franchini et al (2007) reviewed case reports of 65 women treated with Factor VII A for PPH. Although the case reports suggested that Factor VII A reduced bleeding, 30 of the 65 women underwent peripartum hysterectomy. Factor VII A will not work if there is no fibrinogen and effectiveness may also be suboptimal with severe thrombocytopenia (less than $20 \times 10^9/l$). This fact should be kept in mind, since women with PPH are particularly susceptible to severe hypofibrinogenemia.

## Secondary Postpartum Hemorrhage

Secondary hemorrhage occurs in approximately 1 per cent of pregnancies. The specific etiology is often unidentified. The extent of bleeding is usually less than that seen with primary postpartum hemorrhage.

Uterine atony (perhaps secondary to retained products of conception) with or without infection contributes to secondary hemorrhage. Conventional treatment involves antibiotics and uterotonics. The antibiotics usually recommended are a combination of ampicillin (clindamycin, if penicillin allergic) and metronidazole (RCOG 2009). In cases of endomyometritis (tender uterus) or overt sepsis, the addition of gentamicin is recommended. Surgical measures should be undertaken if there is excessive or continuing bleeding, irrespective of ultrasound findings (Alexander et al 2002).

> Antibiotics for secondary PPH:
> - ampicillin (clindamycin, if penicillin allergic) and metronidazole
> - gentamicin can be added in cases of endomyometritis or overt sepsis

A pelvic ultrasound may help to exclude the presence of retained products of conception, although the appearance of the immediate postpartum uterus may be unreliable (Sadan et al 2004). An experienced obstetrician should be involved in decisions and performance of evacuation of retained products of conception, as these women carry a high risk for uterine perforation. Often, the volume of tissue removed by curettage is minimal, yet bleeding subsides promptly. However, patients should be counselled about the possibility of hysterectomy before initiating any operative procedures.

Postpartum hemorrhage may be the first indication for von Willebrand's disease for many patients and should be considered in the differential diagnosis. The prevalence of von Willebrand's disease is reported to be 10 per cent to 20 per cent among adult women with menorrhagia. Hence, testing for bleeding disorders should be considered among pregnant patients with a history of menorrhagia, because the risk of delayed or secondary postpartum hemorrhage is high among women with bleeding disorders (James 2006).

## References

Alexander J, Thomas P, Sanghera J. 2002. Treatments for secondary haemorrhage. *Cochrane Database of Systematic Reviews* Issue 1. Art. No.: CD002867. DOI: 10.1002/14651858.CD002867.

American College of Obstetricians and Gynecologists. 2006. Postpartum hemorrhage. ACOG Practice Bulletin No. 76. American College of Obstetricians and Gynecologists. *Obstet Gynecol.* 108:1039–47.

Anderson J, Etches D. 2008. Postpartum Haemorrhage. In: Damos JD, Eisinger SH, Baxley EG, eds. *Advanced Life Support in Obstetrics Course Syllabus* 4th ed. American Academy of Family Physicians.

B-Lynch C, Coker A, Lawal AH, Abu J, Cowen MJ. 1997. The B-Lynch surgical technique for the control of massive postpartum haemorrhage: an alternative to hysterectomy? Five cases reported. *BJOG* 104:372–5.

Bakri YN, et al. 2001. Tamponade-balloon for obstetrical bleeding. *Int. J. Gynecol. Obstet.* 74: 139–142.

Bhal K, Bhal N, Mulik V, Shankar L. 2005. The uterine compression suture – a valuable approach to control major haemorrhage at lower segment caesarean section. *J Obstet Gynaecol.* 25: 10–14.

Chauleur C, Fanget, C, Tourne, et al. 2008. Serious primary post-partum hemorrhage, arterial embolization and future fertility: a retrospective study of 46 cases. *Hum. Reprod.* 23 (7): 1553—59.

Chesley LC. 1972. Plasma and red cell volumes during pregnancy. *Am J Obstet Gynecol*. 112:440–50

Cho JH, Jun HS, Lee CN. 2000. Hemostatic suturing technique for uterine bleeding during Caesarean delivery. *Obstet Gynecol* 96:129–31.

Combs CA, Murphy EL, Laros RK Jr. 1991. Factors associated with postpartum hemorrhage with vaginal birth. *Obstet Gynecol* 77:69–76

Condous GS, Arulkumaran S, Symonds I, Chapman R, Sinha A, Razvi K. 2003. The tamponade test in the management of massive postpartum hemorrhage. *Obstet Gynecol* 101:767–72.

Drife J. 1997. Management of primary postpartum haemorrhage. *BJOG* 104:275–7.

Franchini M, Lippi G, Franchi M. 2007. The use of recombinant activated factor VII in obstetric and gynaecological haemorrhage. *BJOG* 114: 8–15.

Grotegut CA, Larsen FW, Jones MR, Livingston E. 2004. Erosion of a B-Lynch suture through the uterine wall: a case report. *J Reprod Med* 49:849–52.

Hayman R, Arulkumaran S, Steer P. 2002. Uterine compression sutures: surgical management of postpartum hemorrhage. *Obstet Gynecol* 99:502–6.

Hsu S, Rodgers B, Lele A, Yeh J. 2003. Use of packing in obstetric hemorrhage of uterine origin. *J Reprod Med*. 48:69–71

James AH. 2006. Von Willebrand disease. *Obstet Gynecol Surv.* 61:136–45

Joshi VM, Otive SR, Majumder R, Nikam YA, Shrivastava M.2007. *Internal iliac artery ligation for arresting postpartum haemorrhage. BJOG.* 114:356–61

Joshi VM, Shrivastava M. 2004. Partial ischemic necrosis of the uterus following a uterine brace compression suture. *Br J Obstet Gynecol* 111:279–80.

Kayem G, Kurinczuk JJ, Alfirevic Z, Spark P, Brocklehurst P, Knight M, et al. 2011. Uterine compression sutures for the management of severe postpartum hemorrhage. *Obstet Gynecol* 117:14–20.

Kominiarek MA, Kilpatrick SJ. 2007. Postpartum haemorrhage: a recurring pregnancy complication. *Semin Perinatol* 31(3):159–66.

Maier RC. 1993. Control of postpartum hemorrhage with uterine packing. *Am J Obstet Gynecol*. 169:317–21

Malibary AM. 2004. Modified B-Lynch technique for the control of massive postpartum hemorrhage. An alternative to hysterectomy. *Saudi Med J* 25:1999–2000.

Mathai M, Gulmezoglu AM, Hill S.: 2007. Saving womens lives: evidence-based recommendations for the prevention of postpartum haemorrhage. *Bull World Health Organ*, 85:322-323.

Mousa HA, Alfirevic Z. 2007. Treatment for primary postpartum haemorrhage. *Cochrane Database Syst Rev*(1):CD003249. DOI: 10.1002/14651858. CD003249.pub2.

Nelson GS, Birch C. 2006. Compression sutures for uterine atony and hemorrhage following Caesarean delivery. *Int J Gynecol Obstet* 92:248–50.

Ochoa M, Allaire A, Stitely M. 2002. Pyometria after hemostatic square suture technique. *Obstet Gynecol* 99:506–9.

O'Leary JA. 1995. Uterine artery ligation in the control of postcesarean hemorrhage. *J Reprod Med*. Mar; 40(3):189–93.

Prendiville WJP, Elbourne D, McDonald SJ. 2000. Active versus expected management in the third stage of labour. *Cochrane Database Syst Rev* (3):CD000007.

Rouse DJ, MacPherson C, Landon M, et al. 2006. od transfusion and cesarean delivery. *Obstet Gynecol* 108:891,

Royal College of Obstetricians and Gynecologists. 2009. Prevention and Management of Postpartum Haemorrhage. Green-top Guideline No. 52. London. May

Sadan O, Golan A, Girtler O, Lurie S, Debby A, Sagiv R, et al. 2004. Role of sonography in the diagnosis of retained products of conception. *J Ultrasound Med*. 23:371–4.

*Salomon L.J, deTayrac R, Castaigne-Meary V* et al. 2003. Fertility and pregnancy outcome following pelvic arterial embolization for severe post-partum haemorrhage. A cohort study. *Human Reproduction* Vol.18, No.4 pp. 849±852

Silver RM, Landon MB, Rouse DT, Leveno KJ, Spong CY, Thom EA, et al. 2006. Maternal morbidity associated with multiple repeat cesarean deliveries. *Obstet Gynecol* 07:1226–32.

Stones RW, Paterson CM, Saunders NSTG. 1993. Risk factors for major obstetric haemorrhage. *European Journal of Obstetrics and Gynecology and Reproductive Biology* 48:15–8.

Walker ID, Walker JJ, Colvin BT, Letsky EA, Rivers R, Stevens R. 1994. Investigation and management of haemorrhagic disorders in pregnancy. *J Clin Pathol* 47:100–8

WHO. 2000. Managing Complications in Pregnancy and Childbirth: A Guide for Midwives and Doctors. WHO/RHR/00.7. Geneva: WHO:2000; S25-S34.

World Health Organization (WHO) Department of Reproductive Health and Research. *Maternal Mortality in 2000: Estimates Developed by WHO, UNICEF, and UNFPA*. Geneva: WHO; 2004.

Wu HH, Yeh GP. 2005. Uterine cavity synechiae after hemostatic square suturing technique. *Obstet Gynecol*; 105:1176–78.

You WB, Zahn CM. 2006. Postpartum Hemorrhage: Abnormally adherent placenta, uterine inversion and puerperal hematomas. *Clin Obstet Gynecol* 49:184

Zelop C. 2011. Postpartum Hemorrhage: Becoming More Evidence-Based. *Obstet Gynecol*. January Volume 117, Issue 1, pp 3–5.

# CHAPTER 20

# POSTPARTUM COLLAPSE

*Surabhi Nanda and Leonie K Penna*

The perception in a labour ward is often that maternal and fetal risks end with delivery. While for the majority of mothers this is true, for a small number, conditions may develop after delivery that, without appropriate management, may have serious morbidity and mortality associated with them.

Collapse is a non-specific term implying complete or partial loss of consciousness, either as a primary cerebral event or secondary to a cardio-vascular event leading to cerebral hypo-perfusion. It can range from a simple faint to a catastrophic event heralding imminent death. The term 'postpartum collapse' incorporates the onset of a new condition or the worsening of a pre-existing one within 24 hours of delivery. Fortunately, collapse in a pregnant woman during or just after labour is rare. However, it cannot be overstated that no matter what the cause of collapse, the first few minutes of resuscitation are vital to ensure that the patient remains well oxygenated and perfused.

## Maternal Mortality

The true incidence of postpartum collapse is impossible to estimate, since the definitions and clinical presentations vary enormously and data collection is difficult. In 2005, the World Health Organization estimated that each year there are 529,000 maternal deaths worldwide during pregnancy, childbirth or in the postpartum period (Hill et al 2001; Majhi et al 2001; World Health Organization 2005). In the UK, the Confidential Enquiries into Maternal and Child Health (CEMACH) reports have estimated an incidence of 14 deaths per 100,000 maternities (Lewis 2007), but it is not possible to ascertain the proportion of women who die within the first 24 hours of delivery or those who become acutely unwell during this time. Studies of obstetric morbidity are even more varied in their methodology and variability of definitions, but many of the conditions described may present or become more severe, shortly after delivery (Waterstone et al 2001).

## Maternal Morbidity

Morbidity and long-term disability after an acute event leading to maternal collapse is difficult to quantify, and hence, poorly reported. Effective resuscitation with prompt diagnosis and treatment will minimise this morbidity. The UK Obstetric Surveillance System (UKOSS) is a national system established to study a range of rare disorders of pregnancy, including severe 'near-miss' maternal morbidity (Knight 2008).

## Causes of Postpartum Collapse

Table 20.1 lists the different causes of postpartum collapse, although the incidences are difficult to determine. The leading causes of maternal death in the UK as reported by the CEMACH report for 2003–2005 are listed in Table 20.2.

## Clinical Presentation

The timing, speed of onset and presentation will depend on the underlying pathology and may even suggest the cause. Cardiopulmonary arrest occurs only once in every 30,000 pregnancies, but lesser degrees of collapse are much more common. The average maternity unit will experience a case of cardio-pulmonary arrest only once in 5–10 years, and evidence from CEMACH suggests that when it does occur, staff may be slow to respond despite apparently adequate training. Resuscitation of a recently delivered collapsed woman might need to be undertaken by the community midwife at home, or the Emergency department doctors (18 per cent of all women who die in relation to pregnancy present to the emergency department), or the medical obstetric team. Irrespective of the care provider, an organized time-conscious team approach is the single most important factor for improving the survival chances of the woman.

## Non-Serious Causes of Maternal Collapse

### Hyperventilation

Hyperventilation due to poor analgesia in labour has been reported (Burden et al 1994). Immediately following delivery, symptoms due to hyperventilation may be seen, especially if painful procedures such as perineal suturing are performed with inadequate analgesia. It may be more common in a woman who is very anxious or has a past history of panic attacks. Tetanic spasm of arms and legs may occur, but full collapse is uncommon. Management involves calming the woman and encouraging slower breathing. Oxygen via a facemask will worsen rather than relieve symptoms, which are due to low carbon dioxide levels, resulting in a respiratory alkalosis and an elevated blood pH. Rebreathing of air (for example, from a paper bag) will hasten the recovery from symptoms, but is not usually required.

### Vasovagal syncope

Simple fainting (syncope) may occur at any time and is more common during pregnancy. It is defined as a sudden transient loss of consciousness with concurrent diminution of the postural tone, followed by spontaneous recovery. The exertion combined with emotional factors occurring around the time of delivery may result in a predisposition to syncope in some women. Orthostatic hypotension may occur post-delivery and women should be advised not to stand immediately

> Vasovagal syncope is associated with bradycardia and hypotension. Respiration is not usually affected and the fainting episode is self-limiting.

**Table 20.1** Causes of Postpartum Collapse

| Obstetric causes | Non Obstetric causes |
|---|---|
| **SERIOUS CAUSES** | |
| 1) Hemorrhagic<br>• PPH<br>• Uterine rupture<br><br>2) Non-hemorrhagic<br>• Uterine inversion<br>• Amniotic fluid embolism<br>• Eclampsia<br>• Other hypertensive causes – severe PET, HELLP syndrome, hepatic rupture, intra-cerebral hemorrhage<br>• Peripartum cardio-myopathy<br>• Genital tract sepsis | 1) Thromboembolism<br>• Pulmonary embolism<br>• Cerebral venous thrombosis<br>• Air embolism<br>2) Cardiac Causes<br>• Aortic dissection<br>• Myocardial infarction<br>• Cardiac failure<br>• Arrhythmias<br>3) Respiratory Causes<br>• Asthma<br>• Pneumonia<br>• H1N1 viremia<br>4) Neurological Causes<br>• Epilepsy<br>• Stroke (ischemic or hemorrhagic)<br>5) Metabolic Causes<br>• Hypoglycemia/Hyperglycemia<br>• Hyponatremia<br>• Diabetic ketoacidosis<br>6) Adverse Drug Reactions/Anaphylaxis<br>• Magnesium toxicity<br>• Poisoning<br>• Latex allergy<br>• Local anesthetic toxicity<br>7) Sepsis/septic shock<br>8) Anesthetic causes<br>• General<br>  ♦ Aspiration pneumonitis<br>  ♦ Atelectasis<br>  ♦ Respiratory depression<br>  ♦ Airway obstruction |

Table 20.1 (contd)

|  |  |
|---|---|
|  | • Local<br>   ◆ Hypotension, high block<br>   ◆ Meningitis<br>   ◆ Spinal hematoma/abscess<br>9) Others<br>• Trauma, suicide<br><br>The list is not exhaustive and there is some overlap, i.e. more than one may co-exist. |
| NON SERIOUS CAUSES |  |
| • Hyperventilation<br>• Vasovagal syncope |  |

Table 20.2 Trends in maternal deaths/100,000 maternities 2003–2005

| Causes | Deaths | Rate/100,000 maternities |
|---|---|---|
| **Direct Deaths** | 132 | 6.24 |
| Thrombosis and thromboembolism | 41 | 1.94 |
| Preeclampsia and eclampsia | 18 | 0.85 |
| Hemorrhage | 14 | 0.66 |
| Amniotic fluid embolism | 17 | 0.80 |
| Genital tract sepsis | 18 | 0.85 |
| Anesthetic | 6 | 0.28 |
| **Indirect deaths** | 163 | 7.71 |
| Cardiac | 48 | 2.27 |
| Psychiatric | 18 | 0.85 |
| Late deaths | 82 | — |

after delivery without an attendant, this is particularly true for women on antihypertensive medication. Diagnosis is usually straightforward, as there is bradycardia associated with hypotension. Respiration is not usually affected and the fainting episode is self-limiting. Turning the woman to her side is all that is usually required but if bradycardia persists, atropine 10 mg can be administered subcutaneously. Other causes of collapse should always be considered, particularly if recovery is not rapid from simple measures. Repeated episodes require further investigation (Heaven and Sutton 2000).

## Serious Causes of Postpartum Collapse

The causes of collapse can be broadly divided into hemorrhagic shock and non-hemorrhagic shock. Hemorrhagic complications of pregnancy while uncommon, occur with sufficient frequency that they are anticipated and protocols for their management should exist in all maternity units. Non-hemorrhagic complications are extremely rare and the mortality associated with them is high even in developed countries (NICE 2001).

## Hemorrhagic Causes

***Postpartum hemorrhage (PPH)***: There is rarely any uncertainty regarding hemorrhage as a cause for maternal collapse as postpartum bleeding is usually revealed. On rare occasions, the bleeding may be concealed with the formation of a large paravaginal or broad ligament hematoma. Quoted incidences for PPH vary, but a rate of about 5 per cent occurs in the UK. However, the majority of these are not severe enough to cause maternal collapse. About 0.5 per cent of all deliveries are complicated by a blood loss of more than 1500 ml. Risk factors for PPH include grand multiparity, cesarean and instrumental vaginal delivery, long first stage of labour with prolonged syntocinon use, antepartum hemorrhage, previous postpartum hemorrhage, uterine over-distension (e.g. multiple pregnancies, polyhydramnios, severe macrosomia), and a low-lying placenta.

Prior to collapse, there will usually be symptoms of pain as the hematoma expands. Tachycardia should be seen as the first sign in healthy women and may be wrongly attributed as a response entirely due to pain. The development of hypotension confirms the diagnosis but is a late sign, and thus warrants aggressive treatment to correct hypovolemia and immediate measures to stop further hemorrhage. Coagulopathy may be evident in the event of persistent hemorrhage or where the PPH is secondary to another condition like amniotic fluid embolism. Besides prompt fluid replacement and administration of uterotonics, surgical management includes uterine artery ligation, B-Lynch suture, and insertion of an intrauterine tamponade balloon as well as radiological interventions. In addition, where facilities are available, use of intra-operative cell salvage in select cases can prevent potential crises.

> Tachycardia should be seen as the first sign in healthy women. Hypotension may be a late sign and must be treated aggressively.

***Uterine rupture***: Uterine rupture may become apparent during the first stage of labour with the classic symptoms of abdominal pain, vaginal bleeding, sudden fetal heart rate decelerations or bradycardia and loss of uterine contractions. However, the risk of uterine rupture is high in the second stage and symptoms may not occur prior to spontaneous delivery or instrumental vaginal delivery for fetal heart rate abnormality. A review of cases of ruptured uterus showed that in 7 out of 15 cases, the diagnosis was made postpartum (Gardeil et al 1994). Less dramatic degrees of uterine rupture, in particular, a partial dehiscence of a previous cesarean section scar may cause minimal intrapartum symptoms and only become apparent immediately after delivery when the woman collapses, shocked and hypotensive, with signs suggestive of intra-abdominal bleeding (Webb et al 2000). Delayed dehiscence is extremely rare, but has been reported six weeks postpartum in a woman inadequately treated for endometritis (Kindig et al 1998).

> A partial dehiscence of a previous cesarean section scar may cause minimal intrapartum symptoms and only become apparent immediately after delivery when the woman collapses with hypovolemic shock and signs suggestive of intra-abdominal bleeding.

Uterine rupture needs to be discussed where women with previous cesarean opt for a vaginal birth. Evidence suggests that risk of uterine rupture increases with previous uterine rupture, previous high vertical classical cesarean section, where the uterine incision has involved the whole length of the uterine corpus, three or more previous cesarean deliveries (RCOG Birth after previous caesarean birth guideline No. 45 2007). Other risk factors include prolonged labour with induction with misoprostol or oxytocin.

Treatment of uterine rupture involves prompt resuscitation and laparotomy to repair the uterus and stop hemorrhage. Although repair transvaginally has been described for uterine dehiscence diagnosed postpartum, this should be reserved for asymptomatic women (Philippe et al 1997).

*Other rare causes of hemorrhagic collapse*: Spontaneous hepatic rupture is documented as a cause of postnatal collapse in women with pregnancies complicated by hypertension (Hibbard 1976). Rare cases in women with apparently uncomplicated pregnancies have also been reported (Abdi et al 2001). Diagnosis is extremely difficult, as the symptom of severe pleuritic chest pain associated with hypotension is suggestive of the much more common diagnosis of pulmonary embolism. Unfortunately, anticoagulants if commenced will worsen the bleeding from the hepatic rupture with resulting high mortality. Abdominal ultrasound scanning will reveal the presence of free blood in the abdomen (especially the right upper quadrant). CT or MRI scanning can confirm the diagnosis, which should be suspected in any woman without risk factors for pulmonary embolism, presenting with typical symptoms within 24 hours of delivery, who continues to deteriorate after anticoagulation for a suspected thromboembolism.

Rupture of an aneurysm of the splenic artery is more common during pregnancy and postnatally, due to the increase in cardiac output and hormonal changes in the component structures of vessel walls during this time (Pandian et al 2001). Rupture is characterised by sudden collapse, but with non-specific abdominal signs. Signs of diaphragmatic irritation with shoulder tip pain may be present. Management is surgical with immediate splenectomy required. Splenic rupture and hepatic subcapsular hematoma should be considered as a part of the differential diagnoses when a hemodynamic collapse occurs during or immediately after labour, especially in patients with severe preeclampsia.

Arteriovenous malformations are rare, but may increase in size during pregnancy due to the increase in maternal cardiac output and circulating blood volume resulting in an increased risk of rupture and bleeding. The nature and severity of the symptoms associated with collapse will depend on the site of the malformation. Murray reported a case of hemothorax from a pulmonary arteriovenous malformation at 35 weeks gestation and commented that a third of cases described in the literature occurred in pregnancy (Murray et al 2000).

> Rare causes of hemorrhagic collapse include:
> - Spontaneous hepatic rupture
> - Rupture of a splenic artery aneurysm
> - Splenic rupture and hepatic subcapsular hematoma
> - Arteriovenous malformations

## Non-Hemorrhagic Causes

***Uterine inversion***: Uterine inversion is a rare but extremely dramatic cause of puerperal collapse.

Although rare, it is not completely avoidable and so all labour wards should have guidelines to assist medical and nursing staff in the management of this complication, which they are unlikely to have prior experience of managing. Incidence is variously reported from as high as 1 in 550 to as low as 1 in 27,000. The incidence will vary according to the management of the third stage undertaken, with higher incidences occurring if overly active third stage management is used and lower incidences associated with more physiological third stages. Maternity units with good protocols for third stage management report incidences of about 1 in 2000 (Wendel and Cox 1995) and this probably represents an acceptable rate.

Any management of the third stage that allows cord traction prior to the signs of placental separation will be predisposed to a uterine inversion. Methods of placental delivery that encourage compression of the fundus of the uterus (Credes method), as opposed to waiting for spontaneous uterine contractions, will also increase the risk of inversion. Although inversions may occur with overzealous cord traction on a normal placenta that is slow to separate, cases will occur where there is a complete or partially morbid adherence of the placenta.

Most cases of inversion are acute and occur within 24 hours of delivery. A sub-acute presentation (more than 24 hours but less than four weeks) or a chronic presentation (more than four weeks postnatal) may occur, but they are less likely to be causes of collapse at presentation. For the purposes of description, inversion can be graded according to the level of descent of the fundus. First degree describes an inversion of the fundus within the uterine cavity but not through the cervix, second degree where the uterus is below the cervix but within the vagina; in the third degree the fundus reaches the introitus and in the fourth degree the fundus extends outside the introitus. The grading is not of any great practical application other than to say, the degree of maternal shock increases with increasing grades of inversion (Bhalla et al 2009).

Inversion presents with maternal collapse during the third stage. There is profound hypotension, usually out of proportion to the blood loss (which may be negligible if there has not yet been placental separation). The shock is thought to be neurogenic in origin, resulting from traction on the infundibulopelvic ligaments. Active resuscitation should be commenced with intravenous colloid administration and other differential diagnoses considered. The diagnosis may be self-evident with the presence of a mass in the vagina and a fundus absent from the usual supra-pubic position. However, in lesser degrees of inversion there may be no vaginal mass and the fundus may be still palpable abdominally. In a slim woman, dimpling of the uterus may suggest the diagnosis, but digital examination through the cervix will be required to confirm it. Although there are no studies, ultrasound may assist in the diagnosis of a uterine inversion.

> Uterine inversion presents with maternal collapse during the third stage. There is profound hypotension, usually out of proportion to the blood loss.

Management of inversion involves a rapid attempt at replacing the uterus into its normal position. Adequate analgesia is essential, with general anesthesia being required in most cases. A tocolytic agent, such as terbutaline, can be given to aid replacement by the relaxation of the cervical ring. Manual replacement should be attempted first by placing sustained upward pressure on the fundus to try to push it through the cervical ring. Hydrostatic replacement (O'Sullivan method) involves vulval occlusion and gravity-aided instillation of warm saline into the vagina. A silastic ventouse cup, if available, is very effective for use in this technique (Ogueh and Ayaida 1997). Large volumes of fluid may be required and careful measurement of fluid infused and returned should be made. If these techniques fail, surgical correction will be necessary. In Huntington's technique, Allis forceps are used to gradually try to pull the fundus through the constriction ring from the dimple above (laparotomy). If this fails, Haultain's technique of incising the constriction ring posteriorly and longitudinally should be used. The incision is repaired in layers with Vicryl® and subsequent pregnancies must be managed as a trial of uterine scar (Irani and Jordon 1997).

> Management of inversion involves a rapid attempt at replacing the uterus into its normal position. A tocolytic agent, such as terbutaline, can be given to aid replacement by the relaxation of the cervical ring.

**Amniotic Fluid and Air Embolism**: Amniotic fluid is a rare but catastrophic pregnancy complication; the reported incidence varies between authors. Recent population-based cohort study and nested case-control analysis, using the UK Obstetric Surveillance System, estimated an incidence of 2.0 per 100,000 deliveries (Knight et al 2010). The incidence of the condition is such that no individual or unit will have sufficient experience of the condition and the diagnosis must be considered in all cases of peripartum collapse (Thompson and Greer 2000). An analysis of the American register of cases showed that 70 per cent of amniotic fluid emboli occurred during labour, 11 per cent occurred immediately after vaginal delivery and 19 per cent occurred during or after a cesarean section (Clark et al 1995). In this series, the mortality rate was 61 per cent, but among survivors there was a high risk of neurological impairment with only 15 per cent reporting as having no problem.

In the UKOSS study, amniotic-fluid embolism occurrence was significantly associated with induction of labour and multiple pregnancy: an increased risk was also noted in older, ethnic-minority women. Cesarean delivery was also associated with postnatal amniotic-fluid embolism.

> Amniotic-fluid embolism is associated with:
> - induction of labour
> - multiple pregnancy
> - older women
> - cesarean section

Clinical manifestations of amniotic fluid embolism are similar to those seen in severe anaphylaxis and septic shock, with a sudden onset of profound hypotension and breathlessness, followed rapidly by cardiac arrest. A grand mal seizure, secondary to cerebral hypoxia, may occur with the initial presenting symptoms.

The initial collapse is thought to be due to intense vasospasm in the pulmonary vasculature in response to the presence of amniotic fluid and fetal debris; this results in pulmonary hypertension, profound hypoxia and acute right ventricular failure. This initial collapse with hypoxia and right-sided failure accounts for about 50 per cent of the observed mortality from amniotic-fluid embolism. In women who survive this phase, there is the development of left-sided failure, which may be a consequence of initial severe hypoxia on the myocardium or may be a direct effect of amniotic fluid on the myocardium. Half of all women die within one hour of the onset of symptoms. A consumptive coagulopathy develops in 40 per cent, this usually follows the initial phase of symptoms, but occasionally, a bleeding diathesis can be present from the beginning of collapse (Clark 1986).

Diagnosis is usually made on post-mortem examination, when fetal debris is demonstrated in the pulmonary vasculature. Ante-mortem diagnosis is based upon the clinical picture and further circumstantial evidence comes from an ECG showing right ventricular strain, chest x-ray showing pulmonary edema, abnormal coagulation screen and abnormal blood gases. The presence of fetal debris in blood aspirated from the right atrium (via a central venous pressure line) or from the pulmonary artery (via a pulmonary artery catheter) is more evidence to support the diagnosis, but is not considered completely diagnostic, as fetal cells have been found in the circulation of healthy women.

> The presence of amniotic fluid and fetal debris causes:
> - intense vasospasm in the pulmonary vasculature
> - pulmonary hypertension
> - profound hypoxia
> - acute right ventricular failure

Resuscitation and management involves:

1. Trying to improve oxygen levels by ventilation with 100% oxygen
2. Maintenance of cardiac output and blood pressure by volume expansion with crystalloid and inotropes.
3. Consideration of the use of invasive monitoring with pulmonary artery catheter.
4. Correction of coagulopathy by replacement of specific deficiencies platelets (reduced platelets), fresh frozen plasma (a prolonged prothrombin time), cryoprecipitate (reduced fibrinogen) and blood (if coagulopathy induced bleeding).

High-quality supportive care can result in good maternal outcomes after amniotic-fluid embolism (Gilbert and Danielsen 2009). Clinicians should consider both the risks and benefits of induction and cesarean delivery, because apt patient selection may result in a decrease in the number of women suffering a potentially fatal amniotic-fluid embolism.

Air embolism due to entrapment of air into the venous system, for example, due to manipulation of central venous or peripheral intravenous catheters has been reported as a rare cause of postpartum collapse. Subclinical entry of air into the circulation has been shown to occur up to 50 per cent of cesarean sections, and this is more likely if the uterus is exteriorized and held above the level of the heart; positioning the patient head-up may reduce this. A bolus of 3–5 ml/kg may be associated with mortality, but embolism of this size is rare.

The clinical presentation is similar to that from amniotic-fluid embolism with sudden collapse, but may be associated with symptoms of breathlessness and chest pain prior to collapse (Rogers et al 2000). Chest pain with ST segment depression may suggest air in the coronary circulation. Larger volumes of air may cause reduced cardiac output due to obstruction of right ventricular output. If a patent foramen ovale is present, air can pass into the arterial circulation and cause systemic lesions, such as stroke or myocardial infarction (MI). In the case of massive air embolism, auscultation of the heart may reveal 'mill wheel' or churning noises.

Management involves positioning the patient in the left lateral position to reduce right ventricle outflow obstruction, administration of pure oxygen in addition to general supportive care.

## Genital Tract Sepsis and Septic Shock

The recent CEMACH report noted an increase in deaths due to sepsis, which was the joint second most common direct cause of death in the UK. Severe sepsis with acute organ dysfunction has a 20 per cent to 40 per cent mortality rate. Besides the general immunosuppression known to occur in pregnancy, other risk factors include obesity, impaired glucose tolerance, anemia, prolonged rupture of membranes with subsequent chorioamnionitis or endometritis, cesarean section, vaginal trauma, post-delivery retained products and wound hematoma.

The exact clinical presentation will depend on the extent to which the disease process has evolved, but should be suspected as a cause of collapse in all women with pyrexia.

CEMACH suggests using any two of the following as signs of a systemic inflammatory response syndrome (SIRS):

1) Temperature >38°C or <36°C,

2) Heart rate >90 beats/min,

3) Respiratory rate >20/min or PaCO2 <4.3 kPa and

4) White cell count >12x10⁹/l

Tachycardia and pyrexia occur early in the septic process: with hypotension in the absence of other causes occurring as the disease process becomes more advanced. There may be uterine tenderness, but postpartum women may develop septicemia secondary to chest infections or other usually 'benign' local infections. As septic shock develops, the urine output falls, the blood picture may show a very high or an unusually low white cell count. This may be complicated by hepatic and renal dysfunction, with oliguria and metabolic acidosis in more advanced cases.

Serum lactate, blood gases and blood cultures need to be measured in suspected systemic sepsis. High flow oxygen and aggressive fluid resuscitation are essential with

> Severe sepsis with acute organ dysfunction has a 20 per cent to 40 per cent mortality rate.

> Advancing septic shock is associated with:
> - oliguria
> - very high or an unusually low white cell count
> - hepatic and renal dysfunction
> - metabolic acidosis

> Management of septic shock includes:
> - high flow oxygen
> - aggressive fluid resuscitation
> - appropriate high-dose intravenous antibiotics

targeted appropriate high-dose intravenous antibiotics, the latter should be started empirically whilst awaiting blood cultures, and treatment should be refined once the results are available. Regular monitoring of the patient using charts such as a 'MEOWS' – Modified Early Obstetric Warning System – is essential, and failure to respond to initial resuscitation and antibiotics within 24 hours should trigger critical care referral.

## Septic Shock

The pathophysiology of septic shock is due to the local proliferation of bacteria with a release of toxins and other inflammatory mediators locally, and ultimately, systemically. The inflammatory response is amplified by bacterial toxin-induced release of cytokines from macrophages, which can directly affect organ function and possibly cause the release of secondary mediators. Nitric oxide is one such mediator, causing vasodilatation and hypotension. Interleukins (1, 6 and 8), prostaglandins, leukotrienes, complement, platelet activating factor have all been implicated in the various clinical manifestations of septic shock (Astiz and Rackow 1998). Infections such as pyelonephritis, cholecystitis, appendicitis and pancreatitis are also more likely to cause septic shock in a pregnant than a non-pregnant woman (Faro 1999).

Microorganisms most commonly implicated were beta hemolytic streptococci Lancefield group A (occasionally Group B), *E coli*, Pseudomonas, *Staphylococcus aureus*, *Proteus mirabilis* and *Listeria monocytogenes*.

Tachypnea, tachy-cardia and changes in mental state may occur as early manifestations of severe sepsis with the subsequent development of pyrexia and hypo-tension. Isolated thrombocytopenia is present in 50 per cent of cases of septic shock and disseminated intravascular coagulation is a common sequelae. About 30 per cent to 50 per cent of women will develop adult respiratory distress syndrome (ARDS) (Astiz and Rackow 1998; Lewis 2007). Other potential complications include pulmonary edema and thromboembolism.

> Microorganisms implicated in septic shock:
> - beta hemolytic streptococci Lancefield group A (occasionally Group B)
> - E coli
> - Pseudomonas
> - Staphylococcus aureus
> - Proteus mirabilis
> - Listeria monocytogenes

> Severe sepsis may lead to:
> - thrombocytopenia and disseminated intravascular coagulation
> - adult respiratory distress syndrome (ARDS) pulmonary edema
> - thromboembolism

Fluid resuscitation should be aggressive and unless the response is rapid, invasive monitoring of cardiac function should be considered. Inotropes such as dopamine or dobutamine will usually be required, as myocardial function is often depressed (Lee et al 1989). Choice of antibiotic therapy will depend on the suspected source of infection. The source of infection should be fully investigated and any infective focus such as retained products of conception or abscess, surgically removed. The results from the use of anti-inflammatory therapies (including corticosteroids) have been disappointing, with randomised trials failing to show any improvement in mortality from septic shock (Astiz and Rackow 1998). Further management involves respiratory support with intubation and ventilation if necessary, management of any coagulopathy and renal support.

## Pulmonary Embolism (PE)

In the United Kingdom, pulmonary embolism is the most common cause of maternal death. In the recent Confidential Enquiry, it was the most common direct cause of death with a mortality of 1.56 per 100,000 maternities. There were 33 direct deaths due to PE of which 7 were after a cesarean delivery and 8 after a vaginal birth (Lewis 2007).

Pregnancy is a thrombogenic state and the risk of deep vein thrombosis is increased five-fold compared to non-pregnant women. In women with multiple moderate risk factors such as obesity, labour longer than 12 hours, grandmultiparity, age above 35 years, immobility, preeclampsia, sepsis and gross varicose veins or one major risk factor such as a family history of thrombosis, thrombophilia, anti-phospholipid syndrome or lower limb paralysis, consideration should be given to a prophylactic anticoagulation even after straight forward normal delivery (Greer 1999).

Indications for prophylactic anticoagulation:
- obesity
- labour longer than 12 hours
- grandmultiparity
- age above 35 years
- immobility
- preeclampsia
- sepsis
- varicose veins
- one major risk factor such as a family history of thrombosis, thrombophilia, anti-phospholipid syndrome or lower limb paralysis

Collapse from pulmonary embolism is usually heralded by the sudden onset of pleuritic chest pain. Dyspnea, cyanosis and confusion may occur due to hypoxia.

With large emboli, pulmonary hypertension results in rapid right ventricular failure with tachycardia and hypotension. Massive emboli may result in severe hypoxia with loss of consciousness and cardiac arrest at presentation. The presence of any risk factors for thromboembolism or any history suggestive of deep vein thrombosis increases the likelihood of embolism as a cause for collapse.

Arterial blood gases will reveal hypoxemia and hypocapnia or metabolic acidosis in the event of shock. The ECG may show the presence of large Q-waves and inverted T-waves in lead III or sinus tachycardia, but is often considered unreliable in pregnancy. In massive pulmonary embolism in pregnancy, the features of acute right heart strain are as specific as in the non-pregnant woman. An echocardiogram is often useful, indicating right ventricular size and function, although it is poor at excluding PE (Toglia and Nolan 1997; De Swiet 1999).

Lung imaging with ventilation–perfusion scan or computed tomography pulmonary angiogram depending on local availability and clinical condition is mandatory to confirm the diagnosis, once the woman is stabilised (Macklon 1999; RCOG guideline 37a 2009).

Diagnosis is confirmed by:
- Lung imaging with ventilation–perfusion scan
- CT pulmonary angiogram

Management should involve a multidisciplinary resuscitation team including senior physicians, obstetricians, radiologists and anesthetists. The immediate management of collapse suspected to be due to pulmonary embolism involves resuscitation, analgesia and the commencement of anticoagulation. Volume expansion with crystalloid and oxygen therapy to treat hypoxemia should begin as soon as possible. Pleuritic chest pain may be severe and should be treated preferably with non-opiate analgesia as opiates may increase vasodilatation and exacerbate cardiovascular collapse (Thompson 2000).

Current recommendations for thrombolysis in cases of imminent cardiac arrest include a 50 mg bolus of Alteplase®. Invasive approaches, such as thrombus fragmentation and placement of an inferior vena caval filter, can be considered where facilities and expertise are readily available (Ilsaas et al 1998). In non-massive PE, heparin at therapeutic dosage is recommended instead of thrombolysis, before any imaging is undertaken. One such regimen is an intravenous bolus of heparin 5,000 IU (80 IU/kg) to be given immediately, followed by an infusion of at least 30,000 IU over 24 hours titrated to achieve full anticoagulation (ACOG 2000).

## Eclampsia

With 27 deaths per 100,000 maternities reported by the seventh Confidential Enquiry, pre-eclampsia (and eclampsia) was the second most common direct cause of maternal death. Thirty-eight per cent of eclamptic fits are unheralded by hypertension and proteinuria and 44 per cent occur after delivery (Douglas and Redman 1994). Eclampsia remains a significant cause of maternal mortality with intracerebral hemorrhage frequently found as a cause of death at post-mortem.

Injury should be prevented during the convulsion by placing the woman in a semi-prone position. The airway should be assessed and maintained as necessary.

Intravenous access should be established and monitoring commenced. The initial fit is usually self-limiting and benzodiazepines, such as diazepam, are not usually necessary. The use of diazepam will increase the risk of respiratory depression and should be reserved for uncontrolled fits, and even then, only if with someone skilled in intubation is available.

## Magnesium toxicity

Magnesium sulphate is recommended as a treatment for all women following an eclamptic fit (Duley et al 1995), and increasingly, in women with severe preeclampsia to try to prevent the occurrence of a first fit (Magpie 2002). Magnesium toxicity may arise, particularly in women with renal complications of preeclampsia, resulting in a reduced glomerular filtration rate. Clinical monitoring of patellar reflexes and respiration rate is mandatory in all women receiving magnesium and the infusion should be stopped if abnormality is detected. The Collaborative Eclampsia Trial showed that with this evaluation alone, severe toxicity did not occur (Duley et al 1995). However, laboratory magnesium levels should be performed if possible, when there is loss of patellar reflexes. Respiratory arrest may occur with serum levels of 6.3–7 mmol/l and cardiac arrest at levels greater than 12 mmol/l. Respiratory or cardiac arrest in women receiving magnesium sulphate should be treated with 10 ml of 10 per cent calcium gluconate over ten minutes intravenously as an antidote to magnesium sulphate.

## Anaphylaxis and anaphylactoid reactions

Anaphylaxis is an acute hypersensitivity reaction that can result in asphyxia and cardiac arrest (Jevon 2000). Although the incidence in pregnancy is not known, the incidence of anaphylaxis in the general population appears to be increasing and this is likely to increase the rate seen in pregnant women.

Anaphylaxis involves IgE-mediated reaction of an individual previously sensitised to a particular allergen. An anaphylactoid reaction describes a similar IgG-mediated reaction, but does not require prior sensitisation. Blood products and drugs, such as antibiotics or anesthetics may cause a reaction and these are used relatively frequently in postnatal women. Latex protein allergy may result in a reaction caused by contact with latex-containing products, such as indwelling catheters or examination gloves.

The clinical presentation of anaphylaxis is variable, but it should be suspected in any woman developing tachycardia and hypotension in combination with an urticarial rash or wheezing (bronchospasm).

Management involves removal of the suspected antigen and immediate supportive care with adrenaline 0.5–1 mg boluses IM (or 50 mg increments IV, if the doctor is familiar with this route of injection and there is ECG monitoring), repeated until symptoms improve. Antihistamines (chlorpheniramine 10–20 mg IV) and corticosteroids (hydrocortisone 100–200 mg IV) should be given to lessen the subsequent inflammatory response. Bronchodilators may also be considered. All patients with a suspected anaphylactic reaction should have blood taken 1 h following the start of the reaction followed by a further sample at 6 h. A raised tryptase level will confirm mast cell degranulation, although other measurements (e.g. complement) may also be useful (Jevon and Raby 2001). Both antihistamines and cortisone may cause some degree of hypotension and blood pressure should be monitored. If hypotension persists following these treatments, 1–2 litres of crystalloid should be infused rapidly. All patients should be followed up after the event and allergy testing arranged.

Blood should be discontinued if reaction occurs during transfusion (Michala et al 2008). Further exposure to any suspected trigger should be prevented.

## Drug Toxicity and withdrawal

Unexpected reaction to the drugs used as part of anesthesia or to treat postpartum hemorrhage may be a rare cause of collapse. The administration of epidural and spinal anesthesia may result in rare cases of respiratory arrest although due to the timing of analgesia in labour, these events usually occur prior to delivery (Katsiris et al 1999). This may be the result of a high spinal causing diaphragmatic paralysis or hypersensitivity to opiate analgesia. Intracranial spread results in total spinal, where loss of consciousness occurs as a result of the direct action of local anesthetics on the brain. Toxicity of local anesthetics may occur due to overdose or inadvertent intravenous injection and can cause respiratory, cardiovascular depression or arrhythmias.

Cardiac arrest has been described following the administration of synthetic prostaglandins to treat postpartum hemorrhage at cesarean section, the authors attributing this to coronary artery spasm (Chen et al 1998). Bolus doses of oxytocin have been reported to precipitate peripheral vasodilatation and cardiac arrest in cases with prior hypotension, and when used intravenously, the drug should be given slowly in a maximum bolus of 5IU (NICE 2008). Opioids can cause respiratory depression, hypotension, bradycardia and reduced consciousness. Naloxone can be used to reverse the effects. Ergometrine may cause hypertension and severe vomiting. Antiemetics such as metoclopramide and cyclizine may cause severe tachycardia and rarely, dystonic reactions. Beta-adrenergic agonists used for tocolysis may cause tachycardia and pulmonary edema. Though rare in the immediate postpartum period, opioid withdrawal occurs within 6–12 h of the last dose and may cause problems with postoperative analgesia as well as hypertension, tachycardia, sweating, abdominal pain and vomiting. Myocardial ischemia, arrhythmias and convulsions can occur with both cocaine withdrawal and acute intoxication.

## Cardiomyopathy

Puerperal cardiomyopathy is a dilated cardiomyopathy that typically occurs in the month prior to or up to 5 months after delivery. The estimated incidence of peripartum cardiomyopathy is about 1 in 3500 pregnancies (USA) and identified risk factors include increased maternal age, increasing parity, multiple pregnancy and pre-existing and pregnancy-induced hypertension (Pearson et al 2000). It is a life threatening condition with a maternal mortality of 25 per cent to 50 per cent. The diagnosis can be made following investigations for symptoms suggestive of left ventricular failure, but diagnosis may not be made until cardiovascular collapse occurs or systemic embolism occurs. The latter is seen in 24 per cent to 40 per cent of cases and may result in ischemic stroke. Overall, the symptoms may be very nonspecific and any clinical suspicion warrants echocardiography to exclude the diagnosis (Chan and Hill 1999). Typical symptoms include breathlessness, edema and orthopnea with tachycardia and tachypnea. A wheeze is often mistaken for asthma, but may result from heart failure.

Postnatal treatment involves resuscitation, treatment of heart failure (with diuretics, inotrophs and angiotensin-converting enzyme inhibitors) and thromboprophylaxis. Cardiac transplantation is the only option in cases that do not respond to these conventional measures. The condition often recurs in subsequent pregnancies and carries significant maternal mortality, hence warranting pre-pregnancy counselling of these women.

## Aortic Dissection

Aortic dissection is uncommon in women below 40 years, but the risk is increased in pregnancy with up to 50 per cent of dissections in women of childbearing age occurring during pregnancy. Hemodynamic and hormonal changes of pregnancy contribute to an increased risk in pregnancy. Risk factors include hypertension, increasing age and parity, coarctation of the aorta and connective tissue disorders such as Ehlers-Danlos syndrome and Marfan syndrome.

Marfan syndrome is an autosomal dominant connective tissue disorder with multisystem involvement, including effects on the cardiovascular system. There is

> Risk factors for puerperal cardiomyopathy:
> - increased maternal age
> - increasing parity
> - multiple pregnancy
> - pre-existing and pregnancy-induced hypertension

variable expression of the gene mutation resulting in variable signs and symptoms among sufferers. The prevalence is estimated as 1 in 5000 in the general population. Cardiovascular problems include mitral or tricuspid regurgitation and an aortopathy resulting in aortic dilatation with a risk of dissection. The risk of dissection is increased in pregnancy due to the hemodynamic changes that occur in normal pregnancy resulting in an increased stroke volume. The presence of hypertension increases these risks further. Review of case reports in the literature can lead to the assumption that aortic dissection is a common problem. Uncomplicated cases are under-reported and the true incidence can only be obtained from case series. Lind reviewed 117 pregnancies in 78 women with Marfan's and found five cases of dissection, a rate of 4.5 per cent. All women survived. Aortic diameter and progressive dilatation are the most important predictors of risk in pregnant women with Marfan's. Aortic diameter should be monitored, as it is an indicator of risk in all women known to have the syndrome. Surgical repair is recommended for aortic diameters of 55 mm or more (Mabie and Freire 1995). Most dissections occur as an antenatal event. However, as labour adds a further hemodynamic stress, the possibility of dissection beginning at this time should be remembered. Women remain at risk in the puerperium as demonstrated in Lind's series where two of the five cases presented postnatally. Classic symptoms prior to collapse are severe back pain and dyspnea. The diagnosis can be confirmed by trans-esophageal echocardiography and requires prompt surgical treatment to avoid mortality. As about 15 per cent of cases of Marfan's result from new mutations, not all women will have a family history (Lind and Wallenburg 2001). A suggestive phenotype (skeletal signs, arachnodactyly, ocular problems, cardiac murmur) noted antenatally warrants further investigation.

Dissection of the pulmonary artery has been reported resulting in maternal death, 17 hours postpartum. The authors speculated that the high blood flow rates accompanying parturition or the Valsalva manoeuvre might have precipitated this event (Hankins et al 1985a).

**Cardiac Disease**

Congenital and acquired heart disease is increasing as a cause of maternal death in developed countries and as the incidence of heart disease is higher in developing countries, it constitutes a very significant cause of mortality worldwide. Unfortunately, not all cardiac disease is diagnosed prior to labour and the hemodynamic stresses around delivery may precipitate unexpected cardiovascular collapse. Even women with well-documented cardiac disease are at risk from peri-partum collapse.

Labour is associated with a further increase in cardiac output of about 15 per cent in the first stage and 50 per cent in the second stage. Post delivery, there is an immediate rise in cardiac output due to the relief of pressure on the inferior vena cava, thus increasing venous return. Contraction of the uterus increases the circulating blood volume (Ramsey et al 2001). Overall, immediately postpartum, there is a rise in cardiac output by 60 per cent to 80 per cent, followed by a rapid

> Women with cardiovascular compromise are at highest risk at the end of labour and within one hour after delivery due to a rise in cardiac output by 60 per cent to 80 per cent.

decline to prelabour values by one hour after delivery. Women with cardiovascular compromise are at highest risk at the end of labour and immediately after delivery.

All women with symptoms suggestive of cardiac disease during pregnancy should be investigated. Clinical symptoms such as edema, fatigue, breathlessness and dizziness may easily be attributed to normal pregnancy, but the clinician must maintain a high index of suspicion whilst avoiding over investigation of healthy women.

In women with diagnosed cardiac disease, delivery should be planned and involve discussion with an appropriately trained anesthetist and cardiologist. Women with primary pulmonary hypertension and Eisenmenger syndrome are at greatest risk of deterioration in late pregnancy and the puerperium, with the fluid shifts around delivery resulting in rapid and intractable right ventricular failure or sudden death due to atrial tachyarrhythmias. The avoidance of cardiovascular collapse must be the aim of management by the use of invasive monitoring with pulmonary artery catheters in severe disease (Lupton et al 2002).

### Myocardial infarction

Myocardial infarction has been estimated to occur in only 1 in 10,000 women during pregnancy (Hankins et al 1985b). Acute myocardial infarction in the puerperium is a very rare phenomenon, but is associated with significant mortality. A review by Roth and El Kayam (1996), of all reports of myocardial infarction during pregnancy revealed 125 cases; of these, 17 were described as peri-partum and 30 as postpartum. The overall mortality for infarction in pregnancy was 21 per cent, but was higher (30 per cent) in cases of postpartum infarction.

> Acute myocardial infarction in the puerperium is a very rare phenomenon, but is associated with significant mortality.

Symptoms typically include angina pectoris with crushing retro-sternal pain radiating into the neck, jaw and arm. This pain may be associated with dyspnea, palpitations and vomiting. Collapse denotes the presence of acute complications of infarction such as arrhythmia, ventricular free wall rupture, septum rupture, mitral regurgitation or cardiogenic shock. The electrocardiogram will usually show elevation of the ST segment of the waveform and the development of new Q waves. In combination with a classic history, these are considered diagnostic of acute infarction. Cardiac enzymes are performed to confirm the diagnosis. The levels of creatinine kinase must be interpreted carefully as they may be moderately elevated in women following normal delivery (Leiserowitz et al 1992).

In rare cases, infarction may result from coronary artery spasm caused by the administration of ergometrine to prevent or treat postpartum hemorrhage and drug-related spasm should be considered in the absence of any other risk factor (Ko et al 1998).

## Metabolic Causes

### Hypoglycemia and other causes

Insulin requirements increase during pregnancy and then fall dramatically after delivery. In insulin-dependent diabetes, breastfeeding will reduce insulin requirements further. A poor understanding of these changing requirements and an aim for very tight control may result in loss of consciousness due to hypoglycemia.

The diagnosis is usually suspected due to the knowledge of a diagnosis of insulin-dependent diabetes and is rapidly confirmed by assessment of blood glucose. Other diagnoses must be considered, if the diagnosis is not confirmed or the patient does not respond immediately to intravenous or sublingual glucose. Rare cases of hypoglycemic coma related to insulinoma (Takacs et al 2002) and acute adrenal insufficiency have been reported (Perlitz et al 1999) complicating the puerperium.

Hyperglycemia in a poorly-controlled diabetic can present with a range of symptoms including keto-acidosis and coma. Treatment involves early recognition and treatment with insulin.

Hyponatremia can result from excessive administration of hypotonic intravenous fluids. The woman may be at increased risk because of the dilution of oxytocics in hypotonic solutions and the anti-diuretic action of oxytocin. Rarely, other metabolic causes of collapse like hypo/hypercalcemia or hyperkalemia can be seen on the delivery suite.

### Ischemic stroke

Arterial cerebral ischemia is rare in non-pregnant women of childbearing age, but the risk is increased nine-fold in the puerperium, with incidences of up to 200/100,000 (Kittner et al 1996). A past history of stroke does not increase the risk unless other independent risk factors such a thrombophilia are present. Most strokes in pregnancy occur in the distribution of the carotid and middle cerebral arteries resulting in contra-lateral hemiplegia and sensory loss mainly of the face and arms, there may also be dysphasia.

There are a number of rare causes of stroke that become more common in pregnancy; these include peripartum cardiomyopathy, preeclampsia, sickle cell disease and anti-phospholipid syndrome.

Magnetic resonance imaging (MRI) and computerised tomography (CT) scanning will confirm the diagnosis and exclude a hemorrhagic stroke. Low dose aspirin should be given and anticoagulation may be appropriate (Nelson-Piercy 2002).

### Hemorrhagic Stroke

Like ischemic stroke, hemorrhagic stroke risk is increased by pregnancy, particularly in the puerperium with a relative risk of 28 quoted (Kittner et al 1996). An eclamptic fit is a risk factor for intra-cerebral bleeding and evidence of cerebral haemorrhage is found in 40 per cent of women dying from eclampsia. Intra-cerebral arterio-venous malformations are also a source of bleeding in pregnancy and the puerperium. These are estrogen dependent, resulting in a tendency to increase in dilatation during pregnancy. CT or MRI scanning can confirm diagnosis; treatment is supportive, unless an AV malformation is diagnosed when surgical treatment or embolisation may be required.

### Sub-arachnoid Hemorrhage

There is a 20-fold increase in the risk of subarachnoid hemorrhage in the puerperium. The underlying pathology may be a berry aneurysm or an AV malformation, the latter being a more common cause of subarachnoid hemorrhage in the pregnant compared to the non-pregnant woman.

Collapse with impairment of consciousness is usually preceded by the sudden onset of an occipital headache. There may be associated signs of cerebral irritation, such as neck stiffness and vomiting. Examination may reveal focal neurological signs and papilledema. Urgent CT or MRI scan will confirm the diagnosis. Neurosurgical management is the same as in the non-pregnant patient (Mas and Lamy 1998).

### Cerebral Venous Thrombosis

This is a rare condition, but puerperal cases contribute significantly to the overall numbers. A rate of 11.4/10,00,000 deliveries has been documented with 29 per cent of these occurring postpartum (Laska and Kryscio 1998). Cases can be associated with a thrombophilia, but the hypercoagulable postpartum state increases the risk even in normal women after labour (Cantu and Barinagarrementeria 1993). Infection and dehydration further increase the risk and these factors may account for the higher incidence of this condition seen in developing countries. Presenting features include a headache, vomiting and photophobia, but there may be complete collapse with impaired consciousness, hemiparesis and seizures. Other forms of intracranial pathology must be excluded by MRI or CT scanning prior to treatment with rehydration, anticonvulsants and anticoagulation.

> Cerebral venous thrombosis may present with:
> - intense headache
> - vomiting
> - photophobia
> - complete collapse with impaired consciousness, hemiparesis and seizures

### Drug Overdose, Poisoning and Suicide

Psychiatric illness is common in puerperium with cases of severe postnatal depression, frequently trivialised. Suicide is a relatively common cause of death in the developed world with 10 per cent of maternal deaths in the United Kingdom due to suicide (NICE 2001). Suicide attempts in the puerperium less commonly involve overdose than at other times in women's lives, however, the diagnosis should be considered in any woman returning to hospital with collapse of unknown origin, especially if risk factors for suicide are present.

These risk factors include:

- Documented psychiatric illness since delivery, especially if treated with psychotropic drugs
- History of severe postnatal depression in a previous pregnancy
- Previous history of any psychiatric illness
- Family history of postpartum illness

## Management of postpartum collapse

The Resuscitation Council, UK, recommends starting cardio pulmonary resuscitation (CPR), using adjunct airways and defibrillation within 3 minutes of collapse due to cardiac arrest. Many physiological factors in pregnancy may impede expected response to CPR and thus need to be considered in advance (Nanda and Penna 2009).

Table 20.3 shows the physiological alterations that occur in pregnancy and the puerperium and the implications of these on resuscitation.

### The Structured approach in resuscitation

The standard structured approach in adult resuscitation is recommended as a universal practice in all specialties by the ALSG (Advance Life Support Group). This

**Table 20.3** Alterations in pregnancy and puerperium

| Factors | Physiological changes | Implications on resuscitation |
|---|---|---|
| Cardiovascular | • Increased cardiac output, stroke volume, heart rate<br>• Decreased systemic and peripheral vascular resistance and BP in first and second trimesters, though rises in third.<br>• Decreased serum colloid oncotic pressure<br>• No change in CVP | *Airway*<br>Left lateral tilt:<br>• Suction or aspiration<br>• Removing dentures or foreign bodies<br>• Inserting airways |
| Respiratory | • Increased $O_2$ consumption, metabolic rate, tidal volume<br>• Decreased functional residual capacity<br>• No change in respiratory volume, PEFR, FEV1, vital capacity<br>• Respiratory alkalosis | *Breathing*<br>• Greater oxygen requirement<br>• Reduced chest compliance<br>• More difficult to see rise and fall of chest<br>• More risk of regurgitation and aspiration |
| Hematological | • Hemodilutional anemia<br>• Hypercoagulability<br>• Fall in platelets<br>• Increase plasma volume | |
| Renal | • Increased Renal flow, GFP, creatinine clearance<br>• Proteinuria <300mg/24 hrs<br>• Physiological hydronephrosis<br>• Decreased excretion of sodium, water retention | *Circulation*<br>External chest compression difficult because of anatomical changes |
| GI and Liver | • Decreased gastric motility and emptying, risk of aspiration<br>• Increased liver metabolism | *Monitoring*<br>ECG and insertion of CVP lines might pose difficulty |
| Anatomical | • Enlarged breasts<br>• Peripheral edema<br>• Reduced chest compliance<br>• Raised diaphragm<br>• Laryngeal edema<br>• Vena caval compression due to gravid uterus in supine position (up to 90 per cent) | |

(Adapted from Nanda and Penna, 2009)

includes A, B, C, D, E of resuscitation in addition to primary survey to identify life threatening problems that require immediate attention, followed by a secondary survey to identify other problems that may be causing or contributing to the postnatal collapse. This entire process is one with continuous evaluation and resuscitation till the woman is stable, with the secondary survey delayed until the woman is stable (Grady and Cox 2001).

*Immediate action*

It is important that personal safety and the safety of the support staff are ensured prior to commencing resuscitation. Taking a brief history from the paramedics or the midwife is helpful in beginning to address the possible cause of the collapse and should include a rapid review of antenatal and intrapartum problems and a description of the events around the time of the collapse. This history can be taken simultaneous to the initial assessment of A, B, C. The initial approach should attempt to get a verbal response of some kind from the woman, as the presence or the absence of response will indicate both the extent of cerebral perfusion and respiratory status. A cervical spine injury is rare in postnatal collapse and only needs to be considered if there is a possible history of trauma or a serious fall (e.g. down stairs) during the collapse. If an injury to the neck is a possibility, manual inline stabilisation with avoidance of any head tilt must be employed until a collar can be fitted and the head immobilised by blocks. A left lateral tilt should become an automatic response during the initial resuscitation of any pregnant or recently pregnant woman. In the context of a pregnant woman, high flow oxygen can be administered from the outset whilst assessment is occurring.

> A left lateral tilt should become an automatic response during the initial resuscitation of any pregnant or recently pregnant woman

## A= Airway

Maintenance of patency of airway in a collapsed postnatal woman is of prime importance. It is important to check the airways and remove any form of physical obstruction, like foreign bodies or material such as vomit. If the woman is unconscious, a jaw tilt or thrust may be required to keep the airway patent. An airway adjunct such as a Guedel oropharyngeal airway can be used, but will only be tolerated in a deeply unconscious woman. Naso-pharygeal airways should be avoided in pregnancy, as insertion is often traumatic and bleeding can occur, exacerbating rather than relieving airway problems.

> In an unconscious woman, a jaw tilt or thrust may be required to keep the airway patent.

In a recently delivered woman, there is a higher likelihood of laryngeal edema, which may make intubation difficult and a high risk of chemical pneumonitis secondary to reflux, caused by a lax esophageal sphincter and gastric compression by the gravid uterus, if intubation is not performed. An experienced anesthetist should be called urgently to make a formal assessment of the need and likely difficulty of intubation.

## B=Breathing

Signs of breathing are assessed by looking for chest movements and listening for breath sounds (for no more than 10 seconds). Absence of breathing in the presence of a patent airway can be considered as a marker for absence of circulation. Gasping or agonal breathing is common immediately after a cardiac arrest and should not be taken as a sign for life. It is a sign of imminent death and CPR should be commenced immediately. If breathing is occurring spontaneously but the woman is unconscious, she should be placed in the left lateral position. High dose oxygen should be commenced immediately in all cases of collapse.

The UK Resuscitation Council Guidelines (2010) emphasise the importance of early commencement of effective chest compressions as opposed to deferring this until after administering rescue breaths, in the event of a diagnosed cardiac arrest. If the woman is not breathing and there are no signs of life, CPR (in the form of 30 effective chest compressions at a rate of 100 per minute followed by 2 ventilation breaths) should commence immediately with the woman in lateral tilt. Each ventilatory breath should last for 1 second and chest movement should be observed as in normal breathing. Initially, breathing can be achieved by using airway adjuncts like a pocket mask, these should be readily available in all healthcare settings, including at a homebirth and many non-healthcare settings. A bag and valve mask will be available if the collapse occurs in a hospital setting. High flow oxygen (at 12–15l/min) should be connected as soon as possible. Endo-tracheal intubation is the most effective way of providing adequate ventilation and should be undertaken as soon as an appropriately trained member of staff arrives. Following intubation, ventilation should continue at 10 breaths per minute and does not need to be synchronised with chest compressions. The recent resuscitation guidelines (UK Resuscitation Council Guidelines 2010) acknowledge that CPR can be tiring and each rescuer should take turns (changing after every 2 minutes) for chest compressions. In a hospital setting, mouth-to-mouth breathing is rarely required; nevertheless, all staff should be trained to provide it in an eventuality.

> If the woman is not breathing and there are no signs of life, CPR (in the form of 30 effective chest compressions at a rate of 100 per minute followed by 2 ventilation breaths) should commence immediately with the woman in lateral tilt.

### C=Circulation

Assessment of circulation is made at the same time as assessment of breathing, by checking for carotid or femoral pulse for no more than 10 seconds (the radial or other peripheral pulse is not an adequate check). Once CPR is in progress, the circulation should be reassessed after every 10 ventilation/compression cycles (about 2 minutes), taking no more than 10 seconds each time. A defibrillator should be attached as soon as possible if there is no effective circulation. Automated defibrillators are now available in many units, they can be used to analyse the cardiac rhythm and to defibrillate, if necessary, by any person with minimal training, whilst awaiting the arrest team. After every shock, CPR should restart for two minutes when a rhythm analysis will occur automatically by the automated defibrillator, following a verbal prompt to discontinue CPR.

Assessment of circulation is very important in a newly delivered woman, as hypovolemia secondary to postpartum hemorrhage is one of the leading causes of postpartum collapse. In the absence of obvious hemorrhage, the possibility of a concealed hemorrhage should be considered in a collapsed hypovolemic postpartum woman. A young, usually fit, recently delivered woman will usually not decompensate until she has lost 35 per cent of her total blood volume, following which the signs of hypovolemic shock – tachycardia, cold clammy extremities, hypotension become evident. Two large bore cannulae (16 g or above) should be sited, and blood should be sent for full blood count, group and cross-match, a coagulation screen (including fibrinogen degradation products), baseline urea, electrolytes and liver function. If the cause of the collapse is unknown,

> In a woman with hypovolemic shock two large bore intravenous cannulae (16 g or above) should be sited.

C-reactive protein, blood cultures, glucose, calcium and magnesium should be sent and extra clotted bottles can be taken to send for other targeted investigations. Aggressive fluid replacement should then commence to 'catch up' for any losses. However, caution should be exerted in a woman with collapse of unknown etiology, where fluid replacement should occur according to blood pressure and pulse to avoid overload if preeclampsia is ultimately found to be the underlying cause. The response to fluid administration should be monitored closely in all women, with commencement of a fluid input/output chart to document urine output and to correlate this with frequent pulse and blood pressure measurements. Fluid replacement should commence with crystalloids (Hartmann's solution or normal saline). If the collapse is due to bleeding, this should be followed by red cells as soon as possible (Shierhout and Roberts 1998).

The use of synthetic colloids (Gelofusin or Haemaccel®) is waning in modern practice, as studies have shown it has no added benefit over crystalloids and even suggest a possible worsening of mortality rate when they are administered too early. Ideally, blood replacement should be in the form of cross-matched units, but this will not be immediately available, as the cross-matching procedure takes up to 1 hour (depending on whether a pre-screen has occurred as does in women who have had blood taken in the antenatal period and the presence of abnormal antibodies in the patient). Group-specific blood can be requested if blood is required rapidly and where awaiting a full cross-match incurs too much risk. In cases of heavy rapid blood loss, universal O-negative blood can be given and this should available in all maternity units. All staff working on the labour ward should be aware of its availability and the location of its storage on the delivery suite. The administration of O-negative blood should be carefully considered, as this type of transfusion carries a much greater risk of a transfusion reaction related to other antigens. Transfusion-related acute lung injury can occur in any woman having a large blood transfusion, but the risk of this is greater with incompletely cross-matched blood.

If the circulatory collapse is due to hemorrhage, measures to reduce bleeding in the form of oxytocics and bimanual compression should continue. It is mandatory that every staff member knows the protocol for managing PPH and is aware of the means to escalate the protocol early to involve the consultant obstetrician and a senior anesthetist (even out of hours), in addition to the blood bank and a hematologist. Platelet transfusion, fresh frozen plasma (FFP), cryoprecipitate and even recombinant factor VII may be beneficial and should be considered and requested if needed. Beliefs of those such as Jehovah's Witnesses must be respected; ideally, an advanced directive should be signed antenatally and re-discussed on presentation to the delivery suite if the woman is conscious and competent to do so.

*D=Disability limitation (neurological status)*

Assessment of cerebral perfusion and state of consciousness can be made by a quick neurological examination. Although the Glasgow Coma Scale (GCS) is not widely used in obstetric practice, it is still an excellent indicator of cerebral status and severity (8 or less warranting immediate

> Transfusion-related acute lung injury can occur in any woman having massive blood transfusion.

intubation) or rapidity of deterioration (fall of 2 or more) and is used extensively in other specialities.

### E=Exposure

In the labour ward environment, the risk of hypothermia is low and a collapsed woman can be sufficiently exposed to perform a full examination and rule out any other causes of collapse. This should include a vaginal examination in addition to a detailed system examination.

A secondary survey is rarely needed in the puerperium (unless trauma has occurred), and it should be performed when the woman is clinically stable. This should include a thorough examination of cardiovascular and respiratory systems, a neurological examination including pupillary light reflex, lateralisation of limb weakness and an assessment of consciousness using a scale such as the Glasgow Coma Scale and a careful abdominal and pelvic examination. All findings should be carefully documented. Definitive care can begin when a diagnosis of cause is made and until this time, care is supportive to the woman's condition.

Additional investigations in the form of CT or MR imaging or a cardiac echo might be required and should be requested with appropriate urgency. The recent CEMACH report made the point that there is no place for a consultant-led obstetric unit, without the availability of such facilities, in modern UK practice. Admission to a high dependency unit (HDU) or an intensive care unit (ICU) might be required in a recently collapsed woman. Many obstetric units now have a HDU equipped to undertake basic critical care management. The infrastructure must include both the appropriate equipment, a set of comprehensive guidelines and midwives or nurses trained in HDU management.

A recent study indicated a better prognosis in pregnant and postnatal women admitted to the ITU compared to other ITU inpatients. Obstetric patients were found to have a lower actual mortality ratio (difference between actual and predicted mortality) of 0.25–0.42 compared to the expected mortality ratio of one.

### MEOWS

The early recognition of life-threatening illness can be challenging. Physiological reserves increase in pregnancy, and thereby conceal serious pathology. Use of a Modified Early Obstetric Warning Scoring System (MEOWS) can improve detection of life-threatening illness and has recently been recommended for all maternity units in the UK. In this system, a score is calculated on the basis of five (or six) physiological variables – these include mental response, pulse, blood pressure, temperature, respiratory rate, and urine output if post-operative. The score can be measured by midwifery and nursing staff and, if used correctly, will trigger early referral to a doctor.

> The MEOWS score is based on:
> - mental response
> - pulse
> - blood pressure
> - temperature
> - respiratory rate
> - urine output if post-operative

### Further Management

Admission to a high dependency unit or intensive care unit will be required for most women with serious postnatal collapse. Effective resuscitation will ensure reduction in initial mortality, but even with the best resuscitation, there is a high incidence of complex sequelae, including adult respiratory distress syndrome, renal failure and coagulopathy. Multidisciplinary care involving an obstetrician, anesthetist, hematologist and intensivist will offer the best chance of managing these conditions effectively, reducing mortality and morbidity.

## Preventing Collapse: Issues for future pregnancies

### Antenatal care and risk factor assessment

It is important for the obstetrician or midwife to take a comprehensive history at the first contact with every woman, identifying any risk factors that might warrant review by an obstetrician or another specialist. Early identification of risk factors and multidisciplinary involvement, effective communication and clear documentation of management plans for labour and the post-natal period can help prevent poor outcome. The advice of a specialist obstetric anesthetist should be sought in women with coexistent medical conditions who should be pre-assessed, if possible, before the onset of labour (Nanda and Penna 2009).

Women who experience serious postnatal collapse need careful counselling regarding the risk of a recurrence in a future pregnancy. Three main questions should be addressed:

- Will the problem recur in a future pregnancy?
- If it recurs, will it be worse next time?
- Is there anything that can be done to reduce the chances of a recurrent problem?

A detailed examination, including cardiovascular assessment, for all pregnant women who have recently arrived in the UK and might be at risk of TB, rheumatic heart disease and HIV is recommended as part of a strategy to identify women at high risk of problems (Lewis 2007). Women experiencing domestic violence and drug abusers also need detailed assessment.

Many conditions are spurious in nature, others can be dealt with definitively as part of the management in this pregnancy, but some conditions such as eclampsia or cardiomyopathy carry a significant risk of recurrence in a future pregnancy. These should be frankly discussed, so that the woman and her partner can decide if they wish to have another child. Worsening of a pre-existing disease may be the sequelae to their experience in this pregnancy and, as a result, may further increase the risks of a future pregnancy.

Specific management may be possible in a future pregnancy to reduce the risks of recurrence of some conditions and further investigations may be necessary, such as screening for thrombophilia. Antenatal treatments may be helpful in some conditions, such as administration of heparin to women with a significant risk of thromboembolism. Instituting prophylactic measures, such as those used in the third stage of labour to reduce the risk of postpartum hemorrhage, is essential in future management. The future mode of delivery should be reviewed. The option of an elective cesarean section may be seen by the woman as likely to reduce the risk of recurrence, but should only be advised if risk reduction and not risk increase is the expected outcome.

### Training issues

CEMACH report suggested lack of staff training as one of the contributors of substandard care in the 2003–05 triennia (Lewis 2007). All labour wards should have guidelines for resuscitation in pregnancy and specific guidelines for the management of the more common causes of collapse, such as thromboembolism. It is recommended that drills and skills sessions be organised on labour wards to ensure that all staff are familiar with the practicalities of dealing with emergency situations, where prompt efficient management can make the difference between life and death.

Training of all doctors and midwives who care for women in pregnancy and the puerperium in the techniques of cardiopulmonary resuscitation and in the management of obstetric emergencies is essential to improving maternal outcome. This can be achieved by encouraging attendance at courses such as the Advanced Life Support in Obstetrics (ALSO) courses run in the USA or Managing Obstetric Emergencies and Trauma (MOET) run in the UK (Johanson et al 1999) or The Advanced Labour and Risk Management (ALARM) Course run in Canada. Courses along these lines, emphasising the practical aspects of resuscitation by the use of models and scenarios, can be organised locally, if they are not already available.

> Training of all doctors and midwives who care for women in pregnancy and the puerperium in CPR and in the management of obstetric emergencies is essential to improving maternal outcome.

## Clinical Governance

Enquiries and audit of near misses and serious untoward incidents (SUIs), improvement in communication, senior support (consultant or other senior presence on labour wards), team working, awareness and adoption of clearly documented protocols in managing emergencies and staff training in early recognition and management of the seriously ill pregnant woman with impending maternal collapse has been shown to improve care and outcome.

## Further Training (UK)

MOET: Managing Obstetric Emergencies and Trauma

ALSO: Advanced Life Support in Obstetrics

OATS: Obstetric Anaesthetist Training in the Simulator

MOSES: Multidisciplinary Obstetric Simulated Emergency Scenarios

PROMPT: Practical Obstetric Multi-Professional Training

(www.bartsandthelondon.org.uk)

## References

Abdi S, Cameron IC, Nakielny R, Majeed A. 2001. Spontaneous hepatic rupture and maternal death following an uncomplicated pregnancy and delivery. *Br J Obstet Gynaecol* 108:431–33.

ACOG Practice Bulletin (19). 2000. Thromboembolism in pregnancy. *Int J Gynecol Obstet* 75:203–212.

Astiz M, Rackow E. 1998. Septic shock. *Lancet* 351:1501–1505.

Bhalla R, Wuntakal R, Odejinmi F, Khan RU. 2009. *The Obstetrician & Gynaecologist* 11(1): 13–18.

Birth after previous caeserean sections. 2007. RCOG Press www.rcog.org.uk/files/rcogcorp/uploadedfiles/GT45BirthafterPreviousCeasarean.pdf

Burden RJ, Janke EL, Brighouse D. 1994. Hyperventilation-induced unconsciousness during labour. *Br J Anaes* 73(6):838–39.

Cantu C, Barinagarrementeria F. 1993. Cerebral venous thrombosis associated with pregnancy and puerperium. Review of 67 cases. *Stroke* 24(12):1880–84.

Chan L, Hill D. 1999. ED echocardiography for peripartum cardiomyopathy. *Am J Emerg Med* 17(6):578–80.

Chen FG, Koh KF, Chong YS. 1998. Cardiac arrest associated with sulprostone use during caesarean section. *Anaesth Intensive Care* 26(3):298–301.

Clark S. 1986. Amniotic fluid embolism. *Clin Perinat* 13(4):801–11.

Clark S, Hankins G, Dudley D, Dildy G, Flint Porter T. 1995. Amniotic fluid embolism: Analysis of the National registry. *Am J Obstet Gynecol* 172 (4pt1):1158–69.

De Swiet M. 1999. Management of pulmonary embolus in pregnancy. *Eur Heart J* 20:1372–85.

Douglas KA, Redman CW. 1994. Eclampsia in the United Kingdom. *BMJ* 309:1395–1400.

Duley L, Carroli G, Belizan J. 1995. Which anticonvulsant for women with eclampsia-evidence from the collaborative eclampsia study. *Lancet* 345:1455–63.

Advanced life support working group of the European resuscitation council. 1998. The 1998 European Resuscitation council guidelines for adult advanced life support. *BMJ* 316:1863–70.

Faro S. 1999. Sepsis in obstetric and gynecologic patients. *Curr Clin Top Infect Dis* 19:60–82.

Gardeil F, Daly S, Turner MJ. 1994. Uterine rupture in pregnancy reviewed. *Europ J Obstet Gynecol Reprod Biol* 56(2):107–110.

Gilbert W, Danielsen B. 1999. Amniotic fluid embolism: Decreased mortality in a population based study. *Obstet Gynecol* 93(6):973–77.

Grady K, Cox C. 2001. Structured approach. In *MOET Provider Manual*. RCOG Press: London.

Greer I. 1999. Thrombosis in pregnancy: Maternal and fetal issues. *Lancet* 10(353):1258–65.

Hankins GD, Wendel Jr GD, Leveno KJ, Stoneham J. 1985b. Myocardial infarction during pregnancy; a review. *Obstet Gynecol* 65:139–46.

Hankins GD, Brekken AL, Davis LM. 1985a. Maternal death secondary to a dissecting aneurysm of the pulmonary artery. *Obstet Gynecol* 65(3 suppl):45s–48s.

Heaven D, Sutton R. 2000. Syncope. *Crit Care Med* 28(10):116–20.

Hibbard LT 1976. Spontaneous liver rupture in pregnancy a report of eight cases. *Am J Obstet Gynecol* 126:334–38.

Hill K, Abouzahr C, Wardlaw T. 2001. Estimates of maternal mortality for 1995. *Bull World Health Organisation* 79(3):182–93.

Ilsaas C, Husby P, Koller ME, Segadal L, Holst-Larsen H. 1998. Cardiac arrest due to massive pulmonary embolism following caesarean section. Successful resuscitation and pulmonary embolectomy. *Acta Anaesth Scand* 42(2):264–66.

Irani S, Jordan J. 1997. Management of uterine inversion. *Curr Obstet Gynaecol* 7:232–253.

Jevon P. 2000. Anaphylaxis. *Emer Manage* 96(14):39–40.

Jevon P, Raby M. 2001. *Resuscitation in pregnancy: A practical approach*.

Johanson R, Cox C, Donnell E, Grady K et al. 1999. Managing obstetric emergencies and trauma (MOET). *Obstet Gynaecol* 1(2):46–52.

Katsiris S, Williams S, Leighton B, Halpern S. 1999. Respiratory arrest following intrathecal injection of sufentanil and bipivicaine in a parturient. *Can J Anaesth* 45(9):880–83.

Kindig M, Cardwell M, Lee T. 1998. Delayed postpartum uterine dehiscence. A case report. *J Reprod Med* 43(7):591–92.

Kittner S, Stern B, Feeser B et al. 1996. Pregnancy and the risk of stroke. *N Eng J Med* 335:768–74.

Knight M. 2008. The UK Obstetric Surveillance System. *Obstet Gynaecol Repro Med* 18(7):199–200.

Knight M, Tuffnell D, Brockelhurst P, Spark P, Kurinczuk JJ. 2010. Incidence and risk factors for amniotic-fluid embolism. *Obstet Gynaecol* 115(5):910–917.

Ko W, Ho H, Chu S. 1998. Postpartum mycardial infarction rescued with an intraaortic balloon pump and extracorporeal membrane oxygenator. *Int J Cardiol* 63(1):81–84.

Laska D, Kryscio R. 1998. Stroke and intracranial venous thrombosis during pregnancy and puerperium. *Neurology* 51(6):1622–28.

Lee W, Cotton D, Hankins G, Faro S. 1989. Management of septic shock complicating pregnancy. *Obstet Gynecol Clin North Am* 16(2):431–47.

Leiserowitz GS, Evans AT, Samuels SJ. 1992. Creatinine kinase and its MB iosenzyme in the third trimester and the peripartum period. *J Reprod Med* 37:910.

Lewis G (ed). 2007. The Confidential Enquiry into Maternal and Child Health (CEMACH). Saving Mothers' Lives: reviewing maternal deaths to make motherhood safer- 2003-2005. The Seventh Report on Confidential Enquiries into Maternal Deaths in the United Kingdom. CEMACH: London. www.cemach.org.uk

Lind J, Wallenburg H. 2001. The Marfan syndrome and pregnancy: a retrospective study in a Dutch population. *Eur J Obstet Gynecol* 98:28–35.

Lupton M, Oteng-Ntim, Ayida G, Steer P. 2002. Cardiac disease in pregnancy. *Curr Opin Obstet Gynaecol* 14(2):137–44.

Mabie WC, Freire CM. 1995. Sudden chest pain and cardiac emergencies in the Obstetric patient. *Obstet Gynecol Clin North Am* 22(1):19–37.

Macklon N. 1999. Diagnosis of deep venous thrombosis and pulmonary embolus in pregnancy. *Curr Opin Pulm Med* 5:233–37.

Magpie Trial Collaboration Group. 2002. Do women with pre-eclampsia, and their babies benefit from magnesium sulphate? The Magpie trial: A randomized placebo-controlled trial. *Lancet* 359(9321):1877–90.

Majhi AK, Mondal A, Mukherjee GG. 2001. Safe motherhood: A long way to achieve. *J Ind Med* 99(3):132–37.

Mas JL and Lamy C. 1998. Stoke in pregnancy and the puerperium. *J Neurol* 245:305–13.

Michala L, Madhavan B, Win N, De Lord C, Brown R. 2008. Transfusion-related acute lung injury (TRALI) in an obstetric patient. *Int J Obstet Anesth* 17(1):66–69.

Murray R, Tancredi D, Nadel E, Brown D. 2000. Syncope in pregnancy. *J Emerg Med* 19(1):57.

Nanda S, Penna LK. 2009. Post partum Collapse. *Obstet Gynaecol Repro Med* 19(8):221–228.

Nelson-Piercy C. 2002. *Handbook of obstetric medicine*, 2nd ed. Martin Dunitz Ltd.: London.

NICE. 2008. *Intrapartum care guideline*.

NICE (National Institute for clinical excellence). 2001. *Why mothers die 1997–1999*: The confidential enquiries into maternal deaths in UK. London: RCOG Press.

Ogueh O, Ayaida G. 1997. Acute uterine inversion: a new technique of hydrostatic replacement. *Br J Obstet Gynaecol* 104:951–52.

Pandian Z, Wagaarachchi P, Danelian P. 2001. An unusual case of hypovolemic shock in the postpartum period. *Acta Obstet Gynecol Scand* 80:871–72.

Pearson G, Veille J, Rahimtoola S et al. 2000. Peripartum cardiomyopathy. National heart, lung and blood institute and Office of rare diseases (NIH): Workshop recommendations and review. *JAMA* 283:1183–88.

Perlitz Y, Markovitz VJ, Ami MB, Matilsky M, Oettinger M. 1999. Acute adrenal insufficiency during pregnancy and puerperium: Case report and literature review. *Obstet Gynecol Surv* 54(11):717–22.

Philippe HJ, Karanouh S, Rozenberg P, Dien DT, Nisand I. 1997. Transvaginal surgery for uterine scar dehiscence. *Europ J Obstet Gynecol Reprod Biol* 73(2):135–38.

Project team of the resuscitation council (UK). 1999. The emergency medical treatment of anaphylaxis. *J Anaes Emer* 16(4):243–47.

Ramsey P, Ramin K, Ramin S. 2001. Cardiac disease in pregnancy. *Am L Perinat* 18(5):245–65.

RCOG Greentop guideline No: 45. 2007. *Birth after Previous Cesarean section*. RCOG Press.

RCOG Greentop guideline No. 47. 2008. *Blood transfusion in Obstetrics*. RCOG press. www.rcog.org.uk/files/rcog-corp/uploadedfiles/GT47BloodTransfusions1207amended.pdf

RCOG Greentop guideline No. 52. 2009. *Prevention and management of postpartum haemorrhage*. RCOG press. www.rcog.org.uk/files/rcog-corp/Green-top52PostpartumHaemorrhage.pdf

Resuscitation Council UK. 2005. Adult advanced life support algorithm. www.resus.org.uk/pages/alsalgo.pdf

Rogers L, Dangel-Palmer M, Berner N. 2000. Acute circulatory collapse on obstetrical patients: A case report and review of the literature. *ANNA J* 68(5):444–45.

Roth A, Elkayam U.1996. Acute myocardial infarction associated with pregnancy. *Ann Intern Med* 125:751–57.

Shierhout G, Roberts I. 1998. Fluid resuscitation with crystalloid or colloid in critically ill patients: A systematic review of randomised trials. *BMJ* 316:961–64.

Takacs C, Krivak T, Napolitano P. 2002. Insulinoma in pregnancy: A case report and review of the literature. *Obstet Gynecol Surv* 57(4):229–35.

Thompson AJ, Greer I. 2000. Non-haemorrhagic obstetric shock. *Best Prac Res Clin Obstet Gynaecol* 14(1):19–41.

Toglia M, Nolan T. 1997. Venous thrombo-embolism during pregnancy: a current review of diagnosis and management. *Obstet Gynecol Surv* 52(1):60–72.

Waterstone M, Bewley S, Wolfe C. 2001. Incidence and predictors of severe obstetric morbidity: case control study. *BMJ* 322(7294):1089–94.

Webb JC, Gilson G, Gordon L. 2000. Late second stage rupture of the uterus and bladder with vaginal birth after cesarean section: A case report and review of the literature. *J Mat Fet Med* 9(6):362–65.

Wendel PJ, Cox SM. 1995. Emergency obstetric management of uterine inversion. *Obstet Gynecol* 22:261–74.

# CHAPTER 21

# THE MANAGEMENT OF OBSTETRIC PERINEAL TRAUMA

*Terence Lao*

## Definition

- **First degree tears** involve damage to the fourchette and vaginal mucosa, exposing, but not damaging, the underlying muscles
- **Second degree tears** involve damage to the vaginal and perineal muscles, but anal sphincter is intact
- **Third degree tears** extend to the anal sphincter which is torn, but with the rectal/anal mucosa intact
    - Less than 50 per cent of the external anal sphincter (EAS) thickness is torn
    - More than 50 per cent of the EAS thickness is torn, but the internal anal sphincter (IAS) is intact
    - Both EAS and IAS are torn
- **Fourth degree tears** involve the rectal/anal mucosa in addition, and the anal canal is opened, with possible extension to the rectum.
- **Button-hole tear** refers to the situation where the anal sphincter is intact, but the anal mucosa is torn. This has to be distinguished from a fourth degree tear since the repair is different.

## Epidemiology

The quoted risk is about 1 per cent of all vaginal deliveries. However, it is estimated that a third of women who had vaginal delivery sustained occult anal sphincter trauma, but the diagnosis depends on awareness, training and experience. The prevalence is likely to increase, especially with the availability of anal ultrasound scanning.

Previous anal sphincter tears are associated with increased risk of severe lacerations and sphincter tears in subsequent vaginal deliveries, with a recurrent risk of about three- to four-fold, which is influenced by the birth weight of the baby (Spydslaug et al 2005; Dandolu et al 2005). However, it has also been reported that the rate for recurrent lacerations was significantly lower than the rate for initial lacerations. Previous fourth degree tear has a higher rate of recurrence than previous third degree tear. Forceps delivery with episiotomy had the highest, while ventouse extraction without episiotomy had the lowest risk of recurrence.

Previous pregnancy by itself does not protect against sphincter lacerations in subsequent pregnancies (Walsh et al 1996; Dee Leeuw et al 2001; Lowder et al 2007).

## Pathology

A rigid non-compliant perineum, an excessively big presenting part and rapid forceful stretching of the perineum at delivery, can cause tearing of the vaginal mucosa, perineal skin and underlying muscles. It can be envisaged that weakening of the perineum induced with an episiotomy can make the situation worse. As the anal sphincters (EAS and IAS) are close by, these structures can easily be damaged with a posterior extension of the tear.

> Perineal tears can be caused by
> - a rigid non-compliant perineum
> - an excessively big presenting part
> - rapid forceful stretching of the perineum at delivery

The three dominant factors found in most studies are forceps delivery, nulliparity, and episiotomy (Hudelist et al 2005). Among primiparous women with vaginal delivery, 25 per cent had impaired fecal continence and 45 per cent had abnormal anal physiology (Sultan and Thakar 2002). Instrumental delivery and a second stage prolonged by epidural analgesia posed the greatest risk. On the other hand, parity did not reduce the association between forceps delivery and anal sphincter injuries. For instrumental delivery, the results of most studies indicated that ventouse extraction was associated with a much lower, or an insignificant, risk of anal sphincter injury, although an occasional study reported otherwise.

Ethnicity is apparently a contributory factor, with Indian, Filipino and other Asian women having higher risks, and African-American, Hispanic, and Native American women having lower risk, the underlying explanation remains unknown.

Third and fourth degree tears often involve damage to the neighbouring tissues and organs. Immediate and short-term problems include hemorrhage, hematoma, nerve palsy, perineal pain, and fistulae, while long-term complications include dyspareunia, urinary and fecal incontinence, and urogenital prolapse.

## Etiology

Any situations that result in the rapid overstretching of the perineum, especially in the presence of a defect/weakness in the perineum due to current or prior lacerations, can lead to the occurrence of a third or fourth degree tear (Bodner-Adler et al 2001; Christianson et al 2003).

The known risk factors are listed below:

- Nulliparity
- Fetal macrosomia (birthweight >4.0 kg)
- Persistent occipital posterior position
- Induction of labour
- Epidural analgesia
- Second stage longer than 1 hour
- Shoulder dystocia
- Midline episiotomy
- Instrumental delivery – more likely with forceps
- Third or fourth degree tear in a previous pregnancy

## Prognosis

At three months postpartum, about a third of women with anal sphincter trauma had abnormal anorectal function, and less than 10 per cent had fecal incontinence and/or flatus incontinence (Sultan and Thakar 2002). The long-term result of overlapping repair appeared to deteriorate with time. In a group of patients with a median follow-up period of 77 months, only half were considered to have had a successful outcome, but none was fully continent to both feces and flatus. A pad for incontinence was still required in 52 per cent, life-style restriction was reported in 65 per cent, and 36 per cent had the onset of a new evacuation disorder (Malouf et al 2000). However, recent data suggests that the overlapping technique appears to be associated with better results, although no significant difference in anal continence between these two methods was found on long-term (median 26 months) follow-up (Fernando et al 2002).

> Advantages of overlap repair of EAS:
> - visualisation of the whole length of the EAS
> - greater surface area of contact between the muscles
> - creates a longer anal length
> - decreases chances of fecal incontinence

Pregnancy itself does not appear to reduce the risk of anal sphincter tear in subsequent pregnancies, for the risk in women undergoing a trial of labour after one previous cesarean delivery is similar to that in nulliparous women. Women with prior anal sphincter tear have as much as four-fold increased risk of a recurrence in the subsequent pregnancy. The recurrence risk was reported to be higher with fourth than third degree tears (Payne et al 1999; Dandolu et al 2005). Forceps delivery with episiotomy had the highest risk, while ventouse extraction had slight increased or no increased risk of recurrence. The absolute recurrence risk was also correlated with birthweight, being 1.3 per cent for birthweight <3000 g to 23.3 per cent for birthweight >5000 g (Sau et al 2004; Donnelly et al 1998).

## Clinical approach

### Prevention

It should be realised that the awareness of the presence of risk factors does not necessarily translate into prediction or prevention.

- ❖ Restrictive episiotomy: Irrespective of the presence of other risk factors, restrictive episiotomy can significantly reduce the overall risk of anal sphincter tear and that attributable to episiotomy by up to 50 per cent.
- ❖ Performing a mediolateral episiotomy: A median episiotomy is more likely to extend into the anal sphincter than a mediolateral episiotomy (Clemons et al 2005).
- ❖ Avoid haste in the delivery of the shoulders following instrumental delivery, and involve an assistant to guard the perineum. This will minimise the risk of shoulder dystocia, as well as prevent the extension of the episiotomy towards the anal sphincter caused by the posterior shoulder.
- ❖ In high-risk pregnancies such as fetal macrosomia in the presence of maternal short stature, maternal conditions requiring instrumental delivery, or fetal conditions likely to require operative

delivery, the route of delivery should be reviewed and discussed with the patient, with a detailed explanation of the potential risks. An elective cesarean section may be preferable under the circumstances.

❖ In women with prior third or fourth degree tears and persistent symptoms or evidence of defect in endosonography, an elective cesarean delivery should be offered, especially if associated risk factors are present.

**Repair**

The basic principles of episiotomy repair also apply here, and the general preparations will not be repeated (Handa et al 2001; Williams et al 2006; RCOG Green top guidelines 2007).

1. The repair should take place under general or regional anesthesia in a proper operating theatre, under good lighting and aseptic conditions.

   > The repair should take place under general or regional anesthesia in a proper operating theatre under good lighting and aseptic conditions.

2. The trauma area should be thoroughly cleansed with antiseptic solution prior to the repair. In case of fourth degree tear, the exposed lumen of the rectal/anal canal must be cleansed and all fecal soiling must be removed before repair.

3. Inspection is paramount in identifying the degree of tear and in defining the extent of the wound. The torn muscle fibres of the anal sphincter may be readily identified. If the completely torn muscles have retracted into the fat, the ends cannot be located. Under this situation, evoking the anal reflex by means of stroking gently with the tip of artery forceps radially from the anus towards the posterolateral aspects of the buttocks may be helpful. Normally, this causes the anal sphincter to constrict. If the sphincter is torn, the contracting muscles actually pull the torn edges apart, and the dimples on the skin of either side of the torn edges indicate the sites of attachment of the muscle ends which can be excavated from the fat and held with an Allis forceps. The ends are then brought together with the Allis forceps, for repair.

4. The torn anal/rectal mucosa is repaired with interrupted 2/0 or 3/0 absorbable sutures (PDS or Vicryl) on an atraumatic round body needle. The needle should take up enough of the submucosal tissue to ensure adequate apposition and closure, and everting the torn edges into the lumen of the rectum without excessive tension. The stitches are placed about 5 mm apart and the knots are tied in the anal lumen. This is continued to just beyond the muco-cutaneous junction, so that the gap in the rectal/anal wall is completely closed.

5. The alignment of the wound is inspected again. If all is satisfactory, then the repair is carried out in sections. Early primary repair of the sphincter seems to be better and preferable to secondary repair. The IAS should be identified. It is paler than the EAS and its fibres run in a circular fashion between the EAS and anal epithelium. The torn ends are grasped with an Allis forceps and an end-to-end repair is done with mattress sutures (2/0 or 3/0 PDS or Vicryl). Single

interrupted sutures are more likely to cut through the muscle fibres and cause more damage as the knot is tied.

6. The EAS can be repaired using the overlapping or the end-to-end technique using 2/0 sutures.

### End-to-end repair technique

For this technique, the torn ends are united together with either figure-of-eight or mattress sutures, the latter being preferred as the former may cause ischemia of the muscle ends and affect healing. This method is preferred for a 3a tear in which <50 per cent of the EAS is torn. The disadvantage of this technique is that complete apposition of the torn EAS may not be possible, thus resulting in a shorter anal length.

### Overlapping technique

The overlapping method involves bringing the torn ends of the EAS to overlap each other in a 'double-breast' fashion, using an Allis forceps. The full length of the EAS should be identified to ensure complete approximation and overlap. The muscles of the EAS may need to be mobilised from the surrounding ischio-anal fat by sharp dissection with scissors. Overlap repair ensures visualisation of the whole length of the EAS and greater surface area of contact between the muscles. This will recreate a longer anal length, which is a determinant for fecal incontinence, than is the case with the end-to-end repair. The first (most distal) stitch is inserted through the muscle on one side about 1.5 cm from the torn end and carried to 0.5 cm from the edge of the other side. The needle is then reinserted about 0.5 cm proximally on the other side and carried to the original side, exiting at the same distance from the end, thus forming a loop. The stitch is cut and the ends held with artery forceps. Subsequent stitches are then applied in a similar manner until the entire length of the EAS has been taken up. With an assistant holding the torn ends in place with Allis forceps, the knots are tied, one by one, starting from the most distal loop. This approach will ensure that the tension of the sutures and the approximation of the muscle fibres to be as close to uniform as possible. Further, in a naturally occurring tear of the sphincter, the torn ends are often ragged and of different sizes, and this approach allows the individual stitches to be adjusted to ensure the best anatomical alignment of the torn ends.

7. The rest of the vagina and perineum is repaired in the same way as in the case of an episiotomy. The reconstruction of the perineal muscles is important in ensuring an adequate perineum to reduce the risk of the known long-term complications, including a recurrence of anal sphincter injury in subsequent deliveries. A drain may be necessary for any tunnel or hematoma.

8. A combined rectal and vaginal examination must be performed afterwards to ensure the repair is complete and that no swabs are left behind.

## Postoperative management

The management is similar to that of an episiotomy with the following additions.

❖ Antibiotic cover should be given to prevent infection and breaking down of the repair with the possibility of fistula formation. Intravenous metronidazole (500 mg)

> Antibiotic cover prevents infection and breaking down of the repair/ fistula formation.

- and a cephalosporin (e.g. cefuroxime 1.5 g) should be commenced during the procedure and continued with oral administration after the first 24 hours, for a total of one week.
- If infection is suspected, swabs should be taken from the vagina and rectum, and midstream urine collected, for culture. Meanwhile, an aminoglycoside (e.g. gentamicin 80–120 mg, eight-hourly) should be given in addition.
- Adequate analgesia should be given liberally, since the perineal pain can easily lead to urine retention and constipation.
- A Foley catheter should be inserted routinely for the first 24 hours, since in the majority of the women, the pain and discomfort of the repair, together with the residual effect of any regional or general anesthesia, may impair the sensation and the ability to empty the bladder completely, thus leading to residual urine and urinary infection.
- A stool softener (e.g. lactulose 15 ml bid) and a bulking agent should be prescribed routinely for at least 2 weeks to prevent constipation and the passage of a large bolus of hard stool which can disrupt the repair.
- The operative findings and the repair procedure should be clearly documented in detail in the clinical notes. The patient should receive a complete explanation of the events and the prognosis before discharge.
- Postnatal pelvic floor exercise should be arranged following discharge from hospital.
- Postnatal follow-up should be arranged for as long as necessary, depending on the symptoms and the clinical findings. It is not realistic to expect every hospital to have the expertise and the equipments to perform anorectal physiology tests and endoanal ultrasound. If necessary, the patient should be referred to the appropriate specialist or a colorectal surgeon for secondary sphincter. The mode of delivery for future pregnancies should be discussed. Cesarean delivery should be offered or recommended and documented in the notes if there is residual or persistent symptoms and/or demonstrable defects.
- There are medico-legal concerns. While the occurrence of obstetric anal sphincter injury is not considered substandard care, the failure to recognise such an injury, to perform an adequate repair, or to arrange the appropriate follow-up management and referral where appropriate, especially if healing fails, may be considered substandard care. Careful detailed documentation, and updating the patient on the progress and counselling on management plan, are essential steps in minimising the risk of litigation.

## References

Bodner-Adler B, Bodner K, Kaider A, Wagenbichier P, Leodolter S, Husslein P, Mayerhofer K. 2001. Risk factors for third degree perineal tears in vaginal delivery, with an analysis of episiotomy types. *J Reprod Med*. 46: 752–56.

Christianson LM, Bovbjerg VE, McDavitt EC, Hullfish KL. 2003. Risk factors for perineal injury during delivery. *Am J Obstet Gynecol*. 189: 255–260.

Clemons JL, Towers GD, McClure GB, O'Boyle AL. 2005. Decreased anal sphincter lacerations associated with restrictive episiotomy use. *Am J Obstet Gynecol*. 192: 1260–65.

Dandolu V, Gaughan JP, Chatwani AJ, Harmanli O, Mabine B, Hernandez E. 2005. Risk of recurrence of anal sphincter lacerations. *Obstet Gynecol*. 105: 831–835.

De Leeuw JW, Struijk PC, Vierhout ME, Wallenburg HCS. 2001. Risk factors for third degree perineal ruptures during delivery. *BJOG* 108: 383–87.

Donnelly V, Fynes M, Campbell D, Johnson H, O'Connell R, O'Herlihy C. 1998. Obstetric events leading to anal sphincter damage. *Obstet Gynecol*. 92: 955–61.

Fernando RJ, Sultan AH, Radley S, Jones PW, Johanson RB. 2002. Management of obstetric anal sphincter injury: a systematic review and national practice survey. *BMC Health Services Research* 2:9–18.

Handa VL, Danielsen BH, Gilbert WM. 2001. Obstetric anal sphincter lacerations. *Obstet Gynecol*. 98: 225–30.

Hudelist G, Gelle'n J, Singer C, Ruecklinger E, Czerwenka K, Kandolf O, Keckstein J. 2005. Factors predicting severe perineal trauma during childbirth: role of forceps delivery routinely combined with mediolateral episiotomy. *Am J Obstet Gynecol*. 192: 875–81.

Lowder JL, Burrows LJ, Krohn MA, Weber AM. 2007. Risk factors for primary and subsequent anal sphincter lacerations: a comparison of cohorts by parity and prior mode of delivery. *Am J Obstet Gynecol*. 196: e1–5.

Malouf AJ, Norton CS, Engel AF, Nicholls RJ, Kamm MA. 2000. Long-term results of overlapping anterior anal-sphincter repair for obstetric trauma. *Lancet* 355: 260–65.

Payne TN, Carey JC, Rayburn WF. 1999. Prior third- or fourth-degree perineal tears and recurrence risks. *Int J Gynecol Obstet*. 64: 55–7.

Poen AC, Felt-bersma RJF, Strijers RLM, Dekker GA, Cuesta MA, Meuwissen SGM. 1998. Third degree obstetric perineal tear: long-term clinical and functional results after primary repair. *Br J Surg*. 85: 1433–38.

Royal College of Obstetricians and Gynaecologists. March 2007. Green-top Guideline No.29. www.rcog.org.uk/greentopguidelines

Sau A, Sau M, Ahmed H, Brown R. 2004. Vacuum extraction: is there any need to improve the current training in the UK? *Acta Obstet Gynecol Scand* 83: 466–70.

Spydslaug A, Trogstad LIS, Skrondal A, Eskild A. 2005. Recurrent risk of anal sphincter laceration among women with vaginal deliveries. *Obstet Gynecol*. 105: 307–13.

Sultan AH, Thakar R. 2002. Lower genital tract and anal sphincter trauma. *Best Practice & Research Clinical Obstetrics and Gynaecology* 16: 99–115.

Walsh CJ, Mooney EF, Upton GJ, Motson RW. 1996. Incidence of third-degree perineal tears in labour and outcome after primary repair. *Br J Surg*. 83: 218–21.

Williams A, Adams EJ, Tincello DG, Alfirevic Z, Walkinshaw SA, Richmond DH. 2006. How to repair an anal sphincter injury after vaginal delivery: Results of a randomized controlled trial. *BJOG* 113: 201–7.

Useful websites

www.patient.co.uk

Patient information and contacts

www.rcog.org.uk

Royal College of Obstetricians and Gynecologists

# CHAPTER 22

# PROSTAGLANDINS IN LABOUR

*Uma Ram and Shobana Mahadevan*

Since their discovery in the early 1970s, prostaglandins (PGs) have contributed significantly to the practice of obstetrics. Over the years, many PG compounds have been discovered and the importance of the role of prostaglandins in several reproductive processes including menstruation, ovulation and parturition has become apparent. Significant advances have been made in the application of prostaglandins to common clinical problems in obstetrics.

Prostaglandins are important mediators of uterine activity and play a pivotal role in the contraction of the smooth muscle of the uterus and the biophysical changes associated with cervical ripening. Indeed, prostaglandins seem to play a much larger role in labour than oxytocin.

Prostaglandins are produced by almost every tissue in the body and serve as important messengers or effectors in a wide variety of functions. When efforts are made to accelerate or inhibit the effects of prostaglandins in labour, we also have to deal with their effects on other organs and systems. Attempts to inhibit the production of prostaglandins in an effort to reduce myometrial contractility are limited by the important role of prostaglandins in the maintenance of fetal ductal flow and renal blood flow. Similarly, administration of prostaglandins for the purpose of inducing labour or ripening an unfavourable cervix has to be balanced against the effects of these agents on other systems, including the gastrointestinal tract and brain (O'Brien et al 1995).

The F and E series prostaglandins are the most important for labour, delivery and the postpartum period. In contrast to oxytocin, which requires an induction of receptors that does not usually occur until the later part of pregnancy, prostaglandin receptors are always present in myometrial tissue. This allows for the use of prostaglandins throughout pregnancy.

Although both the F and E series prostaglandins result in uterine contractions, the E series of prostaglandins are relatively more utero-selective and are more effective in producing cervical ripening.

Modification of the naturally-occurring prostaglandins has resulted in products that are longer acting and effective at lower concentrations, with the potential for significant savings in cost. This has allowed their widespread use in developing countries. Problems such as intrauterine fetal death and intractable hemorrhage from postpartum uterine atony, which earlier may have required surgical intervention, can be managed with prostaglandins.

Currently, all prostaglandins used in clinical practice are synthetic. Those like PGE$_2$ and PGF$_2\alpha$ which retain the molecular structure present in nature, are called 'natural' while those synthesised with a different structure are called 'analogues'.

## Structure and Classification

Prostaglandins are members of the eicosanoid family. They are synthesised from arachidonic acid. Each molecule has 20 carbon atoms with a cyclopentane ring and two side chains (Figure 22.1). The position of the side chains and number of multiple bonds determine the group identity and its action. Prostaglandins were designated PG$_1$, PG$_2$, PG$_3$ based on the number of double bonds in the polyunsaturated fatty acids from which they are formed. They were initially divided into classes E and F because of their solubility in ether and phosphate buffer. Subsequently, they have been divided into ten main groups, A to I. The subscripts (alpha, beta) were then added i.e. PGF$_2\alpha$ (Van Dorp et al 1964; Bergström et al 1964)

## Metabolism

Arachidonic acid is metabolised (Figure 22.2) by the enzyme prostaglandin H synthase (PGHS), formerly called fatty-acid cyclooxygenase. The release of arachidonic acid from glycerophospholipids in the plasma membrane has generally been regarded as being the rate-limiting step in prostaglandin biosynthesis (Rice 1995). Prostaglandins act through a number of G-protein coupled receptors. The final pathways involve intracellular cyclic AMP and intracellular calcium. While an increase in intracellular calcium is responsible for contraction, increase in cyclic AMP promotes relaxation. Thus, by modifying these pathways, PGE$_2$ and PGI$_2$ promote uterine quiescence. PGE$_2$ in particular causes cervical ripening. On the other hand, PGF$_2\alpha$ causes uterine contractions. Prostaglandin is catabolised by the enzyme 15-OH PG dehydrogenase to its metabolites, several of which are bioactive. This enzyme is mainly localised in the chorion and prevents the prostaglandins from reaching the myometrium in the non-labouring state.

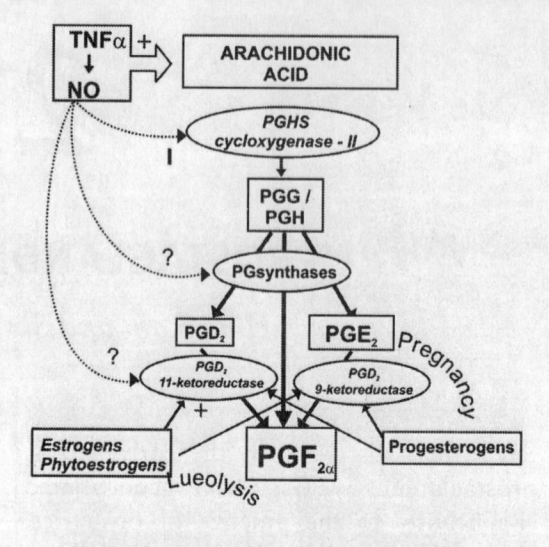

Figure 22.2 Metabolism of prostaglandins

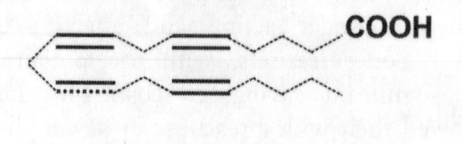

Figure 22.1 Prostaglandin structure

## Distribution in normal tissues

PGE$_2$ is the main prostaglandin product of the fetal membranes. The inner membrane, the amnion, has the highest production rate (Olson et al 1993). PGE$_2$ production by the amnion, chorion, and decidua is increased during labour (Olson et al 1993). Though PGE$_2$ and F$_{2\alpha}$ are detected in the amniotic fluid in all stages of gestation, the major increase occurs with the onset of labour, and they continue to increase with cervical dilatation (MacDonald and Casey 1993). It has been shown that prostaglandin concentrations in amniotic fluid increase early in labour (i.e., <3 cm dilation) before the active stage of labour is reached (Romero 1994)

## Properties and clinical effects

Both PGE$_2$ and PGF$_2\alpha$ stimulate contractions in the pregnant uterus and have similar side effects, especially gastrointestinal, but there are also differences. PGF$_2\alpha$ is a bronchoconstrictor, while PGE$_2$ is not; PGE$_2$ influences thermal regulation, PGF$_2\alpha$ alpha does not; PGE$_2$ is a vasodilator, PGF$_2\alpha$ alpha is a vasoconstrictor.

In the same doses, PGE$_2$ is 10 times more potent on the pregnant uterus (Keirse 1992). Because PGF$_2\alpha$ needs to be administered in larger doses, it causes more side effects, gastrointestinal in particular.

- PGF$_2\alpha$
  - Bronchoconstrictor
  - Vasoconstrictor
- PGE$_2$
  - Influences thermal regulation
  - Vasodilator

Misoprostol is a methyl ester of PGE$_1$. It is inexpensive, easily stored at room temperature and has few systemic side effects. When taken orally or used vaginally, it is rapidly absorbed and converted to misoprostol acid, its active metabolite. Plasma concentrations of misoprostol peak in approximately 30 minutes after oral administration and 80 minutes after vaginal administration and decline rapidly thereafter (Zieman et al 1997). It is primarily degraded in the liver, with less than 1 per cent of the active metabolite excreted in urine (Foote et al 1995). When administered vaginally, there are reduced peak concentrations (227 pg/ml vs 165 pg/ml), longer time to peak concentration of 1 to 2 hours and more area under the misoprostol concentration versus time curve, indicating greater time of exposure than orally administered misoprostol (Zieman et al 1997; Tang et al 2002).

> Plasma concentrations of misoprostol peak in approximately 30 minutes after oral and 80 minutes after vaginal administration and decline rapidly thereafter.

Side effects include nausea, vomiting, diarrhea, abdominal pain, chills and fever. These side effects are more with oral than vaginal use and are dose related. The effect on the reproductive tract is more with the vaginal route. The sublingual route acts as rapidly as the oral, but the effect on uterine contractions is similar to the vaginal route (Aronsson et al 2004).

## Role of prostaglandins in labour

The role of prostaglandins in labour includes softening of the cervix, induction of gap junctions (communication between smooth muscle cells through which conduction of electrophysiological stimuli occur) and direct stimulation of uterine contractions.

## Cervical ripening

The first report of the use of prostaglandin in labour was the use of $PGF_2\alpha$ by Karim et al in 1968. Embrey pioneered the use of $PGE_2$ for induction of labour (Embrey 1969) and cervical ripening (Calder and Embrey 1971).

Many biochemical and functional changes occur in cervical connective tissue during pregnancy (Leppert 1995). The cervix, which is dominated by fibrous connective tissue, is composed of an extracellular matrix consisting predominantly of collagen (70 per cent Type I and 30 per cent Type III), along with elastin and proteoglycans and a cellular portion consisting of smooth muscle, fibroblasts, epithelium and blood vessels (Ludmir and Sehdev 2000). Throughout most of gestation, the cervix remains rigid and closed, to secure the products of conception. This is due to dermatan sulphate which binds to the collagen. At term, the levels of dermatan sulphate decrease. The decrease of progesterone also initiates a cascade that is similar to an inflammatory response with influx of polymorphonuclear cells and the release of the matrix metalloproteins, resulting in the degradation of collagen. Prostaglandins take part in this cervical ripening process, forming a complex network of pathways.

Prostaglandins act synergistically with interleukin-8 to stimulate the fibroblasts to produce hyaluronic acid (Ogawa et al 1998), which in turn alters the composition and structure of the cervix. Besides this, prostaglandins also have an effect on the uterine muscle, inducing contractions. Thus, prostaglandins are involved both in cervical ripening and subsequently, the process of labour.

## Labour

The process of labour is regulated by endocrine factors such as corticoptropin-releasing hormone (CRH), oxytocin as well as paracrine and autocrine factors and cytokines, such as platelet activating factor, endothelin-1 and angiotensin II. Near term, there is a striking increase in the number of oxytocin receptors in the myometrium leading to an increased sensitivity to oxytocin. Therefore, even a small increase in oxytocin (for example, an addition of fetal oxytocin) is sufficient to initiate uterine contractions. Oxytocin also acts on decidual tissue to promote prostaglandin release. At term, free levels of CRH increase in maternal blood, fetal blood, amniotic fluid and the umbilical cord. CRH modulates myometrial response to $PGF2\alpha$. CRH also enhances the fetal production of cortisol, which stimulates the membranes to increase prostaglandin synthesis. Prostaglandins modulate myometrial cell contractility by utilising extracellular calcium.

Prostaglandins soften the cervix, induce gap junctions and further sensitise the myometrium to oxytocin, leading to progressive cervical dilatation. At the end of the first stage of labour, the membranes usually rupture, leading to further increase in prostaglandin synthesis, so that it becomes an irreversible process.

> Prostaglandins soften the cervix, induce gap junctions and further sensitise the myometrium to oxytocin, leading to progressive cervical dilatation.

## The third stage of labour

After the delivery of the fetus, the uterus remains tonically contracted. This helps in separation of the placenta and also prevents postpartum hemorrhage. There is some evidence that there is considerable production of $PGF_2\alpha$ in the decidua and myometrium in the early postpartum period after expulsion of the fetus and placenta. (Husslein et al 1983)

## Induction of labour

Induction is a very common obstetric intervention and failed induction contributes significantly to cesarean sections. The success of induction depends largely on the state of the cervix (which can be assessed with the Bishop's score). When the cervix is unfavourable, preinduction cervical ripening reduces the time required for induction and reduces cesarean delivery. Prostaglandins are the agents of first choice for cervical ripening in comparison to oxytocin, since oxytocin mainly affects the uterine contractions and not the cervix directly.

With intact or absent membranes, prostaglandins are more effective than oxytocin for induction of labour (RCOG 2001).

Dinoprostone is currently the only drug that is approved for preinduction cervical ripening by the US FDA. Dinoprostone has two disadvantages: cost and storage requirements. Misoprostol, a $PGE_1$ analogue, is widely used for cervical ripening and induction of labour. The US FDA has approved it for use in obstetrics since 2002. In view of its cheaper price, stability at room temperature and the ease of administration, it is important to be aware of the efficacy and the safety of misoprostol compared to other induction agents.

> With intact or absent membranes, prostaglandins are more effective than oxytocin for induction of labour.

### Previous scar and prostaglandin use

Studies of the effects of prostaglandins, grouped together as a class of agents, on uterine rupture in women with a prior cesarean delivery have demonstrated inconsistent results (ACOG Practice Bulletin No. 115, 2010).

Evidence from small studies show that the use of misoprostol (prostaglandin $E_1$) in women who have had cesarean deliveries, is associated with an increased risk of uterine rupture (Bennett 1997; Wing et al 1998; Aslan et al 2004)). Therefore, misoprostol should not be used for third trimester cervical ripening or labour induction in patients who have had a cesarean delivery or major uterine surgery.

> Misoprostol should not be used in a woman with a previous cesarean scar as it is associated with scar dehiscence and rupture.

Because of a paucity of hard data, it is difficult to make definitive recommendations regarding the use of prostaglandin $E_2$ for induction in women with a previous cesarean scar (ACOG Practice Bulletin No. 115, 2010).

Macones and colleagues (2005) found an increase in uterine rupture only when oxytocin was used after cervical ripening with prostaglandins. Therefore, it seems logical that avoiding sequential use of prostaglandins and oxytocin will have the lowest risks of uterine rupture.

Women should be counselled adequately about the risk of scar dehiscence and the possible need for an emergency section if they want to undergo an induction with a previous scar (NICE Guideline 70, 2008). It is suggested that in a previous scar, we limit ourselves to one dose of prostaglandin, if it is used.

### Outpatient use of PGE$_2$ and misoprostol for cervical ripening/induction of labour

Several studies have looked at outpatient administration of prostaglandins for the induction of labour in post-dated pregnancies (O'Brien et al 1995; Ohel et al 1996). However, safety data are very limited. Larger studies are necessary before widespread use of outpatient cervical ripening by prostaglandins or other cervical ripening agents (Rath 2009).

## Formulations and routes of administration of prostaglandins

Though initial studies on prostaglandins for induction of labour were largely on PGF$_2\alpha$, today this agent is relegated only to the management of PPH and has been completely superseded by PGE$_2$ for labour induction and pre-induction (Table 22.1). PGE$_2$ (dinoprostone) is available in preparations that differ only in the amount of PGE$_2$ and in the vehicle in which it is contained. Two PGE$_2$ preparations are commercially available: a gel available in a 2.5 mL syringe containing 0.5 mg of dinoprostone and a vaginal insert containing 10 mg of dinoprostone. The vaginal insert releases prostaglandins at a slower rate (0.3 mg/h) than the gel. Both are approved by the US FDA for cervical ripening in women, at or near term. There is currently no evidence to establish the superiority of one PGE$_2$ preparation over the other.

Table 22.1 Preparations and dosages of prostaglandins currently available

| | | |
|---|---|---|
| PGE$_2$ | Vaginal gel | 1 and 2 mg |
| | Endocervical gel | 0.5 mg |
| | Time-release vaginal insert | 3 and 10 mg |
| PGF$_{2\alpha}$ | IM injection | 250/125 mcg |
| Misoprostol tab | Oral, vaginal and rectal administration | 25, 100, 200 mcg |

Misoprostol is available as tablets, in doses of 200, 100 and 25 mcg. It is considerably cheaper and is stable at room temperature. This, therefore, makes it a very useful drug in developing countries. Pulverisation of the tablet and re-suspension as a gel is not recommended, as the stability of the compound and uniformity of dose cannot be guaranteed (Carlan et al 1997). Adding water to the tablet is not necessary, as studies in women with ruptured membranes have not shown any significant difference in efficacy (Ngai et al 1996). Care should be taken with the use of lubricating gel as there is concern about inactivation.

## Prostaglandin E$_2$ (Dinoprostone)

### Routes of administration

*Extra-amniotic*: The effects of prostaglandins on the cervix were initially studied by extra-amniotic infusion of prostaglandins. As less invasive and equally effective routes of administration came into use, this route for administering prostaglandins has been abandoned.

*Oral tablets*: Oral prostaglandin E$_2$ is no more effective than oxytocin for induction of labour and the gastrointestinal side effects, particularly vomiting, has been shown to be higher (Keirse and van Oppen 1989). This route is no longer used for the induction of labour.

*Intracervical PGE$_2$*: Intracervical PGE$_2$ as gel preparation has been widely used and studied. Its usage for cervical ripening is widespread (ACOG 2009).

The gel form is available in a 2.5 ml pre-loaded syringe for intracervical application. It contains 0.5 mg of dinoprostone. With the woman in a dorso-lithotomy position, the cervix is exposed. The tip of the cannula, which is attached to the pre-filled syringe, is inserted gently into the internal os. The gel is then instilled into the cervix. The patient is kept in a reclining position for the next 30 minutes. The dose may be repeated every 6 hours. The manufacturers recommend a maximum cumulative dose of 1.5 mg of dinoprostone (three doses or 7.5 ml of gel) within a 24-hour period. It is good clinical practice to perform a pelvic examination and assess the state of the cervix before the next dose is instilled.

> Intracervical dinoprostone gel for cervical ripening may be used every 6 hours for a maximum of 3 doses in 24 hours.

After using 1.5 mg of dinoprostone in the cervix (3 doses), oxytocin induction should be delayed for 6–12 hours, because the effect of prostaglandins may be heightened with oxytocin (ACOG 2009).

Intracervical PGE$_2$ gel not only ripens the cervix, but also induces labour and reduces the risk of failed induction. About 40 per cent of women do not need further induction of labour.

## Comparison of intracervical PGE$_2$ with placebo or no treatment

In a metanalysis (Boulvain et al 2008), it was shown that compared to placebo, there was a decreased risk of not achieving vaginal delivery within 24 hours and a small and statistically non-significant reduction of the risk of cesarean section when PGE$_2$ was used (RR 0.88; 95 per cent CI 0.77 to 1.00). The finding was statistically significant in a subgroup of women with intact membranes and unfavourable cervix (RR 0.82; 95 per cent CI 0.68 to 0.98). While there was an increase in hyperstimulation rate, there was no significant increase in fetal heart rate changes.

*Vaginal PGE$_2$*: Vaginal prostaglandin E$_2$ is an effective induction agent, as it increases the likelihood of vaginal birth within 24 hours. There is no evidence of an effect on the rate of cesarean section compared to placebo (18.1 per cent versus 98.9 per cent, risk ratio (RR) 0.19, 95 per cent confidence interval (CI) 0.14 to 0.25, two trials, 384 women). The chance of the cervix remaining unfavourable was reduced (21.6 per cent versus 40.3 per cent, RR 0.46, 95 per cent CI 0.35 to 0.62). Requirements for oxytocin augmentation were reduced. Comparing vaginal prostaglandin E$_2$ to placebo or no treatment, the risk of uterine hyperstimulation with fetal heart rate changes was increased (Kelly et al 2009).

Sustained release inserts are associated with a reduction in instrumental vaginal deliveries compared to vaginal PGE$_2$ gel, an effect that was greater in women with an unfavourable cervix (Kelly et al 2009).

Sustained release pessaries are associated with trends of increased hyperstimulation, with and without fetal heart rate changes, compared to gel or tablets. Lower dose regimens, appear as efficacious as higher dose regimens (Kelly et al 2009).

## Comparison of intracervical PGE$_2$ with intravaginal PGE$_2$

Intracervical gel is less effective than intravaginal prostaglandins (Boulvain et al 2008). The risk of not achieving vaginal delivery within 24 hours was increased with intracervical PGE$_2$ (RR 1.26; 95 per cent CI 1.12 to 1.41) when compared to intravaginal PGE$_2$. There was no change in the risk of cesarean section (RR 1.07; 95 per cent CI 0.93 to 1.22) or the risks of hyperstimulation, with and without FHR changes (RR 0.76; 95 per cent CI 0.39 to 1.49) (RR 0.80; 95 per cent CI 0.56 to 1.15) between the two groups.

Trials were too small to provide data for evidence of effectiveness between low and high dose of gels.

In all women, when comparing induction of labour using either oxytocin (alone or in combination with amniotomy) or PGE$_2$ (vaginal or intracervical), overall induction with PGE$_2$ was associated with (RCOG 2001):

- an increase in successful vaginal delivery within 24 hours
- a reduction in cesarean section rate
- a reduction in the risk of the cervix remaining unfavourable/unchanged at 24–48 hours
- a reduction in the use of epidural analgesia
- an increase in the number of women satisfied with the method of induction.

## Prostaglandin E$_1$ (Misoprostol)

Studies with misoprostol have established it as a safe and effective drug for labour induction. Misoprostol has been compared to placebo, oxytocin and prostaglandins (Wing et al 1995; von Gemund et al 2004). Studies have also looked at various routes and doses of misoprostol. Misoprostol use has been controversial (Wagner 2005) and is used 'off label' for preinduction cervical ripening. It may be administered orally or vaginally.

### Vaginal administration

Several investigators have shown that vaginal misoprostol in dosages ranging from 25 mcg 3–6 hourly, to 50 mcg 4 hourly, to 100 mcg 6–12 hourly, appear to be more effective than oxytocin or dinoprostone in the usual recommended doses for induction of labour.

The American College of Obstetricians and Gynecologists recommends the use of the 25 mcg dose. A dose of 25 mcg of misoprostol should be considered as the initial dose for cervical ripening and labour induction. The frequency of administration should not be more than once every 3–6 hours. In addition, oxytocin should not be administered less than 4 hours after the last misoprostol dose. Misoprostol in higher doses (50 mcg every 6

> Misoprostol
> - 25 mcg every 3–6 hours for cervical ripening and induction of labour
> - 50 mcg every 6 hours may be appropriate in some cases
> - Avoid oxytocin for 4 hours after last dose of misoprostol

hours) may be appropriate in some situations, although higher doses are associated with an increased risk of complications, including uterine tachysystole with FHR decelerations (ACOG 2009).

Reviewing the Cochrane database, Hofmeyr and associates, (2003) found that, compared with vaginal prostaglandin $E_2$ or intracervical prostaglandin $E_2$ or oxytocin, vaginal misoprostol was associated with less epidural analgesia use and fewer failures to achieve vaginal delivery within 24 hours. However, misoprostol is associated with increased rates of uterine hyperstimulation, both with and without associated fetal heart rate changes. Compared with vaginal or intracervical prostaglandin $E_2$, oxytocin augmentation was less common with misoprostol. However, the occurrence of meconium-stained liquor was more common.

The occurrence of complications does appear to be dose-dependent (Wing et al 1995; Hofmeyr et al 2005). Lower doses of misoprostol were associated with more need for oxytocin augmentation and less uterine hyperstimulation with and without fetal heart rate changes, when compared to higher doses.

### Oral administration

Oral misoprostol as an induction agent is effective in achieving vaginal delivery. It is more effective than placebo and results in fewer cesarean sections than the current gold standard, vaginal dinoprostone. For women with ruptured membranes, it has similar efficacy to oxytocin. Oral misoprostol, 25 to 50 mcg, is as effective as vaginal misoprostol (Danielsson et al 1999; Souza et al 2008). Wing and associates (2000) reported that a 100 mcg dose was as effective as a 25 mcg intravaginal dose.

The sublingual use of misoprostol has also been studied. Though it may be as effective as the vaginal route, more studies are required before this can be used in clinical practice (Souza et al 2008).

### Optimal dosage of misoprostol

The optimal dose will have to balance the desire for short induction-to-delivery interval with the effect of strong contractions on fetal wellbeing and uterine wall integrity. Though doses as high as 200 mcg have been reported, in view of safety concerns, vaginal doses have been standardised as 25 and 50 mcg. An oral dose of 50 mcg (Alfirevic and Weeks 2006) or 100 mcg (Wing et al 2000) and a vaginal dose of 25 mcg are comparable.

## Prostaglandins and Postpartum hemorrhage (PPH)

Postpartum hemorrhage is one of the leading causes of maternal death in developing countries. It has been well established that active management of the third stage of labour is associated with less blood loss (Prendiville et al 2000). Traditionally, as part of active management, injectable oxytocin and methyl ergometrine are used to prevent PPH. Prostaglandins such as $PGF_2\alpha$, and more recently misoprostol, are an integral part of PPH management. However, they are not superior to ergometrine and oxytocin in prevention of PPH (Villar et al 2002). Neither intramuscular prostaglandin nor misoprostol are preferable to conventional injectable uterotonics as part of management of third stage of labour, especially for low risk women (Gülmezoglu et al 2007).

In the mid 1980s, the US FDA approved PGF$_2\alpha$ for the treatment of uterine atony. The initial recommended dose is 250 mcg given intramuscularly. This dose can be repeated at 15–90 minute intervals for a maximum of eight doses. About 20 per cent of women will experience side effects of PGF$_2\alpha$ use, the commonest being gastrointestinal disturbances, hypertension, fever, flushing and tachycardia (Oleen and Mariano 1990). Bronchoconstriction causing oxygen desaturation has been reported (Hankins et al 1988).

> **PGF$_2\alpha$ in PPH**
> - 250 mcg initially intramuscularly
> - Can be repeated every 15–90 minutes
> - Maximum of 8 doses

Systematic reviews have looked at misoprostol in the treatment of PPH (Hofmeyr et al 2005; Mousa and Alfirevic 2007).

Oral misoprostol in the dose of 600 mcg is not as effective as oxytocin in the prevention of postpartum hemorrhage (Alfirevic et al 2007), but it may be used when the latter is not available, such as the home-birth setting (RCOG Green-top guideline No 52, 2009).

Oral misoprostol given in the high dose that is required to treat PPH is associated with side effects. As an alternative, the rectal route has been proposed. The rectal route is preferred to the vaginal route, because it will not be washed out by blood. Misoprostol given rectally has a lower peak concentration and longer half-life than oral misoprostol. The longer half-life is advantageous to sustain uterine contractions, thus, preventing delayed bleeding and this may be more important than the peak levels. The lack of a sharp rise in levels is responsible for the lower incidence of side effects with the rectal route. Shivering and pyrexia are major side effects in this form of treatment.

Literature supports the use of rectal misoprostol in resource poor settings (Høj et al 2005; Rajbhandari et al 2010). High dose misoprostol (1000 mcg rectally) can bring results comparable to injectable uterotonics.

## Conclusion

Prostaglandins play an important role in the initiation and maintenance of labour. Over the years, they have become the primary pharmacological agents of choice for cervical ripening and induction of labour. As induction of labour is on the rise, the importance of understanding the role of prostaglandins and maximising their therapeutic use cannot be overemphasised.

Today, in most settings, vaginal PGE$_2$ is the agent of choice for preinduction cervical ripening and induction of labour. Misoprostol has been shown to be as effective, but its clinical use is still restricted in many places. As more studies confirm its safety and efficacy, this scenario may change.

Even though prostaglandins are not agents of choice for active management of the third stage, PGF$_2\alpha$ is an essential part of the management algorithm of atonic PPH. Rectal misoprostol may be life-saving in resource-poor settings.

# References

Alfirevic Z, Blum J, Walraven G, Weeks A, Winikoff B. 2007. Prevention of postpartum hemorrhage with misoprostol. *Int J Gynaecol Obstet* 99 Suppl 2:S198–201.

Alfirevic Z, Weeks A. 2006. Oral misoprostol for induction of labour. *Cochrane Database of Systematic Reviews* Issue 2. Art. No.: CD001338. DOI: 10.1002/14651858.CD001338.pub2.

American College of Obstetricians and Gynecologists 2009. Practice Bulletin No. 107 Induction of Labor. *Obstet Gynecol* 114: 386–97.

American College of Obstetricians and Gynecologists. 2010. Practice Bulletin No. 115. Vaginal Birth After Previous Cesarean Delivery *Obstet Gynecol*

American College of Obstetricians and Gynecologists. 1999. Induction of labor with misoprostol. ACOG Committee Opinion No. 228. Washington, DC: American College of Obstetricians and Gynecologists; November

American College of Obstetricians and Gynecologists. 1999b. Induction of labor with misoprostol. Committee Opinion No. 228, November

Aslan H, Unlu E, Agar M, Ceylan Y. 2004. Uterine rupture associated with misoprostol labor induction in women with previous cesarean delivery. *Eur J Obstet Gynecol Reprod Biol* 113:45–8

Aronsson A, Brydeman M, Gemzell- Danielsson K. 2004. Effects of misoprostol on uterine contractility following different routes of administration. *Hum Reprod*. 19:81–4.

Bennett BB. 1997. Uterine rupture during induction of labor at term with intravaginal misoprostol. *Obstet Gynecol*. 89:832–3.

Bergström S, Danielsson H, Samuelsson B. 1964. The enzymatic formation of $PGE_2$ from arachidonic acid. *Biochim Biophys Acta*. 90:207–10.

Boulvain M, Kelly AJ, Irion O. 2008. Intracervical prostaglandins for induction of labour. *Cochrane Database of Systematic Reviews* Issue 1. Art. No.: CD006971. DOI: 10.1002/14651858.CD006971.

Calder AA, Embrey MP. 1971. Prostaglandins and the unfavourable cervix. *Lancet*. 1973; 2:1322–23. 1:152–55.

Carlan SJ, Bouldin S, O'Brien WF. 1997. Extemporaneous preparation of misoprostol gel for cervical ripening: a randomized trial. *Obstet Gynecol*. 90:911–15.

Cochrane Database of Systematic Reviews. 2009, Issue 4. Art. No:CD003101. DOI:10.1002/14651858.CD003101.pub2.

Danielsson KG, Marions L, Rodriguez A, et al. 1999. Comparison between oral and vaginal administration of misoprostol on uterine contractility. *Obstet Gynecol*. 93:275–80.

Embrey MP. 1969. The effect of prostaglandins on the human pregnant uterus. *J Obstet Gynaecol Br Commonw*. 76:783–89.

Foote EF, Lee DR, Karim A, et al. 1995. Disposition of misoprostol and its active metabolite in patients with normal and impaired renal function. *J Clin Pharmacol*. 35:384–89.

Gülmezoglu AM, Forna F, Villar J, Hofmeyr GJ. 2007. Prostaglandins for prevention of postpartum haemorrhage. *Cochrane DatabaseSyst Rev* (3): CD000494.

Hankins GDV, Berryman GK, ScottRT Jr, et al. 1988. Maternal arterial desaturation with 15-methyl prostaglandin F2 alpha for uterine atony. *Obstet Gynecol*. 72:367,

Høj L., Cardoso P., Nielsen B.B., Hvidman L., Nielsen J., Aaby P. 2005. Effect of sublingual misoprostol on severe postpartum haemorrhage in a primary health centre in Guinea-Bissau: randomised double blind clinical trial. *BMJ* 331:723

Hofmeyr GJ, Walraven G, Gülmezoglu AM, Maholwana B, AlfirevicZ, Villar J. 2005. Misprostol to treat postpartum haemorrhage: a systematic review. *BJOG* 112:547–53.

Hofmeyr GJ, Gülmezoglu AM. 2003. Vaginal misoprostol for cervical ripening and induction of labour. *Cochrane Database of Systematic*

*Reviews* Issue 1. Art. No.: CD000941. DOI: 10.1002/14651858.CD000941.

Husslein P, Fuchs AR, Fuchs F. 1983. Oxytocin- and prostaglandin plasma concentrations before and after spontaneous labor: evidence of involvement of prostaglandins in the mechanism of placental separation] *Wien Klin Wochenschr.* May 27; 95(11):367–71.

Karim SMM, Trussell RR, Patel RC, et al. 1968. Response of pregnant human uterus to PGF2a-induction of labour. *Br Med J.* 4:621–23.

Keirse MJNC, van Oppen ACC. 1989. Comparison of prostaglandins and oxytocin for inducing labour. In: Chalmers I, Enkin M, Keirse MJNC, eds. *Effective Care in Pregnancy and Childbirth.* Oxford: Oxford University Press; 1080–1111.

Keirse MJNC. 1992. Therapeutic uses of prostaglandins. Bailliere's Clin Obstet Gynaecol. 6:787–808.

Kelly AJ, Tan B. 2001.,Intravenous oxytocin alone for cervical ripening and induction of labour. *Cochrane Database Syst Rev.* Art. No.: CD003246.DOI: 10.1002/14651858.CD003246.

Kelly AJ, Malik S, Smith L, Kavanagh J, Thomas J. 2009. Vaginal prostaglandin (PGE$_2$ and PGF$_2\alpha$) for induction of labour at term. *Cochrane Database of Systematic Reviews* Issue 4. Art. No.:CD003101. DOI: 10.1002/14651858.CD003101.pub2.

Leppert PC. 1995. Anatomy and physiology of cervical ripening. *Clinical Obstet Gynecol.* 38:267–79.

Ludmir J, Sehdev HM. 2000. Anatomy and physiology of the uterine cervix. *Clin Obstet Gynecol.* 43:433–39.

Macones GA, Peipert J, Nelson DB, Odibo A, Stevens EJ,Stamilio DM, et al. 2005. Maternal complications with vaginal birth after cesarean delivery: a multicenter study. *Am J Obstet Gynecol* 193:1656–62. (Level II-3)

MacDonald PC, Casey ML. 1993. The accumulation of prostaglandins (PG) in amniotic fluid is an aftereffect of labour and not indicative of a role for PGE$_2$ and PGF$_2$ alpha in the initiation of parturition. *J Clin Endocrinol Metab* 76:1332,.

Mousa HA, Alfirevic Z. 2007. Treatment for primary postpartum haemorrhage. *Cochrane Database Syst Rev.* (1):CD003249. DOI: 10.1002/14651858.CD003249.pub2.

Ngai SW, To WK, Lao T, et al. 1996. Cervical priming with oral misoprostol in prelabor rupture of membranes at term. *Obstet Gynecol.* 87:923–26.

NICE. 2008. Guideline 70 – induction of labour. July

O'Brien JM, Mercer BM, Cleary NT, Sibai BM. 1995. Efficacy of outpatient induction with low-dose intravaginal prostaglandin E2: a randomized, double-blind, placebo-controlled trial. *Am J Obstet Gynecol.* Dec; 173(6):1855–9.

O'Brien WF. 1995. The role of prostaglandins in labor and delivery. *Clin Perinatol.* Dec; 22(4):973–84.

Ogawa, M., Hirano, H., Tsubaki, H., Kodama, H., and Tanaka, T. 1998 The role of cytokines in cervical ripening: correlations between the concentrations of cytokines and hyaluronic acid in cervical mucus and the induction of hyaluronic acid production by inflammatory cytokines by human cervical fibroblasts. *Am. J. Obstet. Gynecol.*, 179, 105–110.

Ohel G, Rahav D, Rothbart H, Ruach M. 1996. Randomised trial of outpatient induction of labor with vaginal PGE$_2$ at 40–41 weeks of gestation versus expectant management. *Arch Gynecol Obstet.* 258(3):109–12.

Oleen MA, Mariano JP. 1990. Controlling refractory atonic postpartum hemorrhage with Hemabate sterile solution. *Am J Obstet Gynecol.* 162:205.

Olson DM, Zakar T, Mitchell BF. 1993. Prostaglandin synthesis regulation by intrauterine tissues. In: GE Rice, SP Brennecke, eds. *Molecular Aspects of Placental and Fetal Autocoids.* London: CRC Press, 54–95

Plaut MM, Schwartz ML, Lubarsky SL. 1999. Uterine rupture associated with the use of misoprostol in the gravid patient with a previous cesarean section. *Am J Obstet Gynecol.* 180:1535–42.

Prendiville WJP, Elbourne D, McDonald SJ. 2000. Active versus expectant management in the third stage of labour. *Cochrane Database Syst Rev*; (3):CD000007.

Rajbhandari S, Hodgins S, Sanghvi H, et al. 2010. Expanding uterotonic protection following childbirth through community-based distribution of misoprostol: operations research in Nepal. *Int J Gynecol Obstet* 108: 282–88.

Rath W H. 2009. Journal of Perinatal Medicine. Volume 37, Issue 5, 461–67.

RCOG. 2001. Evidence-based clinical guideline No 9 – Induction of Labour,

RCOG. 2009. Green-top guideline No 52.

Rice GE. 1995. Glycerophospholipid metabolism and human labour. *Reprod Fertil Dev.*7:613 622.

Romero R, Baumann P, Gonzales R, et al. 1994. Amniotic fluid prostanoid concentrations increase early during the course of spontaneous labor at term. *Am J Obstet Gynecol*. 171:1613–20.

Souza A, Amorim M, Feitosa F. 2008. Comparison of sublingual versus vaginal misoprostol for the induction of labour: a systematic review. *BJOG*. 115:1340–49.

Tang OS, Schweer H, Seyberth HW, et al. 2002. Pharmacokinetics of different routes of administration of misoprostol. *Hum Reprod*. 17:332–36.

Van Dorp DA, Beerthuis RK, Nugteren DH, et al. 1964. The biosynthesis of prostaglandins. *Biochim Biophys Acta* 90:204–7.

Villar J, Gülmezoglu AM, Hofmeyr GJ, et al. 2002. Systematic review of randomized controlled trials of misoprostol to prevent postpartum hemorrhage. *Obstet Gynecol*. 100:1301,

Von Gemund N, Scherjon S, LeCessie S, et al. 2004. A randomised trial comparing low dose vaginal misoprostol and dinoprostone for labour induction. *Br J Obstet Gynaecol* 111:42.

Wagner M. 2005. Off-label use of misoprostol in obstetrics: A cautionary tale. *BJOG*, 112: 266.

Wing DA, Lovett K, Paul RH. 1998. Disruption of prior uterine incision following misoprostol for labor induction in women with previous cesarean delivery. *Obstet Gynecol*. 91:828–30.

Wing DA, Jones MM, Rahall A, Goodwin TM, Paul RH. 1995. A comparison of misoprostol and prostaglandin E2 gel for preinduction cervical ripening and labor induction. *Am J Obstet Gynecol* 172:1804.

Wing DA, Park MR, Paul RH. 2000. A randomized comparison of oral and intravaginal misoprostol for labor induction. *Obstet Gynecol* 95:905.

Zieman M, Fong SK, Benowitz NL, et al. 1997. Absorption kinetics of misoprostol with oral or vaginal administration. *Obstet Gynecol*. 90:88–92.

# CHAPTER 23

# INDUCTION OF LABOUR

*Duru Shah and Sudeshna Ray*

Induction of labour can be defined as an intervention intended to artificially initiate uterine contractions resulting in progressive effacement and dilatation of the cervix. This should ideally result in the birth of the baby through the vaginal route (RCOG 2001). When it is believed that the clinical course and outcome of the pregnancy would be better if the pregnancy was interrupted rather than allowed to carry on in its natural course, induction of labour is carried out (RCOG 2008).

Induction of labour is one of the most common interventions practiced in modern obstetrics. Overall, throughout the world, up to 20 per cent of women have labour induced by one method or the other. Induction is indicated before the spontaneous onset of labour when the benefit to the mother or the fetus is perceived to outweigh continuation of pregnancy. Induction rates vary with practices and cultural backgrounds. Elective inductions for the convenience of either the obstetrician or the patient are on the rise. Due to the attendant risk of severe, though infrequent, adverse maternal outcomes, elective inductions are not routinely recommended. Recent opinions, however, tend to veer towards the idea that elective inductions before 41 weeks may not be as bad as obstetricians have traditionally believed (Macones 2009).

The reasons for the rising rates of induction of labour can be complex and multifactorial (Rayburn and Zhang 2002). Some of them are:

- Improved ability of physicians to determine gestational age accurately with early dating scans, thus avoiding the possibility of iatrogenic prematurity
- Widespread availability of cervical ripening agents
- Improved knowledge of methods and indications for induction
- More relaxed attitudes towards marginal/elective indications, both of the physician and the patient
- Litigation constraints

Certain unspoken reasons like the financial gain of the provider and conveniences of the physician may also have contributed to the rise.

## Criteria of an ideal inducing agent

An ideal inducing agent is one which:

- Achieves onset of labour within the shortest possible time
- Does not result in greater pain and hence does not require greater analgesics as compared to spontaneous labour
- Has a very low incidence of failure to induce labour
- Does not increase the rate of cesarean or operative vaginal deliveries as compared to spontaneous labour
- Does not increase perinatal morbidity compared to spontaneous labour

Clearly, obstetricians are yet to find an ideal inducing agent. Hence, the decision for induction should be well thought out and communicated to the woman concerned.

## Counselling the couple prior to induction

It is essential to have good communication with the woman and her family prior to induction; wherever possible, this should be supported by evidence-based and preferably, written information. While counselling, the following need to be discussed (RCOG 2008):

- The indications for induction; more specifically, the risk associated with continuing the pregnancy
- The time and procedure of induction
- Arrangements for support during labour
- Pain relief measures since induced labour may be more painful than spontaneous labour
- The need for close monitoring of the fetal heart rate (including electronic fetal monitoring in labour)
- Alternative options available to the mother if she refuses induction
- The risks associated with induction of labour, specifically with the inducing agent used
- The chances of failure of induction and the options available in case of failure

In summary, the woman and her family should be offered to be made a part of the decision-making process and her views respected, whatever they may be. A positive attitude imparted to the woman when she is actively involved in the decision making, not only increases the chances of success of induction but also enables her to better face the consequences (Nuutila et al 1999).

### Women's attitudes towards induction

Studies show variable results about the attitudes of women towards induction. One study showed that 78 per cent of women following an induction prefer not to be induced in the next pregnancy (Cartwright 1977). More recent studies show a better response. Sandhu and Sandhu (1995) showed that 65 per cent of women opted for induction for the next pregnancy. Roberts and Young (1991) found that when perception after the event was compared with anxieties of continuing the pregnancy beyond term in uncomplicated pregnancies, more women opted for elective induction than conservative management.

> When perception after the event was compared with anxieties of continuing the pregnancy beyond term in uncomplicated pregnancies, more women opted for elective induction than conservative management.

They also reiterated that 'most pregnant

women are unwilling to accept the conservative management of prolonged pregnancy and become more reluctant to do so if undelivered by 41 weeks' gestation. Women are not as favourably disposed towards the conservative management of prolonged pregnancy as has been suggested previously.'

**Table 23.1** Elective induction: advantages and disadvantages

**Advantages:**
- Relieves anxiety of continuing the pregnancy further
- Benefits both the mother and the fetus in situations where continuing the pregnancy might pose more problems
- Allows the woman to plan her delivery

**Disadvantages:**
- May increase the risk of CS or operative vaginal deliveries although evidence is not conclusive
- Might increase perinatal morbidity in the form of fetal distress, birth asphyxia, and increased release of meconium
- Studies show a greater use of epidural analgesia and pain perception in induced labour
- Mobility of the woman may be restricted and some women perceive it as more dissatisfactory than spontaneous labour

## Indications for induction

Induction of labour should be considered when continuation of the pregnancy is more hazardous for the mother and/or the baby than terminating the pregnancy. As is evident from the criteria, there is no absolute indication for induction. The common indications are listed in Table 23.2.

### Post-term/prolonged pregnancy

This is the commonest indication worldwide for induction of labour and perhaps the most definitive indication. Pregnancies that reach beyond 294 days (42 gestational weeks) are defined as post-term. About five to ten per cent of all pregnancies maybe post-term, depending on the diagnostic criteria, dating policy and population investigated (Roberto et al 1992). Risks to both the mother and the infant increase as pregnancy progresses beyond 40 weeks of gestation (Caughey and Musci 2004). Hilder et al (1998) demonstrated that the risks of stillbirth and infant mortality increase significantly in prolonged pregnancy when expressed per 1000 ongoing pregnancies. In their study, the combined risk of delivery and subsequent infant death per 1000 ongoing pregnancies was found to be low before 37 weeks and increased 11-fold from 0.34 per 1000 ongoing pregnancies at 37 weeks to 3.72 per 1000 ongoing pregnancies at 43 weeks of gestation. The risk is greater with primiparas (Ingemarsson and Källén 1997) and those with intrauterine growth restriction (Divon et al 1998). Associated morbidity includes an increased risk of fetal distress, shoulder dystocia, labour dysfunction, obstetric trauma and perinatal complications like meconium aspiration syndrome (MAS), asphyxia, fractures, nerve injuries, septicemia and pneumonia (Olesen et al 2003).

Studies showed varied results when expectant management is compared to induction of labour. Runa et al (2007) included 508 women randomly assigned to induction of labour at 289 days or antenatal fetal surveillance every third day until spontaneous labour. No differences of clinical importance were observed in women in whom labour was induced compared to those managed expectantly with regard to the following outcomes: neonates whose five-minute Apgar score was less than 7; prevalence of operative

**Table 23.2** Indications for induction

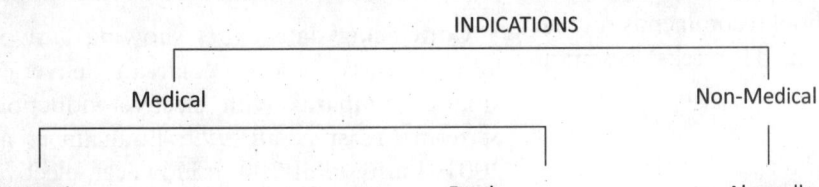

INDICATIONS

**Medical**

Maternal
- Hypertensive disorders of pregnancy
- Diabetes
- Other medical disorders in which continuation of pregnancy is more hazardous to both mother and baby than ending the pregnancy
- PROM
- SROM

Fetal
- Post-term
- Intrauterine growth restriction
- Oligohydramnios
- Isoimmunisation
- IUFD

**Non-Medical**

Also called elective Induction due to maternal social or geographical factors.
e.g distance from hospital and psychosocial conditions

---

vaginal delivery or prevalence of cesarean delivery. This finding was different from the Canadian Multicenter Post-term Pregnancy Trial (Hannah et al 1992) that showed that in post-term pregnancy, induction of labour results in a lower rate of cesarean section than serial antenatal monitoring; the rates of perinatal mortality and neonatal morbidity are similar with the two approaches.

A recent systematic review (Caughey et al 2009) showed that women at or beyond 41 completed weeks of gestation who were managed expectantly had a higher risk of cesarean delivery. It also suggests that elective induction of labour at 41 weeks of gestation and beyond is associated with a decreased risk of cesarean delivery and meconium-stained amniotic fluid. A systematic review of the Cochrane database (Gülmezoglu et al 2006) found that a policy of labour induction after 41 completed weeks or later compared to awaiting spontaneous labour either indefinitely or at least one week was associated with fewer perinatal deaths.

The policy of inducing labour at 41 weeks and 4 days (291 days of gestation) in uncomplicated pregnancies appears to be beneficial in the Indian population too (James et al 2001). Fetal monitoring should begin at 41 weeks of gestation. In their study of expectant management versus induction of labour in post-term pregnancies, James et al (2001) found that 57 per cent of women went into spontaneous labour by 41 weeks and 4 days (291 days) of gestation and only 14 per cent developed fetal compromise before that. However, when the gestational age was more than 41 weeks and 4 days (291 days), the incidence of meconium staining of amniotic fluid and evidence of uteroplacental insufficiency increased significantly. The rate of cesarean section, instrumental delivery, fetal distress and duration of labour did not differ significantly between the two groups.

The American College of Obstetricians and Gynecologists recommends that women with post-term gestations who have unfavourable cervices can either undergo labour induction or be managed expectantly. Many authorities recommend prompt delivery in a post-term patient with a favourable cervix and no other complications

(ACOG 2004). The Department of Obstetrics and Gynecology and Reproductive Biology at Harvard Medical School recommends routine induction of labour at 41 weeks' gestation (Rand et al 2000).

## Elective induction

An elective induction is one that has no medical indication, either maternal or fetal. This issue needs to be addressed especially because it has contributed significantly to the current rise in induction rates. The rising rates may be the result of more autonomy being offered to women concerning their delivery, and may represent convenience for physicians and patients. It may also just be apparent due to a decrease in indicated inductions when compared to the overall increase in numbers. Zhang et al (2002), reviewing national trends in labour induction in the United States, found that the increase in clinically indicated induction was significantly lower than the overall increase, suggesting that elective induction had risen much more rapidly.

By definition, elective induction does not provide any benefits from a strictly medical standpoint; hence, it is important to evaluate whether the induction has definite benefits which outweigh any risk to the mother and the baby. Elective induction allows better planning of daytime deliveries with a less fatigued patient and presence of more staff to provide care. The argument for an elective induction is stronger when there is a risk of rapid labour (history of previous precipitate labour); when the woman lives at a distance or at a geographically inconvenient place; or for psychosocial indications. A few studies show a modest increase in instrumental delivery with elective induction, possibly because of a higher rate of epidural analgesia (Crowley 2004; Cammu et al 2002).

Convincing data exists showing a two-fold increased risk of cesarean deliveries among nulliparas with elective induction at term (Yeast et al 1999; Boulvain et al 2001; Luthy et al 2002). However, elective induction at term does not appear to increase risk among multiparous women with a favourable cervix (Crowley 2004).

No significant change in perinatal outcome was observed in women undergoing elective induction of labour with appropriately calculated gestational age (Dublin et al 2000; Van Gemund et al 2003; Glantz et al 2005).

Fisch and colleagues (2009) have reduced the rate of cesarean sections following inductions in their institution by insisting on strict protocols. Considering the potential risks associated with elective induction of labour at term, the mandatory prerequisites while offering the option are:

❖ Calculation of an accurate gestational age with early first or second trimester scans
❖ A detailed discussion of the potential risks and outcome with the woman concerned, empowering her to make an informed choice
❖ A Bishop score of 8 in nulliparas and 6 in multiparas
❖ 39 completed weeks of gestation

## Intrauterine growth restriction

Intrauterine growth restriction results mostly from chronic placental insufficiency (Haram 2006). These fetuses are identified by the presence of growth below the 10th centile with umbilical artery Doppler abnormalities and reduced amniotic fluid volume (Tan 2005). Infants with growth restriction have a higher risk of perinatal morbidity and mortality, which usually results from placental insufficiency. The placental insufficiency is likely to be aggravated by labour. Because of a low placental reserve as compared to a fetus of normal growth and weight, these fetuses, as a group, might require intervention with delivery before the onset of spontaneous labour.

There is little evidence of benefit by inducing labour in severe fetal growth restriction. The NICE guidelines (RCOG 2008) consider that labour in the presence of fetal growth restriction may result in perinatal loss and that, in such cases, induction of labour should be avoided.

### Isolated oligohydramnios

Isolated oligohydramnios may not be an absolute indication for induction of labour as there is no difference in fetal tolerance to labour and neonatal outcome when isolated oligohydramnios is compared to normal fluid volume. Conway et al (1998) in a case-control study of 183 women found that the women who were induced had significantly more cesarean deliveries. They concluded that isolated oligohydramnios at term, in the absence of hypertension, diabetes, fetal anomalies or suspected fetal growth restriction, may not be a marker for fetal compromise, and induction of labour may not be warranted in most cases.

### Macrosomia in the diabetic and non-diabetic patient

Macrosomia is defined as a fetus with a birth weight above 4000 g (Delpapa and Mueller-Heubach, 1991). Chauhan and colleagues (2005), in a literature review of 20 studies, reported that the probability of detecting a macrosomic fetus in an uncomplicated pregnancy is variable, ranging from 15 per cent to 79 per cent with sonographic estimates of birth weight and from 40 per cent to 52 per cent with clinical estimates.

There is no evidence that induction of labour is beneficial in women with suspected fetal macrosomia. Because accurately assessing the fetal weight is difficult and the diagnosis of fetal macrosomia is problematic, induction of labour in this group of women is not to be recommended (RCOG 2008).

### Previous cesarean section

Induction of labour for maternal or fetal indications remains an option for women undergoing trial of labour after a cesarean section (TOLAC). However, the potential increased risk of uterine rupture associated with any induction, and the potential decreased possibility of achieving a successful vaginal birth, should be discussed clearly with the patient (ACOG 2010). The rate of uterine rupture may depend on whether labour was spontaneous (0.52 per cent), was induced without prostaglandins (0.77 per cent) or was induced with prostaglandins (2.24 per cent) (Lydon-Rochelle et al 2001).

Uterine rupture is more likely to be associated with induction of labour in women with no previous vaginal birth than in women with previous vaginal birth (Kayani 2005).

The NICE guidelines development group (RCOG 2008) suggests that in women with a previous cesarean section, vaginal $PGE_2$ followed by amniotomy may prove a more effective method of induction of labour than with amniotomy plus intravenous oxytocin.

Vaginal misoprostol is associated with a high frequency of uterine rupture compared with intravenous oxytocin. The American College of Obstetricians and Gynecologists (2010) states that misoprostol should not be used for third trimester cervical ripening or labour induction in patients who have had a cesarean delivery or major uterine surgery.

**Preterm prelabour rupture of membranes**

Preterm prelabour rupture of membranes (PPROM) is defined as rupture of the amniotic membranes prior to 37 weeks of gestation (Simhan 2005). It is associated with significant maternal and neonatal morbidity and mortality and effective treatment consists of an early diagnosis and gestation-dependent management.

Conservative management of PROM at 34–36 weeks prolongs pregnancy by only a few days and significantly increases the risk of chorioamnionitis. Therefore, PROM at 34–36 weeks should be actively managed. There is limited evidence on the preferred method of induction, but as with induction for other indications, intravaginal prostaglandins is the preferred agent. Before 34 weeks, however, the policy of immediate induction might be inappropriate considering the risk of prematurity unless the pregnancy is complicated with chorioamnionitis (ACOG 2007).

**Prelabour rupture of membranes at term**

Prelabour rupture of membranes at term occurs in eight per cent of pregnancies (ACOG 2007).

Merrill and Zlatnik (1999), in a large randomised study, found that oxytocin induction reduced the time interval between premature rupture of membranes and delivery as well as the frequencies of chorioamnionitis, postpartum febrile morbidity and neonatal antibiotic treatments, without increasing cesarean deliveries or neonatal infections. The data supports labour induction at the time of presentation for women with premature rupture of membranes at term. This reduces the risk of chorioamnionitis. An adequate time for the latent phase of labour to progress should be allowed (ACOG 2009).

**Intrauterine fetal death**

Intrauterine fetal death (IUFD) is estimated to occur in one per cent of all pregnancies. Though 90 per cent of women will deliver spontaneously within three weeks of intrauterine death (Silver 2007), women might not prefer to wait for an indefinite period. There is also a 25 per cent risk of disseminated intravascular coagulopathy four weeks after IUFD.

The method and timing of delivery after a fetal death depends on the gestational age at which the death occurred, the maternal history of a previous uterine scar and the maternal preference.

For women with IUFD at or after 24 weeks of gestation, evidence from RCTs suggested that oral misoprostol is more effective than placebo as an induction agent to achieve labour. Vaginal misoprostol was associated with a shorter induction-to-birth duration than oral misoprostol. However, very high oral doses (400 mcg every four hours) are more effective in terminating labour within 48 hours compared with lower vaginal doses.

Most women may opt for induction of labour. For women with IUFD at or after 24 weeks of gestation, evidence from RCTs suggested that oral misoprostol is more effective than placebo as an induction agent to achieve labour. Vaginal misoprostol was associated with a shorter induction-to-birth duration than oral misoprostol (RCOG 2008). Evidence from case-series studies also suggests that the combination of oral mifepristone and vaginal misoprostol for induction of labour is effective and safe (Wagaarachchi et al 2002).

## Contraindications for induction of labour

Generally, they are the same as those that preclude spontaneous labour and vaginal delivery. Maternal contraindications are prior uterine incision type, abnormal placentation and active genital herpes. Fetal contraindications include multifetal gestation, significant macrosomia, severe hydrocephalus, malpresentations or non-reassuring fetal status.

## Preinduction cervical ripening

Starting with a favourable cervix ensures the success of labour induction. The goal of cervical ripening is to facilitate the process of cervical softening, effacement and dilatation, thus reducing the induction-to-delivery time. When there is an indication for induction and the cervix is unfavourable, agents for cervical ripening may be used. The status of the cervix can be determined by the Bishop pelvic scoring system (Table 23.3). An unfavourable cervix has generally been defined as a Bishop score of 6 or less in most randomised trials. If the total score is more than 8, the probability of vaginal delivery is more likely and is comparable to that after spontaneous onset of labour.

**Table 23.3** Bishop's score and Modified Bishop's score

**Bishop's Score (Bishop 1964)**

|  | 0 | 1 | 2 | 3 |
|---|---|---|---|---|
| Dilation (cm) | 0 | 1–2 | 3–4 | 5–6 |
| Effacement (%) | 0–30 | 40–60 | 60–70 | 80+ |
| Station (cm) | -3 | -2 | -1/0 | +1/+2 |
| Consistency | Firm | Medium | Soft | |
| Position | Posterior | Mid-position | Anterior | |

**Modified Bishop's Score (Calder 1974)**

|  | 0 | 1 | 2 | 3 |
|---|---|---|---|---|
| Dilation (cm) | <1 | 1–2 | 2–4 | >4 |
| Effacement (%) | >4 | 2–4 | 1–2 | <1 |
| Station (cm) | -3 | -2 | -1/0 | +1/+2 |
| Consistency | Firm | Average | Soft | |
| Position | Posterior | Mid-anterior | | |

### Mechanical methods

*Sweeping of membranes*: Also called stripping of membranes, this is a simple procedure performed at the time of a vaginal examination. The clinician's finger is introduced into the os and moved in a circular fashion to separate the membranes from the lower uterine segment. Separating the chorion from the decidua increases prostaglandin ($PGF_2$) secretion from the latter and initiates labour (McColgin et al 1993). Women undergoing sweeping of membranes face few adverse effects like discomfort, vaginal bleeding and contractions which are unassociated with labour. Technically, the procedure needs a cervical scoring of at least greater than 4 (Cammu and Haitsma 1998). A large meta-analysis of 22 trials involving

277 women was performed to compare the effect of sweeping of membranes with the use of oxytocin or prostaglandins (Boulvain et al 2001). It was found that sweeping of membranes in women at term reduces the duration of pregnancy and there is a decline in the frequency of pregnancies continuing beyond 41 weeks. However, the author's recommendation was that routine use of sweeping of membranes from 38 weeks of pregnancy onwards does not seem to produce clinically important benefits. In another RCT involving 195 women beyond 40 weeks, sweeping of membranes was found to induce labour within 72 hours in two-thirds of women compared to one-third in the control group (Allot and Palmer 1993).

Another RCT from the Netherlands (De Miranda et al 2006) evaluated the effects of membrane sweeping, repeated every 48 hours (n = 375) and no sweeping (n = 367) in low-risk pregnancies at 41 weeks of gestation. Serial sweeping caused a significant decline in the proportion of post-term pregnancies in both multiparous and nulliparous women.

The RCOG recommends membrane sweeping as an integral part of preventing prolonged pregnancy that should be offered to all women before formal induction of labour: to all nulliparas at 40 and 41 weeks and to all parous women at 41 weeks. Repeated attempts may be beneficial.

*Transcervical catheter and extra-amniotic saline infusion (EASI)*: The methods available for mechanical dilatation include transcervical Foley catheter (Foley) and transcervical Foley catheter with extra-amniotic saline infusion (EASI). The transcervical Foley catheter is used for cervical ripening in an inpatient setting, and the addition of extra-amniotic saline infusion supposedly promotes endogenous prostaglandin release by stripping of membranes and by supplying additional mechanical force.

There are conflicting reports on the efficacy of adding extra-amniotic saline infusion to Foley insertion (Guinn et al 2004; Karjane et al 2006). However, a systematic review of the Cochrane database (Boulvain et al 2001) stated that 'there is insufficient evidence to evaluate the effectiveness, in terms of likelihood of vaginal delivery in 24 hours, of mechanical methods compared with placebo/no treatment or with prostaglandins. The risk of hyperstimulation was reduced when compared with prostaglandins (intracervical, intravaginal or misoprostol). Compared to oxytocin in women with unfavourable cervix, mechanical methods reduce the risk of cesarean section. There is no evidence to support the use of extra-amniotic infusion.

## Amniotomy (artificial rupture of membranes)

Amniotomy is the deliberate rupture of membranes used for induction of labour (provided the membranes are accessible), thus avoiding the need for pharmacological intervention. It is theoretically supposed to release endogenous prostaglandins and thus result in labour. The drawbacks are that labour might not ensue with amniotomy alone, the time taken to deliver might not be acceptable and a risk of maternal and fetal infection exists if labour becomes prolonged. Used alone for inducing labour, amniotomy may be associated with unpredictable and sometimes long intervals before the onset of contractions. Bricker and Luckas (2000) found insufficient evidence for the efficacy and safety of amniotomy alone for labour induction. Moldin and Sundell (1996), in a trial of amniotomy combined with early oxytocin infusion compared with amniotomy alone, found that the induction-to-delivery interval was shorter with the amniotomy-plus-oxytocin method.

Based on available evidence, RCOG does not recommend amniotomy alone for primary induction of labour, except when other pharmacological interventions are contraindicated (RCOG 2008)

## Pharmacological Interventions for Induction

### Prostaglandins (PGE$_2$)

Prostaglandins have been used to induce labour since the 1960s. Initial work focused on prostaglandin $F_{2\alpha}$, as prostaglandin $E_2$ was considered unsuitable for a number of reasons. Prostaglandins can stimulate uterine contractions, resulting in labour. With the development of alternative routes of administration, comparisons were made between various formulations of vaginal prostaglandins. They can be administered through various routes: vaginal, oral, intravenous, extra-amniotic and intracervical.

Intracervical PGE$_2$ as gel preparation has been widely used and studied. Its use for cervical ripening is widespread (ACOG 2009).

The gel form is available in a 2.5-ml pre-loaded syringe for intracervical application. It contains 0.5 mg of dinoprostone. With the woman in a dorso-lithotomy postion, the cervix is exposed and held. The tip of the cannula, which is attached to the pre-filled syringe, is inserted gently to just below the internal os. The gel is then instilled into the cervix. The patient is kept in a reclining position for the next 30 minutes. The dose may be repeated every six hours. The manufacturers recommend a maximum cumulative dose of 1.5 mg of dinoprostone (three doses or 7.5 ml of gel) within a 24-hour period. It is good clinical practice to perform a pelvic examination and assess the state of the cervix before the next dose is instilled.

> Intracervical dinoprostone gel for cervical ripening may be used every 6 hours for a maximum of 3 doses in 24 hours.

After using 1.5 mg of dinoprostone in the cervix (three doses), oxytocin induction should be delayed for 6–12 hours because the effect of prostaglandins may be heightened with oxytocin (ACOG 2009).

Intracervical PGE$_2$ gel not only ripens the cervix but also induces labour and reduces the risk of failed induction. About 40 per cent of women do not need further induction.

A systematic review of the Cochrane database (Kelly et al 2009) showed that vaginal prostaglandin E$_2$ compared with placebo or no treatment reduces the likelihood of vaginal delivery not being achieved within 24 hours. The risk of the cervix remaining unfavourable or unchanged was reduced and the need for oxytocin augmentation was reduced (35.1% versus 43.8%, RR 0.83, 95% CI 0.73 to 0.94, 12 trials, 1321 women) when PGE$_2$ was compared to placebo. There was no evidence of a difference between cesarean section rates, although the risk of uterine hyperstimulation with fetal heart rate changes was increased (4.4% versus 0.49%,

RR 4.14, 95% CI 1.93 to 8.90, 14 trials, 1259 women).

The review also found that the $PGE_2$ tablet, gel and pessary are all equally efficacious and the use of sustained release $PGE_2$ inserts appear to be associated with reduced instrumental vaginal delivery rates when compared to vaginal $PGE_2$ gel or tablet.

The authors concluded that $PGE_2$ increases successful vaginal delivery rates in 24 hours and cervical favourability with no increase in operative delivery rates. Sustained release vaginal $PGE_2$ is superior to vaginal $PGE_2$ gel for some outcomes studied.

Evidence suggests that oral $PGE_2$ may be more effective than placebo in inducing labour and reducing cesarean rates. However, French (2001) in a systematic review found no clear advantages to oral prostaglandin over other methods of induction of labour. Oral prostaglandin consistently results in more frequent gastrointestinal side effects, in particular vomiting, compared to the other treatments.

## Oxytocin

Oxytocin is the commonest induction agent used worldwide. It has been used alone, in combination with amniotomy or following cervical ripening with other pharmacological or non-pharmacological methods. Intravenous oxytocin was the most commonly used agent for induction before the advent of prostaglandins. In modern obstetrics, it is more commonly used for augmentation of labour.

To determine the effects of oxytocin alone for third-trimester cervical ripening and induction of labour, in comparison with other methods of induction of labour or placebo/no treatment, Alfirevic et al (2009) reviewed the Cochrane database. They found that intracervical prostaglandins were more successful in bringing about vaginal delivery within 24 hours than oxytocin alone. There was also an increase in cesarean sections (19.1% versus 13.7 %) in the oxytocin group.

Intravenous oxytocin and amniotomy compare well with other methods used at term to bring on labour. Compared to oxytocin alone, amniotomy and intravenous oxytocin results in more vaginal births in women with unfavourable cervix and significantly fewer instrumental vaginal deliveries than placebo. However, this method is associated with significantly more postpartum hemorrhage and dissatisfaction with treatment (Howarth and Botha 2001). In women with an unfavourable cervix, the maternal and fetal outcomes are no different between the amniotomy plus intravenous oxytocin group and the intravaginal $PGE_2$ group. These trials are small in number and not sufficient for recommendation of one over another.

### Regimens for induction with oxytocin

Varied regimens are used for oxytocin infusion. It should be started with a lower dose (1–2 mu/minute) and increased at intervals of 30 minutes; as soon as physiological contractions are achieved (3–4 contractions in 10 minutes) or an absolute maximum of 32 milliunits per minute is reached, further increments should be stopped. The volume infused should be minimum to deal with the antidiuretic effect of oxytocin (RCOG 2001a).

In some obstetric departments, five units of synthetic oxytocin are added to 500 ml of normal saline. This gives a concentration of 10 mu/ml (ACOG 2009). This allows for an optimal dose of oxytocin to be given without the risk of fluid overload, which is, however, rare. The use of an infusion pump increases the safety of oxytocin delivery to the patient and may avoid inadvertent increase in dosage.

## Misoprostol

Misoprostol is an inexpensive synthetic analogue of prostaglandin $E_1$. In most countries, misoprostol is marketed for use in the prevention and treatment of peptic ulcer disease. Misoprostol has been widely used for obstetric and gynecological indications, such as induction of abortion and of labour. It is more stable and easier to store than other prostaglandins. It has few systemic side effects. It is rapidly absorbed orally and vaginally. Several studies have evaluated the efficacy of misoprostol as an inducing agent and it has been compared with other prostaglandins. These studies suggest that it is effective for both cervical ripening and induction of labour (Young et al 1999; Hofmeyr and Gülmezoglu 2003).

Several investigators have shown that vaginal misoprostol in doses ranging from 25 mcg 3–6 hourly, to 50 mcg 4 hourly, to 100 mcg 6–12 hourly appear to be more effective than oxytocin or dinoprostone in the usual recommended doses for induction of labour. Doses not exceeding 25 mcg 4 hourly appeared to have similar effectiveness and risk of uterine hyperstimulation as conventional labour inducing methods (Hofmeyr and Gülmezoglu 2003).

The American College of Obstetricians and Gynecologists (ACOG 2009) recommends the use of the 25-mcg dose by the vaginal route. Twenty five mcg of misoprostol should be considered as the initial dose for cervical ripening and labour induction. The frequency of administration should not be more than every 3–6 hours. In addition, oxytocin should not be administered less than 4 hours after the last misoprostol dose.

Oral misoprostol (25 mcg) has been found to be as effective as vaginal misoprostol and results in fewer cesarean sections than vaginal prostaglandins in women with ruptured membranes (Souza 2008). Oral misoprostol causes an increase in meconium-stained liquor compared to intravenous oxytocin. An oral dose of 50 mcg (Alfirevic and Weeks 2006) or 100 mcg (Wing et al 2000) and a vaginal dose of 25 mcg are comparable.

There is insufficient data on buccal and sublingual misoprostol for clinical recommendations (Muzonzini and Hofmeyr 2004).

There are several challenges with misoprostol. First, there is the concern of uterine hypercontractility, and second, the administration of the appropriate dose of 25 mcg is difficult as current preparations come as 100–200 mcg tablets (Alfirevic and Weeks 2008). Misoprostol is unlicensed for use in induction of labour in the UK and USA/Canada. Both ACOG and RCOG recommend the use of misoprostol in clinical trials, because of concerns of hyperstimulation and because the best dose regimen is yet to be determined.

## Mifepristone

Mifepristone (RU 486) is a progesterone receptor antagonist. The rationale behind its use for induction of labour is that in spontaneous labour, a fall in progesterone is one of the main factors leading to onset of labour. A number of studies have looked at the efficacy of RU 486 in cervical ripening. When compared to placebo, it is more effective in increasing the chances of spontaneous labour and reducing the need for prostaglandins (Lelaidier et al 1993). However, a systematic review of the Cochrane database (Neilson 2000) found insufficient information available from clinical trials to support the use of mifepristone to induce labour.

## Non-pharmacological methods of labour induction

### Sexual intercourse and breast stimulation

The rationale behind sexual intercourse being an inducing agent is that human semen contains a high natural prostaglandin concentration (Benvold et al 1987); this might induce contractions when the cervix is receptive to prostaglandins. A systematic review of the Cochrane database compared a group who had regular intercourse with a group who abstained from it (Kavanagh et al 2001). There was no observed benefit of sexual intercourse as an induction agent.

Breast stimulation causes the uterus to contract, though the mechanism remains unclear. Nipple stimulation has been a subject of a number of observational and randomised studies. A Cochrane review (Kavanagh et al 2005) reveals that it causes a decline in the number of women remaining undelivered after 72 hours and also a reduction in the rate of postpartum hemorrhage. Though it seems to be an effective option as it is inexpensive and leaves the woman in control, there are many questions which remain largely unanswered such as the time taken for induction, the adequacy of the procedure to bring about the contractions and its effectiveness in 'at risk' pregnancies.

## Complications of induction of labour

The main risks of induction of labour are uterine hyperstimulation, failed induction and uterine rupture (Table 23.4).

### Uterine hyperstimulation

The chances of uterine hyperstimulation with any inducing agent vary from 1 to 5 per cent. Uterine hyperstimulation may result in prolonged, tonic or too frequent contractions; this may be associated with abnormal fetal heart rate (FHR) patterns.

If oxytocin has caused tachysystole, it should be promptly discontinued. The woman should be turned to her side. Tocolysis with beta-adrenergic drugs (a single dose of terbutaline 250 mcg given subcutaneously) has been found to be effective in normalising hyperstimulation and reversing abnormal FHR patterns (ACOG 2009). There is no evidence of any benefit obtained by the administration of magnesium sulphate or by vaginal irrigation in an attempt to wash out vaginal $PGE_2$. In case tocolysis fails to

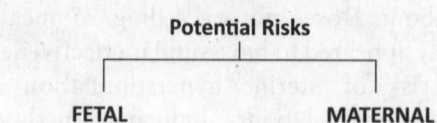

**Table 23.4** Potential risks

| FETAL | MATERNAL |
|---|---|
| • Fetal distress | • Uterine hypercontractility |
| • Umbilical cord prolapse | • Uterine rupture |
| • Hyperbilirubinmia | • Hyponatremia |
|  | • Operative delivery |
|  | • Postpartum hemorrhage |

correct the hyperstimulation, emergency delivery may be needed.

### Failed induction

There is no universally agreed definition of the criterion of a failed induction; hence, the actual rates are difficult to determine. An estimate of 15 per cent in the presence of an unfavourable cervix has been quoted by the RCOG. Induction of labour with a good cervical score might reduce the cesarean section rate for failed induction of labour (Arulkumaran et al 1985).

Failed induction is failure to establish labour and needs to be differentiated from failure of progress of labour. A timeframe needs to be set (usually 24–48 hours) after adequate induction, after which the indication and the situation needs to be reviewed. There is no evidence to recommend treatment for failed induction but usually delivery by cesarean section will be required.

It therefore becomes imperative to start induction for an indication that justifies operative delivery in case of failure. For elective induction, the attempt can be repeated after a few days if the situation permits it.

### Uterine rupture

Uterine rupture is an unusual event during induction of labour, particularly in an unscarred uterus. The condition is associated with very high maternal and fetal morbidity and mortality. It is more common in a previously scarred uterus (cesarean scar, myomectomy or uterine curettage with an undiagnosed perforation). It can also occur in multigravidas with previous vaginal deliveries; rarely, it has been reported in primigravidas (Selo-Ojemo and Ayida 2002).

There is no specific management of uterine rupture following an induction. With immediate resuscitation and simultaneous laparotomy, maternal mortality can be avoided in an institutional delivery but the fetus is extremely difficult to salvage following a uterine rupture (Bujold and Gauthier 2002)

### Other complications

a) **Iatrogenic prematurity** can occur if the gestational age has not been confirmed adequately by dates and first-trimester sonography. This may be justified in cases where the induction has been done for a medical reason, for example, preeclampsia but amounts to negligence in case of an elective ('social') induction.

b) **Umbilical cord prolapse** is a complication which follows artificial rupture of membranes. As a prerequisite for this procedure, therefore, it is important to assess the engagement of the presenting part and ARM should be avoided in case of a high floating head.

c) **Maternal hyponatremia** may occur following prolonged use of intravenous oxytocin in high doses owing to the antidiuretic nature of oxytocin. The dose of oxytocin and the volume of fluid infused should be limited to avoid this rare complication.

d) Evidence suggests an increased risk of **postpartum hemorrhage** following induction of labour. Active management of the third stage of labour is recommended for all women.

e) **Neonatal hyperbilirubinemia**, though clinically insignificant, has been reported following oxytocin infusion but the evidence is not strong enough.

### Cervical scoring system

Bishop originally described this in 1964; he showed that there is an inverse relationship between the cervical score and the time taken for the women to be in established labour. The modern scoring system used is the Calder's modified Bishop's score.

When the natural process of ripening does not begin, the cervix is said to be unfavourable (scores below 6). Induction is quicker in those whose cervical score is more, depicting the beginning of the latent phase; the risk of failed induction is also lower in these women (Arulkumaran et al 1985).

Prostaglandins can be used for both unfavourable and favourable cervix as an inducing agent but scores above 6 allow for easier artificial rupture of membranes.

### Summary of Recommendations for Induction of Labour

- Healthcare professionals should explain to the woman the reasons, when, where and how induction could be carried out, the alternative options and the risks and benefits of induction of labour.
- The benefits of induction of labour must be weighed against the potential maternal or fetal risks associated with this procedure.
- If induction is indicated and the status of the cervix is unfavourable, agents for cervical ripening may be used. The status of the cervix can be determined by the Bishop pelvic scoring system. If the total score is more than 8, the probability of vaginal delivery after labour induction is similar to that after spontaneous labour.
- Women with uncomplicated pregnancies should usually be offered induction of labour between 41+0 and 42+0 weeks to avoid the risks of prolonged pregnancy.
- If delivery is indicated, women who have had a previous cesarean section may be offered induction of labour with vaginal $PGE_2$, cesarean section or expectant management on an individual basis, taking into account the woman's circumstances and wishes. Women should be informed of the increased risks with induction of labour, that is, increased risk of need for emergency cesarean section and increased risk of uterine rupture.
- Induction of labour should not routinely be offered on maternal request alone.
- If there is severe fetal growth restriction with confirmed fetal compromise, induction of labour is not recommended.

**Table 23.5** Prerequisites for IOL

- Communication about the indication, procedure, potential benefits and risks
- Informed consent
- Thorough assessment for possibility of vaginal delivery. Any other indication that may favour a cesarian delivery should be reconsidered before induction
- Assessment of cervical status
- Hospital set up with facilities for emergency operational delivery, neonatal care unit and blood transfusion facilities

- If a woman who has had an intrauterine fetal death chooses to proceed with induction of labour, oral mifepristone, followed by vaginal PGE$_2$ or vaginal misoprostol, should be offered.
- In the absence of any other indications, induction of labour should not be carried out simply because a healthcare professional suspects a baby is large for gestational age (macrosomic).
- Vaginal prostaglandin E$_2$ (PGE$_2$) is the preferred method of induction of labour, unless there are specific clinical reasons for not using it (in particular, the risk of uterine hyperstimulation).
- Wherever induction of labour is carried out, facilities should be available for continuous electronic fetal heart rate and uterine contraction monitoring
- Tocolysis should be considered if uterine hyperstimulation occurs during induction of labour.
- If induction fails, the subsequent management options include either a further attempt to induce labour or delivery by cesarean section

## References

Alferevic Z, Weeks A. 2008. Oral misoprestol for IOL. *Cochrane Database of Systematic Reviews*; Oxford Update service.

Alfirevic Z, Kelly AJ, Dowswell T. 2009. Intravenous oxytocin alone for cervical ripening and induction of labour. *Cochrane Database of Systematic Reviews*, Issue 4.

Alfirevic Z, Weeks A. 2006. Oral misoprostol for induction of labour. *Cochrane Database of Systematic Reviews*, Issue 2. Art. No.: CD001338. DOI: 10.1002/14651858.CD001338.pub2.

Allott HA, CR Palmer. 1993. Sweeping the membranes: a valid procedure in stimulating the onset of labour? *Br J Obstet Gynaecol* 100:898–903.

American College of Obstetricians and Gynecologists. 2004. Management of postterm pregnancy. ACOG Practice Bulletin No. 55. *Obstet Gynecol* 104:639–46.

American College of Obstetricians and Gynecologists. 2007. Premature rupture of membranes. Practice Bulletin No. 80. *Obstet Gynecol* 109:1007–19.

American College of Obstetricians and Gynecologists. 2009. Induction of Labor. ACOG Practice Bulletin No. 107. *Obstet Gynecol* 114:386–97.

American College of Obstetricians and Gynecologists. 2010. Vaginal birth after previous cesarean delivery. Practice Bulletin No. 115. *Obstet Gynecol* 116:450–63.

Arulkumaran S, DMF Gibb, RI Tambyraja, SH Heng, SS Ratnam. 1985. Failed induction of labour. *Aust NZ J Obstet Gynaecol* 25:190–93.

Benvold E, C Gottlieb, K Svanborg, M Bygdeman, P Eneroth. 1987. Concentartion of prostaglandins in seminal fluid of fertile men. *Intl J Androl* 10: 463–69

Boulvain M, Marcoux S, Bureau M, Fortier M, Fraser W. 2001. Risks of induction of labour in uncomplicated term pregnancies. *Paediatric Perinatal Epidemiology* 15:131–139.

Boulvain M, Stan C, Irion O. 2001. Membrane sweeping for induction of labour (Cochrane Review). *Cochrane Database Systematic Reviews* 2005(1) CD 000451.

Boulvain M, Kelly A, Lohse C, Stan C, Irion O. 2001. Mechanical methods for induction of labour. *Cochrane Database Systematic Reviews* (4): CD001233.

Bricker L, Luckas M. 2000. Amniotomy alone for induction of labour. *Cochrane Database of Systematic Reviews*, Issue 4. Art. No.: CD002862. DOI: 10.1002/14651858. CD002862.

Bujold E. Gauthier RJ. 2002. Neonatal morbidity associated with uterine rupture: What are the risk factors? *Am J Obstet Gynecol* 186(2):311–14.

Cammu H, Martens G, Ruyssinck G, Amy JJ. 2002. Outcome after elective labor induction in nulliparous women: A matched cohort study. *Am J Obstet Gynecol* 186:240–244.

Cammu H, V Haitsma. 1998. Sweeping of the membranes at 39 weeks in nulliparous women: a randomized controlled trial. *Br J Obstet Gynaecol* 105(1):41–44.

Cartwright A. 1977. Mother's experience of induction. *BMJ* 2:745–49.

Caughey AB, Sundaram V, Kaimal AJ, et al. 2009. Systematic Review: Elective Induction of Labor Versus Expectant Management of Pregnancy; *Annals of Internal Medicine* vol. 151 no. 4 252–263.

Caughey AB, Musci TJ. 2004. Complications of term pregnancies beyond 37 weeks of gestation. *Obstet Gynecol* 103:57–62.

Chauhan SP, Grobman WA, Gherman RA et al. 2005. Suspicion and treatment of the macrosomic fetus: a review. *Am Obstet and Gynecol* 193(2):332–46.

Conway DL, Adkins WB, Schroeder B, Langer O. 1998. Isolated oligohydramnios in the term pregnancy: is it a clinical entity? *J Matern Fetal Med* Jul–Aug; 7(4):197–200.

Crowley P. 2004. Interventions for preventing or improving the outcome of delivery at or beyond term (Cochrane review). In: *The Cochrane Library*, Issue 2.

Delpapa EH, Mueller-Heubach E. 1991. Pregnancy outcome following ultrasound diagnosis of macrosomia. *Obstetrics and Gynecology* 78:340–3.

Divon MY, Haglund B, Nisell H, Otterblad PO, Westgren M. 1998. Fetal and neonatal mortality in the postterm pregnancy: the impact of gestational age and fetal growth restriction. *Am J Obstet Gynecol* Apr; 178(4):726–31.

De Miranda, E Van Der Bom JG, Bonsel GJ et al. 2006. Membrane sweeping and preventing of post term pregnancy. *A RCT BJOG* 113(4):402–8.

Dublin S, Lydon-Rochelle M, Kaplan RC, Watts DH, Critchlow CW. 2000. Maternal and neonatal outcomes after induction of labor without an identified indication. *Am J Obstet Gynecol* 183:986–94.

French L. 2001. Oral prostaglandin E2 for induction of labour. *Cochrane Database of Systematic Reviews*, Issue 2. Art. No.: CD003098. DOI: 10.1002/14651858.CD003098

Gabriel R, T DArnaud, F Chalot, N Gonzalez, F Leymarie, C Quereux. 2002. Transvaginal sonographyof the uterine cervix prior to labour induction. *Ultrasound Obstet Gynaecol* 19(3):254–57.

Glantz JC. 2005. Elective induction vs. spontaneous labor: associations and outcomes. *J Reprod Med* 50:235–40.

Guinn DA, Davies JK, Jones RO, Sullivan L, Wolf D. 2004. Labor induction in women with an unfavorable Bishop score: randomized controlled trial of intrauterine Foley catheter with concurrent oxytocin infusion versus Foley catheter with extra-amniotic saline infusion with concurrent oxytocin infusion. *Am J Obstet Gynecol* 191:225–9. 277:1794–801.

Gülmezoglu AM, Crowther CA, Middleton P. 2006. Induction of labour for improving birth outcomes for women at or beyond term. *Cochrane Database of Systematic Reviews*, Issue 4. Art. No.: CD004945.

Hannah ME, Hannah WJ, Hellmann J, Hewson S, Milner R, Willan A. 1992. Induction of labor as compared with serial antenatal monitoring in post-term pregnancy. A randomized controlled trial. The Canadian Multicenter Post-term Pregnancy Trial Group. *N Engl J Med* 11; 326(24):1587–92.

Haram K. 2006. Intrauterine growth restriction. *International Journal of Gynaecology and Obstetrics* 93(1):5–12.

Hilder, L., Costeloe, K. and Thilaganathan, B. 1998. Prolonged pregnancy: evaluating gestation-specific risks of fetal and infant mortality. *BJOG:* 105: 169–173. doi: 10.1111/j.1471-0528.1998.tb10047.x

Hofmeyr GJ, Gülmezoglu AM. 2003. Vaginal misoprostol for cervical ripening and induction of labour. *Cochrane Database Systematic Reviews* (1):CD000941.

Howarth G, Botha DJ. 2001. Amniotomy plus intravenous oxytocin for induction of labour. *Cochrane Database of Systematic Reviews*, Issue 3. Art. No.: CD003250. DOI: 10.1002/14651858.CD003250.

Ingemarsson I, Källén K. 1997. Stillbirths and rate of neonatal deaths in 76,761 postterm pregnancies in Sweden, 1982-1991: a register study. *Acta Obstet Gynecol Scand* Aug; 76(7):658–62.

James C, George SS, Gaunekar N, Seshadri L. 2001. Management of prolonged pregnancy: A randomized trial of induction of labour and antepartum foetal monitoring. *Natl Med J India* SepOct; 14(5):270–3.

Karjane NW, Brock EL, Walsh SW. 2006. Induction of labor using a Foley balloon, with and without extraamniotic saline infusion. *Obstet Gynecol* 107:234–9.80-mL.

Kavanagh J, Kelly AJ, Thomas J. 2001. Sexual intercourse for cervical ripening and induction of labour. *Cochrane Database of Systematic Reviews*, Issue 2. [DOI: 10.1002/14651858.CD003093].

Kavanagh J, Kelly AJ, Thomas J. 2005. Breast stimulation for cervical ripening and induction of labour. *Cochrane Database of Systematic Reviews*, Issue 3. [DOI: 10.1002/ 14651858.CD003392.pub2: CD003392].

Kayani SI. 2005. Uterine rupture after induction of labour in women with previous caesarean section. [erratum appears in BJOG 112(4):528]. *BJOG* 112(4):451–5.

Kelly AJ, Malik S, Smith L, Kavanagh J, Thomas J. 2009. Vaginal prostaglandin (PGE2 and PGF2a) for induction of labour at term. *Cochrane Database of Systematic Reviews*, Issue 4. Art. No.: CD003101. DOI: 10.1002/14651858.CD003101.pub2

Kiss H, R Ahner, M Hohlagschwander, H Leitich, P Husslein. 2000. Fetal fibronectin as predictor of term labour:a literature review. *Acta Obstet et Gynaecol Scand* 79(1): 3–7.

Lelaidier C, Benifla JL, Fernandez H, Baton C, Bourget P, Bourrier MC, Frydman R 1993. The value of RU-486 (mifepristone) in medical indications of the induction of labor at term. Results of a double-blind randomized prospective study (RU-486 versus placebo). *J Gynecol Obstet Biol Reprod* 22(1):91–100.

Luthy DA, Malmgren JA, Zingheim RW. 2002. Increase CS rates associated with elective induction in nulliparous women. *Am J Obstet Gynecol* P87:S106.

Lydon-Rochelle M, Holt VL, Easterling TR, Martin DP. 2001. Risk of uterine rupture during labor among women with a prior cesarean delivery. *N Engl J Med* 345:3–8.

Macones GA. 2009. *Elective Induction of Labor: Waking the Sleeping Dogma?* vol. 151 no. 4 281–282.

McColgin SW, WA Bennett, H Roach, BD Cowan, JN Martin, JC Morrison. 1993. Parturitional factors associated with membrane stripping. *Am J Obstet Gynaecol* 169:71–77.

Merrill DC, Zlatnik FJ. 1999. Randomized, double-masked comparison of oxytocin dosage in induction and augmentation of labor. *Obstet Gynecol* 94:455–63.

Moldin PG, Sundell G. 1996. Induction of labour: a randomised clinical trial of amniotomy versus amniotomy with oxytocin infusion. *Br J Obstet Gynaecol* 103:306–12.

Muzonzini G,.Hofmeyr GJ. 2004. Buccal or sublingual misoprostol for cervical ripening and induction of labour. *Cochrane Database Systematic Reviews* CD004221.

NICE guidelines. 2001. *RCOG*. Induction of labour.

NICE guidelines. 2008. *RCOG*. Induction of labour.

Neilson, JP. 2000. Mifepristone for induction of labour. Cochrane Database *Systematic Reviews* CD002865.

Nuutila M, Halmesmaki E, Hiilesmaa V et al. 1999. Women's anticipations of and experiences with induction of labor. *Acta Obstet Gynecol Scand* 78:8, 704–709.

Olesen, AW, Basso, O, Olsen, J. 2003. Risk of recurrence of prolonged pregnancy. *BMJ* 326:476.

Pandis A, Papageorghiou V, Ramanathan M, Thompson, KH Nicolaides, 2001. Pre-induction sonographic measurement of cervical length in the prediction of successful induction of labor. *Ultrasound Obstet Gynecol* 18(6):623–28.

Rand L, Robinson JN, Economy KE, Norwitz ER. 2000. Post-term induction of labor revisited. *Obstet Gynecol* 96:779–783.

Rayburn WF, Zhang J. 2002. Rising Rates of Labor Induction: Present Concerns and Future Strategies. *Obstetrics & Gynecology* 100: 1, 164–167.

Roberts L, Young K. 1991. The management of the prolonged pregnancy – an analysis of women's attitudes before and after term. *Br J Obstet Gynaecol* 98(1):1102–06.

Sandhu SK, H Sandhu. 1995. Psychological aspects of planned induction of labour. *J Ind Med Assoc.* 93(8):297–98.

Schaffir J. 2002. Survey of folk beliefs about induction of labour. *Birth* 29(1):47–51.

Selo-Ojemo DO, GA Ayida. 2002. Uterine rupture after a single vaginal 2mg prostaglandin gel application in a primiparous woman.*Europ J Obstet Gynaecol Reprod Biol* 101(1):88.

Simhan HN. 2005. Preterm premature rupture of membranes: diagnosis, evaluation and management strategies. *BJOG: an International Journal of Obstetrics and Gynaecology;*112 Suppl 1:32–7.

Silver RM. 2007. Fetal death. *Obstetrics and Gynecology* 109(1):153–67.

Souza A, Amorim M, Feitosa F. 2008. Comparison of sublingual versus vaginal misoprostol for the induction of labour: a systematic review. *BJOG* 115:1340–1349.

Tan TYT. 2005. Intrauterine growth restriction. *Current Opinion in Obstetrics and Gynecology* 17(2):135–42.

Van Gemund N, Scheryon S, Lecessie S, Van Roosmalan, J, Kanhai HH. 2003. An RCT comparing perinatal outcome in Elective IOL vs Expectant Management of Labour. *BJOG* III; 42–49.

Wagaarachchi PT, Ashok PW, Narvekar NN et al. 2002. Medical management of late intrauterine death using a combination of mifepristone and misoprostol. *BJOG* 109(4):443–7.

Wing DA, Park MR, Paul RH. 2000. A randomized comparison of oral and intravaginal misoprostol for labor induction. *Obstet Gynecol* 95:905.

Yeast JD, Jones A, Poskin M. 1999. Induction of labor and the relationship to cesarean delivery: A review of 7001 consecutive inductions. *Am J Obstet Gynecol* 180:628–33. Young DC, Crane JMG, Hutchens D, Bennett KA, Butt KD. 1999. Misoprostol use in pregnancy: an update. *J Society Obstet Gynaecol Can*. 21:239–45.

Zhang J, Yancey MK, Henderson CE. 2002. U.S. national trends in labor induction, 1989–1998. *J Reprod Med* 47:120–4.

# CHAPTER 24

# PRELABOUR RUPTURE OF MEMBRANES

*Mirudhubashini Govindarajan*

Rupture of fetal membranes occurring prior to the onset of labour is termed prelabour rupture of membranes (PROM), irrespective of whether this rupture occurs before term, at term or post term. Preterm prelabour rupture of membranes (PPROM) refers to the occurrence of this event prior to 37 weeks' gestation and before the onset of labour. This accounts for about one-fourth of all cases of ruptured membranes.

## Terminology

The term *prelabour rupture of membranes* is considered to be more appropriate, compared to *premature rupture of membranes,* since the latter may lead to confusion about the timing of the event.

It is clinically relevant to differentiate PROM into:

PROM
- Beyond 36 completed weeks of gestation

PPROM
- PPROM – near term
  32 to 36 weeks of gestation
- PPROM – remote from term
  24 to 31 weeks of gestation
- PPROM – pre-viable
  Before 24 weeks of gestation

## Incidence

The reported incidence of PROM in the literature varies widely between 3–18.5 per cent (Gunn et al 1970). This large variation in incidence may be secondary to differing ethnic and socio-economic factors. Prelabour rupture of membranes (PROM) is a complication in approximately one third of preterm births (ACOG 2007). This is a leading cause of preterm birth and perinatal morbidity and has a tremendous socio-economic impact worldwide.

## Fetal membrane: Structure, development and pathophysiology

The fetal membrane comprises of the *amnion, chorion* and an *intermediate layer*. The amnion is the innermost thin epithelial layer that lines the amniotic cavity. The outer chorion consists of multilayered trophoblasts. An intermediate layer of acellular connective tissue, binding these two layers, is composed of type I and III collagen giving the membranes their tensile strength.

The amnion, chorion and the intermediate layer fuse together at about 12 weeks of gestation. The resulting amnio-chorion fuses with the maternal decidua at 20 to 25 weeks' gestation.

PROM can result either from inherited intrinsic weakness of the collagen matrix or an acquired degradation. Increased local levels of matrix metalloproteinases (MMP-2, MMP-3, MMP-8 and MMP-9) or decreased levels of tissue inhibitors of MMP (TIMP-1, TIMP-3) contribute to PROM (Maymon et al 2000; Park et al 2003). Bacterial invasion facilitates membrane rupture through direct secretion of proteases and also through stimulation of host inflammatory response resulting in elaboration of local cytokines and prostaglandins (Gomez et al 1997; Goncalves et al 2002).

> Pathogenesis of PROM:
> - Inherited intrinsic weakness
> - Acquired degradation of collagen matrix
> - Increased local levels of MMP
> - Decreased levels of TIMP
> - Bacterial invasion

## Clinical risk factors

Preterm prelabour rupture of membranes (PPROM) is a complex and multifactorial entity. A large number of clinical risk factors are associated with PPROM.

### Infection

The greatest risk factor for PPROM is infection (Gomez et al 1997; Mercer 2003). Bacterial proteases decrease the strength and elasticity of the chorioamniotic membranes. Infections with *gonococcus*, *Trichomonas*, *Chlamydia*, or colonisation with Group B β-hemolytic *Streptococcus* (GBS), or *Gardenella vaginalis*, have an increased risk of PROM (Edwards et al 1978; Minkoff et al 1984). These bacteria produce phospholipases, break down arachidonic acid and stimulate the release of prostaglandins, leading to preterm contractions. Infection also releases pro-inflammatory cytokines and mediators that cause weakening of the fetal membranes by disrupting extracellular matrix and releasing MMPs (Maymon et al 2000; Park et al 2003).

### Genetics

Genetic susceptibility may be a risk factor for PPROM. Association of MMP-9 gene promoter activity with ROM has been described. Several genetic polymorphisms with distinct racial distributions are associated with an increased risk of PPROM (Wang 2006; Anum et al 2009). Inherited conditions such as Ehlers-Danlos syndrome with defects in collagen structure also have an increased risk of PPROM.

### Previous preterm delivery

Women who have had previous PPROM are estimated to have a 21 per cent (Naeye 1982) to 32 per cent (Asrat et al 1991) recurrence risk in subsequent pregnancies. This may be due to endogenous maternal genetic factors or persistence of exogenous environmental factors.

### Nutrition

Vitamin C acts as a co-enzyme for collagen cross linking in the extra cellular matrix of fetal membranes. Low ascorbate levels often found in smokers may be a contributory factor for PPROM.

## Iatrogenic causes

Rupture of the fetal membranes can be secondary to iatrogenic procedures. Fluid leakage has been described after 1 per cent of genetic amniocentesis and 3 per cent to 5 per cent of diagnostic fetoscopies (Rodeck 1980; Gold et al 1989). Predisposing factors which may lead to PPROM are listed in Table 24.1.

**Table 24.1** Predisposing Factors for PPROM

| | |
|---|---|
| Social Factors | • Low socio-economic status<br>• Racial factor<br>• Single motherhood<br>• Low education level |
| General Health Factors | • Extremes of age (<18 and >40 years)<br>• Low BMI<br>• Poor nutrition<br>• Corticosteroid usage<br>• Collagen diseases<br>• Chronic infections<br>• Tobacco use, smoking<br>• Substance abuse |
| Local Factors | • Uterine anomaly<br>• Excessive uterine distension<br>• In-utero DES exposure<br>• Previous cervical surgery<br>• Sexually transmitted diseases<br>• Urinary tract infections |

## PROM/PPROM: Clinical Diagnosis

Diagnosis of PPROM should be prompt. The patient's history alone has a sensitivity of 90 per cent for the diagnosis of PPROM (Gold et al 1989). A sterile speculum examination should be performed to look for gross pooling of amniotic fluid in the posterior fornix and/or for passage of amniotic fluid through the cervical os. If no fluid is seen, the woman should be instructed to cough or perform a Valsalva manouevre to further evaluate for any leakage from the cervix. *Digital examination should be avoided* unless the woman is in active labour or imminent delivery is planned, since very little information is obtained from this examination. Digital examination increases the risk of infection and preterm labour (Munson et al 1985; Alexander et al 1998).

Other investigative modalities have also been utilised to assist in the evaluation of PPROM.

> Diagnosis of ROM:
> • Patient's history
> • Sterile speculum examination
> • Digital examination to be avoided

### Nitrazine test

The normal pH of the vagina during pregnancy is 4.5–5.0. When membranes rupture and the vaginal mucosa is bathed in amniotic fluid with a pH of 7.3, the vaginal pH increases to above 6.0. Nitrazine paper turns from yellow to blue in colour at this pH. The nitrazine test may be false-positive if semen, blood, lubricants or infection are present in the vagina (ACOG 2007).

### Fern test

Vaginal fluid is smeared on a glass slide and allowed to air dry for 10 minutes. Microscopic examination of the smear shows arborisation or *fern* pattern in a positive test. Specificity of the fern test for PROM has been reported to be 84–100 per cent (Bennett et al 1993).

> A combination of the patient's history, a speculum examination, nitrazine test, and fern test for evaluation of a patient with symptoms suggestive of PROM yields a sensitivity of 93.1 per cent (Gold et al 1989).

## Dye test

If the diagnosis of ruptured membranes cannot be confirmed with non-invasive tests, ultrasound-guided invasive testing is possible (ACOG 2007). A 22-gauge needle is inserted under ultrasound guidance into the amniotic cavity and 1 ml of indigo carmine or Evans blue in 10 ml of normal saline is instilled. A tampon placed in the vagina is checked after 30 to 60 min. A blue-tinged tampon may be seen if the woman has ruptured membranes. This is an invasive test and may promote rupture of membranes, and hence, not used in clinical practice.

## Ultrasound imaging

Ultrasound examination of amniotic fluid volume may be useful in documenting oligohydramnios, but is not diagnostic of PROM. Ultrasound examination in suspected PPROM is useful in assessing fetal viability, presentation, fetal weight, placental location and cervical length, funneling or dilatation.

## Other tests

All women with PPROM should have a baseline complete blood count.

Cervical cultures for gonococcus, Chlamydia and a vaginal culture for group B streptococcus should also be done.

## PROM/PPROM: Clinical Course

The latency period between rupture of membranes and delivery is inversely related to the gestational age (Carroll et al 1995).

At term, 95 per cent of women with PROM will deliver within 24 hours of membrane rupture (Hannah et al 1996). The median interval between membrane rupture and delivery at term is 12 to 18 hours, with 90 per cent of deliveries occurring within 24 hours.

- Between 28 and 34 weeks, the median latency is 24 hours with 90 per cent of deliveries occurring within 7 days.
- In PPROM at less than 26 weeks, the median latency interval ranges from 10.6 to 21.5 days, with 57 per cent of women giving birth within 1 week (Schucker and Mercer 1996).

The likelihood of spontaneous resealing of the membranes is usually low, between 2.8 and 13 per cent (Johnson et al 1990). However, in iatrogenic PPROM occurring after amniocentesis, the prognosis is much better, with 86 per cent to 94 per cent resealing spontaneously (Gold et al 1989; Borgida et al 2000).

## PROM/PPROM: Potential Complications

A range of complications can occur both in the mother and the fetus as a result of PROM/PPROM. It is essential to monitor both for these potential complications (Table 24.2).

Table 24.2  Potential complications

| | |
|---|---|
| Maternal Complications | • Risk of infection<br>• Risk of placental abruption<br>• Risk of operative delivery |
| Fetal/ Neonatal Complications | • Infection<br>• Intrauterine fetal demise<br>• Musculoskeletal morbidity<br>• Pulmonary hypoplasia<br>• Necrotising enterocolitis (NEC)<br>• Neurological damage<br>• Neonatal Infection |

## Maternal Complications

### Risk of infection

Conservative management of PROM/PPROM provides the opportunity for subclinical decidual infection to progress to overt ascending infection. The risk of intrauterine infection increases with the duration of membrane rupture and with declining gestational age (ACOG 2007). Twenty-five per cent of all cases of PPROM develop chorioamnionitis. At less than 24 weeks, the incidence of chorioamnionitis increases to 40 per cent.

> Prolonged rupture of membranes can lead to:
> - Chorioamnionitis
> - Endometritis
> - Maternal sepsis

In women who have clinical chorioamnionitis, about 40 per cent will also develop postpartum endometritis. The incidence of postpartum maternal sepsis in PPROM has been reported to be between 0 per cent and 3 per cent (Moretti and Sibai 1988; Morales and Talley 1993; Shumway et al 1999). Sepsis leading to death (0.14 per cent) is an uncommon complication of PPROM remote from term.

### Risk of placental abruption

Placental abruption affects 4–12 per cent of pregnancies with preterm PROM (Gonen et al 1989). Placental abruption and hemorrhage occur secondary to uterine decompression and inflammation in 10 per cent of cases with PPROM, as opposed to 1 per cent of the general obstetric population. Placental abruption occurs in up to 50 per cent of PPROM prior to 20 weeks' gestation (Rotschild et al 1990; Fortunato et al 1994).

### Risk of operative delivery

Cesarean delivery rates significantly increase in PROM, secondary to obstetric complications such as fetal malpresentations, non-reassuring fetal heart patterns, cord compression and placental abruption.

## Fetal/Neonatal Complications

### Infection

Fetal infection is a major complication of mid-trimester PPROM. Neonatal mortality for mid-trimester PPROM (<26 weeks' gestation) is approximately 35–40 per cent. In the majority of cases, this occurs secondary to infection (Moretti and Sibai 1988; Major and Kitzmiller 1990; Dinsmoor et al 2004).

The risk of perinatal mortality has been correlated with the residual volume of amniotic fluid. In pregnancies with PPROM between 20 and 25 weeks' gestation, the group with the largest vertical pocket of amniotic fluid ≥ 2 cm had a greater neonatal survival rate than those with a fluid pocket of <2 cm. Hadi et al (1994) studied women with PPROM at between 20 and 25 weeks' gestation. They found that virtually all women with oligohydramnios delivered before 25 weeks, whereas the women with adequate amniotic fluid volume delivered in the third trimester. In the group of women with severe oligohydramnios, the incidence of chorioamnionitis was also significantly higher.

Studying very low birth weight infants, Alexander et al (1998) found that neonates born with infection had a higher incidence of sepsis, respiratory distress syndrome, early onset seizures, intraventricular hemorrhage (IVH) and periventricular leukomalacia. It is therefore obvious that very low birth weight infants are susceptible to neurological injury in the presence of chorioamnionitis. In 1999, Yoon et al described a condition known as fetal inflammatory response syndrome (FIRS), defined as elevated IL-6 in fetal plasma obtained by cordocentesis. An association of periventricular white matter lesions to the cytokines released in FIRS was established. A three-year follow-up showed an association between FIRS and cerebral palsy.

> Chorioamnionitis in very low birth weight neonates can lead to:
> - Sepsis
> - Respiratory distress syndrome
> - Early onset seizures
> - Intraventricular hemorrhage
> - Periventricular leukomalacia

### Intrauterine fetal demise

The incidence of intrauterine fetal demise decreases as gestational age increases (Bengtson et al 1989; Morales and Talley 1993). The risk of placental abruption with PROM at term is only 0.4–1.3 per cent (Yoon et al 1999).

Most fetal demises are attributable to placental abruption, cord prolapse, cord compression or fetal infection. Placental abruption occurs in up to 50 per cent of PPROM prior to 20 weeks' gestation (Rotschild et al 1990; Fortunato et al 1994). Cord prolapse is not common, with the incidence reported to be around 1.9 per cent. The main risk factor for cord prolapse is a non-cephalic presentation of the fetus, especially before 26 weeks (Lewis et al 2007).

> Fetal demise in PPROM could result from:
> - Placental abruption
> - Cord prolapse
> - Cord compression
> - Fetal infection

### Musculoskeletal morbidity

In chronic oligohydramnios, the intrauterine pressure becomes asymmetric and fetal growth and movements are restricted. This leads to limb position deformities and craniofacial defects. The reported incidence for these deformities varies between 3.5 per cent and 50 per cent in mid-trimester PPROM with severe oligohydramnios. The risk increases when the duration of PPROM exceeds 14 days (Rotschild et al 1990).

### Pulmonary hypoplasia

In PPROM, the pressure gradient between the amniotic cavity and the alveoli is altered, leading to loss of fetal lung fluid into the amniotic cavity and resultant pulmonary hypoplasia. The incidence of pulmonary hypoplasia varies with the gestational age at PPROM. Blott and Greenough (1988) reported an incidence of 50 per cent at 19 weeks, 10 per cent at 25 weeks and rare after 26 weeks. In this study, all fetuses with pulmonary hypoplasia were born to mothers with a median amniotic fluid pocket of less than 2 cm. Lethal pulmonary hypoplasia rarely occurs with membrane rupture subsequent to 24 weeks of gestation, presumably because alveolar growth that is adequate to support postnatal development has already occurred (Rotschild et al 1990).

### Neurological damage

Hypoxia, inflammation and gross prematurity contribute to neurological damage in approximately 6–12 per cent of all PPROM infants (Yoon et al 1999). As mentioned earlier, the presence of chorioamnionitis increases the risk of neurological complications in the neonate.

**Neonatal infections**

In the newborn, infections ranging from localised conjunctivitis and ear infections to congenital pneumonia and sepsis can occur. Long-term morbidities are uncommon with deliveries after 32 weeks' gestation, highlighting the need for conservative management at an earlier gestation.

## Prediction and Prevention of PPROM

Prevention of PPROM requires screening for clinical markers and ameliorating these underlying risk factors. Potentially modifiable risk factors include poor nutrition, urinary tract and sexually transmitted infections, acute pulmonary diseases and cigarette smoking. Identification of a cervical length shorter than 25 mm on transvaginal ultrasound confers increased risk of subsequent PROM (Guinn et al 1995). A combination of short cervical length and positive fetal fibronectin test increases the risk of PPROM and preterm delivery 9–10-fold (Mercer et al 2000).

Unfortunately, most cases of PPROM still occur in low-risk women. Although there is an association between short cervix and preterm delivery, there is no data to support routine screening for all women. An effective screening protocol for assessing the risk of preterm birth that combines cervical measurements and other risk factors has not been

> Routine screening of cervical length by transvaginal ultrasound, to predict PROM/preterm labour, is not recommended in women at low risk of preterm labour.

developed (ACOG 2009). Tests such as fetal fibronectin screening and transvaginal sonography need not be incorporated into routine antenatal care for low-risk women since effective interventional strategies have not been identified so far.

## Management

### Hospitalisation and monitoring

In view of the potential for acute complications (intrauterine and fetal infection, umbilical cord compression), outpatient management of PPROM is not recommended (ACOG 2007). Hospitalisation for the duration of pregnancy should be standard management for these women. This approach is justified because, if chorioamnionitis is diagnosed, expedient delivery will be required to reduce the risk of neonatal sepsis and morbidity. Institutions providing care for PPROM should have resources for emergency operative deliveries and neonatal intensive care.

Frequent examinations for fever, maternal tachycardia, uterine tenderness, fetal tachycardia and blood-stained or purulent discharge are mandatory. However, there is no consensus in the contemporary literature regarding the type or frequency of fetal monitoring necessary. Many institutions use daily non-stress testing to assess the fetus.

### Antenatal corticosteroid therapy in PPROM

The National Institutes of Health Consensus Development Conference (2000) and The American Congress of Obstetricians and Gynecologists (ACOG 2007) recommend the use of a single course of antenatal corticosteroids with PPROM without evidence of chorioamnionitis, between

24 and 32 weeks' gestation. This has been shown to decrease the incidence of respiratory distress syndrome (RDS), intraventricular hemorrhage (IVH), necrotising enterocolitis (NEC) and neonatal death. Although corticosteroids may potentially increase the risk of perinatal infection, it should be administered to patients with PPROM of less than 32 weeks' gestation, since the neonatal benefits may outweigh the risks. There is no consensus for treatment between 32 and 34 weeks.

Two doses of 12 mg betamethasone should be administered parenterally to the mother, 24 hours apart. The last dose should be at least 24 hours and preferably 48 hours prior to delivery. The current consensus is that there is no benefit in repeating this course of betamethasone if the pregnancy continues. Currently, there is evidence that both dexamethasone and betamethasone are comparable in reducing the rates of major neonatal complications in preterm infants.

Repeated weekly antenatal corticosteroid therapy is not recommended. This approach may carry potential risks. The benefits and risks of a single *rescue dosage* remote from the initial dose remain to be determined.

### Use of tocolytics in PPROM

The use of prophylactic tocolysis after PPROM has been shown to prolong latency in the short term (Christensen et al 1980). However, Garite et al (1987) showed that the use of aggressive therapeutic tocolysis after contractions have begun did not prolong latency. The majority of women with PPROM have intrauterine infection at the onset of labour. The use of tocolytics is of concern since the incidence of perinatal infection is high and prolongation of these pregnancies may not be ideal. A retrospective study by Wolfensberger et al (2006) using prolonged tocolysis for more than 48 hours concluded that a latency of greater than one week could be achieved, but was negated by the incidence of chorioamnionitis.

If tocolysis is used, it must be given only to enable the use of corticosteroids to improve pulmonary maturity. The rationale in this situation is to forestall delivery sufficiently so that the antenatal corticosteroids have time to work. Tocolysis may also have a role to play where an in-utero transfer to a high-risk unit with NICU facilities becomes necessary. However, the use of tocolytics to permit the administration of antibiotics and corticosteroids has not been conclusively evaluated.

Tocolysis should not be used repeatedly to inhibit labour as it may mask infection. If betamimetic drugs are combined with corticosteroids, there is a risk of acute pulmonary edema. Strict control of fluid balance is necessary to prevent this

---

Corticosteroids in PPROM:
- 24–32 weeks' gestation
- 12 mg of betamethasone
- 2 doses, 24 hours apart
- Last dose at least 24 hours before delivery
- No benefit in repeating the dose if pregnancy continues

Tocolysis in PPROM:
- Not recommended routinely
- Used only to forestall delivery, thus allowing antenatal corticosteroids time to work
- Not to be used repeatedly
- Betamimetic agents combined with corticosteroids can lead to maternal pulmonary edema

complication. Prostaglandin synthetase inhibitors are to be avoided, because they can mask early signs of intrauterine infection and affect neonatal cardiovascular adaptation to extra-uterine life.

### Antibiotic prophylaxis

The purpose of prophylactic antibiotics in patients with PPROM is to decrease the risk of perinatal infections and to increase the latency period. Mercer and Arheart (1995) in a meta-analysis showed that antimicrobials reduced the rate of chorioamnionitis, reduced newborn sepsis and prolonged pregnancy by seven days.

Two large, multicentre clinical trials have demonstrated the usefulness of antibiotics for PPROM. The National Institute of Child Health and Human Development Maternal Fetal Medicine Unit (NICHD-MFMU) Research Network (Mercer et al 1997) and the Oracle 1 Randomised Trial (Kenyon et al 2001) found that the combination of initial intravenous therapy (48 hours) with ampicillin and erythromycin, followed by oral therapy of limited duration (five days) with amoxicillin and enteric-coated erythromycin-base at 24–32 weeks of gestation, decreased the likelihood of chorioamnionitis and delivery for up to three weeks. In both studies, the incidence of severe respiratory distress syndrome (RDS), severe IVH, neonatal sepsis, pneumonia and necrotising enterocolitis (NEC) were reduced with the use of ampicillin or erythromycin. However, they reported an increased incidence of NEC in fetuses whose mothers were treated with amoxicillin/clavulanic acid. Prolonged treatment with antibiotics may generate drug-resistant microorganisms. McDuffie et al (1993) reported the development of resistant Enterobacteriaceae after prophylactic ampicillin or amoxicillin was used. The potential benefits of antimicrobials are well described, but there is no consensus on the duration of therapy. Both three-day and seven-day courses of either ampicillin or ampicillin-sulbactam seem to be effective in reducing perinatal infection (Lewis et al 2003; Segel et al 2003).

Women with PPROM should have genital tract cultures obtained for GBS, since these are the most common microorganisms causing neonatal pneumonia, meningitis and sepsis. Penicillin G should be started after cultures are obtained with a loading dose of $5 \times 10^6$ units intravenously followed by a maintenance dose of $2.5 \times 10^6$ units every 4 hours. If penicillin G is not available, a 2 g loading dose of intravenous ampicillin should be started, followed by 1 g every 4 hours. The purpose of this management is to decrease the vertical transmission of GBS and the severe neonatal morbidity that may occur. Women with chorioamnionitis should receive broadspectrum antibiotics. For those who are allergic to penicillin, erythromycin is recommended.

### Timing of delivery

***PROM at term (37–40 weeks)***: There is no substantial fetal benefit from expectant

---

Antibiotics in PPROM:
- Latency period is increased to 7 days
- Incidence of severe RDS, severe IVH, neonatal sepsis, pneumonia and NEC reduced with ampicillin or erythromycin
- Ampicillin, ampicillin-sulbactam, or erythromycin recommended
- Amoxicillin/clavulanic acid can cause NEC so should be avoided
- 3- or 7-day regimens equally effective

management at term and hence the best approach is early delivery. If spontaneous labour is not established, induction is recommended. Hannah et al (1996), in a multi-centre study comparing induction and expectant management in women with PROM at term, found that induction of labour with oxytocin or prostaglandin E$_2$ and expectant management resulted in similar rates of neonatal infection and cesarean section. Induction of labour with intravenous oxytocin resulted in a lower risk of maternal infection than did expectant management. In the study, it was found that women viewed induction of labour more positively than expectant management. If the cervix is unfavourable, prostaglandin use is justifiable. In cases of hind water leak, the forewater may need to be ruptured. Some authors recommend expectant management for 24 hours if the cervix is not favourable. Vaginal examination should be avoided during the expectant management phase. In general, antibiotics are not recommended although some advocate selective use in known carriers of group B streptococci.

*PPROM at 34–36 completed weeks' gestation*: Infants born at 34–36 weeks' gestation have a slightly higher risk of complications than term infants. However, severe acute morbidity and mortality are uncommon. Conservative management of

> PROM at term:
> - Induction of labour with oxytocin or prostaglandins recommended
> - Rates of maternal infection less with oxytocin induction as compared to expectant management
> - Cesarean section rates similar between induction and expectant management
> - Antibiotics are not recommended

PROM at 34–36 weeks prolongs pregnancy by only a few days and significantly increases the risk of chorioamnionitis. Therefore, PROM at 34–36 weeks should be actively managed. Antenatal corticosteroids for fetal lung maturation are not recommended at this gestational age.

> PROM at 34–36 weeks:
> - Induction recommended since prolongation of pregnancy may lead to chorioamnionitis
> - Antenatal corticosteroids not recommended
> - Antibiotics are not recommended

*PPROM at 32–33 completed weeks' gestation*: The management for PPROM at 32–33 weeks of gestation should be individualised. It is recommended that pregnancy be managed conservatively till 33 completed weeks if no maternal or fetal contraindications exist (ACOG 2007). Administration of antenatal corticosteroids is an appropriate choice. Concurrent antibiotic treatment should be given to reduce the risk of intrauterine infection.

*PPROM at 24–31 completed weeks' gestation*: Between 24 and 31 weeks, the greatest threat to the fetus is from prematurity, and therefore a policy of expectant management is the norm. Delivery may need to be expedited where there is chorioamnionitis or signs of fetal compromise.

Prolongation of the pregnancy, especially where liquor is re-accumulating, is likely to improve the outcome in terms of survival and neurological development. In PROM under 28 weeks, more than 60 per cent of fetuses survive, because the mean time between PROM and the onset of labour is four weeks, allowing delivery at a gestational age with a better prognosis. After 26 weeks, and especially after 28 weeks, fetal lung maturity can be induced with corticosteroids. There is strong evidence to support antenatal treatment with corticosteroids to significantly reduce the incidence of RDS in infants at 28–34 weeks' gestation.

> PROM at 24–31 weeks:
> - Expectant management
> - Prolongation of pregnancy improves outcome
> - Antibiotics recommended to increase latency period
> - Antenatal corticosteroids recommended

*Previable PPROM before 24 weeks*: Previable PPROM with persistent second trimester bleeding, oligohydramnios or elevated maternal serum α-fetoprotein is more likely to be associated with abnormal placentation and carries a poor prognosis.

Persistent severe oligohydramnios after PPROM before 20 weeks is the strongest predictor for subsequent lethal pulmonary hypoplasia (Blott and Greenough 1988). Serial fetal biometric evaluation, thoracic circumference, fetal breathing movements and Doppler studies (ductus arteriosus, pulmonary artery) can demonstrate fetal pulmonary growth over time. Repeat ultrasound evaluation can be performed weekly for amniotic fluid volume and assessment of fetal lung growth.

With previable PPROM and prolonged bed rest, in addition to the known maternal risks, muscle wasting, bone demineralisation and deep venous thrombosis can also occur. Prolonged hospitalisation also has significant financial and social implications.

Delivery in previable PROM can be accomplished with vaginal prostaglandin $E_2$, high-dose oxytocin infusion or by dilatation and evacuation. The optional approach depends on the gestational age, presence of chorioamnionitis, prior cesarean delivery, available facilities and the physician's experience.

### Use of sealants for treatment

Attempts to seal the membrane defect have included sealing with fibrin, platelet, cryoprecipitate or gelatin sponges (O'Brien et al 2001). Restoration of normal amniotic fluid volume has been attempted with transabdominal amnioinfusion. The maternal risks and fetal benefits of these interventions have not been adequately evaluated and the data is inadequate to recommend that any of these approaches be incorporated into routine clinical practice.

## PPROM in Special Circumstances

### Cervical cerclage

PPROM complicates one-fourth of all pregnancies with cervical cerclage and half of the pregnancies requiring an emergency cerclage. In PPROM with cervical cerclage occurring prior to 24 weeks' gestation, most agree on removing the cerclage and counselling the patient about termination of pregnancy. In PPROM with cervical cerclage after 24 weeks, the dilemma of whether or not to remove the cervical cerclage prevails. The few available studies have shown no statistical difference in the incidence of chorioamnionitis, latency period and neonatal outcome between the two approaches (Major and Kitzmiller 1990).

## Iatrogenic mid-trimester PPROM

Amniotic fluid leakage complicates 1.0–1.2 per cent of genetic amniocentesis and the associated pregnancy loss is 0.06 percent (Eddleman et al 2006). The outcome of iatrogenic mid-trimester PPROM is different from that of spontaneous mid-trimester PPROM with the exception of iatrogenic PPROM occurring after cervical cerclage. In most patients, the membranes tend to reseal and the amniotic fluid volume is restored (Gold et al 1989).

## PPROM in patients who are HIV positive

A major risk factor for vertical transmission of HIV is the duration of ruptured membranes prior to delivery. There is a significant increase in vertical transmission rate if the duration of rupture of membranes is greater than four hours in patients with low CD4+ levels. Studies have confirmed that ruptured membranes greater than four hours prior to delivery significantly increases the rate of vertical transmission to 25 per cent as compared to 14 per cent among mothers with a shorter length of ruptured membranes.

## Herpes genetalis (HSV) and PPROM

Congenital herpes is a major perinatal infection with the possibility of a fatal disease in the neonate. It may be acquired if a mother has PPROM with active genital lesions.

Few studies have looked at the risk of perinatal transmission after PPROM when expectant management is implemented. A case series studied expectant management for women with active recurrent herpes simplex virus lesions and PROM before 32 weeks of gestation (Major et al 2003). None of the infants developed neonatal herpes infection.

## Management protocols – PROM/PPROM

| | |
|---|---|
| 37 weeks to term | • Proceed to delivery<br>• Induction of labour<br>• Group B streptococcal prophylaxis if necessary |
| 34 weeks to 36 weeks | • Proceed to delivery – induction if needed<br>• Corticosteroids not necessary |
| 32 weeks to 34 weeks | • Expectant management unless fetal pulmonary maturity is documented<br>• Group B streptococcal prophylaxis is recommended<br>• Corticosteroids – some experts recommend but no consensus<br>• Antimicrobials to prolong latency if no contraindications |
| 24 weeks to 31 completed weeks | • Expectant management<br>• Group B streptococcal prophylaxis is recommended<br>• Single-course corticosteroid use is recommended<br>• Tocolytics – no consensus<br>• Antimicrobials to prolong latency if no contraindications |
| Before 24 weeks | • Patient needs extensive counselling<br>• Group B streptococcal prophylaxis is not recommended<br>• Corticosteroids are not recommended<br>• Antimicrobials – incomplete data on use in prolonging latency<br>• Induction of labour by the appropriate method |

## Summary

There is potential for significant perinatal morbidity and mortality with term or preterm PROM, which can be reduced by timely obstetric intervention. Expeditious delivery of the patient with term and late preterm PROM can reduce the risk of perinatal infection without increasing the likelihood of operative delivery. Conservative management of PROM remote from term can reduce gestational age–dependent morbidities. Attention to early diagnosis and management of complications can lead to good perinatal outcomes in most cases.

## Key Points for Clinical Practice

- Patients at 34 or more weeks' gestation with PPROM should be delivered.
- Patients at less than 32 weeks' gestation with PPROM should be managed conservatively with corticosteroid and antimicrobial prophylaxis unless there is an indication for delivery.
- The management of patients with PPROM between 32 and 34 weeks' gestation is controversial.
- Patients with PPROM and either HIV or genital HSV require individual evaluation and treatment.

## References

Alexander JM, Gilstrap LC, Cox SM et al. 1998. Clinical chorioamnionitis and the prognosis for very low birthweight infants. *Obstet Gynecol*. 91:725–29.

American College of Obstetricians and Gynecologists. 2007. Premature rupture of membranes. Practice Bulletin No. 80. *Obstet Gynecol* 1007–19

American College of Obstetricians and Gynecologists. 2009. Ultrasonography in Pregnancy. Practice Bulletin No. 101. *Obstet Gynecol* 113: 451–61.

Anum EA, Hill LD, Pandya A et al. 2009. Connective tissue and related disorders and preterm birth: clues to genes contributing to preterm birth. *Placenta* 30(3): 207.

Asrat T, Lewis DF, Garite TJ, Major CA, Nageotte MP, Towers CV et al. 1991. Rate of recurrence of preterm premature rupture of membranes in consecutive pregnancies. *Am J Obstet Gynecol* 165:1111–5.

Bengtson JM, VanMarter LJ, Barss VA et al. 1989. Pregnancy outcome after premature rupture of the membranes at or before 26 weeks' gestation. *Obstet Gynecol* 73: 921–27.

Bennett SL, Cullen JB, Shere DM et al. 1993. The ferning and nitrazine tests of amniotic fluid between 12 and 41 weeks gestation. *Am J Perinatol* 10: 101–4.

Blott M, Greenough A. 1988. Neonatal outcome after prolonged rupture of the membranes starting in the second trimester. *Arch Dis Child* 63; 1146–50.

Borgida AF, Mills AA, Feldman DM, Rodis JF, Egan JF. 2000. Outcome of pregnancies complicated by ruptured membranes after genetic amniocentesis. *Am J Obstet Gynecol* 183:937–9.

Carroll SG, Blott M, Nikolaides KH. 1995. Preterm prelabor amniorrhexis: Outcome of live births. *Obstet Gynecol* 86:18.

Christensen KK, Ingemarsson I, Leideman T, Solum H, Svenningsen N. 1980. Effect of ritodrine on labor after premature rupture of the membranes. *Obstet Gynecol* 55: 187–90.

Dinsmoor MJ, Bachman R, Haney EI et al. 2004. Outcomes after expectant management of extremely preterm premature rupture of the membranes. *Am J Obstet Gynecol* 190: 183–7.

Edwards LE, Barrada MI, Hamman AA et al. 1978. Gonorrhea in pregnancy. *Obstet Gynecol* 132: 637–41.

Eddleman K, Malone F, Sullivan L, Dukes K, Berkowitz R, Kharbutli Y, et al. 2006. Pregnancy loss rates after mid-trimester amniocentesis. *Obstet Gynecol* 108: 1067–72.

Fortunato SJ, Welt SI, Eggleston Jr MK, Bryant EC. 1994. Active expectant management in very early gestations complicated by premature rupture of membranes. *J Reprod Med* 39: 13–16.

Garite TJ, Keegan KA, Freeman RK, Nageotte MP. 1987. A randomized trial of ritodrine tocolysis versus expectant management in patients with premature rupture of membranes at 25 to 30 weeks of gestation. *Am J Obstet Gynecol* 157:388–93.

Gold RB, Goyert N, Schwartz DB et al. 1989. Conservative management of second-trimester post-amniocentesis fluid leakage. *Obstet Gynecol* 74: 745–47.

Gomez R, Romero R, Edwin SS, et al. 1997. Pathogenesis of preterm labor and preterm premature rupture of membranes associated with intraamniotic infection. *Inf Dis Clin North Am* 11:135–76.

Goncalves LF, Chaiworapongsa T, Romero R. 2002. Intrauterine infection and prematurity. *Ment Retard Dev Disabil Res Rev* 8:3–13.

Gonen R, Hannah ME, Milligan JE. 1989. Does prolonged preterm premature rupture of the membranes predispose to abruptio placentae? *Obstet Gynecol* 74:347–50.

*Gunn GC, Mishell DR, Morton DG. 1970. Premature rupture of the fetal membranes*: A review. *Am J Obstet Gynecol* 106:469–483.

Guinn DA, Goldenberg RL, Hauth JC, Andrews WW, Thom E, Romero R. 1995. Risk factors for the development of preterm premature rupture of the membranes after arrest of preterm labor. *Am J Obstet Gynecol* Oct; 173(4):1310–5.

Hadi HA, Hodson CA, Strickland D. 1994. Premature rupture of the membranes between 20 and 25 weeks' gestation, role of amniotic fluid volume in perinatal outcome. *Am J Obstet Gynecol*; 39 13–16.

Hannah ME, Ohlsson A, Farine D, et al. 1996. Induction of labor compared with expectant management for prelabor rupture of the membranes at term. TERMPROM Study Group. *N Engl J Med* 334:1005–10.

Johnson JW, Egerman RS, Moorhead J. 1990. Cases with ruptured membranes that "reseal". *Am J Obstet Gynecol* Sep; 163(3):1024–30.

Kenyon SL, Taylor DJ, Tarnow-Mordi W. 2001. Broad spectrum antibiotics for preterm, prelabor rupture of fetal membranes: the ORACLE I randomized trial. ORACLE Collaborative Group *Lancet* 357:979–88.

Lewis DF, Adair CD, Robichaux AG et al. 2003. Antibiotic therapy in preterm premature rupture of membranes: Are seven days necessary? A preliminary randomized clinical trial. *Am J Obstet Gynecol* 188:1413–1416.

Lewis DF, Robichaux AG, Jaekle RK et al. 2007. Expectant management of preterm premature rupture of membranes and non-vertex presentation: What are the risks? *Am J Obstet Gynecol* 196:566.

Major CA, Kitzmiller JL. 1990. Perinatal survival with expectant management of midtrimester rupture of membranes. *Am J Obstet Gynecol* 163: 838–44.

Major CA, Towers CV, Lewis DF et al. 2003. Expectant management of preterm premature rupture of membranes complicated by active recurrent genital herpes. *Am J Obstet Gynecol* 188: 1551–54.

Maymon E, Romero R, Pacora P et al. 2000. Matrilysin (matrix metalloproteinase 7) in parturition, premature rupture of membranes, and intrauterine infection. *Am J Obstet Gynecol* 182: 1545–53.

McDuffie R, McGregor J, Gibbs R. 1993. Adverse perinatal outcome and resistant Enterobacteriaceae after antibiotic usage for premature rupture of the membranes and group B streptococcus carriage. *Obstet Gynecol* 82: 487–89.

Mercer BM, Arheart KL. 1995. Antimicrobial therapy in expectant management preterm premature rupture of membranes. *Lancet* 346:1271.

Mercer BM, Goldenberg RL, Meis PJ, Moawad AH, Shellhaas C, Das A, et al. 2000. The Preterm Prediction Study: prediction of preterm premature rupture of membranes using clinical findings and ancillary testing. The National Institute of Child Health and Human Development Maternal–Fetal Medicine Units Network. *Am J Obstet Gynecol* 183:738–45.

Mercer BM, Miodovnik M, Thurnau GR, Goldenberg RL, Das AF, Ramsey RD, et al. 1997. Antibiotic therapy for reduction of infant morbidity after preterm premature rupture of the membranes. A randomized controlled trial. National Institute of Child Health and Human Development Maternal–Fetal Medicine Units Network. *JAMA* 278: 989–95.

Mercer BM. 2003. Preterm premature rupture of the membranes. *Obstet Gynecol* 101: 178–93.

Minkoff H, Grunebaum AN, Schwarz RH et al. 1984. Risk factors for prematurity and premature rupture of membranes: a prospective study of the vaginal flora in pregnancy. *Am J Obstet Gynecol* 150: 965–72.

Morales WJ, Talley T. 1993. Premature rupture of membranes at <25 weeks: a management dilemma. *Am J Obstet Gynecol* 168: 503–7.

Moretti M, Sibai BM. 1988. Maternal and neonatal outcome of expected management of premature rupture of membranes in the midtrimester. *Am J Obstet Gynecol* 159: 390–96.

Munson LA, Graham A, Koos BJ, Valenzuela GJ. 1985. Is there a need for digital examination in patients with spontaneous rupture of the membranes? *Am J Obstet Gynecol* 153:562–3.

Naeye RI. 1982. Factors that predispose to premature rupture of membranes. *Obstet Gynecol* 60:93–8.

National Institutes of Health Consensus Development Conference. 2000. Statement on Repeat Courses of Antenatal Corticosteroids. Bethesda MD. August 17–18.

O'Brien JM, Mercer BM, Barton JR et al. 2001. An *in vitro* model and case report that used gelatin sponge to restore amniotic fluid volume after spontaneous premature rupture of the membranes. *Am J Obstet Gynecol* 185: 1094–97.

Park KH, Chaiworapongsa T, Kim YM et al. 2003. Matrix metalloproteinase 3 in parturition, premature rupture of the membranes, and microbial invasion of the amniotic cavity. *J Perinat Med* 31: 12–22.

Rodeck CH. 1980. Fetoscopy guided by real-time ultrasound for pure fetal blood samples, fetal skin samples, and examination of the fetus *in utero*. *Br J Obstet Gynaecol* 87: 449–56.

Rotschild A, Ling EW, Puterman ML, Farquharson D. 1990. Neonatal outcome after prolonged preterm rupture of the membranes. *Am J Obstet Gynecol* 162: 46–52.

Schucker JL, Mercer BM. 1996. Midtrimester premature rupture of the membranes. *Semin Perinatol* 20:389–400.

Segel SY, Miles AM, Clothier B, et al. 2003. Duration of antibiotic therapy after preterm premature rupture of fetal membranes. *Am J Obstet Gynecol* 189:799–802.

Shumway JB, Al-Malt A, Amon E et al. 1999. Impact of oligohydramnios on maternal and perinatal outcomes of spontaneous premature rupture of the membranes at 18 – 28 weeks. *J. Matern Fetal Med* 8:20–23.

Wang H, Parry S. Macones G, et al. 2006. A functional SNP in the promoters of SERPINH1 gene increases risk of preterm premature rupture of membranes in African Americans. *PNAS* 103:13463–467.

Wolfensberger A, Zimmermann R, von Mandach U. 2006. Neonatal mortality and morbidity after aggressive long-term tocolysis for preterm premature rupture of the membranes. *Fetal Diagn Ther* 21:366–73.

Yoon BH, Romero R, Kim KS et al. 1999. A systemic fetal inflammatory response and the development of bronchopulmonary dysplasia. *Am J Obstet Gynecol* 181: 773–79.

# CHAPTER 25

# PRETERM LABOUR AND DELIVERY—MANAGEMENT ISSUES

*T P Baskaran*

## Introduction

Preterm labour complicates approximately 10 per cent of pregnancies. It contributes to significant neonatal morbidity and mortality. Children who are born prematurely have a higher risk of cerebral palsy, sensory deficits, learning disabilities and respiratory illness compared with those born at term (Wang 2004). Beck and colleagues (2010) estimated that 9.6 per cent of all births were preterm in 2005, which translates to about 12.9 million births definable as preterm. Approximately 85 per cent of this burden was concentrated in Africa and Asia, where 10.9 million births were preterm. In Malaysia, 50 per cent of neonatal deaths are due to preterm birth (World Health Organization 2006).

> Children who are born prematurely have a higher risk of cerebral palsy, sensory deficits, learning disabilities and respiratory illness than those born at term.

> Approximately 85 per cent of preterm births occur in Africa and Asia.

Very often, the diagnosis of preterm labour is made at too advanced a stage in labour to effectively stop it or act upon it. This appears to be true both in developed and in developing nations. However, in recent years, neonatal outcome appears to have improved. The change in the trend of improved neonatal outcome associated with preterm labour is not related to better prediction, diagnosis or management of the problem but due to improvements in neonatal intensive care.

## Definition

A simplistic definition of preterm delivery would be any birth before 37 completed weeks or 259 days of gestation (World Health Organization 1992). This definition indicates the maturity of the fetus as does that of the American College of Obstetricians and Gynecologists, which defines preterm labour as regular contractions associated with cervical change before 37 weeks' gestation (ACOG 2003). Preterm labour can be more specifically described as the presence of uterine contractions of sufficient

> Preterm labour is defined as the presence of uterine contractions of sufficient strength and frequency to cause progressive effacement and dilation of the cervix between 20 and 37 weeks.

strength and frequency to cause progressive effacement and dilatation of the cervix between 20 and 37 weeks. This definition illustrates the extended period of gestation during which preterm delivery may be detrimental to the survival of the newborn. It must be recognised that, in practice, most neonatal morbidly and mortality occurs in the subset of children born before 32 weeks. Hence, it would be prudent to pay greater attention to pregnancies at the lower end of the spectrum rather than those at the upper end. Though fewer deliveries occur in this group, the associated morbidity is exponentially greater. On a practical note, every centre has to recognise its lower limit for salvaging babies in the event of such a delivery.

## Incidence

Preterm birth rates available from some developed countries, such as the United Kingdom, the United States and the Scandinavian countries, show a dramatic rise over the past 20 years (Callaghan 2006).

Some factors that may contribute to this rise may be the increasing rates of multiple births, greater use of assisted reproduction techniques, increase in the proportion of births among women over 34 years of age and changes in clinical practices, such as greater use of elective cesarean section. Changes in the definitions of fetal loss, stillbirth and early neonatal death may have also contributed

> Factors contributing to increase in preterm birth
> - Increasing rates of multiple births
> - Greater use of assisted reproduction techniques
> - Births among women over 34 years of age
> - Greater use of elective cesarean section

to the significant increase in preterm birth rates recorded in developed countries in the past two decades (Stanton et al 2006).

On the other hand, in developing countries, it is difficult to extract data about preterm births because of the lacunae in accurate medical record-keeping. Estimates of the rate of preterm births in developing countries are influenced by many factors, including varying procedures used to determine gestational age, national differences in the birth registration process, heterogeneous definitions used for preterm birth and differences in the perception of the viability of preterm. These issues make measurement of preterm birth and comparisons across and between developing countries difficult (Beck et al 2010).

## Risk factors

Various risk factors have been identified to be associated with or contributing to the occurrence of preterm labour. This list is not exhaustive, and as we investigate each case of preterm labour, it would be apparent that some risk factors would have a greater association to a particular population.

### Iatrogenic factors

Developments in the fields of antenatal diagnosis, maternal fetal medicine and neonatalogy have lead to increased early interventions by obstetricians. Medical conditions which threaten maternal well-being, such as preeclampsia, are aggressively managed by operative deliveries which results in babies being delivered earlier. Similarly, any pregnancy with a maternal medical condition which may adversely affect fetal well-being is at risk of being delivered before term. This number is on the rise with the availability of advanced fetal surveillance and imaging technology such as the cardiotocograph and high-end ultrasound machines. The practice of 'defensive medicine' as a result of the increase in litigation has only increased the burden.

### Social factors

The universal effect of low socio-economic status on health appears to directly affect the incidence of preterm labour (Moutquin 2003). This is due to an intricate web of inter-related factors such as social habit, religion-based beliefs, financial circumstances and rapid changes taking place in our social environment. Issues such as easy, early and affordable access to specialist care, socials ills such as smoking, consumption of alcohol and substance abuse and economic compulsion for women to work may all contribute to the increase in preterm labour and delivery. Psychological stress in this group of women is often not recognised, and when recognised, not addressed appropriately. However, it is not clear if these factors are a cause or merely an association with the occurrence of preterm labour. At present, there is no clear evidence to show that appropriate social support would reduce the preterm delivery rates.

### Ethnic origin

There is evidence that there may be variations in duration of gestation among various ethnic groups (Patel et al 2004). Higher rates of preterm labour have been reported among women of African origin. This may not be purely related to ethnic origin but may be due to other contributing socio-economic conditions. In Malaysia, in the management of post-date pregnancies, some clinicians take into consideration the fact that the population of Indian origin may have a shorter gestational period.

### Previous obstetric history

Past obstetric history may be one of the strongest predictors of recurrent preterm birth. A previous occurrence of preterm birth before 34 weeks may increase the risk of recurrence (Krymko et al 2004). In a study of almost 16,000 women, there was a three-fold increase in risk with a previous preterm birth compared to a previous term pregnancy (Bloom et al 2001). However, it should be remembered that though prior preterm birth is a risk factor, only 10 per cent of all preterm births will occur in women with a previous preterm birth.

> Past obstetric history may be one of the strongest predictors of recurrent preterm birth.

### Interval between pregnancies

A short interval between pregnancies is known to be associated with preterm birth. In a meta-analysis (Conde-Agudelo 2006), it was shown that intervals shorter than 18 months and longer than 59 months were associated with preterm birth and small-for-gestational age infants.

### Cervical insufficiency (incompetence)

Cervical insufficiency is the term currently used to describe what was previously referred to as 'cervical incompetence', as the latter was considered to be inappropriate. Cervical insufficiency is characterised by recurrent, painless cervical dilatation and spontaneous mid-trimester birth in the absence of spontaneous membrane rupture, bleeding or infection (Cunningham et al 2010). The reported incidence of cervical insufficiency is approximately 1–2 per cent. Diagnosis is often made in a subjective manner using a clinical history of painless preterm birth. Harger (2002) lists the following as features of cervical insufficiency:

- Two or more second trimester pregnancy losses (excluding those resulting from preterm labour or abruption)
- History of losing subsequent pregnancies at an earlier period of gestation
- History of painless cervical dilation of up to 4–6 cm
- Absence of clinical findings consistent with placental abruption
- History of cervical trauma due to cone biopsy
- History of cervical laceration during previous delivery
- History of excessive forced cervical dilation during termination of a pregnancy

In contrast to a clinical history–based diagnosis, measurement of the cervical length may be a more objective alternative. In a clinical trial conducted by the National Institute of Child Health and Human Development Maternal Fetal Medicine Unit (NICHD-MFMU) Network (Iams et al 1996), the relation of cervical length measurement to the risk of spontaneous preterm delivery was assessed. Patients with singleton pregnancies had their cervical length measured transvaginally at 24 and 28 weeks of gestation. The study defined the fifth, tenth and fiftieth per centile for cervical lengths as 22 mm, 26 mm and 35 mm, respectively.

> Most women with a shortened cervix are unlikely to deliver preterm, in the absence of a clinical history of preterm delivery.

This study noted that the relative risk of preterm delivery increased six-fold when the cervical length was less than 26 mm. Though it showed that there was a correlation between the cervical length and risk of preterm delivery, the positive predictive value was only 17.8 per cent for a cervical length of less than 25 mm at 24 weeks. Therefore, most women with shortened cervix on ultrasound are unlikely to deliver preterm, in the absence of a clinical history of preterm delivery.

### Infection (vaginal/intrauterine)

The presence of infection in the genital tract, either as a result of overgrowth of normal bacterial flora or abnormal vaginal flora, at 26–32 weeks' gestation, has been shown to be associated with preterm labour (Kiss et al 2004). Though it may appear reasonable to screen all pregnant women for vaginal infection, screening and treating of low-risk women has not been shown to be beneficial.

*Group B streptococcus (GBS)*: This has been shown to be associated with preterm rupture of membranes resulting in preterm labour. Population screening has not been useful in identifying women at high risk of PPROM. The current practice in Malaysia is to screen only women at high risk and to provide intrapartum intravenous antibiotics.

*Bacterial vaginosis*: This condition has been shown to increase preterm delivery (Flynn et al 1999). The risk appears to be almost double when detected in early pregnancy (21 per cent) compared to later in pregnancy (11 per cent) (Joesoef et al 1993; Leitich et al 2003). Bacterial vaginosis is caused by anerobes such as *Gardenerella vaginalis* and *Mycoplasma hominis*. Affected women generally complain of thin, watery non-itchy discharge per vagina, with a fishy odour. However, it is known that as many as 50 per cent who are afflicted may be asymptomatic.

Studies have been carried out to look at the benefits of screening and treating both the low- and the high-risk groups. The results have been contradictory.

### Uterine anomalies

Uterine anomalies are seen in less than 1 per cent of the population. Any structural anomaly which alters the uterine cavity is likely to cause miscarriage, preterm labour or malpresentation of the fetus (Michalas 1991; Raga 1997).

### Birth defects

Fetal structural anomalies are seen in about 3 per cent of pregnancies. Dolan and colleagues (2007) found that birth defects were associated with preterm labour. Conditions which increase the uterine size beyond what is normal for a particular gestation are likely to initiate preterm labour. These include conditions that cause polyhydramnios and fetal structural anomalies such as lymphatic malformation, sacro-coccygeal tumour and conjoint twins.

### Multiple pregnancy

Preterm delivery occurs in 43.6 per cent of all twin deliveries, compared to 5.6 per cent in singleton pregnancies (Patel et al 1983). In addition, monochorionicity is noted to have a greater association with preterm labour. Multiple pregnancy is associated with a higher risk of almost every potential obstetric complication, the most serious being preterm labour. Preterm delivery occurs in 43.6 per cent of all twin deliveries compared to 5.6 per cent in singleton pregnancies (Patel et al 1983). Higher orders of pregnancies are exponentially at greater risk of earlier delivery. Triplet pregnancies managed conservatively in Hospital Kuala Lumpur had a reported average gestation of 31 weeks.

> Preterm delivery occurs in 43.6 per cent of all twin deliveries compared to 5.6 per cent in singleton pregnancies. Monochorionicity has a greater association with preterm labour.

### Other factors

Some of the other clinical history and findings which may be relevant in risk scoring include:

1. Abdominal surgery during pregnancy
2. Placenta previa
3. Premature rupture of membranes
4. An underweight mother
5. Smoking

## Predicting preterm labour

The risk assessment for preterm delivery remains difficult, particularly among women with no history of preterm birth. The fact remains that a large proportion cases of preterm labour have no known cause. In the absence of an accurate and objective means of identifying it early, it is important to recognise that every pregnant woman is at risk of preterm labour. Prediction of preterm birth is an important strategy in reducing neonatal morbidity and mortality. However, predicting preterm labour continues to be a difficult task. Various means have been used to identify the woman at risk, including:

## Risk scoring

Risk scoring is based on the risk factors mentioned earlier. One of the strongest risk factors is a history of preterm labour. Other factors that have strong predictive values include bleeding, multiple pregnancy and cervical insufficiency. Several studies have failed to show any benefit from risk-scoring systems (Hueston 1995; Mercer 1996). Screening for risk of preterm labour, other than risk factors elicited in the history, is not beneficial in the general obstetric population (ACOG 2008).

## Screening tests

*Testing for salivary estriol*: In a normal pregnant woman, serum estriol levels increase throughout pregnancy. This increase accelerates about five weeks prior to uneventful term delivery. This is supported by animal studies which have shown that the onset of labour results in the increased production of estriol by the placenta. This appears to be moderated by the fetal hypothalamo-pituitry-adrenal axis. Hence, it has been postulated that similar occurrence in human pregnancy will be reflected in an increase in salivary and serum levels of estriol. Estriol levels greater than 2.1 ng/ml of saliva are considered positive. However, diurnal variation and other factors such as suppression of salivary estriol levels by antenatal betamethasone administration (Leff and Goldkrand, 2002) make this test unsuitable for routine use.

> Salivary estriol screening is unsuitable for routine use.

*Testing for fetal fibronectin*: Fibronectins are proteins found in the plasma and extracellular matrix. Fetal fibronectin (FFN) is differentiated from other fibronectins by the presence of a specific region known as the 3CS domain (connecting segment), which can be recognised by the monoclonal antibody FDC-6 (Metsurah et al 1988). Fetal fibronectin is known as the 'glue' between the fetal membranes and the uterine decidua. It is usually present in vaginal and cervical secretions up to 20 weeks' gestation and again at term. Hence, it has been suggested that its detection between 22 and 37 weeks' gestation would imply a disruption of the chorio-decidual interface. Sampling for fetal fibronection is obtained from the posterior fornix prior to a digital examination. Sample contamination by amniotic fluid and blood should be avoided.

Lockwood et al (1991) proposed that this may be an effective tool to identify women at risk of preterm labour. Any level higher than 50 ng/ml, after 22 weeks' gestation, would be considered a positive test. A negative test appears to be useful in ruling out onset of preterm labour within two weeks. A negative test is more useful than a positive test in a high-risk population. This test is not to be performed before 24 weeks or after 34 weeks and has a limited role in a low-risk population.

The usefulness of FFN testing along with transvaginal ultrasound evaluation of the cervical length has been assessed (Krupa et al 2006) and found effective in predicting preterm labour. In a study by Goldenberg et al (2008), high-risk women with a positive fetal fibronectin result and a short cervix were at substantially increased risk of spontaneous preterm birth; women with either marker alone

> High-risk women with a positive FFN result and a short cervix on ultrasound are at increased risk for preterm birth.

had intermediate and approximately equal risks of spontaneous preterm birth, and women without either marker had a low risk of spontaneous preterm birth. These two tests in combination may be useful in predicting preterm labour in a high-risk population.

***Assessment of cervical length***: Assessment of the cervical length is best done using transvaginal ultrasound. The length of the cervix is measured from the internal to the external os. In addition, dilatation of the internal os and funnelling (ballooning of the membranes into the dilated internal but with a closed external os), if present, is recorded. Transvaginal ultrasound is currently recommended as the most reliable method which is reproducible as opposed to the trans-abdominal and trans-labial methods (Berghella and Berghella 2005). The distance of the probe, obstruction of view by the symphysis pubis and an overdistended bladder causing distortion of the cervical length are some of the reasons to avoid a trans-abdominal ultrasound assessment of the cervix.

The advantage of an ultrasound examination over a clinical digital examination is the ability to assess the internal os in addition to accurately measuring the cervical length (the distance between the internal and external os). Zilanti et al (1995) described the progression of cervical effacement in four stages and denoted them with the alphabets 'T', 'Y', 'V' and 'U'.

'T': Closed uneffaced cervix

'Y': Partial effacement from internal os

'V': Further progression of effacement

'U': Membranes exposed through the internal os into the vagina (funnelling)

Funnelling is ultrasound evidence of ballooning of the membranes into a dilated internal os, but with a closed external os (Owen et al 2003). A shortened cervix in association with 'funnelling' has been shown to be an indicator of greater risk of preterm delivery (Rust et al 2005).

A cervical length greater than 25 mm would be considered normal. The presence of a cervix of normal length makes interventions unnecessary, even in the presence of symptoms.

Newer imaging techniques such as volume by 3D scanning (Rozenberg et al 2003) and length assessment by magnetic resonance imaging (Brandao 2010) have not been found to be superior to transvaginal ultrasound.

The measurement of the cervical length has no role for general population screening. Berghella et al (2009) in a systematic review of the Cochrane database stated that there is insufficient evidence to recommend routine screening of asymptomatic or symptomatic pregnant women with transvaginal ultasound measurement of the cervical length. In addition, this screening modality is not recommended before 14 weeks or after 35 weeks of gestation.

> Currently there is insufficient evidence to recommend routine screening of asymptomatic or symptomatic pregnant women with transvaginal ultasound measurement of the cervical length.

***Monitoring uterine activity***: Home uterine activity monitoring (HUAM) is based on the principle of tocodynamometry. This involves the telemetric recording and transmission of uterine contractions to a monitoring centre.

Based on the information received, the patient is provided with feedback from the healthcare worker. Though initial studies showed that HUAM was effective in predicting preterm labour, results of subsequent large-scale randomised studies have not been conclusive. The Americn College of Obstetricians and Gynecologists (1995) concluded that the use of this expensive and time-consuming system does not reduce preterm rates. It is interesting to note that HUAM had the opposite effect in monitoring twin pregnancies (Dyson et al 1997). The increased contact with the health care worker resulted in increased unplanned antenatal visits and use of tocolytic therapy.

> HUAM is an expensive and time-consuming modality that does not reduce preterm birth rates.

## Diagnosis of preterm labour

Most women seeking medical attention for preterm labour will present with a history of painful or painless uterine contractions. However, this is not diagnostic of labour and may be merely Braxton-Hicks contractions. Other symptoms which may indicate impending preterm birth include pelvic pressure, menstrual-like cramps, watery vaginal discharge and lower back pain. The signs and symptoms of labour may appear only within 24 hours of preterm labour (Iams et al 1994).

Specific details regarding the length and strength of contractions, in addition to the duration of the interval between contractions, may be indicative of labour. Cervical changes in the presence of uterine contractions is the strongest indicator of preterm labour. Positive history of leaking of liquor, vaginal bleeding and risk factors may further assist in clinching the diagnosis.

| Clinical Examination | |
|---|---|
| Abdominal examination | Uterine contractions at regular intervals |
| Speculum examination (sterile procedure to minimise risk of infection) | To determine the length of the cervix and extent of dilatation of cervical os |
|  | To determine the presence of amniotic fluid |
| Digital examination | To be avoided if membranes have ruptured, unless sufficient information was not obtained during speculum examination. Cervical effacement and dilatation are looked for. |

## Prevention of preterm labour

Many methods have been described to predict the onset of preterm labour, yet none seem to be effective or accurate. Hence, prevention is an important strategy in the management of a patient at high risk of preterm labour. This has been attempted by the use of *cervical cerclage*, *antibiotics* and *progesterone*.

### Cervical cerclage

Cervical cerlage placement as a 'treatment' for cervical insufficiency remains controversial. It was first introduced by VN Shirodkar in 1955 at Grant Medical College in Mumbai, India. Two years later, a variation of this technique was published by Prof Ian McDonald of the Royal Melbourne Hospital.

> **Primary cerclage:** Prophylatically in women considered at high risk of preterm birth based on their obstetric history.
> **Secondary cerclage:** When ultrasound findings are indicative of cervical insufficiency in a high-risk woman.
> **Tertiary cerclage:** An emergency procedure in the presence of positive clinical examination findings.

Primary cerclages are placed prophylatically in women considered at high risk of preterm birth based on their obstetric history. Secondary cerclages are placed when ultrasound findings are indicative of cervical insufficiency in a high-risk woman. Tertiary cerclages are performed as an emergency procedure in the presence of positive clinical examination findings.

The 1993 MRC/RCOG Multicentre Randomised Trial of Cervical Cerlage concluded that clear benefit was seen only in patients with a history of three or more spontaneous births or preterm deliveries (MacNaughton et al 1993). In 2001, the Cervical Incompetence Prevention Randomized Cerclage Trial (CIPRACT Trial) showed that patients with cervical insufficiency and cerclage placement (as compared to bed rest only) had a lower incidence of preterm delivery prior to 34 weeks in addition to lowered neonatal morbidity (Althuisius et al 2001). Patients were enrolled in this study based on obstetric history followed by ultrasound findings. Another study which had enrolled and randomised patients based only on ultrasound findings concluded that cerclage failed to alter any perinatal outcome variable (Rust et al 2000). To et al (2004) concluded a randomised controlled study with similar findings. Daskalakis et al (2006) compared two groups of patients who met the criteria for an emergency cerclage. The study compared a group of 29 patients who opted for the procedure, against 17 patients who chose bed rest. The former benefitted with prolongation of pregnancy. All patients received tocolytics and antibiotics. Elective prophylatic cerclage has been studied in multiple gestation. No benefit has been noted in twins (Dor et al 1982) or in triplets (Roman et al 2005).

> Elective prophylactic cerclage has no benefit in twin or triplet pregnancy.

## Antibiotics

About 25–40 per cent of preterm births are estimated to result from intrauterine infections (Cunningham et al 2010). It has been postulated that intrauterine infections may trigger labour by activating the innate immune system (Goldenberg et al 2008). Though it seems to be an attractive proposition to give antibiotics to women at high risk of preterm birth, studies have not been conclusive as to its efficacy. A meta-analysis by Morency and Bujold (2007) seemed to indicate that antibiotics given in the second trimester to women with a history of preterm labour would be effective in preventing recurrence of preterm labour. However, Andrews et al (2006) found that using azithromycin and metronidazole between pregnancies in high-risk women did not prevent preterm labour.

> Treatment of bacterial vaginosis or trichomonas vaginalis does not decrease the rate of preterm birth.

Carey et al (2000) used oral metronidazole to treat bacterial vaginosis, but did not find a reduction in preterm birth. In a systematic review, Okun et al (2005) found that women with bacterial vaginosis had a reduction in persistent infection with antibiotics, but did not have a reduction in the risk of preterm birth. On the other hand, in women with trichomonas vaginalis, metronidazole reduced the risk of persistent infection but increased the incidence of preterm birth.

## Progesterone

Progesterone appears to maintain pregnancy, and lack or withdrawal of it tends to initiate labour. Hence, it has been hypothesised that the administration of progesterone should prevent preterm labour. A large randomised placebo-controlled trial was conducted investigating the use of 17α-hydroxy-progesterone caproate therapy (250 mg administered intramuscularly) for the prevention of preterm birth (Meis et al 2003). The study group included high-risk women with a documented history of a spontaneous singleton preterm birth at less than 37 weeks of gestation. A total of 459 women were enrolled between 16 weeks and 20 weeks of gestation. The study group received weekly intramuscular injections of 17α-hydroxyprogesterone caproate (the controls received a placebo) from 16–20 weeks' gestation to 37 weeks. A significant decrease in preterm birth in the study group led to the trial being stopped early. The trial showed significant reductions in preterm and early preterm birth, low birth weight, as well as significant reductions in infant complications (intraventricular hemorrhage, necrotising enterocolitis, neonatal intensive care unit admissions, and the need for supplemental oxygen therapy). Four-year follow-up found no adverse health outcomes of surviving children.

However, a randomised trial of 17α-hydroxyprogesterone caproate in women with twin gestations found no benefit in progesterone supplementation for the prevention of preterm delivery in that high-risk group (Rouse et al 2007).

Micronised progesterone capsules (200 mg vaginally daily) have been used in a trial of progesterone for asymptomatic women with a very short cervix (less than 15 mm),

> Progesterone for preventing preterm labour:
> - Weekly intramuscular injections of 17α-hydroxy-progesterone caproate from 16–20 weeks' gestation to 37 weeks.
> - Not beneficial in twin pregnancies

and appear to be effective for this indication (da Fonseca et al 2007). Progesterone is not recommended as a supplementary treatment to cervical cerclage for suspected cervical insufficiency, as a preventive agent for asymptomatic women with a positive fetal fibronectin screen result or as a tocolytic agent (ACOG 2008).

> Progesterone is not recommended
> - as supplementary treatment to cervical cerclage for suspected cervical insufficiency
> - as a preventive for asymptomatic women with a positive fetal fibronectin screen result, or
> - as a tocolytic agent

## Management of preterm labour

### Inhibiting preterm labour

Once preterm labour is established, there is little the clinician can offer to stop the contractions. Bed rest, abstention from intercourse, and oral or parenteral hydration have traditionally been used in the management of preterm birth. The effectiveness of these interventions is uncertain. Bed rest, being the most frequently prescribed intervention, has been investigated in several studies. A systematic review of the Cochrane database (Sosa et al 2004) found no evidence to support or refute bed rest in preventing preterm birth. The study recommends that routine advice of bed rest for preventing preterm birth not be given to pregnant women.

> There is no evidence to support or refute bed rest in preventing preterm birth. However, routine advice of bed rest for preventing preterm birth should not be given to pregnant women.

## Tocolytics

Tocolytic drugs have been used in an attempt to inhibit preterm labour. Tocolysis may be required to administer antenatal steroid therapy, transfer the patient to a tertiary care centre, prepare for neonatal care or prepare the patient for an operative delivery.

A variety of drugs which act on the uterine smooth muscle to inhibit contractions are available. These include ethanol, magnesium sulphate, calcium channel blockers, oxytocin antagonists, non-steroidal anti-inflammatory drugs (NSAIDs) and beta-mimetic agonists. Tocolytics can be administered either parenterally or orally. Tocolytic drugs may prolong gestation for 2–7 days, which can provide time for the administration of antenatal steroids and transfer of the mother to a tertiary unit (Merkatz et al 1980; Guinn et al 1997). There appears to be a limited role for the use of tocolysis beyond 34 weeks for the inhibition of preterm birth (Goldenberg 2002). Moreover, there is no clear evidence that it improves outcome in the management of preterm labour (RCOG 2002). There is no clear first-line tocolytic drug. The choice should be individualised and is usually based on the maternal condition, potential drug side effects and gestational age (ACOG 2003).

> There is no clear first-line tocolytic drug. The choice of tocolytic should be individualised and is usually based on the maternal condition, potential drug side effects and gestational age.

### Beta sympathomimetic drugs

The commonly used beta sympathomimetic drugs are ritodrine, terbutaline and salbutamol. These are often associated with serious maternal side effects, namely arrhythmia and pulmonary edema. Beta-mimetics are potent cardiovascular stimulants and can cause serious complications, such as maternal myocardial ischemia, metabolic derangements (for example, hyperglycemia and hypokalemia) and fetal cardiac effects (ACOG 2003). Hence, prior to initiating medication, the patient's cardiac status must be assessed by performing an ECG and a blood test for electrolytes. The RCOG no longer recommends ritodrine as the first drug of choice (RCOG Clinical Guidelines 2002).

### Calcium channel blockers

The most common calcium channel blocker used is nifedipine. Nifedipine functions by inhibiting the influx of calcium ions into the myometrial and other cells and in turn reduces muscle contractility. It achieves peak plasma levels within an hour following oral intake. Its ability to inhibit preterm labour was recognised in the 1980s. It appears to be safer and more effective than beta sympathomimetics (King et al 2003). Its main advantages include fewer metabolic and cardiovascular complications. This is particularly useful in cases such as multiple pregnancy, diabetes mellitus and cardiac disease in pregnancy.

Though more clinical trials are available to substantiate the efficacy of atosiban, the cost consideration tips the choice in favour of nifedipine, especially in developing countries. Different doses of nifedipine have being used by various groups.

*Dosage of nifedipine:* One of the commonly recommended protocols consists of 20 mg orally stat, followed by 20 mg orally after 30 minutes if contractions persist. This is followed by a maintenance dose of 20 mg orally every 3–8 hours for 48–72 hours. The maximum dose is 160 mg/

day. After 72 hours, if maintenance is required, patients can be given a daily dose of 30–60 mg of a sustained-release preparation.

It is important to remember that calcium channel blockers may predispose to pulmonary edema and when used with magnesium sulphate can cause hypotension and collapse (Ben-Ami 1994).

> **Dosage of nifedipine:**
> - 20 mg orally stat
> - Followed by 20 mg orally after 30 minutes if contractions persist
> - Maintenance dose of 20 mg orally every 3–8 hours for 48–72 hours.
> - Maximum dose is 160 mg/day

### Atosiban

Atosiban is an oxytocin antagonist. Since oxytocin initiates labour, it seems logical that its antagonist would prevent it. Valenzuela et al (2000) compared subcutaneous atosiban with placebo. Atosiban delayed the next episode of threatened labour but there is insufficient evidence for firm conclusions about effects on other outcomes.

*Dosage*: The recommended dose and administration schedule for atosiban is a three-step procedure. The initial bolus dose is 6.75 mg over one minute, followed by an infusion of 18 mg/hour for three hours and then 6 mg/hour for up to 45 hours. Treatment should not last longer than 48 hours and the total dose given during a full course should preferably not exceed 330 mg of atosiban (RCOG Clinical Guidelines 2002). Numerous clinical trials have been conducted to compare its efficacy and safety with that of other commonly used tocolytic agents. It has been shown to be as effective as beta sympathomimetics but with milder side effects. The high cost of atosiban is a factor limiting its use in developing countries.

> **Dosage of atosiban:**
> - Initial bolus dose of 6.75 mg over one minute
> - Followed by an infusion of 18 mg/hour for three hours
> - Then 6 mg/hour for up to 45 hours

### Corticosteroids in preterm labour

Recognising that the most common cause of neonatal mortality after preterm labour is respiratory distress syndrome (RDS), the obstetrician should ensure that antenatal corticosteroids are administered prior to delivery. The reduction of RDS in preterm neonates of mothers who were administered betamethasone prior to delivery was observed in the early 1970s (Liggins and Howie 1972). The National Institutes of Health Consensus Development Conference Statement in 1995, in part stated that 'antenatal corticosteroid therapy is indicated for women at risk of premature delivery with few exceptions and will result in a substantial decrease in neonatal morbidity and mortality, as well as substantial savings in health care costs'. A systematic review of the Cochrane Database (Crowley 2003) confirmed that antenatal corticosteroids significantly reduced the incidence and severity of neonatal respiratory distress syndrome.

> Antenatal corticosteroids reduce respiratory distress syndrome and reduce the incidence and severity of necrotising enterocolitis and intraventricular hemorrhage.

All women who are at risk of preterm delivery between 24 weeks and 34 weeks of gestation are potential candidates for corticosteroid therapy (Ballard and Ballard

1995). Its effects on the fetal intestine appear to be responsible for the reduction in the risk of necrotising enterocolitis (NEC). In addition, these neonates also have a reduced risk of intraventricular hemorrhage (IVH). These and other benefits are independent of the effects seen on the pulmonary tissue (Ballard and Ballard 1995).

**Betamethasone or dexamethasone?**

Liggins and Howie (1972) pioneered the use of antenatal betamethasone in the prevention of RDS. Baud et al (1999) found betamethasone to be superior to dexamethasone in preventing RDS and periventricular leukomalacia. However, Elimian and colleagues in the Betacode trial (2007) found that the two drugs were comparable in reducing in major neonatal morbidities in premature infants.

*Dosage*: The most extensively studied regimens of corticosteroid treatment for the prevention of RDS are two doses of betamethasone 12 mg, given intramuscularly 24 hours apart and four doses of dexamethasone 6 mg, given intramuscularly 12 hours apart (RCOG 2004).

> Betamethasone
> - 2 doses of 12 mg, given IM 24 hours apart
>
> Dexamethasone
> - 4 doses of 6 mg, given IM 12 hours apart

Should a corticosteroid dose ('rescue therapy') be given if delivery becomes imminent more than seven days after the last dose? Though the American College of Obstetricians and Gynecologists (2008) recommends that a rescue dose be restricted to trials, McEvoy et al (2010) showed that a rescue dose >/=14 days after the last dose increased respiratory compliance in the treated infants.

*Single or multiple courses?*: Roberts and colleagues (2006) reviewed the Cochrane Database and recommended the continued use of a single course of antenatal corticosteroids to accelerate fetal lung maturation in women at risk of preterm birth. According to the review, a single course of antenatal corticosteroids should be considered routine for preterm delivery with few exceptions.

> A single course of antenatal corticosteroids is still considered standard of care. Further studies are required before multiple/repeat doses can be recommended.

The American College of Obstetricians and Gynecologists (Committee opinion 402, 2008) recommends a single course of antenatal corticosteroids in preterm labour.

Crowther and Harding in a systematic review (2007) stated that repeat dose(s) of prenatal corticosteroids reduce the occurrence and severity of neonatal lung disease and the risk of serious health problems in the first few weeks of life. The review, however, stated that there is insufficient evidence on the longer-term benefits and risks.

## Labour and delivery

Preterm labour which continues on to a delivery is an obstetrician's dilemma. This is especially true when preterm labour occurs at the lower limits of viability. Both a vaginal delivery and an emergency cesarean section have risks and benefits,

> Neonatal outcome is dependent on several factors which include the period of gestation, successful completion of antenatal steroid therapy, fetal weight, fetal well-being prior to delivery, the presence or absence of membranes and the place and mode of delivery.

but the risk/benefit balance depends on the gestational age (Drife 2006). Though advanced neonatal care has improved survival rates for early gestation, cesarean section before 28 weeks' gestation, solely for fetal indications, is still controversial. Neonatal outcome is dependent on several factors which include the period of gestation, successful completion of antenatal steroid therapy, fetal weight, fetal well-being prior to delivery, the presence or absence of membranes and the place and mode of delivery.

As neonatal survival rates are primarily due to good quality neonatal care, it is important that the delivery is carried out in an appropriate tertiary care obstetric unit. As pointed out earlier, one of the objectives of suppressing preterm labour is to enable in-utero transfer. However, it is important to note that the maternal condition must be given due consideration before proceeding with an in-utero transfer, lest the transfer is detrimental to maternal well-being.

## The role of ultrasound in preterm labour

Table 25.1 lists the uses of ultrasound in preterm labour. Information obtained during an ultrasound scan prior to delivery will be useful in counselling the parents with regards to prognosis. The information obtained will also be useful to the neonatologist in preparing to manage the neonate. Needless to say, the information will assist the obstetrician in deciding on the mode of delivery.

**Table 25.1** Role of ultrasound in preterm labour

| Standard fetal biometry |
|---|
| Confirmation of gestation |
| Estimation of fetal weight |
| Determine growth pattern (looking for IUGR): plot biometry on growth graphs |
| **Amniotic fluid volume** |
| Amniotic fluid index |
| Maximum vertical pool |
| **Fetal activity** |
| **Doppler studies** |
| Umbilical artery |
| Middle cerebral artery |
| Ductus venosus |
| **Rule out gross structural anomalies** |
| Non viable fetal conditions |
| Markers for chromosomal abnormalities |

## Mode of delivery

The optimal mode of delivery in preterm labour is still debatable. An episiotomy may be necessary for a vaginal delivery in the absence of a relaxed vaginal outlet. The routine use of forceps is not recommended (Cunningham et al 2010).

Grant et al reviewed the Cochrane Database (2001) and found no significant differences between elective and selective policies for cesarean delivery for fetal, neonatal or maternal outcomes. They did not find enough evidence to evaluate the use of a policy for elective cesarean

> It should be borne in mind that lack of conclusive evidence in favour of cesarean section does not mean there is clear evidence in favour of vaginal delivery in preterm labour.

delivery for small babies. Ghi and colleagues (2010), in a retrospective study, found that in severely premature infants born after spontaneous onset of labour, the risk of adverse perinatal outcome did not seem to depend upon the mode of delivery, whereas the risk of maternal complications is significantly increased after cesarean section. In a statement of the prematurity working group of the World Association of Perinatal Medicine, Skupski and colleagues (2009) state that the available scientific evidence does not support a recommendation for cesarean delivery for improving survival or decreasing morbidity for the extremely premature fetus. However, it should be borne in mind that lack of conclusive evidence in favour of cesarean section does not mean there is clear evidence in favour of vaginal delivery (Drife 2006).

Murphy and Twaddle (2005) state that the consensus is that cesarean section before 25 weeks of gestation confers little benefit in terms of survival, even for breech presentation. For breech infants with an estimated fetal weight of 1.5 kg and above, delivery by cesarean section is usually recommended. It is good clinical practice to involve the patient and her partner in the decision making.

## References

Althuisius SM, Dekker GA, Hummel P, Bekedam DJ, van Geijin HP. 2001. Final results of the Cervical Incompetence Prevention Randomized Cerclage Trial (CIPRACT): Therapeutic cerclage with bed rest versus rest alone. *Am J Obstet Gynecol* 185:1106–1112.

American College of Obstetricians and Gynecologists. 2003. Management of preterm labor. ACOG Practice Bulletin No. 43. *Obstet Gynecol* 101:1039–47.

American College of Obstetricians and Gynecologists. 2008. Antenatal corticosteroid therapy for fetal maturation. Committee Opinion No. 419. *Obstet Gynecol* 112:963–965.

American College of Obstetricians and Gynecologists. 1995. Preterm Labor. Technical Bulletin No. 206, June 1995.

American College of Obstetricians and Gynecologists. 2008. Antenatal Corticosteroid Therapy for Fetal Maturation. ACOG Committee Opinion No. 402. *Obstet Gynecol* 111:805.

Andrews WW, Goldenberg RL, Hauth JC et al. 2006. Interconceptional antibiotics to prevent spontaneous preterm birth: a randomized clinical trial. *Am J Obstet Gynecol* 194(3): 617.

Ballard PL, Ballard RA. 1995. Scientific basis and therapeutic regimens for use of antenatal glucocorticoids. *Am J Obstet Gynecol* 173:254.

Baud O, Foix-L'Helias L, Kaminski M, Audibert F, Jarreau P, Papiernik E et al. 1999. Antenatal glucocorticoid treatment and cystic periventricular leukomalacia in very premature infants. *N Engl J Med* 341:1190–6.

Beck S, Wojdyla D, Say L et al. 2010. The worldwide incidence of preterm birth: a systematic review of maternal mortality and morbidity. *Bulletin of the World Health Organization* 88:31–38.

Ben-Ami M, Giladi Y, Shalev E. 1994. The combination of magnesium sulphate and nifedipine: a cause of neuromuscular blockade. *Br J Obstet Gynaecol* 101:262.

Berghella V, Baxter JK, Hendrix NW. 2009. Cervical assessment by ultrasound for preventing preterm delivery. *Cochrane Database of Systematic Reviews*, Issue 3. Art. No.:CD007235.

Berghella V, Berghella M. 2005. Cervical length assessment by ultrasound. *Acta Obstet Gynecol Scand* 84(6):543–4.

Bloom SL, Yost NP, McIntire DD, Leveno KJ. 2001. Recurrence of preterm birth in singleton and twin pregnancies. *Obstet Gynecol* 98(3):379–85.

Brandao RS et al. 2010. Magnetic Resonance Imaging vs. Transvaginal Ultrasound for Cervical Length Assessment in the Second Half of Pregnancy. *Ultrasound in medicine and biology*. 36(4):571–5.

Callaghan WM, MacDorman MF, Rasmussen SA, Qin C, Lackritz EM. 2006. The contribution of preterm birth to infant mortality rates in the United States. *Pediatrics* 118: 1566–73.

Carey JC, Klebanoff MA, Hauth JC, Hillier SL, Thom EA, Ernest JM et al. 2000. Metronisazole to prevent preterm delivery in pregnant women with asymptomatic bacterial vaginosis. *N Engl J Med* 342:534–40.

Conde-Agudelo A, Rosas-Bermúdez A, Kafury-Goeta AC. 2006. Birth Spacing and Risk of Adverse Perinatal Outcomes: A Meta-analysis. *JAMA* 295(15):1809–1823.

Crowley P. 2003. Prophylactic corticosteroids for preterm birth (Cochrane Review). In: *The Cochrane Library*, Issue 1.

Crowther CA, Harding JE. 2007. Repeat doses of prenatal corticosteroids for women at risk of preterm birth for preventing neonatal respiratory disease. *Cochrane Database of Systematic Reviews*, Issue 3. Art. No.: CD003935.

Cunningham FG, Leveno KJ. Bloom SL et al. 2010. *Williams' Obstetrics*, 23rd ed. McGraw-Hill.

da Fonseca EB, Celik E, Parra M, et al, for the Fetal Medicine Foundation Second Trimester Screening Group. Progesterone and the risk of preterm birth among women with a short cervix. N Engl J Med 2007; 357:462-9.

Daskalakis G, Papantoniou N, Mesogitis S, Antsaklis A. 2006. Management of cervical insufficiency and bulging fetal membranes. *Obstet Gynecol* 107:221–226.

Dolan, S M, Gross, S J, Merkatz, I R et al 2007. The First and Second Trimester Evaluation of Risk (FASTER) Trial Research Consortium: The Contribution of Birth Defects to Preterm Birth and Low Birth Weight. *Obstetrics & Gynecology* 110(2, Part 1):318–324.

Dor J, Shalev J, Blankstein J, Serr DM. 1982. Elective cervical suture of twin pregnancies diagnosed ultrasonically in the first following induced ovulation. *Gynecol Obstet Invest* 13:55–60.

Drife J. 2006. Mode of delivery in the early preterm infant (<28 weeks) *BJOG* 113: (3) 81–85.

Dyson D, Danbe K, Bamber J et al. 1997. A multicentre randomised trial of three levels of surveillance in patients at risk for preterm labour—twin gestation subgroup analysis. *Am J Obstet Gynecol* 176:S118.

Elimian A, Garry D, Figueroa R, Spitzer A, Wiencek V, Quirk JG. 2007. Antenatal betamethasone compared with dexamethasone (Betacode trial): a randomized controlled trial. *Obstet Gynecol* 110:26–30.

Flynn C, Helwig A, Meurer L. 1999. Bacterial vaginosis in pregnancy and the risk of prematurity: a meta-analysis. *J Fam Pract* 48:885–892.

Ghi T Maroni, E, Arcangeli, T et al. 2010. Mode of delivery in the preterm gestation and maternal and neonatal outcome. *J Matern Fetal Neonatal Med*, Volume 23, Number 12, 1424–1428.

Goldenberg RL. 2002. The management of preterm labor. *Obstet Gynecol* 100:1020.

Goldenberg RL, Culhane JF, Iams JD et al. 2008. Preterm birth 1. Epidemiology and causes of preterm birth. *Lancet* 371:75.

Grant A, Glazener CM. 2001. Elective versus selective caesarean section for delivery of the small baby (Cochrane Review). In: *The Cochrane Library*, Issue 1. Oxford: Update Software.

Guinn DA, Goepfert AR, Owen J, Brumfield C, Hauth JC. 1997. Management options in women with preterm uterine contractions: a randomized clinical trial. *Am J Obstet Gynecol* 177:814.

Harger JH. 2002. Cerclage and cervical insufficiency: an evidence-based analysis. *Obstet Gynecol* 100:1313–1327.

Hueston WJ, Knox Mark A, Eilers G, Pauwels J, Lonsdorf D. 1995. The Effectiveness of Pretermbirth Prevention Educational Programs for High-Risk Women: A Meta-Analysis. *Obstet Gynecol* 86(4, Part 2):705–712.

Iams JD, Johnson FF, Parker M. 1994. A prospective evaluation of the signs and symptoms of preterm labor. *Obstet Gynecol* 84:227.

Iams JD, Goldenberg RL, Meis PJ et al. 1996. NICHD HHD MFM Network. The length of the cervix and the risk of spontaneous premature delivery. *N Engl J Med* 334:567–572.

Joesoef RM, Hillier SL, Utomo B, Wiknjosastro G, Linnan M, Kandun N. 1993. BV and prematurity in Indonesia: Association in late and early pregnancy. *Am J Obstet Gynecol* 169: 175–8.

King JF, Flenady V, Papatsonis D et al. 2003. Calcium channel blockers for inhibiting preterm labour: a systematic review of the evidence and protocol for administration of nifedipine. *Aust N Z J Obstet Gynecol* 43:192–8.

Kiss H, Petricevic L, Husslein P. 2004. Preospective randomised controlled trial of an infection screening programme to reduce the rate of preterm delivery. *BMJ* 329:371.

Krymko H, Bashiri A, Smolin A, Sheiner E, Bar-David J, Shoham-Vardi I, Vardi H, Mazor M. 2004. Risk factors for recurrent preterm delivery. *Eur J Obstet Gynecol Reprod Biol* Apr 15; 113(2):160–3.

Krupa FG, Faltin D, Cecatti JG, Surita FG, Souza JP. 2006. Predictors of preterm birth. *Int J Gynaecol Obstet* Jul; 94(1):5–11. *Epub* May 24.

Leff RP, Goldkrand JW. 2002. Suppression of salivary estriol by betamethasone. *J Matern Fetal Neonatal Med* 11:195–9.

Leitich H, Bodner-Adler B, Brunbauer M, Kaider A, Egarter C, Husslein P. 2003. Bacterial vaginosis as a risk factor for preterm delivery: a meta-analysis. *Am J Obstet Gynecol* Jul; 189(1):139–47.

Liggins GC, Howie RN. 1972. A controlled trial pf antepartum glucocorticoid treatment for prevention of the respiratory distress syndrome in premature infants. *Pediatrics* 50:515.

Lockwood CJ, Senyei AE, Dische R et al. 1991. Fetal fibronectin in cervical and vaginal secretions as a predictor of preterm delivery. *N Engl J Med* 325:669–74.

MacNaughton MC, Chalmers IG, Dubowitz V et al. 1993. Final report of the Medical Research Council/ Royal College of Obstetricans and Gynaecologist Multicentre Randomised Trial of Cervical Cerclage. *Br J Obstet Gynaecol* 100:516–523.

McEvoy C, Schilling D, Peters D et al. 2010. Respiratory compliance in preterm infants after a single rescue course of antenatal steroids: a randomized controlled trial. *Am J Obstet Gynecol* 202:544.e1–9.

Mercer BM, Goldenberg RL, Das A, Moawad AH, Iams JD, Meis PJ, et al. 1996. The *Preterm Prediction Study*: a clinical risk assessment system. *Am J Obstet Gynecol* 174:1885.

Merkatz IR, Peter JB, Barden TP. 1980. Ritodrine hydrochloride: a betamimetic agent for use in preterm labor. II. Evidence of efficacy. *Obstet Gynecol* 56:7.

Michalas SP. 1991. Outcome of pregnancy in females with uterine malformations. *Int J Gynecol Obstet* 35:215–9.

Meis PJ, Klebanoff M, Thom E, Dombrowski MP, Sibai B, Moawad AH et al. 2003. Prevention of recurrent preterm delivery by 17 alpha hydroxyprogesterone caproate. National Institute of Child Health and Human Development Maternal-Fetal Medicine Units Network. *N Engl J Med* 348:2379.

Metsurah H, Takio K, Greene T et al. 1988. The oncal fetal structure of human fibronectin defined by monoclonal antibody FDC-6. Unique requirements for antigen specificity provided by aglycosylhexaptide. *J Biol Chem* 263:3314–22.

Morency AM, Bujold E. 2007. The effect of second-trimester antibiotic therapy on the rate of preterm birth. *J Obstet Gynaecol Can* 29(1):35–44.

Moutquin JM. 2003. Socio-economic and psychosocial factors in the management and prevention of preterm labour. *BJOG* Apr;110 Suppl 20:56–60.

Murphy K, Twaddle S. 2005. Organisation of high-risk obstetric and neonatal services. *In:* NormanJ, GreerI, editors. Preterm Labour: Managing Risk in Clinical Practice. Cambridge, UK: University Press, 307–28.

National Institutes of Health Consensus Development Conference Statement. 1995. Effect of corticosteroids for fetal maturation on perinatal outcomes. *Am J Obstet Gynecol* 173:246–252.

Okun N, Gronau KA, Hannah ME. 2005. Antibiotics for bacterial vaginosis or Trichomonas vaginalis in pregnancy: a systematic review. *Obstet Gynecol* 105(4):857.

Owen J, Iams JD, Hauth JC. 2003. Vaginal sonography and cervical incompetence. *Am J Obstet Gynecol* 188:586.

Patel N, BarrieW, Campbell Det al. 1983. Scottish twin study 1983—preliminary report. Glasgow: University of Glasgow, Departments of Child Health and Obstetrics, Social Paediatric and Obstetric Research Unit.

Patel RR, Steer P, Doyle P et al. 2004. Does gestation vary by ethnic group? A London-based study of over 122 000 pregnancies with spontaneous onset of labour. *Int J Epidemiol* 33(1):107–113.

Raga F, Bausel C, Remohi J. 1997. Reproductive impact of congenital mullerian anomalies. *Human Reproduction* 12 (10):2277–81.

Roberts D, Dalziel SR. 2006. Antenatal corticosteroids for accelerating fetal lung maturation for women at risk of preterm birth. *Cochrane Database of Systematic Reviews*, Issue 3. Art.No.: CD004454.

Roman AS, Rebarber A, Pereira L, Sfakianaki AK, Mulholland J, Berghella V. 2005. The efficacy of sonographically indicated cerclage in multiple gestations. *J Ultrasound Med* 24:763–768.

Rouse DJ, Caritis SN, Peaceman AM, Sciscione A, Thom EA, Spong CY et al. 2007. A trial of 17 alpha-hydroxyprogesterone caproate to prevent prematurity in twins. National Institute of Child Health and Human Development Maternal-Fetal Medicine Units Network. *N Engl J Med* 357:454.

Royal College of Obstetricians and Gynaecologists. 2002. Greentop Guideline 1(B). Preterm Labour, Tocalytic Drugs. October 2002.

Royal College of Obstetricians and Gynaecologists. 2004. Greentop Guidelines No 7 Antenatal Corticosteroids to Prevent Respiratory Distress Syndrome (revised February 2004).

Rozenberg P, Rafii A, Senat M, Dujardin A, Rapon J, Ville Y. 2003. Predictive value of two-dimensional and three-dimensional multiplanar ultrasound evaluation of the cervix in preterm labour. *J Matern Fetal Neonatal Med* 13:237–241.

Rust OA, Atlas RO, Jones KJ, Benham BN, Balducci J. 2000. A randomized trial of cerclage versus no cerclage among patients with ultrasonographically detected second trimester preterm dilation of the internal os. *Am J Obstet Gynecol* 183:830–835.

Rust OA, Atlas RO, Kimmel S, Roberts WE, Hess LW. 2005. Does the presence of a funnel increase the risk of adverse perinatal outcome in a patient with a short cervix? *Am J Obstet Gynecol* 192:1060–1066.

Sosa C, Althabe F, Belizán JM, Bergel E. 2004. Bed rest in singleton pregnancies for preventing preterm birth. *Cochrane Database of Systematic Reviews*, Issue 1. Art. No.: CD003581.

Skupski DW, Greenough A, Donn, SM et al. 2009. Delivery mode for extremely premature fetus: a statement of the prematurity working group of the World Association of Perinatal Medicine. *J Perinatal Med* 37(6):583–586.

Stanton C, Lawn JE, Rahman H, Wilczynska-Ketende K, Hill K. 2006. Stillbirth rates: delivering estimates in 190 countries. *Lancet* 367: 1487–94.

To MS, Alfirevic Z, Heath VCF et al. 2004. Cervical cerclage for prevention of preterm delivery in women with short cervix: randomized controlled trial. *Lancet* 363:1849–1853.

*Valenzuela* G., Sanchez-Ramos L., Romero R., et al. 2000. Maintenance. treatment of preterm labor with the oxytocin antagonist *atosiban*. *Am J Obst. Gynec.*

Wang ML, Dorer DJ, Fleming MP, Catlin EA. 2004. Clinical outcomes of near-term infants. *Pediatrics*; 114: 372–6.

World Health Organization.1992. *International classification of diseases and related health problems*. 10th revision. WHO, Geneva.

World Health Organization.2006.Neonatal and perinatal mortality: country, regional and global estimates. WHO, Geneva

Zilianti M, Azuaga A, Calderon F et al. 1995. Monitoring the effacement of the uterine cervix by transplacental sonography: A new prespective. *J Ultrasound Med* 14:719–724.

# CHAPTER 26

# PROLONGED PREGNANCY

*Amarnath Bhide*

The normal gestation length in humans is 37–42 completed weeks from the time of the last menstrual period. A pregnancy of duration over 294 days (42 weeks) is referred to as a post-term pregnancy. However, there are several other terminologies in use.

*Prolonged pregnancy*: A pregnancy that lasts for more than 41 weeks.

*Post-maturity*: A pregnancy that lasts for more than 42 weeks and when signs of placental insufficiency in the newborn such as loss of subcutaneous fat and passage of meconium are present.

## Incidence of post-term pregnancy

The reported frequency of post-term pregnancy varies from 4 per cent to 14 per cent (Bakketeig and Bergsjo 1989). This can depend on variables within different populations, the proportion of women who undergo elective delivery and the criteria used to assess the gestational age. It is well known that the last menstrual period (LMP), even when recalled with confidence, can result in considerable dating error. The more accurate determination of gestational age made possible by routine early pregnancy ultrasound reduces the number of women who receive induction of labour for apparently post-term pregnancy.

> Routine early pregnancy ultrasound is a more accurate determinant of gestational age than LMP and reduces the number of women who receive induction of labour for apparently post-term pregnancy.

## Does this alteration in pregnancy dating have any effect on perinatal outcome?

Tunon and co-authors (1999) looked at fetal outcome in pregnancies defined as post-term according to the last menstrual period, but not according to the ultrasound estimate. They found that in this group, compared to women delivering at term, there was no significant increase in low five-minute Apgar score (<7) or of transfer to the neonatal intensive care unit. In the two groups of women who were either post-term according to the ultrasound estimate but not according to the last menstrual period estimate or who were post-term according to both estimates, there were increased risks for low Apgar score and transfer to the neonatal unit. There was no significant difference in perinatal mortality between any of the groups. Although this was a retrospective study with surrogate measures of outcome, it would suggest that using ultrasound biometry is a safe method of dating a pregnancy.

## Risks in post-term pregnancy

It is well recognised that prolonged pregnancy is associated with increased risk of perinatal mortality. Part of this increase is due to congenital malformations, which are more frequent among post-term births, and part due to asphyxia. Perinatal morbidity is also increased. This may be secondary to intrapartum events like birth trauma or meconium aspiration syndrome. The incidence of early neonatal seizures, a marker for perinatal asphyxia, is higher in infants born after 41 weeks.

> Prolonged pregnancy is associated with increased risk of:
> - congenital malformations
> - asphyxia
> - birth trauma
> - meconium aspiration syndrome
> - early neonatal seizures

## Pathophysiology of prolonged pregnancy

The risks associated with prolonged pregnancy can be grouped as follows (Table 26.1):

### Ageing of the placenta

Placental ageing is thought to lead to deficient function and progressive fetal hypoxemia. This mechanism is thought to lead to the post-maturity syndrome, and also partly accounts for the increase in the risk of stillbirths.

### Continued growth of the baby

A large proportion of fetuses will continue to grow with advancing gestational age. This leads to an increase in the prevalence of fetal macrosomia with the attendant risks of fetopelvic disproportion and shoulder dystocia.

### Reduction in amniotic fluid volume

The amniotic fluid volume gradually reduces with advancing gestation, most likely due to progressive placental dysfunction. Oligohydramnios increases the risk of cord compression during labour, resulting in a higher risk of fetal heart rate abnormalities and fetal blood sampling. Higher rates of meconium staining of the amniotic fluid due to increased bowel maturity lead to a higher risk of meconium aspiration syndrome. Higher rates of induction of labour lead to higher rates of emergency cesarean section.

Table 26.1 Risk in post-term pregnancies (data from Eden et al 1987)

| | Post-dates (born after 42 weeks) | Control (born at 40 weeks) |
|---|---|---|
| Oxytocin stimulation | 14.2% | 2.8% |
| Shoulder dystocia | 2.8% | 0.8% |
| Meconium-stained liquor | 17.6% | 8.3% |
| Cesarean section | 26.5% | 19.4% |

## Prevention of Mortality and Morbidity

### Membrane sweeping

One way of avoiding these risks is to ensure that pregnancies do not extend beyond 42 completed weeks. Stripping or sweeping of membranes (digital separation of the fetal membranes from the lower pole of the uterus) in pregnancies at term reduces the frequency of the pregnancy continuing beyond 42 weeks and also reduces the incidence of formal induction of labour (Boulvain et al 2003). Women have reported increased discomfort during vaginal examination with 'sweeping', but this practice does not appear to have any effect on the subsequent mode of delivery or on the risk of infection.

> Stripping or sweeping of membranes in pregnancies at term reduces the frequency of the pregnancy continuing beyond 42 weeks.

## Induction of Labour

In 1993, the publication of a large Canadian multicentre study (Hannah et al) suggested that, in the management of post-term pregnancy, induction of labour after 41 weeks' gestation results in a lower rate of cesarean section than serial antenatal monitoring. A subsequent meta-analysis by the Cochrane Collaboration (Crowley 2006) suggests that routine induction of labour after 41 completed weeks reduces the risk of perinatal death in normally formed babies.

The Cochrane Review (2006) concluded that routine induction after 41 weeks reduces perinatal mortality without any increase in cesarean section rate. The National Institute of Health and Clinical Excellence guidelines on antenatal care recommend an offer of induction of labour to all women after 41 weeks. It would be prudent to discuss the risks and benefits of labour induction versus expectant management at 41 weeks so that the woman can make an informed choice. If the woman chooses to wait for spontaneous labour onset beyond 42 weeks, twice-weekly fetal monitoring is recommended.

> Routine induction after 41 weeks reduces perinatal mortality without any increase in cesarean section rate.

## Timing of Induction

Induction of labour between 41 and 42 weeks is in essence a very crude strategy for reducing term and post-term stillbirth rates. Although the risk of fetal death increases after 42 weeks, the absolute risk of stillbirth is still low. It must be stated that many more fetuses die in utero between 37 and 42 weeks than after 42 weeks.

Timing of induction is an artificially and arbitrarily decided point. With increasing gestation, there is an increase in the 'risk' of stillbirth, but it is gradual, without a clearly defined shoulder. The exact timing of any planned induction is still debatable. If one's prime objective is to reduce the fetal death rate, then clearly the earlier the induction date, the greater the number of antepartum stillbirths prevented, and therefore, the greater the effect of the intervention.

The problem with early induction of labour is that the number of inductions (false positive rate) will also be large (Mongelli et al 2001). The intervention also 'medicalises' pregnancy, which is essentially a natural process. Any chosen time-point will therefore be a compromise between these two variables. What is needed are better methods of identifying the term or near-term fetus at risk.

## Risk versus Rate of Stillbirth

Most studies on term stillbirth assess the gestation-specific stillbirth rate. This is expressed as the number of stillbirths per

1000 total births at each week of gestation. In a retrospective analysis of all deliveries in Sweden occurring from 1987 to 1992, Divon and co-authors (1998) noted a statistically significant rise in the odds ratios for fetal death detected from 41 weeks' gestation onwards. Using fetal mortalities at 40 weeks' gestation as a reference level, they found odds ratios for fetal death of 1.5, 1.8 and 2.9 at 41, 42 and 43 weeks, respectively.

Hilder and co-workers (1998) argue that the gestation-specific rate of stillbirth does not equate to the risk of stillbirth. They state that as only women who are still pregnant are at risk of stillbirth, it would be more appropriate to calculate the risk of stillbirth as a proportion of the ongoing pregnancies at a particular gestation (Fig. 26.1). In a retrospective analysis of 171,527 notified births, they found similar rates for stillbirth at term and in the post-term period. When calculated per 1000 ongoing pregnancies, however, the risk of stillbirth increases six-fold from 37 weeks to 43 weeks' gestation.

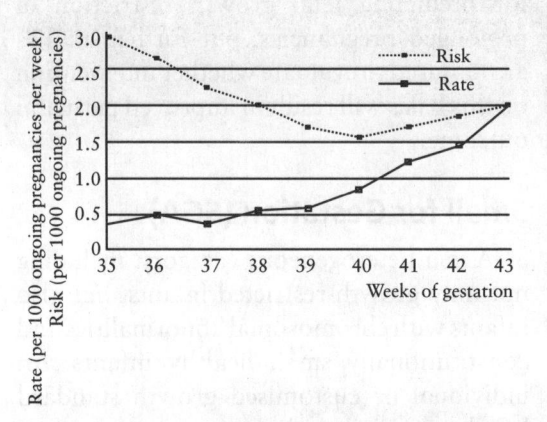

**Figure 26.1** Calculating risk of still birth (*Source*: Cotzias CS, Paterson Brown S, Fisk NM. Prospective risk of unexplained stillbirth in singleton pregnancies at term: population based analysis. BMJ 999; 319:2878.)

Whichever denominator is chosen, it would appear that there is a statistically significant increase in the relative risk of fetal mortality in accurately dated pregnancies that extend beyond 41 weeks of gestation. The absolute risk, however, remains fairly low.

## The Impact of Fetal Weight

Divon and co-authors (1998) examined the impact of gestational age and fetal growth restriction on the perinatal mortality rates of more than 180,000 Swedish women. They found an overall increase in fetal mortality in pregnancies that extended beyond 41 weeks' gestation and reported that fetal growth restriction (defined as birth weight under two standard deviations below the mean for gestational age) was independently associated with increased perinatal mortality in these pregnancies.

Campbell and co-authors (1997), in a retrospective cohort of over 440,000 Norwegian women, found that post-dated fetuses whose birth weight was below the tenth per centile were at a significantly increased risk of both 'fetal distress' in labour (risk ratio 1.7) and perinatal mortality (risk ratio 5.7).

> Post-dated fetuses whose birth weight is below the tenth per centile are at a significantly increased risk of both 'fetal distress' in labour and perinatal mortality.

Clausson and co-authors (2001) performed a population-based study of 510,029 singleton term and post-term births recorded in the Swedish Birth Register to evaluate the risk of adverse pregnancy outcomes among small for gestational age (SGA) and appropriate for gestational age

(AGA) births. They found that compared to term AGA births, term SGA births were at an increased risk of stillbirth (risk ratio 8.02) and infant death (risk ratio 7.57). Among post-term SGA births, the risk ratios were 10.56 for stillbirth and 5.00 for infant death. When births with congenital malformations were excluded, however, the risk of infant death decreased considerably.

In addition to an increased risk of perinatal mortality, SGA fetuses born at term or post-term would appear to carry an increased risk of perinatal morbidity. In a case-control study of SGA fetuses born at term to an otherwise uncomplicated pregnancy, Minior and Divon (1998) found that when compared to AGA infants, SGA newborns were more likely to be admitted to the neonatal intensive care unit. They were also more likely to have respiratory distress, hypoglycemia, thrombocytopenia and hyperbilirubinemia, and significantly more likely to require delivery by cesarean section.

This increased risk of perinatal morbidity has been corroborated by Sylvestre and co-authors (2001) in a prospective study on 792 patients at or beyond 41 weeks' gestation, who were managed expectantly. In their study, patients were tested twice-weekly with non-stress testing (NST) and amniotic fluid index (AFI) evaluation until delivery. Induction of labour was recommended when at least one of the following abnormal findings was detected: oligohydramnios (AFI <5 cm), fetal heart rate decelerations or a persistently non-reactive NST.

Following delivery, fetuses were retrospectively categorised as small (birth weight <10th per centile), average (between the 10th and 90th per centile) or large (birth weight >90th per centile). The incidence of abnormal antepartum fetal testing results and that of cesarean delivery for intrapartum non-reassuring fetal status was then calculated for these three birth weight categories. They found a significant inverse relationship between the incidence of abnormal antepartum fetal testing (36 per cent, 14 per cent and 9 per cent) and birth weight category (small, average and large fetuses, respectively, P < 0.001). In addition, there was a significantly higher incidence of cesarean delivery for non-reassuring fetal status in small fetuses (12.3 per cent vs. 5.3 per cent for small vs average/large, respectively, P = 0.024).

> There is a significantly higher incidence of cesarean delivery for non-reassuring fetal status in post-dated small fetuses.

From these studies one can conclude that for a term or post-term fetus, being too small carries a greater risk of asphyxia-related complications of pregnancy and labour than does being too large. The report from O'Reilly-Green and Divon (1999) suggests that an ultrasound is a useful tool for predicting fetal growth restriction in prolonged pregnancies, but further studies are required to evaluate whether intervention on this basis will result in improved perinatal outcome.

## Small for Gestation (SGA)

SGA is a heterogeneous category, including not only growth-restricted infants, but also infants with chromosomal abnormalities and constitutionally small healthy infants. An individual or customised growth standard has been developed that sets an optimal fetal growth rate for each pregnancy, based on maternal anthropometrics, parity and ethnic background (Gardosi et al 1995). This attempts to separate intrauterine growth restriction from the small, healthy infant.

In a population-based, cohort study looking at deliveries at all gestational ages, Clausson and co-authors (2001) found that the risks of stillbirth and neonatal death were consistently higher if SGA was classified by a customised, rather than by a population-based birth weight standard. Compared with infants who were not SGA by both standards, the risk ratio for stillbirth was 6.1 for SGA babies by customised standard only, whereas it was 1.2 for SGA babies as defined by a population standard only. They suggested that the use of a customised growth standard probably allows improved identification of fetal growth restriction.

A more recent study found that a non-customised but intrauterine-based standard has a similar ability to predict the risk of stillbirth and early neonatal mortality as a customised birth weight standard. Contrary to previous studies, Hutcheon et al (2008) found that the process of customising population-weight-for-gestational-age standards to account for maternal characteristics does little to improve the prediction of perinatal mortality. Further randomised studies are needed in this area.

## Large for Gestation (LGA)

A potential problem of prolonged pregnancy is fetal macrosomia with an increased risk of shoulder dystocia in the event of a vaginal delivery. However, the ability at term to estimate fetal weight either clinically or by means of ultrasonography is limited (Weiner et al 2002). Moreover, most cases of shoulder dystocia occur in non-macrosomic infants. The recent Cochrane review suggests that induction of labour for suspected fetal macrosomia does not reduce the risk of cesarean section. Neither does induction of labour alter neonatal or maternal morbidity rates (Irion and Boulvain 2003). There is thus no compelling evidence to support the practice of cesarean section to prevent shoulder dystocia in ultrasonographically suspected macrosomic infants. It has been estimated that 2000–3000 cesarean sections would be needed to prevent one permanent brachial plexus injury from shoulder dystocia (Rouse and Owen 1999).

> There is no compelling evidence to support the practice of cesarean section to prevent shoulder dystocia in ultrasonographically suspected macrosomic infants.

## Appropriate Tests for Fetal Well-being in Prolonged Pregnancy

Currently, fetal movement counting, antepartum cardiotocography, amniotic fluid volume and fetal Dopplers are some of the tests used to monitor fetuses in prolonged pregnancy. Very few tests have been shown to be predictive of stillbirth in prolonged/post-term pregnancy. The mechanism of increased stillbirth risk in prolonged pregnancy is not clear, which is reflected in the lack of a satisfactory test.

### Fetal movement counting

A randomised trial published in 1989 evaluated the effect of fetal movement counting on the risk of antenatal stillbirth in normally formed singleton pregnancies (Grant et al 1989). There was no difference in the rate of stillbirth in the two groups. Although a beneficial effect

> A history of sudden reduction in fetal movements reported by the mother should be taken seriously.

could not be ruled out, there was also the possibility of harm. Formal fetal movement counting is seldom practised as a routine test for fetal well-being at present. However, educating the mother on the importance of fetal movements is beneficial. A history of sudden reduction in fetal movements reported by the mother should be taken seriously, and induction of labour or fetal surveillance should be considered.

## Antepartum cardiotocography

A Cochrane review of antepartum cardiotocography (Pattinson and McCowen 2000) concluded that there was no evidence of benefit by the use of antepartum cardiotocography in monitoring high-risk pregnancy. However, this practice continues because of the lack of an effective alternative.

## Amniotic fluid estimation

Expectant management of prolonged pregnancy has traditionally involved antepartum fetal surveillance. This usually consists of a non-stress cardiotocograph and a four-quadrant amniotic fluid index (AFI) performed twice weekly. Magann et al (2000) questioned the ability of an AFI to identify actual abnormal amniotic fluid volumes. They performed ultrasound estimations of amniotic fluid volume using the AFI and single deepest pocket techniques on 179 women with singleton pregnancies. Each woman subsequently had ultrasound-directed amniocentesis with dye-dilution and spectrophotometric calculation of their actual amniotic fluid volume. Actual amniotic fluid volumes were low in 62 women. They found that an AFI up to 5 cm (sensitivity 10 per cent, specificity 96 per cent) and a single deepest pocket of up to 2 cm (sensitivity 5 per cent, specificity 98 per cent) were both inadequate in identifying true amniotic fluid volumes.

In an earlier paper, Magann et al (1999) looked at the role of the AFI estimate in 1001 high-risk patients. They found no significant differences in the incidence of non-reactive non-stress test results, meconium-stained amniotic fluid, cesarean delivery for fetal distress, low Apgar scores and infants with a cord pH of <7.10 between groups of women with oligohydramnios and normal amniotic fluid volume. These two papers strongly question the validity of using AFI as a means of surveillance in post-term pregnancy. A low AFI may be specific for true oligohydramnios, but the poor sensitivity suggests that its use as a screening test is suboptimal.

## Fetal Doppler

Umbilical artery Doppler is an important tool for monitoring intrauterine growth restriction (IUGR) in the preterm fetus. However, its role in the diagnosis and monitoring of IUGR in late gestation is controversial since abnormal umbilical artery Doppler waveforms are rare and perinatal morbidity attributable to IUGR may occur even when umbilical artery blood flow is normal. The fetal response to mild arterial hypoxemia includes redistribution of cardiac output to the brain at the expense of the body. This process is identified by the demonstration of low-impedance Doppler waveforms from the middle cerebral artery.

Two recent studies examined fetal arterial Doppler parameters in term and post-term pregnancies. Hershkovitz et al (2000) performed a small study on 47 structurally normal small fetuses at or near term. Thirty-one fetuses had normal middle cerebral blood flow and 16 had cerebral blood flow redistribution. There were no significant differences in the maternal characteristics between the two groups. They found that the cesarean section rate and the number of infants requiring special care admission were both higher in the redistribution group. These fetuses were, however, delivered two weeks earlier on average and were therefore also smaller, which may account for some of the observed differences.

The second study, performed by Selam and co-authors (2000) was only on 38 pregnancies beyond 41 weeks' gestation. They found evidence of fetal arterial redistribution present in pregnancies with oligohydramnios. There is evidence therefore, that suggests that fetuses may undergo redistribution of their arterial blood flow in response to a failing uteroplacental unit in late pregnancy before marked changes occur in the umbilical artery waveform. Whether this information can be utilised in an effective manner to bring about significant changes in fetal morbidity or mortality needs further evaluation.

## Conclusion

There is a well-recognised increased risk of fetal mortality and morbidity in pregnancies that extend into the post-term period. At the present time, it is not possible to predict pregnancies that are likely to experience a complication. Therefore, induction of labour between 41 and 42 weeks' gestation appears to be an effective strategy to reduce the risk of late intrauterine death. We should not, however, become complacent as more late fetal intrauterine deaths occur between 37 and 41 weeks' gestation than after this period. It appears that smaller term fetuses run a greater risk than their larger counterparts, although current methods of antepartum assessment of term fetus are still inadequate. Improvement in the efficiency of induction of labour is needed.

### Practice Points

1. Routine dating of pregnancy using early ultrasonography reduces the rate of prolonged pregnancy.
2. The risk of stillbirth in prolonged pregnancy increases with increasing gestational age, but the absolute risk remains small.
3. Appropriate fetal well-being tests in prolonged pregnancy are unknown.
4. Small fetuses are a particularly high-risk group at risk of fetal compromise and adverse outcomes.
5. Currently, the only policy of benefit is routine induction of labour after 41 weeks, but the exact timing is arbitrary.

## References

Bakketeig LS, P. Bergsjo 1989. Post-term pregnancy: Magnitude of the problem. In *Effective care in pregnancy and childbirth*, ed M Enkin, MJ Keirse, I Chalmers, 772. Oxford: Oxford University Press.

Boulvain M, C Stan, O Irion. 2003. Membrane sweeping for induction of labour. (Cochrane review) In *The Cochrane Library*, Issue 2. Oxford: Update Software.

Campbell MK, T Obstye, LM Irgens. 1997. Post-term birth: risk factors and outcomes in a 10–year cohort of Norwegian births. *Obstet Gynecol* 89:543–48.

Clausson B, J Gardosi, A Francis, S Cnattingius. 2001. Perinatal outcome in SGA births defined by customised versus population-based birthweight standards. *Br J Obstet Gynaecol* 108: 830–34.

Crowley P. 2006. Interventions for preventing or improv-ing the outcome of delivery at or beyond term. *Cochrane Database of Systematic Reviews* Issue 4.

Divon MY, B Haglund, H Nisell, PO Otterblad, M Westgren. 1998. Fetal and neonatal mortality in the postterm pregnancy: The impact of gestational age and fetal growth restriction. *Am J Obstet Gynecol* 178:726–31.

Eden R, L Seifert, A Winegar, W Spellacy. 1987. Perinatal characteristics of uncomplicated postterm pregnancies. *Obstet Gynecol* 69:34–8.

Gardosi J, M Mongelli, M Wilcox, A Chang. 1995. An adjustable fetal weight standard. *Ultrasound Obstet Gynecol* 6:168–74.

Grant A, D Elbourne, L Valentin, S Alexander. 1989. Routine formal fetal movement counting and risk of antepartum late death in normally formed singletons. *Lancet* 8659:345–49

Hannah ME, WJ Hannah, J Hellman, S Hewson, R Milner, A Willan. 1993. Induction of labor as compared with serial antenatal monitoring in post-term pregnancy – A randomised controlled trial. *N Engl J Med* 32:1587–92.

Hershkovitz R, JCP Kingdom, M Geary, CH Rodeck. 2000. Fetal cerebral blood flow redistribution in late gestation: Identification of compromise in small fetuses with normal umbilical artery Doppler. *Ultrasound Obstet Gynecol* 15:209–12.

Hilder L, K Costeloe, B Thilaganathan. 1998. Prolonged pregnancy: evaluating gestation-specific risks of fetal and infant mortality. *Br J Obstet Gynaecol* 105:169–73.

Hutcheon J, Zhang X, Cnattingius S, Kramer M, Platt R. Customised birthweight percentiles: does adjusting for maternal characteristics matter? BJOG 2008;115:1397–1404.

Irion O, M Boulvain. 2003. Induction of labour for suspected fetal macrosomia (Cochrane Review). In *The Cochrane Library*, Issue 1. Oxford: Update Software

Magann EF, SP Chauhan, PS Barrilleaux, NS Whitworth, JN Martin. 2000. Amniotic fluid index and single deepest pocket: Weak indicators of abnormal amniotic volumes. *Obstet Gynecol* 96:737–40.

Magann EF, SP Chauhan, MJ Kinsella, MF McNamara, NS Whitworth, JC Morrisin. 1999. Antenatal testing among 1001 patients at high risk: The role of ultrasonographic estimate of amniotic fluid volume. *Am J Obstet Gynecol* 180:1330–36.

Minior VK, MY Divon. 1998. Fetal growth restriction at term: myth or reality? *Obstet Gynecol* 92:57–60.

Mongelli M, YC Wong, A Venkat, TM Chua. 2001. Induction policy and missed post-term pregnancies: A mathematical model. *Aus NZ J Obstet Gynaecol* 41:38–40.

O'Reilly-Green CP, MY Divon. 1999. Receiver operating characteristic curves of ultrasonographic estimates of fetal weight for prediction of fetal growth restriction in prolonged pregnancies. *Am J Obstet Gynecol* 181:1133–38.

Pattinson N, L McCowan. 2000. Cardiotocography for antepartum fetal assessment. (Cochrane review) In *The Cochrane Library*, Issue 2. Oxford: Update Software.

Rouse D and J Owen. 1999. Prophylactic Caesarean delivery for fetal macrosomia diagnosed by means of ultrasonography – a Faustian bargain? *Am J Obstst Gynecol* 181:332–38

Selam B, R Koksal, T Ozcan. 2000. Fetal arterial and venous Doppler parameters in the interpretation of oligohydramnios in postterm pregnancies. *Ultrasound Obstet Gynecol* 15:403–6.

Sylvestre G, M Fisher, M Westgren, MY Divon. 2001. Non-reassuring fetal status in the prolonged pregnancy: The impact of fetal weight. *Ultrasound Obstet Gynecol* 18:244–47.

Tunon K, SH Eik-Nes, P Grottum. 1999. Fetal outcome in pregnancies defined as post-term according to the last menstrual period estimate, but not according to the ultrasound estimate. *Ultrasound Obstet Gynecol* 14:12–16.

Weiner Z, I Ben-Shlomo, R Beck-Fruchter, Y Goldberg, E Shalev. 2002. Clinical and ultrasonographic weight estimation in large for gestational age fetus. *Eur J Obstst Gynecol Reprod Biol* 105: 20–24.

# CHAPTER 27

# PROLONGED AND OBSTRUCTED LABOUR

*Pankaj Desai and Purvi Patel*

## Prolonged Labour

Normal labour usually progresses in a predictable fashion once the diagnosis of labour has been made. The progress of labour is evaluated primarily through estimates of cervical dilatation and descent of the fetal presenting part, that is, by using a partogram. In developing countries, the focus of a partogram in managing labour is on preventing maternal and fetal death related to prolonged labour, whereas in developed countries, the focus is on earlier identification and management of dystocia to offer interventions and avoid cesarean sections (WHO 1988, 1994). Dystocia (poor progress of labour) in women accounts for approximately 50 per cent of all primary cesarean sections (Fraser et al 1995; Shields et al 2007).

Poor progress of labour is a sign of an underlying pathology. If the causative pathology can be identified, specific management can be employed. Though this is not always possible in clinical practice, proper understanding of the problem will go a long way in reducing the morbidities associated with prolonged labour.

## Incidence

The overall incidence of dystocia in women in labour is difficult to determine, partly due to ambiguities in definition. Also, the clinical diagnosis of dystocia is often retrospective. If the outcome is uneventful and a spontaneous vaginal delivery occurs, dystocia may go unreported.

About 20 per cent of labours involve either *protraction* or *arrest disorders* (Zhu et al 2006). A prospective Danish study reported an incidence of 37 per cent when only low-risk nulliparous women at term were considered; almost two-thirds of these cases occurred in the second stage (Kjaergaard et al 2009). However, the reported incidence varies among studies secondary to differences in the definition of dystocia. Dystocia in the second stage is more common in nulliparas (5–10 per cent) than in multiparas (<2 per cent).

## Etiology

Progress in labour results from the interaction of three factors:

- Power
- Passage

❖ Passenger

## Power

Efficient uterine activity is essential to promote the formation of the lower uterine segment and to impart flexion and rotation to the fetal presenting part. Intrauterine pressure monitoring has not been found to have any extra advantage over abdominal palpation in monitoring uterine activity. If progressive cervical dilatation is taking place, there is no need for a lower limit to be placed on acceptable uterine activity. The adequacy of uterine activity should be questioned only when there is poor progress of labour.

> A contraction frequency of three to four contractions every 10 minutes is optimal, and palpable contractions should last for at least 40 seconds.

## Passage

The bony pelvis and the soft tissues are both important for progress of labour. Soft tissues include the cervix, lower uterine segment and the pelvic floor. While an android pelvis favours the occipito-posterior position, it can also lead to deep transverse arrest. An anthropoid pelvis is likely to be associated with persistent occipito-posterior position. A platypelloid pelvis is associated with deep transverse arrest. Gross pelvic abnormalities are usually identified early in labour. Relative cephalopelvic disproportion accounts for most cases of dystocia.

> Type of dystocia associated with pelvic shape:
> - Android pelvis: occipito-posterior position, deep transverse arrest
> - Anthropoid pelvis: persistent occipito-posterior position
> - Platypelloid pelvis: deep transverse arrest

## Passenger

Apart from fetal macrosomia, abnormal fetal presentations (brow, face), abnormal positions (occipito-posterior, occipito-transverse) and attitude (deflexion, asynclitism) are contributory factors to labour progress. Major flexion abnormalities like face and brow presentation are diagnosed in active labour but mild deflexion of the fetal head may not be diagnosed at times. Most cases respond with flexion and rotation with enhanced uterine activity. Some may result in prolonged labour despite the use of oxytocin. There are no safe and effective measures to correct flexion abnormalities of the fetal head. When asynclitism occurs, the second stage of labour is prolonged and arrest of descent is common. This increases the chances of operative vaginal delivery. Fetal abnormalities such as hydrocephalus, fetal ascites and fetal tumours may also be associated with dystocia.

> Deflexion of the head and asynclitism may lead to prolonged labour.

The labour characteristics of a nulliparous and a multiparous woman are fundamentally different. A multiparous woman requires less uterine force to overcome the resistance of the reproductive tract as it has already been stretched by previous delivery. The uterine musculature also retains effective contractility. Nulliparous women, on the other hand, are more likely to develop labour abnormalities that require some form of intervention.

## Assessment of labour progress

The mean duration of each phase of labour has been tabulated in Table 27.1. Since 1954, when Emanuel Friedman (1954) first reported a graphic representation of progress of labour, the concept of a 'partogram' has been used in the management of labour. The normal labour curve, developed by Friedman, based on observations, show that the first stage of labour is divided into an *acceleration phase*, an *active phase* and a *deceleration phase*.

The acceleration phase is at the onset of the active phase of labour (effaced cervix at 3–4-cm dilatation). In the active phase, cervical dilatation occurs at the rate of 1 cm/hour. The deceleration phase is a likely aberration of the mathematical analysis of Friedman's original data and not a physiologic event as such. In the second stage of labour, the fetal head descends by 1 cm/hour in the maternal pelvis.

**Table 27.1** Mean duration of the various phases and stages of labour

| Parity | Latent phase (hour) | Active phase (hour) | Maximum dilatation (cm/hour) | Second stage (hour) |
|---|---|---|---|---|
| Nulliparous | | | | |
| Mean | 6.4 | 4.5 | 1.0 | 1.0 |
| Upper limit | 20.0 | 12.0 | 3.0 | 3.0 |
| Multiparous | | | | |
| Mean | 4.8 | 2.5 | 1.5 | 0.5 |
| Upper limit | 13.5 | 5.0 | 6.0 | 1.0 |

Subsequently, Philpott and Castle (1972) and Beazley and Kurjak (1972) modified the partogram. In England, Studd et al (1975) studied 741 consecutive spontaneous labours to identify high-risk labours that needed

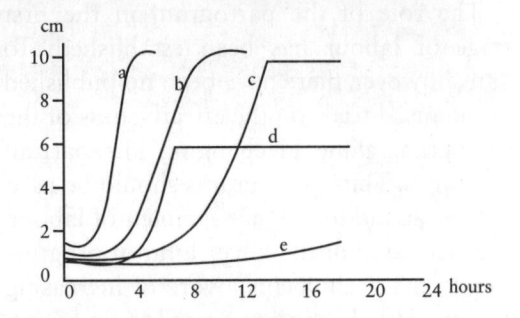

a: Normal cervicogram (multigravida)
b: Normal cervicogram (primigravida)
c: Prolonged active phase
d: Secondary arrest of dilatation
e: Prolonged latent phase

**Figure 27.1** Cervicograms of normal and abnormal labour patterns

oxytocin augmentation. Uterine contractions were augmented if progress extended two hours past the limit indicated by the partogram. This resulted in shorter labours, fewer instrumental deliveries and cesarean sections, and higher neonatal Apgar scores than in labours that were not augmented. This study, building on the reports of Philpott and Castle (1972), was followed by the increased use of the partogram in the United Kingdom, and its use subsequently spread throughout the world.

Partograms attempt to define a boundary that can be used to diagnose slow progress, as indicated in Fig. 27.1. However, they have been devised using data from specific populations with individual characteristics. There are clinically significant ethnic differences (Lim et al 1997) and hence, they cannot be generalised to different populations (Greenberg et al 2006). The positive predictive value for operative delivery from an *alert line* set at 1 cm/hour gradient and an *action line* two hours later is only 43 per cent.

The role of the partogram in the first stage of labour has been established. To date, however, there have been no published randomised trials on the effectiveness of the partogram alone in changing intrapartum outcomes. Thus, partograms should be used only as an aid to the management of labour. Transgression of the lower limit of progress should make clinicians aware of increasing risk and should prompt a need to find out a cause for the slow progress of labour.

## Classification of prolonged labour

Friedman described three abnormal patterns of labour:

* Prolonged latent phase
* Primary dysfunctional labour
* Secondary arrest

A more practical classification is to characterise labour abnormalities as:

* **Prolongation disorder:** Prolonged latent phase
* **Protraction disorders** (slower than normal progress)
    * Protracted active phase dilatation
    * Protracted descent
* **Arrest disorders** (complete cessation of progress)
    * Prolonged deceleration phase
    * Arrest of descent
    * Failure of descent

## Prolongation disorder

### Prolonged latent phase

Diagnosis of the onset of labour is crucial because if the diagnosis of labour has been erroneously made, all subsequent actions will be inappropriate. The latent phase begins with the onset of regular uterine contractions and extends to the beginning of the active phase of cervical dilatation. The duration of the latent phase averages 6.4 hours in nulliparas and 4.8 hours in multiparas. Based on the 95$^{th}$ per centile limit of distribution of latent phase duration, the latent phase is considered abnormally prolonged if it lasts *more than 20 hours in nulliparas and more than 14 hours in multiparas.*

The true incidence of prolonged latent phase is difficult to determine, but it is approximately 3.5 per cent for nulliparas. Prolongation of the latent phase occurs less commonly in multiparas. Though the precise cause is unclear, some believe this is a type of primary dysfunctional labour. A prolonged latent phase may be secondary to ineffective uterine contractions.

Treatment options include therapeutic rest regimes or augmentation of labour with oxytocin. Both have been found to be associated with similar outcomes. Friedman preferred therapeutic narcosis to oxytocin augmentation. It has been found that after 6–12 hours of rest with sedation and hydration, 85 per cent of women spontaneously enter the active phase of labour. About 10 per cent will have been in false labour as sometimes it is difficult to ascertain the difference between false labour and prolonged latent phase. Onset of true labour can be awaited in these women. In the remaining 5 per cent, uterine contractions remain ineffective and augmentation with oxytocin may be effective in the progression to the active phase of labour. Some authorities, especially proponents of active management of labor, recommend oxytocin infusion as the primary treatment for all women with prolonged latent phase. Oxytocin is the treatment of choice if an immediate delivery is required as in severe preeclampsia or chorioamnionitis.

Holmes et al (2001) have demonstrated that women who present to the hospital at less than 3 cm dilatation are more likely to undergo cesarean section or an operative vaginal delivery than those presenting with advanced cervical dilatation. Their results imply that women who present with less than 3 cm cervical dilatation could have intrinsically different labours from those who present with more advanced dilatation. Although earlier studies suggested that prolonged latent phase is not associated with increased perinatal mortality and is not the harbinger of other labour abnormalities, subsequent studies (Maghoma and Buchmann 2002; Simon and Grobman 2005) have shown otherwise. Chelmow et al (1993) found that a prolonged latent phase is associated with an increased risk of subsequent labour abnormalities, cesarean delivery, low Apgar scores, need for neonatal resuscitation, third- and fourth-degree perineal lacerations, febrile morbidity and intrapartum blood loss.

## Protraction disorders

Protraction disorders are of two types:
* Protracted active phase dilatation
* Protracted descent

*Protracted active phase dilatation* is characterised by an abnormally slow rate of dilatation in the active phase of less than 1.2 cm/hour in nulliparas or less than 1.5 cm/hour in multiparas. *Protracted descent* of the fetus is characterised by a rate of descent of less than 1 cm/hour in nulliparas or less than 2 cm/hour in multiparas. Protracted second stage is said to occur when the second stage exceeds two hours in nulliparas (three hours with epidural analgesia) or one hour in multiparas (two hours with epidural analgesia). It has an incidence of 26 per cent in nulliparas and 8 per cent in multiparas.

The underlying pathogenesis of protracted labour is multifactorial. Genuine cephalopelvic disproportion may be responsible in about one-third of women. Other factors include relative disproportion due to occipito-posterior position and epidural analgesia. Pelvic tumours are rare. Factors found to be associated with failure to progress in the first stage of labour include nulliparity, prelabour rupture of membranes, labour induction, maternal age more than 35 years, fetal weight more than 4 kg, hypertensive disorders and hydramnios (Sheiner et al 2002). Factors associated with prolonged second stage are longer first stage of labour, nulliparity, short maternal stature, birth weight and high station at full cervical dilatation.

### Treatment

Treatment depends on the presence or absence of cephalopelvic disproportion, adequacy of uterine contractions and the fetal status. A useful test to assess the presence of cephalopelvic disproportion is the Mueller–Hillis manoeuvre. It consists of the application of fundal pressure at the peak of a uterine contraction and assessing, with a hand placed in the vagina, if such pressure produces downward mobility of the fetal head. If there is no movement of the fetal head, the possibility of cephalopelvic disproportion is high.

***Oxytocin augmentation***: In the absence of cephalopelvic disproportion, conservative management with close monitoring, especially for fetal well-being, and treatment with amniotomy and oxytocin infusion has a good prognosis for vaginal delivery. About 80 per cent of nulliparas and 90 per cent of multiparas respond to oxytocin. However, an improved cervical dilatation rate does not always culminate in an uncomplicated vaginal delivery. O'Driscoll and Meagher (1986) suggest that an early, more active use of oxytocin, as described in the 'Active Management of Labour' protocol, effectively corrects most protraction disorders, although these authors do not specifically separate protraction disorders from arrest disorders. It seems to be a safe option to try oxytocin in nulliparous women with suboptimal progress of labour, to determine whether the labour will progress to completion.

Usually 2.5 units of oxytocin in 500 ml of normal saline is started at a rate of 10 drops/minute or 2.5 mU/minute. It is advisable to start with 2.5 mU/minute of oxytocin drip and increase the rate at half-hourly intervals along with monitoring of uterine activity. For active management and better response to oxytocin, amniotomy is recommended when the cervical dilatation is >3 cm.

In some obstetric departments, 5 units of synthetic oxytocin are added to 500 ml of normal saline. This gives a concentration of 10 mU/ml (ACOG Practice Bulletin No. 107, 2009). This allows for an optimal dose of oxytocin to be given without the risk of fluid overload, which is, however, rare. The use of an infusion pump increases the safety of oxytocin delivery to the woman and may avoid inadvertent increase in dosage.

A meta-analysis of clinical trials of oxytocin augmentation shows an increase in the rate of cervical dilatation, but no reduction in cesarean section rates (Thornton and Lilford 1994) and instrumental delivery rates (Hinshaw et al 2008; Dencker et al 2009).

*Amniotomy*: It is usually stated that amniotomy augments uterine activity. Randomised controlled trials of routine amniotomy have shown that there is no improvement in clinical outcome, but labour is shortened. There is no reduction in surgical interventions and there are no benefits for the neonate (Group 1994; Fraser et al 1993; 2000).

However, amniotomy should be considered in the presence of prolonged labour with intact membranes and inadequate uterine contractions. Rupture of the membranes stimulates the decidua to release prostaglandins. Prostaglandins cause cervical ripening and augment uterine activity. It allows the fetal head, rather than the otherwise intact amniotic sac, to be the dilating force. If the fetal heart rate pattern is non-reassuring, amniotomy can also allow early detection of meconium. However, if the labour parameters are normal, there is no clinical benefit from amniotomy (Neilson 2008).

*Cesarean section*: Cesarean section is indicated for cases of cephalopelvic disproportion after a proper trial of labour.

## Arrest disorders

There are two patterns of arrest in labour:

- ❖ Secondary arrest of dilatation, with no progressive cervical dilatation in the active phase of labour for two hours or more
- ❖ Arrest of descent, with descent failing to progress for an hour or more

In their pure form, arrest disorders differ from protraction disorders in that, prior to the arrest of progress, the rate of cervical dilatation or descent of the fetal head is normal. Arrest of progress can also complicate a protraction disorder. The incidence is 6 per cent in nulliparas and 2 per cent in multiparas.

Approximately 50 per cent of women with arrest disorders demonstrate cephalopelvic disproportion when inadequate uterine contractions have been treated. Other causative factors include fetal malpositions (occipito-posterior, occipito-transverse, face, brow) and epidural analgesia.

In the presence of arrest disorders, it is prudent to evaluate for cephalopelvic disproportion. Cesarean section is warranted in the presence of cephalopelvic disproportion. In the absence of cephalopelvic disproportion, consider oxytocin if uterine contractions are inadequate. Although Friedman (1978) found that 80 per cent of women with arrest disorders who did not have cephalopelvic disproportion delivered following oxytocin augmentation, cesarean section rates are around ten-fold greater than normal labour. O'Driscoll and Meagher (1986) suggest that a trial of oxytocin augmentation is indicated in all protraction and arrest disorders. With careful maternal and fetal monitoring, oxytocin augmentation is continued for 4–6 hours. If there is no progress with signs of disproportion lik excessive caput and moulding and CTG changes within this time, oxytocin is discontinued and operative delivery should be considered.

In the presence of adequate uterine contractions, arrest disorders have poor prognosis for vaginal delivery. These are associated with increased perinatal mortality if allowed to continue.

## Second stage abnormalities

In the past, arbitrary limits on the duration of the second stage of labour resulted in traumatic mid-cavity forceps deliveries or unnecessary cesarean deliveries. New research has demonstrated that after excluding patients with fetal distress, the duration of the second stage bears no relationship to perinatal outcome (Myles and Santolaya 2003). The evidence is in favour of delayed pushing (Hansen et al 2002). If labour progresses with oxytocin and the head descends low enough into the pelvis, instrumental vaginal delivery should be undertaken. If there is no descent, cesarean section is indicated.

Collectively, the studies on a prolonged second stage of labour suggest that there is little risk to the fetus (2–4 hours) provided the fetal condition is carefully monitored, but that this is associated with an increase in *maternal postpartum hemorrhage*, *perineal tears* and *postpartum pyrexia*. These may in part be attributed to or associated with instrumental delivery.

A subtle variant of secondary arrest is a delay of labour between 7 cm and 10 cm cervical dilatation. After the cervix is dilated more than 7 cm, descent or rotation of the fetal head can be expected. If this does not occur, uterine contractions, if they are not adequate, should be augmented with oxytocin. Even though full dilatation may be achieved in such cases, there is an increased risk of difficult instrumental delivery (Davidson et al 1976). *Posterior presentation*, *face presentation*, *marked degrees of asynclitism* and *fetal macrosomia* are associated with longer labours, even with adequate contractions.

## Consequences of prolonged labour

Prolonged labour is associated with an increased incidence of cesarean section. Dumont et al (2001) reported a cesarean section rate of 22 per cent in cases of protracted labour, which was defined as a labour lasting over 12 hours. WHO partographic studies (1994) demonstrated that when the labour remained on the left of the alert line, the cesarean section rate was 0.6 per cent, and when the action line was reached, the cesarean section rate was 21.8 per cent.

Other consequences of prolonged labour are chorioamnionitis, atonic postpartum hemorrhage, obstructed labour, ruptured uterus and puerperal sepsis. The fetal consequences include hypoxia, intracranial injury, pneumonia and delayed milestones.

### Conclusion

Whatever the pattern of delay, identification of a clear single causative factor is often not possible. This could be due to multifactorial causes, an inability to detect the contributory factor due to imprecise diagnostic tools, lack of knowledge of other factors or all these factors in combination. Treatment is more likely to be successful when the diagnosis of a single causative factor is possible.

If the progress of labour is inadequate, prompt intervention (augmentation of powers) is required. Early medical intervention can correct the underlying problem in a larger proportion of cases as compared to late medical therapy. In spite of medical intervention, if the expected labour progress cannot be achieved, medical therapy should be abandoned and surgical therapy should be considered to prevent maternal or fetal compromise.

## Obstructed Labour

Labour is considered obstructed when the presenting part of the fetus cannot progress into the birth canal in spite of strong uterine contractions, due to mechanical obstruction. There is usually a mismatch between fetal size, or more accurately, the size of the presenting part of the fetus, and the mother's pelvis. Some malpresentations, especially a brow or a shoulder presentation, will also cause obstruction. The obstruction can only be alleviated by an operative delivery: cesarean section, instrumental delivery (forceps or vacuum extraction) or symphysiotomy.

Neglected obstructed labour is a major cause of both maternal and neonatal morbidity and mortality. The incidence of obstructed labour is 4.6 per cent of all live births globally (AbouZahr 1988; 2003). Obstructed labour is common in developing countries (Ozumba and Uchegbu 1991; Jayaram 1993). It accounts for 11.4 per cent of maternal deaths in the Eastern part of India (Dutta and Pal 1978). Approximately 8 per cent of all maternal deaths in developing countries are due to obstructed labour (Liljestrand 2002). This figure is an underestimation of the problem, because deaths due to obstructed labour are often classified under other associated complications such as sepsis, postpartum hemorrhage or ruptured uterus. Obstructed labour is responsible for 80 per cent of genito-urinary fistulae in developing countries (Mala and Rao 2002; Biswas et al 2007). Delayed management of obstructed labour causes fistulae in surviving women, which if not treated, may make them social outcasts for the rest of their lives (Muleta 2006; Roush 2009). This may also lead to constant depression, physical illness and infections.

## Causes of obstructed labour

- *Cephalopelvic disproportion (contracted pelvis or large fetus)*: Two major evolutionary forces have made the human female susceptible to cephalopelvic disproportion: the assumption of an erect bipedal posture, which leads to structural constraints on the pelvic architecture, and the increasing size of the human brain over a period of time
- *Malpresentations*, for example, brow, shoulder, mento-posterior, and after-coming head in breech presentation
- *Fetal malformations*, for example, hydrocephalus, locked twins, conjoint twins, fetal ascites
- *Abnormalities of the reproductive tract*, for example, pelvic tumour, stenosis of the cervix or vagina
- *Rare causes*, for example, *a vesical calculus, an ovarian cyst* or even *a hydatid cyst in the pelvis* find mention in case reports as causing obstructed labour

## Risk factors for obstructed labour

- Age <17 years (because the pelvis is not fully developed)
- Grand multigravidae who commonly have abnormal presentations, large babies due to increasing parity, subluxation of the sacroiliac joints pushing the sacral promontory forward and affecting the antero-posterior diameter of the pelvic inlet)
- Height <145 cm (usually associated with malnutrition and small pelvis)
- Previous cesarean section, stillbirths and previous prolonged labour
- Diseases like rickets, osteomalacia and poliomyelitis.
- Community risk factors include poor antenatal care, poor intrapartum monitoring (partogram not used), traditional beliefs and practices regarding prolonged/obstructed labour, custom of early marriage, lack of transport and communication and delay in referral to higher level of care for cesarean sections

## Course of labour

### Early (developing) stage

Obstruction usually occurs at the pelvic brim, but occasionally it may occur in the cavity or at the outlet of the pelvis. There is misfit of the presenting part to the brim and this hinders the descent of the presenting part. Membranes rupture early. The presenting part is not well-applied to the cervix and the cervix dilates slowly or there is no further cervical dilatation. Even when the cervix is well dilated, it is not closely applied to the presenting part and hangs loose like a thick curtain. The cervix becomes edematous as the woman continues to push. In a vertex presentation, a large caput succedaneum may form and the moulding may be excessive. Sometimes, the large caput and excessive moulding, elongate the head. The vertex may be visible at or just above the introitus when, actually, most of the head is well above the brim. This can be quite misleading and an inexperienced obstetrician may feel that delivery is imminent. If the diagnosis is not made at this stage and early intervention instituted to deliver the woman, she will progress to late fully developed obstructed labour.

### Late (fully developed) stage

The woman will look exhausted. Signs of maternal exhaustion may include dehydration, rapid pulse, raised temperature and increased respiratory rate. There may be edema of the vulva.

Abdominal examination may reveal an ileus (due to electrolyte imbalance). The upper part of the uterus (upper segment) will be hard. The uterine wall is closely applied to the fetus as all amniotic fluid would have drained out. Mobility of the fetal parts will be restricted and the fetal outline becomes obscure. *Bandl's ring* forms and will be visible: the junction of the thick upper segment and thin lower segment will be well demarcated and seen as a groove between the two segments. The Bandl's ring may rise to the level of the umbilicus. The stretched round ligaments may also be felt.

These findings develop since the upper segment continues to contract and retract. There is no full relaxation between uterine contractions. Due to obstruction, the presenting part does not move down the uterus. The passive lower segment gradually becomes stretched to accommodate the body of the fetus. At this stage, the lower segment becomes quite tender and is likely to rupture.

Soon, uterine exhaustion may occur and contractions may become weaker. This is more likely in a primigravida. If intervention is not carried out at this stage, after a lapse of time, strong uterine contractions resume and uterine rupture occurs. On the other hand, in a multigravida, uterine contractions tend to persist till uterine rupture occurs. When labour is obstructed, the fetal head impacts against the soft tissues of the pelvic floor, pinning the bladder base and the urethra against the pelvic bone. This leads to ischemic necrosis and ultimately a fistula. It is the duration of impaction without relief, rather than the magnitude of the pressure, which determines the degree of tissue necrosis. The fistula site depends greatly on the degree of cervical effacement and dilatation, and the level at which the presenting part impacts.

## Clinical features and diagnosis

### In early cases

Abdominal examination will reveal stretching of the lower uterine segment and an edematous, drawn-up bladder. Contractions are hypertonic. The presenting part is not engaged. There may be fetal distress. In vertex presentation, a large caput and excessive moulding may be seen. Though the scalp may be seen at the introitus, both poles of the head are felt on abdominal palpation.

### In late cases

The woman looks exhausted and dehydrated (dry tongue, tachycardia, ketonuria). She may be febrile. Abdominal examination reveals the fetal head above the brim or there may be an abnormal presentation. The urinary bladder is distended. Usually frequent, strong uterine contractions are present but if the woman has been in labour for a long time, contractions may have stopped due to uterine exhaustion. The uterus is contracted and moulded over the fetus and no relaxation of the uterus is felt. Bandl's' ring may be seen near the umbilicus and may be palpated (normally the junction between the upper uterine segment and the lower segment is not felt/seen during labour). Distended bowel loops may be seen. Vaginal examination indicates absence of liquor with foul-smelling meconium. Urinary catheterisation is difficult. Urine is concentrated and often blood stained. The vulva and vagina appear edematous. The vagina is hot and dry. The cervix is edematous, not well-applied over the presenting part and may hang loose like a thick curtain. The cervix may be partially or fully dilated. A large caput succedaneum is felt. The cause of obstruction can be made out, that is, cephalopelvic disproportion (severely moulded head with a large caput succedaneum), shoulder presentation with or without arm prolapse, brow or face (mento-posterior) presentation.

*Ruptured uterus* is common in multiparas but rare in nulliparas. Warning signs include Bandl's ring and tenderness of the lower segment of the uterus. Rupture of the uterus should be suspected in the presence of shock, abdominal distension/free fluid, abnormal uterine contour, tender abdomen, easily palpable fetal parts, absent fetal movements and fetal heart sounds.

Diagnosis could be more difficult if the rupture is incomplete or the tear is small. In this case, the fetus will remain at least partially in the uterus and signs of shock in the mother are delayed until after delivery because the pressure of the fetus prevents bleeding to some extent. Symptoms in this case could be initially very slight, and labour may even continue. Suspect rupture if there is sudden onset of fetal distress and the mother's pulse rate starts rising.

The partogram for this particular labour would indicate a prolonged first stage with secondary arrest with poor cervical dilation in spite of strong contractions or a prolonged second stage with evidence of fetal distress.

## Consequences of obstructed labour

The consequences of obstructed labour include atonic as well as traumatic PPH, uterine rupture, peritonitis and puerperal sepsis that contribute to maternal mortality in about 5–10 per cent of cases. Delayed complications include urinary fistulae and obstetric palsy (peroneal nerve injury and foot-drop). Fetal complications include an increased incidence of stillbirths and neonatal deaths, birth asphyxia, intracranial hemorrhage and delayed complications such as delayed milestones, convulsive disorders and mental retardation.

## Management

Management includes preventive measures and management after diagnosis.

### Prevention

*Antenatal*: The risk factors mentioned earlier should be identified during antenatal care. Contracted pelvis, cephalopelvic disproportion and abnormal presentations should be detected early. Such cases should have timely referral to a hospital with operating facilities for delivery. External version at term can reduce malpresentations at labour.

*Partogram*: Almost all obstructed labours can be prevented by adequate intrapartum care. A partogram aids in early detection and timely intervention before labour becomes obstructed (Lennox et al 1998, Mathai 2009). A protracted active phase can be detected at an early stage and appropriate management can be instituted. Non-descent of the head in spite of good uterine action and satisfactory cervical dilatation indicates cephalopelvic disproportion and requires referral. Oxytocin augmentation should be used judiciously in labour.

### Management after diagnosis

Complications resulting from obstructed labour can be avoided if a woman in obstructed labour is identified early and appropriate action is taken. Management after diagnosis includes correction of dehydration with crystalloids, intravenous broadspectrum antibiotics including coverage for anaerobic organisms, and blood transfusion if required. Oxygen and inotropic support may also be required if shock is present. Urinary catheterisation is to be carried out. This may be difficult but can be accomplished by straightening the urethra with two fingers in the vagina pushing the presenting part upwards. Immediate delivery must be carried out.

*Cesarean section*: Cesarean section remains the mainstay of treatment in obstructed labour. An immediate cesarean section is indicated if the fetus is alive and the fetal station is high, there is a gross cephalopelvic disproportion, or malpresentations like brow or shoulder presentation are seen. It may also be indicated even if the fetus is dead. Cesarean section of obstructed labour is rendered difficult by an advanced bladder, a thinned-out lower segment that is lifted high and a deeply impacted presenting part. The peritoneum should be opened at a higher level to avoid bladder injury. The incision on the lower segment should not be placed low, to prevent inadvertent entry into the vagina. The fetus can be delivered by reverse breech extraction or by the shoulders first technique (Desai et al 2001) to prevent uterine extensions. After delivery of the fetus, the lower edge of the uterine incision may retract down and one may mistakenly suture the upper edge of the uterine incision to the posterior uterine wall.

*Instrumental vaginal delivery*: Instrumental vaginal delivery is used in cases with fetal malpositions, soft tissue obstruction or ineffective maternal bearing down efforts due to obstetric analgesia.

*Symphysiotomy*: Symphysiotomy is carried out as an alternative to cesarean section in borderline cephalopelvic disproportion in many African countries (Bergstrom et al 1994; Bjorklund 2002; Liljestrand 2002). The arguments in favour of symphysiotomy are both clinical and cultural.

Cesarean section is seen as a sort of failure of maternal achievement, especially in African culture. A modest permanent enlargement of the pelvis post-symphysiotomy (together with the absence of a scarred uterus) may facilitate subsequent vaginal delivery. Symphysiotomy is particularly suitable when the mother is going to return to her remote locality and perhaps may not receive supervision in subsequent births. The procedure involves division of the fibrocartilage of the pubic symphysis, usually under local anesthesia, to widen the birth canal. The separation of the joint should not be more than 3.5 cm. Bladder drainage, pelvic strapping and bed rest is advisable for three weeks following delivery.

*Destructive operations*: Destructive procedures may play a role in cases with a dead fetus with a fully dilated cervix, when the pelvis is not grossly contracted and there is no impending uterine rupture. These procedures should be undertaken only if the operator is sufficiently skilled in the procedures. Craniotomy for an unengaged head, decapitation for a shoulder presentation and evisceration for fetal ascites or conjoint twins can be performed.

In hydrocephalus, craniocentesis is carried out either vaginally (preferable) or abdominally after fixing the head with suprapubic pressure in early labour. This is possibly the only indication acceptable today. The cerebrospinal fluid is drained to reduce the head circumference of the fetus to a normal size and then labour is allowed to progress. Occasionally draining of brain matter through a perforation may be required to conduct a vaginal delivery.

Occasionally, an elongated cervix of a prolapsed uterus can obstruct the fetal presenting part. If the dilatation is more than 7 cm with the presenting part adequately descended, Duhrssen's cervical incision may be used to deliver the presenting part. Three incisions at the 2, 6 and 10 o'clock positions are made on the cervix. This procedure may also be used in case of an entrapped after-coming head in breech delivery. Though this procedure is rarely used in modern obstetrics, it is only mentioned as a procedure in situations where immediate cesarean section is not possible or transfer to another hospital may not be feasible.

The use of internal version for shoulder presentation is mentioned only to be condemned in obstructed labour.

Postpartum atonic hemorrhage is likely with any method of delivery for obstructed labour and prevention with uterotonic drugs should always be employed. Post-operative ileus may take a longer time to resolve and intravenous fluids should be continued till that time. Postoperative indwelling bladder catheteristion may be indicated for 5–7 days in advanced obstruction.

## Conclusion

Prolonged, obstructed labour is an expression usually used in one breath. The two can take place independent of each other. It is very critical to predict these conditions accurately and in time. Accurate prediction will help in preventing the conditions of prolonged and obstructed labour rather than struggling to manage them once they occur. With better provision of antenatal care and wider coverage of women receiving antenatal care in any society, these conditions will become rarer. The mainstay of treatment is indeed cesarean section, but even in cesarean section, the dexterity of the obstetrician and control over technique is tested. Thus, prolonged, obstructed labours are rightly termed a challenge for both the mother and the obstetrician.

## References

ACOG Practice Bulletin No. 107. 2009. Induction of Labor. American College of Obstetricians and Gynecologists. *Obstet Gynecol* 114: 386–97.

AbouZahr C.1998. Prolonged and obstructed labour. In: Murray CJL and Lopez AD, eds. *Health dimensions of sex and reproduction: the global burden of sexually transmitted diseases, maternal conditions, perinatal disorders, and congenital anomalies.* WHO.

AbouZahr C. 2003. Global burden of maternal death and disability. *Br Med Bull* 67:1–11.

Beazley JM, Kurjak A. 1972. Influence of a partograph on the active management of labour. *Lancet* Aug 19; 2(7773):348–51.

Bergstrom S, Lublin H, Molin A. 1994. Value of symphysiotomy in obstructed labor management and follow up of 31 cases. *Gynaecol Obstet Invest* 38:31–35.

Biswas A, Bal R, Alauddin M, Saha S, Kundu MK, Mondal P. 2007. Genital fistula-our experience. *J Indian Med Assoc* Mar; 105(3):123–6.

Bjorklund. 2002. Review of symphysiotomy for obstructed labor. *Br J Obstet Gynaecol* 109:227–231.

Chelmow D, Kilpatrick SJ, Laros RK. 1993. Maternal and neonatal outcomes after prolonged latent phase. *Obstet Gynecol*. 81:486-91.

Davidson AC, Weaver JB, Davies P, Pearson JF. 1976. The relationship between ease of forceps delivery and speed of cervical dilatation. *Br J Obstet Gynaecol*. 83:279–283.

Dencker A, Berg M, Bergqvist L, Ladfors L, Thorsen LS, Lilja H. 2009. Early versus delayed oxytocin augmentation in nulliparous women with prolonged labor-a randomized controlled trial. *Br J Obstet Gynaecol* Mar; 116(4):530–6.

Desai P, Desai P, Shah A et al. 2001. Preventing complications by "shoulder first" method of delivery in cases of obstructed labor. *J Obstet Gynaecol Ind* 51:91–4.

Dumont A, L de Bernis, M Bouvier-Colle et al. 2001. Caesarean section in sub-Saharan Africa. *Lancet* 358:1328–34.

Dutta DC, Pal SK. 1978. Obstructed labor: A review of 307 cases. *J Obstet Gynaecol India* 28:55–58.

Fraser WD, Marcoux S, Moutquin JM, Christen A. 1993. effect of early amniotomy on the risk of dystocia in nulliparous women. The Canadian Early Amniotomy Study Group. *N Engl J Med* 328(16), 1145–1149.

Fraser WB, Krauss I, Boulvain M, Oppenheimer L, Milne KJ, Liston, RM,Lalonde B. 1995. Dystocia. Society of Obstetricians and Gynaecologists Canada (SOGC) Policy Statement, No. 40, October *J Soc Obstet Gynaecol Can* 17:985–1001.

Fraser WD, Turkot L, Krauss I, Brisson-Carrol G. 2000. Amniotomy for shortening spontaneous labor. *Cochrane Database Syst Rev* (2), CD000015(4).

Friedman EA.1954. The graphic analysis of labor. *Am J Obstet Gynecol* 68:1568–75.

Friedman EA. 1978.Ed. *Labor clinical evaluation and management*, 2nded. Appleton-Century-Crofts: New York.

Greenberg MB, Cheng YW, Hopkins Lm, Stotland NE, Bryant AS, Caughey AB. 2006. Are there ethnic differences in the length of labor? *Am J Obstet Gynecol Sep*; 195(3):743–8.

Group UA. 1994. A multicentre randomized trial of amniotomy in spontaneous first labor at term. *Br J Obstet Gynaecol* 101: 307–309.

Hansen SL, Clark SL, Foster JC. 2002. Active pushing versus passive fetal descent in the second stage of labor: A randomized trial. *Obstet Gynecol* 99(2):29–34.

Hinshaw K; Simpson S; Cummings S; Hildreth A; Thornton J. 2008. A randomised controlled trial of early versus delayed oxytocin augmentation to treat primary dysfunctional labour in nulliparous women. *Br J Obstet Gynaecol* Sep; 115(10):1289–95.

Holmes P, Oppenheimer L, Wen S.2001. The relationship between cervical dilatation at initial presentation in labour and subsequent intervention *Br J Obstet Gynaecol* 108: 1120–1124.

Jayaram, Kamala V. 1993. Obstructed labor, an analysis of 126 cases. *J Obstet Gynaecol India* 43:60–63.

Kjaergaard H, Olsen J, Ottesen B, Dykes AK. 2009. Incidence and outcomes of dystocia in the active phase of labor in term nulliparous women with spontaneous labor onset. *Acta Obstet Gynecol Scand*; 88:402.

Lennox CE, Kwast BE, Farley TM. 1998. Breech labor n the WHO partograph. Int J Gynec *Obstet* 62(2): 117–127.

Liljestrand J. 2002. The value of symphysiotomy. *Br J Obstet Gynaecol* 109:225–26.

Lim AM, Wong WP, Sinnathuray, TA. 1997. Characteristics of normal labour among different racial groups in Malaysia. BJOG. 84:8 600–604.

Maghoma J, Buchmann EJ. 2002. Maternal and fetal risks associated with prolonged latent phase of labor. *J Obstet Gynecol* Jan; 22(1):16–19.

Mala V, Rao KB. 2002. Incontinence in women. In *Obstetrics and Gynaecology for postgraduates*, Ed SS Ratnam, KB Rao, S Arulkumaran, vol 2, 2nd ed. Orient Longman.

Mathai M. 2009. The partograph for the prevention of obstructed labor. *Clin Obstet Gynecol* Jun; 52(2):256–69.

Muleta M. 2006. Obstetric fistula in developing countries: a review article. *J Obstet Gynaecol Can*. Nov; 28(11):962–6.

Myles TD, Santolaya J. 2003. Maternal and neonatal outcomes in patients with a prolonged second stage. *Obstet Gynecol* 102(1):52–8.

Neilson JP. 2008. Amniotomy for shortening spontaneous labor. *Obstet Gynecol*. Jan; 111(1):201–4.

O'Driscoll K, Meagher D. 1986. *Active management of labour*. 2nd Ed. Eastbourne, Sussex, UK: Bailli_re Tindall:1–12.

Ozumba BC, Uchegbu H. 1991. Incidence and management of obstructed labor in eastern Nigeria. *Aust NZ J Obstet Gynaecol* 31:213–16.

Philpott RH, Castle WM.1972. Cervicographs in the management of labor in primigravidae. I. The alert line for detecting abnormal labour. *J Obstet Gynaecol Br Commonw*; 79:592–8.

Roush KM. 2009. Social implications of obstetric fistula: an integrative review. *J Midwifery Womens Health* Mar-Apr; 54(2):e21–33.

Sheiner E, Levy A, Feinstein U, Hallak M, Mazor M. 2002. Risk factors and outcome of failure to progress during the first stage of labor: a population-based study. *Acta Obstet Gynecol*. Mar; 81(3):222–6.

Shields SG, Ratcliffe SD, Fontaine P, Leeman L. 2007. Dystocia in nulliparous women. *Am Fam Physician* Jun1; 75(11):1671–8.

Simon CE, Grobman WA. 2005. When has an induction failed? *Obstet Gynecol* 105: 705–709.

Studd J, Clegg DR, Sanders RR, Hughes AO. 1975. Identification of high risk labours by labour nomogram. *Br Med J* 7:545–7.

Thornton JG, Lilford RJ. 1994. Active management of labor: Current knowledge and research issues. *Br Med J* 309: 366–369.

World Health Organization. 1988. The partograph: a managerial tool for the prevention of prolonged labor. Section I. The principle and strategy. 89.2.

World Health Organization. 1994. Partograph in management of labor. *Lancet* 343:1399–1404.

Zhu BP, Grigrescu V, Le T et al. 2006. Labor dystocia and its association with inter-pregnancy interval. *Am J Obstet Gynecol* 195:121.

# CHAPTER 28

# PERIPARTUM HYSTERECTOMY

*Anita Dutta and Edwin Chandraharan*

## Introduction

Primary postpartum hemorrhage (PPH) denotes blood loss in excess of 500 ml from the genital tract within 24 hours of the birth of a baby (Mousa and Alfirevic 2007). Secondary PPH is defined as abnormal or excessive bleeding from the birth canal between 24 hours and 6 weeks postnatally (Alexander et al 2002). The incidence of PPH is 15–19 per cent of pregnancies in developed countries. Obstetric hemorrhage contributes 11–33 per cent of maternal deaths worldwide and is the commonest cause of maternal mortality in developing countries. The World Health Organization (WHO) estimates a 1 per cent case fatality rate for the 14 million annual cases of obstetric hemorrhage (UNICEF 2001). The estimated mortality rate from hemorrhage in sub-Saharan Africa is 300 per 100,000 live births (Geller et al 2006).

In the 7th Confidential Enquiries into Maternal Deaths in the United Kingdom (CEMACH 2007), hemorrhage was the third most common direct cause of maternal death. This illustrates that even in the developed world, obstetric hemorrhage contributes to significant maternal morbidity and mortality. Massive postpartum hemorrhage (bleeding >2 l of blood within a short time or more than 30 per cent of blood volume) is a life-threatening obstetric emergency. The causes of such massive hemorrhage include uterine atony, genital tract trauma, retained placental tissue and membranes and coagulopathy. When conservative measures fail to arrest the hemorrhage, surgical measures such as peripartum hysterectomy may help save lives.

Over the years, the 'art' of obstetrics has changed significantly and there has been an increase in the incidence of cesarean sections worldwide. Currently in the United Kingdom, an estimated 23 per cent of women undergo a cesarean section (CS) (approximately 160,000 women per year) (NHS Maternity Statistics 2006). Similarly, in the United States, this figure is 31.1 per cent (Hamilton et al 2007) and the incidence is reported to be rising possibly due to increasing body mass index (BMI), assisted reproduction techniques and rising incidence of primary (previous) cesarean sections.

An association has been noted between a previous CS and abnormal placentation (such as placenta previa and morbidly adherent placentae – placenta accreta, increta and percreta) and uterine rupture. In the presence of these conditions, there is a significant risk of having a peripartum hysterectomy (PH). The incidence of placenta accreta is as high as 67 per cent in patients with placenta previa and multiple previous cesareans (Clark et al 1985). The number of previous cesareans is also related to an increased risk of placenta accreta, from 0.19 per cent for one previous cesareans to 9.1 per cent for four previous cesareans (Kwee et al 2006).

> The risk of having a peripartum hysterectomy increases with:
> • placenta previa
> • morbidly adherent placentae (placenta accreta, increta and percreta)
> • uterine rupture

Studies have shown that the associated risk of peripartum hysterectomy extends beyond the initial CS to subsequent deliveries; women who have had one previous CS have more than double the risk of peripartum hysterectomy in the next pregnancy, and women who have had two previous cesareans have 18 times the risk (Kinght et al 2008). The prevalence rates of uterine rupture in pregnancy and labour is between 0.1 per cent and 1 per cent, and in women with a previous CS scar, the prevalence of ruptured uterus is about 1 per cent (Hofmeyr et al 2005).

> The risk of having a peripartum hysterectomy is 18 times the risk in women who have had 2 previous cesarean sections.

## Peripartum Hysterectomy

### Definition and causes

Peripartum hysterectomy (PH) includes hysterectomies that are performed at the time of CS or postpartum following either vaginal birth or CS. Emergency PH is performed mostly as a life-saving procedure for massive obstetric hemorrhage that is unresponsive to conservative or medical methods. PH is an uncommon, but well-described surgical procedure that is typically used as the last resort for refractory obstetric hemorrhage (Barclay 1970). However, if the patient is hemodynamically unstable, it is recommended that this procedure be undertaken sooner rather than later (Chandraharan and Arulkumaran 2008). Such a decision should be made by the most senior obstetrician.

Various algorithms have been suggested to aid in the systematic management of PPH. One such algorithm 'HAEMOSTASIS' (Chandraharan and Arulkumaran 2005) is given in Table 28.1. Emergency PH is indicated when the PPH is unresponsive to conservative measures such as bimanual compression, medical management (use of oxytocics or ecbolics), use of a tamponade of the uterus (with a gauze pack or fluid-filled catheters, including a 'condom catheter' in low-resource countries), conservative surgical procedures such as uterine compression sutures and ligation of the uterine or internal iliac arteries (systematic pelvic devascularisation) and/or radiographic interventions (uterine artery embolisation).

The earliest documented human PH was performed in 1868 by Horatio Robinson Storer of Boston (Bixby 1869). The first successful operation was performed in 1876 by Eduardo Porro, Professor of Obstetrics at Pavia, who advocated hysterectomy during a CS to control uterine hemorrhage and prevent peritonitis. The incidence of PH quoted in the recent literature is 0.24–1.4 per 1000 births (Todman 2007; Sakse et al 2007).

**Table 28.1** Management algorithm of PPH 'HAEMOSTASIS' (Chandraharan and Arulkumaran 2005)

| H | Ask for **H**elp and **h**ands on the uterus (uterine massage) |
|---|---|
| A | **A**ssess and resuscitate |
| E | **E**stablish the cause, **e**nsure availability of blood and **e**cbolics |
| M | **M**assage the uterus |
| O | **O**xytocin infusion/prostaglandins- IV/IM/per rectal |
| S | **S**hift to the theatre – aortic pressure or anti-shock garment/bimanual compression as appropriate |
| T | **T**amponade balloon/uterine packing, after exclusion of tissue and trauma |
| A | **A**pply compression sutures – B-Lynch/ modified |
| S | **S**ystematic pelvic devascularisation – uterine/ ovarian/quadruple/internal iliac |
| I | **I**nterventional radiology and, if appropriate, uterine artery embolisation |
| S | **S**ubtotal/total abdominal hysterectomy |

Despite variations in the literature, it is estimated that the rate of PH is 1 per 1000 deliveries or less (Kastner et al 2002; Bai et al 2003; Eniola et al 2006; Glaze et al 2008).

## Indications for peripartum hysterectomy

Peripartum hysterectomy is a radical surgical option to save the life of the mother, when all other conservative measures to arrest hemorrhage have failed or if the patient is hemodynamically unstable (Mishra and Chandraharan 2009). In the above mentioned situations, it is important to consider this option early to improve maternal outcome as 'too little being done too late' has been found to be associated with increased maternal morbidity and mortality. It is essential to balance the need for future fertility against the need for timely radical intervention to save a life.

The most senior obstetrician managing a case of massive PPH should be involved in making this decision, preferably in consultation with another senior obstetrician. It is a good practice to keep the patient and her immediate family involved in making this decision. Early recourse to PH is advisable in women who decline blood and blood products as any further delay is likely to compromise maternal well-being. The indications for PH are listed in Table 28.2.

**Table 28.2** Indications for peripartum hysterectomy

- Massive obstetric hemorrhage
- Morbidly adherent placentae such as placenta accreta (isolated accreta or previa accreta), placenta increta or percreta.
- Placenta previa
- Uterine atony not responding to conservative measures
- Uterine rupture: spontaneous or traumatic
- Uterine inversion
- Cervical lacerations
- Broad ligament hematoma (Fig. 28.1)
- Septicemia with coagulopathy, not responding to medical treatment
- Trauma
- Cancer: cervical
- Others: large or multiple fibroids with continuous bleeding

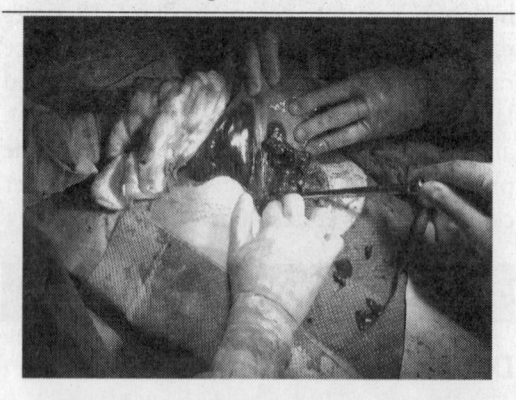

**Figure 28.1** A broad ligament hematoma following cesarean section

## Technique

The operative technique for PH is similar to the surgical principles used during a hysterectomy for benign gynecological conditions in a non-pregnant woman. However, due to the physiological and anatomical changes of pregnancy, there may be 'distortion' of normal pelvic anatomy. This is due to changes in the size and position of the gravid uterus and neighbouring organs, especially the ovaries, bladder and ureters, as well as to increased blood supply. These changes may increase the likelihood of surgical complications.

The UK Obstetric Surveillance System (UKOSS) recently published data regarding women in the UK who underwent a PH between February 2006 and February 2007 (Knight 2007). A total of 318 women had peripartum hysterectomy, most commonly secondary to uterine atony (53 per cent) and morbidly adherent placenta (39 per cent). The case fatality rate was 0.6 per cent, with two women dying. The study also highlighted the consequences of PH, with 20 per cent of women suffering damage to other structures, 20 per cent requiring further surgery to control bleeding and nearly 20 per cent reporting additional significant morbidity.

Increased morbidity and complications may be caused by several factors: hemostasis may be difficult due to tissue edema, and increased vascularity and dissection of the urinary bladder may be difficult following uterine incision or due to scarring from a previous CS. Therefore, bladder and ureteric injury is relatively common with PH. Due to enlargement of the gravid uterus, the ovarian ligament may become 'shortened' during pregnancy. Hence, it is important to apply the upper uterine clamps medially, very close to the cornua to avoid inadvertent injury to the ovaries (which may necessitate an oophorectomy). Table 28.3 lists the practical steps taken during a PH.

> Increased morbidity and complications may be due to:
> - tissue edema and increased vascularity leading to increased bleeding
> - difficult bladder dissection

**Table 28.3** Practical steps taken during a peripartum hysterectomy

- Exteriorise the uterus and inspect for injuries; active bleeders to be held by Green Armytage clamps
- Lift the uterus and maintain traction
- Upper uterine clamp (to the Fallopian tubes and round ligaments) should be applied as medially as possible
- Round ligament should be clamped, cut and transfixed (Fig. 28.2a)
- Medial portion of tube and branch of the ovarian vessel supplying the uterus should be double-clamped, cut, transfixed and ligated (Fig. 28.2b)
- Urinary bladder separated from the lower segment of the uterus by sharp dissection to expose 2–3 cm of the cervix
- The avascular portion of the broad ligaments are incised and the uterine vessels identified, clamped and ligated (Fig. 28.3)
- Clamps are placed tightly along the lateral aspect of the uterus to prevent injury to the ureter and hematoma formation.
- If the cervix is amputated (subtotal hysterectomy), it is closed with figure-of-eight sutures.
- In total abdominal hysterectomy, the bladder should be mobilised downwards to free the upper vagina, prior to the application of clamps.

A subtotal hysterectomy is safer, quicker and easier to perform than a total abdominal hysterectomy, especially if the bleeding is from the upper segment. In uterine rupture, placental abnormalities (placenta previa or morbidly adherent placenta) and genital tract trauma (upper vaginal or cervical), the bleeding would be from the lower uterine segment. In this situation, a total abdominal hysterectomy is inevitable to control bleeding.

> A subtotal hysterectomy is safer, quicker and easier to perform as compared to a total abdominal hysterectomy

During a total hysterectomy, the cervical stump is elevated with traction and is separated from the cardinal and uterosacral ligaments. Figure 28.4 demonstrates the importance of mobilising the urinary bladder downwards to 'free up' the cervix and the upper vagina for the application of clamps.

The vagina is then entered anteriorly or at the lateral angle above a curved clamp and the complete removal of the cervix is ensured, as shown in Fig. 28.5.

Excess removal of the superior vagina causes vaginal shortening. This can be prevented by inserting a finger through an

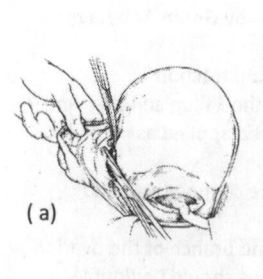

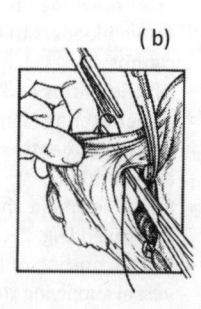

**Figure 28.2** Application of the upper clamps as medially as possible to avoid inadvertent injury to the ovary

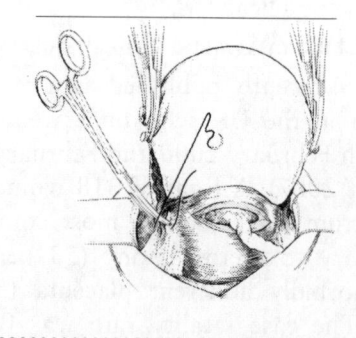

**Figure 28.3** Application of uterine artery clamps close to the lateral uterine wall to avoid inadvertent injury to the ureters

**Figure 28.4** Mobilising of the bladder and freeing up of the upper vagina prior to application of clamps. The cervico-vaginal junction can be identified by inserting a finger through the uterine incision.

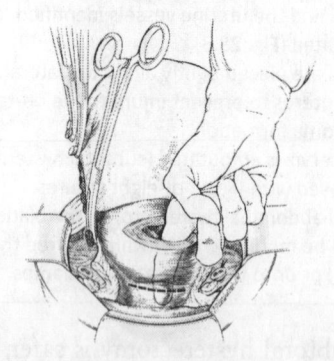

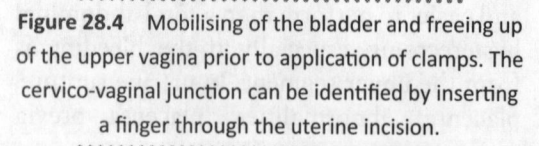

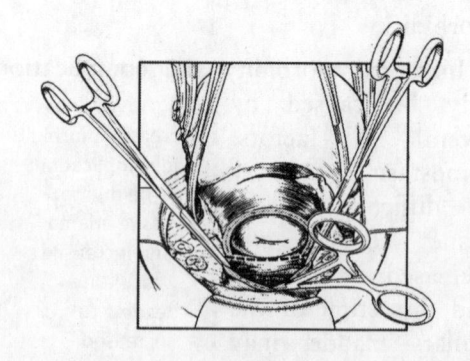

**Figure 28.5** Complete removal of the cervix after application of vaginal clamps

incision in the lower uterine segment to identify the cervico-vaginal junction before excising the cervix, after mobilising the bladder (Fig. 28.4).

The vaginal cuff is then supported by approximation to the cardinal and uterosacral ligament pedicles as in a standard abdominal hysterectomy. This can be either left open or closed in an interrupted or running locking continuous suture. If significant bleeding is a concern, the cuff may be left open for dependent drainage or placement of a drain.

## Total or subtotal hysterectomy

There has been much debate regarding the benefits of subtotal vs total hysterectomy.

Total hysterectomy is effective in arresting bleeding due to uterine atony and placenta previa. The lower limit of the cervix could be identified by exploring the endocervical canal downwards and feeling for the external os (lip) of the cervix.

A subtotal hysterectomy may not control the bleeding arising from the lower uterine segment (placenta previa, morbidly adherent placenta to the previous uterine scar, upper vaginal or cervical tears) as the cervical branch of the uterine artery is still intact. Studies have shown that there is no difference in blood loss or transfusion rates between total and subtotal PH (Selo-Ojeme 2005; Smith and Mousa 2007). However, the operative time and hospital stay is reduced in subtotal hysterectomy (Yucel 2006; Smith and Mousa 2007). Hence, it is a quicker and a technically easier procedure, especially in cases of atonic PPH, when the placental site is in the upper segment.

> A subtotal hysterectomy may not control the bleeding arising from the lower uterine segment (placenta previa, morbidly adherent placenta to the previous uterine scar, upper vaginal or cervical tears)

## Complications

As mentioned earlier, recent data from UKOSS has shown that increased morbidity and mortality is associated with PH. Table 28.4 shows the complications associated with PH.

Urologic complications may be reduced by careful sharp dissection of the bladder in the midline to mobilise the bladder flap, placing the clamps and sutures directly against the side walls of the uterus and cervix, perioperative cystoscopy with ureteral stent placement and ensuring urinary bladder integrity by filling with a methylene blue solution (Roopnarinesingh et al 2003).

**Table 28.4** Complications associated with PH

- Bleeding: coagulopathy
- Infection: sepsis
- Paralytic Ileus, hypokalemia
- Pulmonary: edema, effusion and emboli
- Ureteric injury: 1 in 2002 (Mickal et al 1969)
- Urinary bladder injury : 5–9 per cent (Eisenkep et al 1982)
- Urinary retention, hydronephrosis, acute tubular necrosis
- Cardiovascular complications: cardiomyopathy, pericardial effusion
- Psychiatric: depression
- Neurologic: hypoxic encephalopathy
- Others: multiple re-operations, re-admissions, wound dehiscence
- Pelvic hematoma
- Ovarian vein thrombosis
- Loss of fertility
- Death (case fatality rate 0.6 per cent)

## Strategies to reduce the incidence of peripartum hysterectomy

Peripartum hysterectomy is associated with significant maternal morbidity and mortality and hence, steps should be taken to avoid this procedure by:

1. **Identifying the risk factors for massive obstetric hemorrhage** (RCOG Guidelines 2009)
    - Previous PPH, obesity, bleeding disorder; grand multiparity, fetal macrosomia, polyhydramnios, multiple pregnancy, placenta previa, placenta accreta or precreta.
    - Intrapartum factors such as prolonged labour (>12 hours)
    - Prolonged third stage of labour (retained placenta)
    - Trauma: genital tract injury, instrumental delivery

2. **Instituting prophylactic measures**

If massive PPH is anticipated in view of the presence of above risk factors, then appropriate preventive measures may be instituted. These include a multi-disciplinary approach involving the senior obstetrician, anesthetists and hematologist to ensure correction of anemia with hematinics with or without erythropoietin.

In placenta previa or morbidly adherent placenta, an interventional radiology team may be contacted for placement of prophylactic uterine artery balloon catheters. Such prophylactic uterine artery balloon placement prior to planned surgery allows immediate inflation of balloons after delivery to provide a temporary occlusion. Should occlusion be required for a period longer than 12 hours, uterine artery embolisation is recommended. This may allow replacement of blood and blood products and correction of coagulopathy, thereby, reducing the risk of PH. Indeed, at St George's Healthcare NHS Trust, London, the use of the 'Maternity Dashboard' (2008) to monitor clinical outcomes has shown that prophylactic uterine artery balloon placement prior to planned surgery in major degree placenta previa and morbidly adherent placentae reduced the need for PH. Cell savers may also be arranged for autologous blood transfusion.

Active management of the third stage of labour as well as early recognition of PPH and institution of timely and appropriate measures to control bleeding may help avoid the need for further radical measures. Timely correction of blood volume and arrest of bleeding during the 'golden hour' (the first hour of severe shock) may prevent the development of coagulopathy and hemodynamic instability that may preclude conservative measures and necessitate radical measures such as PH.

It is also essential that senior obstetricians should be directly involved in the care of patients who are at increased risk of PPH, such as major degree placenta previa, morbidly adherent placentae or women who decline blood and blood products. This will not only enable institution of conservative measures to avoid a hysterectomy and to preserve future fertility but will also enable timely recourse to PH, when indicated, to save lives.

## Conclusion

Massive PPH is an acute, life-threatening obstetric emergency. It is associated with increased maternal morbidity and mortality worldwide. Management involves effective communication, resuscitation, monitoring and investigation as well as arresting the bleeding. In addition, prompt diagnosis of the cause, a 'multi-disciplinary' approach, appropriate post-PPH care in the ITU or HDU setting and communication with relatives and debriefing of patient, form the cornerstones of good clinical care to optimise outcome.

When conservative measures fail to control bleeding or when the patient is hemodynamically unstable, radical measures such as PH should be considered. Preservation of future fertility should be balanced against the need for timely intervention to arrest bleeding to optimise maternal outcome. 'Too little done too late' may result in maternal deaths and hence, despite its associated risks, PH can be a life-saving procedure.

## Acknowledgements

We would like to gratefully acknowledge Ms. Sunita from Printon, India for figures 28.2 to 28.5.

## References

Alexander J, Thomas PW, Sanghera J. 2002. Treatments for secondary postpartum haemorrhage. *Cochrane Database Syst Rev* (1):CD002867. DOI: 10.1002/14651858.CD002867.

Bai SW, Lee HJ, Cho JS et al. 2003. Peripartum hysterectomy and associated factors. *J Reprod Med* 48:148–152.

Barclay DL. 1970. Cesarean hysterectomy: thirty years experience. *Obstet* Gynecol 35:120–31.

Bixby GH. 1869. Extirpation of the puerperal uterus by abdominal section. *J Gynae Soc Boston* 1:223.

Chandraharan E & Arulkumaran S. 2005. Management algorithm for atonic postpartum haemorrhage. *J Paediatrics Obstet Gynaecol* June: 106–112.

Chandraharan E, Arulkumaran S. 2008. Surgical aspects of postpartum haemorrhage. Review Article. *Best Pract Res Clin Obstet Gynaecol* Dec; 22(6):1089–102.

Clark SL, Koonings PP, Phelan JP. 1985. Placenta praevia/accreta and prior caesarean section. *Obstet Gynecol* 66:89–92.

Eisenkep SM, Richman R, Platt LD et al. 1982. Urinary tract injury during cesarean section. *Obstet Gynecol* 60:591.

Eniola OA, Bewley S, Waterstone M et al. 2006. Obstetric hysterectomy in a population of south east England. *J Obstet Gynaecol* 26:104–109.

Geller E, Adams MG, Kelly PJ, Kodkany BS, Derman RJ. 2006. Postpartum hemorrhage in resource-poor settings: *International Journal of Gynecology & Obstetrics*, Vol 92, Issue 3, March; 202–211S.

Glaze S, Ekwalanga P, Roberts G et al. 2008. Peripartum hysterectomy: 1999 to 2006. *Obstet Gynecol* 111:732–738, 36.

Hamilton BE, Martin JA, Ventura SJ. 2007. Births: preliminary data for 2006. *Natl Vital Stat Rep* 56:1–18.

Hofmeyr JG, Say L, Gülmezoglu AM. 2005. WHO systematic review of maternal mortality and morbidity: the prevalence of uterine rupture. *BJOG* 112:1221–1228.

Kastner ES, Figueroa R, Garry D, Maulik D. 2002. Emergency peripartum hysterectomy: experience at a community teaching hospital. *Obstet Gynecol* 99:971–5.

Knight M on behalf of UKOSS. 2007. Peripartum hysterectomy in the UK: management and outcomes of the associated haemorrhage. *BJOG* Nov; 114(11):1380–1387.

Knight M, Kurinczuk JJ, Spark P, Brocklehurst P for the UKOSS. 2008. Cesarean delivery and peripartum hysterectomy. *Obstet Gynecol* 111:97–105.

Kwee A, Bots ML, Visser GHA, Bruinse HW. 2006. Emergency peripartum hysterectomy: a prospective study in The Netherlands. *Eur J Obstet Gynecol* 124:187–92.

Maternity Dashboard: Clinical Performance and Governance Score Card. 2008. Royal College of Obstetricians and Gynaecologists. Good Practice Series No. 7. RCOG Press.

Mickal A, Begneaud WP, Hawes Jr TP. 1969. Pitfalls and complications of cesarean section hysterectomy. *Clin Obstet Gynecol* 12:660.

Mishra N, Chandraharan E. 2009. Postpartum Haemorrhage. Chapter In: Best Practice in Labour and Delivery. Warren R and Arulkumaran S (eds). Cambridge University Press.

Mousa HA, Alfirevic Z. 2007. Treatment for primary postpartum haemorrhage. *Cochrane Database Syst Rev*(1):CD003249. DOI:10.1002/14651858. CD003249.pub2.

NHS Maternity Statistics, England, 2004–5. Leeds (UK): Information Centre for Health and Social Care, 2006. Available at: http://www.ic.nhs.uk/statistics-and-data-collections/hospital-care/maternity/nhs-maternity-statistics England-2004-05. Accessed Oct. 18, 2007.

RCOG Guidelines. 2009. Prevention and Management of Postpartum Haemorrhage. Green-top guideline No 52. RCOG Press.

Roopnarinesingh R, Fay L, McKenna P. 2003. A 27-year review of obstetric hysterectomy. *J Obstet Gynaecol* 23:252–4.

Sakse A, Weber T, Nickelsen C, Secher NJ. 2007. Peripartum hysterectomy in Denmark 1995–2004. *Acta Obstet Gynecol Scand* 86:1472–5.

Selo-Ojeme DO, Bhattacharjee P, Izuwa-Njoku NF et al. 2005. Emergency peripartum hysterectomy in a tertiary London hospital. *Arch Gynecol Obstet* 271:154–159.

Smith J, Mousa HA. 2007. Peripartum hysterectomy for primary postpartum haemorrhage: Incidence and maternal morbidity. *J Obstet Gynaecol* 27:44–47.

Todman D. 2007. A history of caesarean section: from the ancient world to the modern era. *Aust N Z J Obstet Gynaecol* 47:357–61.

UNICEF. 2001. The Progress of the Nations 2001. United Nations Children's Fund:New York.

Yucel O, Ozdemir I, Yucel N et al. 2006. Emergency peripartum hysterectomy: A 9-year review. *Arch Gynecol Obstet* 274:84–87.

# CHAPTER 29

# RUPTURE UTERUS

*Muralidhar V Pai and K N Sreelakshmi*

Uterine rupture is an obstetric emergency that is increasing in incidence. The most common cause is the giving way of a previous cesarean or hysterotomy scar. Kieser and Baskett (2002) reviewed all cases of uterine rupture in Nova Scotia in a 10-year period, and found that 92 per cent occurred in women with a previous cesarean scar. This is a change from earlier years, when grand multiparity was more often the cause of uterine rupture.

Uterine rupture is defined as a non-surgical disruption of some or all the layers of the uterus (serosa, myometrium and endometrium). Although maternal and perinatal outcome has appreciably improved over the years, uterine rupture still accounts for 20 per cent of maternal deaths from hemorrhage and three per cent of total maternal deaths. In rural India, maternal mortality from uterine rupture has been reported to be as high as 30 per cent (Chatterjee and Bhaduri 2007).

## Definition

*Complete uterine rupture* is the disruption of all layers of the uterus; thus, the uterine cavity communicates with the peritoneal cavity. All or part of the fetus is in the peritoneal cavity with significant bleeding from the edges of the scar or from extension of the rent. There can be fetal distress, stillbirth and significant maternal morbidity, with a potential for maternal mortality.

In *incomplete rupture* of the uterus, the visceral peritoneum is intact or the rent may have extended to the broad ligament. In this case, the fetus will be within the uterus and minimal bleeding is noticed from the edges.

It is important to differentiate between uterine rupture and *uterine scar dehiscence*. This distinction is clinically relevant because dehiscence most often represents an occult scar separation observed at laparotomy in women with a prior cesarean section. The serosa of the uterus is intact, and hemorrhage, with its potential for fetal and maternal sequelae, is absent.

- Complete uterine rupture: disruption of all uterine layers
- Incomplete uterine rupture: visceral peritoneum is intact
- Uterine scar dehiscence: occult scar separation with intact serosa

## Incidence and risk factors

The overall incidence of uterine rupture is 1 in 2000 births. Most often reported following prior cesarean section, uterine rupture can also occur in an unscarred uterus (1 in 8000 to 1 in 15,000 deliveries). The risk factors are listed in Table 29.1

**Table 29.1** Risk factors for uterine rupture

**Risk Factors**

Previous cesarean section or hysterotomy

Myomectomy (through or to the endometrium)

Cornual resection of interstitial Fallopian tube, adenomyomectomy, metroplasty

Induction of labour (use of oxytocin, prostaglandins or misoprostol)

Obstructed labour

Previous minor procedures

Trauma
- External or internal version
- Breech extraction
- Instrumental delivery (forceps application)
- Manual removal of placenta in adherent placenta
- Manipulations in shoulder dystocia

Müllerian duct anomalies

Spontaneous
- Multiparity

### Previous cesarean section

The most common predisposing factor for uterine rupture is separation of a previous cesarean scar. The rate of uterine rupture depends on both the type and the location of the previous uterine incision (Table 29.2). Women with an unknown type of scar do not appear to be at increased risk of uterine rupture.

**Table 29.2** Risk of uterine rupture with trial of labour (TOL)

| Prior incision type | Rupture rate (%) |
| --- | --- |
| Low transverse | 0.5–1.0 |
| Low vertical | 0.8–1.1 |
| Classic or T | 4.0–9.0 |

Multiple prior cesarean sections are associated with an increased risk of uterine rupture. In a large single-centre study of more than 1,000 women with multiple prior cesarean deliveries undergoing a trial of labour (TOL), Miller and colleagues (1994) reported uterine rupture in 1.7 per cent of women with two or more previous cesarean deliveries as compared to a frequency of 0.6 per cent in those with one prior operation (odds ratio 3.06; 95 per cent confidence interval, 1.95 to 4.79). Interestingly, the risk of uterine rupture was not increased further for women with three prior cesarean deliveries.

Prior vaginal delivery appears to be protective against uterine rupture following TOL. In a study of 3,783 women undergoing TOL, Zelop and colleagues (1999) noted the rate of uterine rupture among women with a prior vaginal birth to be 0.2 per cent (2/1021) compared to 1.1 per cent (30/2,762) among women with no prior vaginal deliveries.

A large observational cohort study identified an approximate four-fold increased rate of rupture following the use of the single closure technique of uterine incision, when compared to the previous double-layer closure (Bujold et al 2002).

Shipp and colleagues (2001) reported an incidence of rupture of 2.3 per cent (7/311) in women with an interdelivery interval less than 18 months as compared to 1.1 per cent (22/ 2,098) with a longer interdelivery interval. After controlling for demographic characteristics and oxytocin use, women with a shorter interpregnancy interval were found to be three times more likely to experience uterine rupture.

Induction of labour after a prior cesarean delivery appears to be associated with an increased risk of uterine rupture. Zelop et al (1999) found that the rate of uterine rupture in 560 women who underwent labour induction after a single previous cesarean delivery was 2.3 per cent compared with 0.72 per cent for 2,214 women who had gone into labour spontaneously.

The American College of Obstetricians and Gynecologists (ACOG 2009) discourages the use of prostaglandins to induce labour in most women with a previous cesarean delivery. There is substantial evidence for an increased risk of uterine rupture associated with prostaglandins. Lydon-Rochelle and co-workers (2001) reported a 15.6-fold increased risk of uterine rupture when prostaglandins were used in gravidas who underwent a TOL after a previous cesarean section. The uterine rupture rate was 2.45 per cent versus 0.77 per cent without prostaglandin use, in 366 women with scars from a previous cesarean delivery who underwent labour induction with prostaglandins.

## Myomectomy

Uterine rupture can occur in cases of previous myomectomy, especially when the uterine cavity has been entered, but the incidence is not as high as following a cesarean. The majority of uterine ruptures that involved uteri with myomectomy scars have occurred during the third trimester of pregnancy or during labour. The difference here lies in the fact that the uterus, after a myomectomy, does not undergo involution with rhythmical contractions, which happens after a cesarean section. The myometrium, after a myomectomy, heals better because it is at rest.

It is difficult to assess published reports of uterine rupture because they do not always specify the number, size and locations of leiomyomata, the number and locations of uterine incisions, entry of the uterine cavity and type of closure technique. Variations in these may need to be studied to determine the actual risk of uterine rupture following a myomectomy.

### Other uterine surgeries

The risk of rupture is also high after deep cornual resection of an interstitial Fallopian tube, metroplasty or an adenomyomectomy.

### Induction of labour (use of oxytocin, prostaglandins or misoprostol) in a scarred uterus

Induction of labour in a scarred uterus may be associated with an increased risk of uterine rupture. In a population-based retrospective cohort analysis, Lydon-Rochelle and colleagues (2001) reported a 15-fold increase in the rate of rupture in women undergoing induction with prostaglandin

> Factors increasing the risk of rupture after previous cesarean section:
> - Single-layer closure of uterine incision
> - Interdelivery interval of < 18 months

> The use of prostaglandins is not safe for cervical ripening, induction or augmentation of labour in the presence of a previous cesarean scar.

for trial of labour after cesarean (TOLAC). They found that elective repeat cesarean section was safer than prostaglandin induction.

Rupture in a scarred uterus has been reported with misoprostol, even with a dose as low as 25 mcg. Uterine rupture in an unscarred uterus is reported with higher doses, but studies are not available comparing scarred and unscarred uteri. Bucket-handle tears on the cervix are common after misoprostol induction, and it should be emphasised that rupture of the uterus should be considered if the apex of the cervical tear is not accessible.

> Rupture in a scarred uterus has been reported with misoprostol, even with a dose as low as 25 mcg. Misoprostol therefore should not be used in the presence of a previous cesarean scar.

Landon and co-workers (2004) noted the risk of uterine rupture to be nearly three-fold (OR 2.86, 95 per cent CI, 1.75 to 4.67) with induction with oxytocin in women with a previous cesarean scar (1.1 per cent versus 0.4 per cent) (Table 29.3). On the other hand, a meta-analysis (Rosen and co-authors 1991) concluded that oxytocin use does not appear to influence the risk of dehiscence or uterine rupture in TOLAC. However, excessive use of oxytocin may be associated with uterine rupture, and careful labour augmentation should be practiced in women attempting TOL.

### Previous repair of uterine rupture

The incidence of recurrent rupture is high in a previously repaired uterine rupture. There is a 6 per cent chance of recurrence in

> Women with a previous uterine rupture should be delivered by an elective cesarean section once fetal pulmonary maturity is assured.

**Table 29.3** Risk of uterine rupture following labour induction after previous cesarean

|  | Lydon-Rochelle (%) | Landon (%) |
| --- | --- | --- |
| All inductions | 24/2,326 (1.0) | 48/4,708 (1.1) |
| Spontaneous | 56/10,789 (0.5) | 24/6,685 (0.4) |
| Prostaglandins | 9/366 (2.5) | 0/227 (0.0) |
| Prostaglandin + Oxytocin | — | 13/926 (1.4) |

those who have had a low-segment rupture. Recurrence can be as high as 32 per cent when the prior rupture was in the upper segment (Reyes-Ceja et al 1969; Ritchie 1971).

### Obstructed labour

Obstructed labour due to various reasons results in ischemia of the lower uterine segment consequent to pressure of the presenting part. Uterine rupture due to obstructed labour has an especially high incidence of infection and long-term sequelae like genitourinary fistulae. In this situation, there are ragged tears and there may also be annular separation of the cervix. A hysterectomy may be considered to control the bleeding.

### Uterine rupture after previous minor procedures

A uterine wall weakened by previous wounds like brisk curettage, manual removal of the placenta or perforation after curettage is at risk of rupture.

### Trauma

Direct trauma on the maternal abdomen leading to rupture is extremely rare. Obstetric manipulations such as external cephalic version, internal podalic version for the second twin, breech extraction, manual removal of the placenta, manipulations for shoulder dystocia, and fundal pressure in a normal delivery increase the risk of rupture. Instrumental delivery before full cervical dilatation may result in tears in the cervix that may extend upwards to an uncontrollable degree. These tears are more dangerous; hence at cervical exploration, if the apex of the tear is not seen, rupture of the uterus should be the provisional diagnosis.

> Obstetric manipulations that may lead to uterine rupture:
> - External cephalic version
> - Internal podalic version for the second twin
> - Breech extraction
> - Manual removal of the placenta
> - Manipulations for shoulder dystocia
> - Excessive fundal pressure in a normal delivery

### Spontaneous rupture in pregnancy

Spontaneous rupture in pregnancy is rare, but when it does occur, is more common in the third trimester. This is also more common in a grand multipara. There are reports of second-trimester uterine rupture after misoprostol induction for termination of pregnancy with a previous cesarean (Goyal 2009), but there are no randomised controlled trials comparing uterine rupture in cases with or without previous cesarean delivery. The risk is also noticed with a combination of misoprostol and mifepristone. Uterine rupture in a primigravida is a rare event, without typical signs and symptoms. The morbidity and mortality of the mother and child are directly related to a high index of suspicion and prompt treatment by the clinician (Walsh and Baxi 2007). Probable risk factors are uterine anomalies, unmonitored injudicious administration of oxytocin, direct trauma, induction of labour with misoprostol and excessive fundal pressure during labour.

### Uterine rupture in Müllerian anomalies

There is an increased incidence of rupture in Müllerian anomalies. Although the uterine rupture rate in anomalous, unscarred uteri during pregnancy appears to be increased relative to that for normal uteri, the precise risk of different uterine malformations remains uncertain. The rupture classically presents in the late second and early third trimester. Many are diagnosed as a Müllerian anomaly only at laparotomy. Usually, the decision for a laparotomy is made late because they are misdiagnosed as preterm labour and undergo an emergency laparotomy only after they become hemodynamically unstable. This leads to high perinatal morbidity and mortality. This diagnosis should be considered in patients with recurrent undiagnosed vague abdominal pain throughout pregnancy. Rupture is more often seen in a unicornuate uterus and uterus didelphys. This occurs most often in the early third trimester. The risk is further increased if a metroplasty has been performed.

> Though there is a risk of uterine rupture in Müllerian anomalies, successful pregnancy outcomes of 60–70 per cent have been reported with unicornuate uterus and uterus didelphys.

Pregnancies in a rudimentary horn are usually disastrous, resulting in rupture prior to 20 weeks in most reported cases.

### Diagnosis of uterine rupture

Obstructive rupture has a distinct premonitory phase (prior to rupture).

Signs and symptoms of this phase include abdominal pain or tenderness, and vaginal bleeding. However, abdominal pain is an unreliable and uncommon sign of uterine rupture. Fetal heart rate abnormalities are more common than abdominal pain. Johnson and Oriol (1990) found that only 22 per cent of complete uterine ruptures presented with abdominal pain, whereas 76 per cent presented with signs of fetal distress diagnosed by continuous electronic fetal monitoring.

Epidural analgesia does not mask the pain caused by uterine rupture. There is no absolute contraindication to epidural anesthesia for a trial of labour with a previous cesarean scar because epidurals rarely mask the signs and symptoms of uterine rupture (ACOG 2004).

The fetal heart tracing may show sudden variable decelerations or abrupt and prolonged bradycardia. Bujold and colleagues (2002) showed that abnormal patterns in fetal heart rate were the first manifestations of uterine rupture in 87 per cent of patients. Leung and colleagues (1993) found prolonged decelerations in fetal heart rate in 79 per cent of cases, and this was the most common finding associated with uterine rupture.

Additional complaints include epigastric or shoulder pain, abdominal distension and constipation. Classically, the patient complains of continuous pain in the abdomen with no relief between contractions. At the time of rupture, the patient has a sense of something giving way at the height of a uterine contraction. The constant pain changes to dull aching pain with cessation of uterine contractions. General examination reveals features of exhaustion and shock. Abdominal examination reveals the absence of a uterine contour, superficial fetal parts, absence of fetal heart sounds, and two separate swellings: the contracted uterus and the fetal ovoid. Vaginal examination reveals recession of the presenting part and varying degrees of bleeding.

In the second stage of labour, the receding of the presenting part is a characteristic sign. Sometimes, after delivery of the fetus, the cord recedes back due to extrusion of the placenta into the abdominal cavity. This is almost pathognomonic of uterine rupture. Uterine rupture is quite often diagnosed only after the third stage, when the patient has suddenly collapsed with only minimal vaginal bleeding. The diagnosis of rupture should be considered in cases of unexplained severe shock and when the patient is far more anemic than warranted.

In vaginal birth after previous cesarean, it is unclear whether the uterine scar should be explored to check for its integrity. Most clinicians, however, document the integrity of a prior scar by palpation. The clinical consensus is that the scar needs to be surgically corrected only if there is significant bleeding. A scar dehiscence (uterine serosa intact) does not need any intervention.

In silent rupture, which is also more common with a previous scar, the patient may not have abdominal pain and the features are not as dramatic as those following obstructed labour.

## Management of uterine rupture

The patient should be prepared for a laparotomy at the earliest suspicion of rupture. Resuscitation is carried out simultaneously. The site, extent of rupture and hemodynamic stability will determine the treatment. A clean rupture of a previous scar requires surgical repair, with or without tubal ligation. The differential diagnosis for uterine rupture is listed in Table 29.4.

Hysterectomy should be considered the treatment of choice when intractable uterine bleeding occurs or when the uterine rupture sites are multiple, longitudinal or low lying. Ragged tears, a rupture involving the broad ligament or the uterine artery, extension to the cervix, or a broad fundal rupture also necessitate a hysterectomy, either total or subtotal. Great care should be taken to identify the ureters (especially when the tears have extended to the lower segment) and avoid injury to them. Although anterior wall rupture is more common, posterior wall rupture can also occur. This may be more difficult to repair and may be associated with high morbidity and mortality. Instances of posterior wall rupture have been reported even in cases of previous cesarean delivery.

> Indications for hysterectomy in uterine rupture:
> - Ragged tears
> - Rupture involving the broad ligament or the uterine artery
> - Extension to the cervix
> - Broad fundal rupture

## Maternal and perinatal complications

The most serious sequelae of uterine rupture include hypoxic-ischemic encephalopathy, perinatal death and hysterectomy. It is unclear from published studies how often uterine rupture results in perinatal death. Perinatal mortality is significantly different between developing and developed countries. Guise and colleagues (2004) calculated 0.14 additional perinatal deaths per 1000 trials of labour. This figure is similar to the National Institute of Child Health and Human Development (NICHD) MFMU Network study, in which there were two neonatal deaths among 124 ruptures, for an overall rate of rupture-related perinatal death of 0.11 per 1,000 cases where trial of labour was attempted after a previous cesarean section (Landon et al 2004). An all-inclusive review of 880 maternal uterine ruptures in studies of varying quality during a 20-year period showed 40 perinatal deaths in 91,039 trials of labour, for a rate of 0.4 per 1,000 (Chauhan et al 2003) (Table 29.5).

**Table 29.4** Differential diagnosis for uterine rupture

**Differential diagnosis for uterine rupture**

Obstetric
    Placental abruption
    Preterm labour
    Other causes of postpartum collapse like inversion and broad ligament hematoma

Surgical
    Appendicitis
    Biliary colic
    Pancreatitis
    Peptic ulcer disease
    Intestinal obstruction
    Ovarian torsion
    Urinary tract disorders

**Table 29.5** Risk of perinatal death related to uterine rupture

| Author | No. of ruptures | Perinatal deaths/TOL |
| --- | --- | --- |
| Guise (pooled data) | 74 | 0.14/1,000 |
| Landon | 123 | 0.11/1,000 |
| Chauhaun (pooled data) | 880 | 0.4/1,000 |

A high incidence of acidosis is also seen in the fetus at birth, leading to hypoxic-ischemic encephalopathy (Table 29.6). Perinatal hypoxic brain injury is recognised as an under-reported adverse outcome related to uterine rupture.

Table 29.6 Perinatal outcomes after uterine rupture in term pregnancies

| Outcome | Term pregnancies with uterine rupture (N = 114) |
|---|---|
| Intrapartum stillbirth | 0 |
| Hypoxic-ischemic encephalopathy | 7 (6.2) |
| Neonatal death | 2 (1.8) |
| Admission to the neonatal intensive care unit | 46 (40.4) |
| 5-minute Apgar score ≤5 | 16 (14.0) |
| Umbilical artery blood pH ≤7.0 | 23 (33.3) |

Adapted from Landon MB, Hauth JC, Leveno KJ, MFMU Network

Maternal hysterectomy may be a complication of uterine rupture, if the defect cannot be repaired or is associated with uncontrollable hemorrhage. Maternal mortality is three per cent and may be more in the rupture of an unscarred uterus.

Following a uterine rupture, there is a high incidence of complications of blood component therapy, genitourinary tract injury and hysterectomy.

## Pregnancy after surgical repair of rupture

Most cases of massive rupture will lead to a hysterectomy as a life-saving measure. In selected cases, surgical repair of the rupture and tubal ligation may be performed. In extremely selected cases, surgical repair of the rent alone, with uterine preservation, is done. Sheth (1968) described a series of 66 women where the uterine rupture was repaired rather than a hysterectomy performed. In 25 women, tubal sterilisation was done along with the repair. Thirteen women who were not sterilised had a subsequent pregnancy. Of these, 25 per cent had a recurrence of uterine rupture.

Pregnancy after surgical repair can be successful with impeccable obstetric care. Frequent antenatal check-ups, prophylactic steroids for pulmonary maturity and elective cesarean section may result in a successful pregnancy outcome. Admission to a hospital at least a week before the gestational age at which labour started in the previous pregnancy is definitely advised. The gestational age at which cesarean delivery should be performed can be individualised, based on data about the gestational age at which the woman went into labour in previous pregnancies, type of scar and gestational age at which the rupture occurred.

## Prevention

All cases of prolonged labour should be shifted from a primary healthcare facility to a tertiary care facility. Partogram should be made mandatory for all cases. Birth attendants should be aware of the small possibility of rupture even in a primigravida. Selection of cases for vaginal birth after cesarean should be judicious and a senior obstetrician should be involved in the decision making. The hospital should follow strict protocol for oxytocin administration during labour. Misoprostol should be avoided for inducing labour in women with a previous cesarean or hysterotomy scar. Early diagnosis and intervention definitely reduces both maternal and perinatal morbidity and mortality.

## Practice points

1. Uterine rupture is a catastrophic obstetric event accounting for 20 per cent of maternal deaths because of hemorrhage and 3 per cent of overall maternal deaths.
2. The most common cause of uterine rupture is rupture of the scar of a previous cesarean scar.
3. A primigravida has a low risk of uterine rupture but injudicious administration of oxytocin and induction of labour with misoprostol are the most important risk factors for rupture.
4. Rupture of the rudimentary horn in pregnancy is seen in late second and early third trimesters of pregnancy.
5. Infection and genitourinary fistulae are more common in rupture after obstructed labour. There may also be annular separation of the cervix, necessitating total hysterectomy.
6. Uterine rupture should be suspected if the apex of a cervical tear is not definable after difficult instrumentation or internal podalic version.
7. Spontaneous rupture in pregnancy is more common in a grand multipara.
8. A non-reassuring fetal heart rate pattern with variable rate decelerations in labour is the first, and often the only, sign of uterine rupture.
9. Fetal parts being easily felt per abdomen, receding of either the presenting part in the second stage of labour or of the cord in the third stage are pathognomonic signs of rupture.

## References

American College of Obstetricians and Gynecologists. 2009. Induction of Labor. ACOG Practice Bulletin No. 107. *Obstet Gynecol* 114:386–97.

American College of Obstetricians and Gynecologists. 2004. Vaginal birth after previous cesarean. ACOG Practice Bulletin No. 54. *Obstet Gynecol* Jul;104 (1):203–12.

Bujold E, Bujold C, Hamilton EF et al. 2002. The impact of a single-layer or double-layer closure on uterine rupture. *Am J Obstet Gynecol* 186:1326.

Bujold E, Mehta SH, Bujold C, Gauthier RJ. 2002. Interdelivery interval and uterine rupture. *Am J Obstet Gynecol* Nov;187 (5):1199–202.

Chatterjee SR, Bhaduri S. 2007. Clinical analysis of 40 cases of utrine ruptureat Durgapur Subdivisional Hospital: An observational study. *J Indian Med Assoc* 105:510.

Chauhan SP, Martin Jr JN, Henrichs CE et al. 2003. Maternal and perinatal complications with uterine rupture in 142,075 patients who attempted vaginal birth after caesarean delivery: a review of the literature. *Am J Obstet Gynecol* 189:408.

Goyal V. 2009. Uterine rupture in second-trimester misoprostol-induced abortion after caesarean delivery: A systematic review. *Obstet Gynecol* 113; (5):1117–23.

Guise JM, McDonagh MS, Osterweil P et al. 2004. Systematic review of the incidence and consequences of uterine rupture in women with previous caesarean section. *BMJ* 329:19.

Johnson C, Oriol N. 1990. The role of epidural anesthesia in trial of labor. *Reg Anesth* Nov–Dec;15(6):304–8.

Kieser KE, Baskett, TF. 2002. A 10-year population based study of uterine rupture. *Obstet Gynecol* 100:749.

Landon MB, Hauth JC, Leveno KJ for the National Institute of Child Health and Human Development Maternal-Fetal Medicine Units Network et al. 2004. Maternal and perinatal outcomes associated with a trial of labor after prior caesarean delivery. *N Engl J Med* 351:2581.

Leung AS, Leung EK, Paul RH. 1993. Uterine rupture after previous cesarean delivery: maternal and fetal consequences. *Am J Obstet Gynecol* Oct;169(4):945–50.

Lydon-Rochelle M, Holt V, Easterling TR, Martin DP. 2001. Risk of uterine rupture during labor among women with a prior caesarean delivery. *N Engl J Med* 345:36.

Miller DA, Diaz FG, Paul RH. 1994. Vaginal birth after caesarean: a 10 year experience. *Obstet Gynecol* 84:255.

Reyes-Ceja,L, Cabrera R, Insfran E et al. 1969. Pregnancy following previous uterine rupture: Study of 19 patients. *Obstet Gynecol* 34:387.

Ritchie EH. 1971. Pregnancy after rupture of the pregnant uterus: A report of 36 pregnancies and a study of cases reported since 1932. *J Obstet Gynecol Br Commonw* 78:642.

Rosen MG, Dickinson JC, Westhoff CL. 1991. Vaginal birth after caesarean: A meta-analysis of morbidity and mortality. *Obstet Gynecol* 77:465.

Sheth SS. 1968. Results of treatment of rupture of the uterus by suturing. *J Obstet Gynecol Br Commonw* 75:55.

Shipp TD, Zelop CM, Repke JT et al. 2001. Interdelivery interval and risk of symptomatic uterine rupture. *Obstet Gynecol* 97:175.

Walsh C, Baxi LV. 2007. Primigravida rupture uterus: A review of literature. *Obstetrics and Gynaecological Survey* 62, (5) 327–334.

Zelop CM, Shipp TD, Repke JT et al. 1999. Uterine rupture during induced or augmented labor in gravid women with one prior caesarean delivery. *Am J Obstet Gynecol* 181:882.

# CHAPTER 30

# MANAGEMENT OF SEVERE PREECLAMPSIA AND ECLAMPSIA

*Evita Fernandez and Nuzhat Aziz*

## Introduction

Hypertension, the most common medical complication during pregnancy, occurs in approximately 5–10 per cent of all pregnancies (NHBPEP 2000). Worldwide, hypertensive disorders of pregnancy are responsible for 12 per cent of maternal mortality during pregnancy and puerperium (World Health Report, WHO 2005). The First Report of Confidential Review of Maternal Deaths, Kerala (Paily 2009) found that hypertensive disorders in pregnancy were the second most common cause of deaths in the state of Kerala, India. About 13.35 per cent of maternal deaths were caused by hypertensive disorders during 2004–05.

The National High Blood Pressure Education Program Working Group on High Blood Pressure in Pregnancy (NHBPEP 2000) classifies hypertension in pregnancy as follows (Table 30.1):

- Chronic hypertension
- Gestational hypertension
- Preeclampsia
- Preeclampsia superimposed on chronic hypertension

Approximately 15–25 per cent of women initially diagnosed with gestational hypertension will develop preeclampsia, and this is more likely with earlier presentation or if the woman has had a prior miscarriage. However, women with gestational hypertension diagnosed after 36 weeks have only about 10 per cent risk of developing preeclampsia (Saudan et al 1998).

## Preeclampsia

Preeclampsia is a pregnancy-specific syndrome that usually occurs after 20 weeks of gestation and is characterised by increased blood pressure and proteinuria. Increased blood pressure (BP) is defined as a BP higher than 140/90 mmHg, measured on at least two occasions, six hours apart. An accurate diagnosis of preeclampsia is

> Criteria for diagnosis of preeclampsia:
> - Blood pressure of 140 mmHg systolic or higher or 90 mmHg diastolic or higher that occurs after 20 weeks of gestation in a woman with previously normal blood pressure
> - Proteinuria, defined as urinary excretion of 0.3 g protein or higher in a 24-hour urine specimen

Table 30.1  Classification of hypertension in pregnancy

| | |
|---|---|
| Chronic Hypertension | Chronic hypertension is defined as hypertension that is present and observable before pregnancy or that is diagnosed before the 20th week of gestation |
| Gestational Hypertension | Gestational hypertension is a provisional diagnosis for women with new-onset, non-proteinuric hypertension after 20 weeks of gestation |
| Preeclampsia | Preeclampsia is the development of new-onset hypertension with proteinuria after 20 weeks of gestation |
| Superimposed Preeclampsia | Development of new onset proteinuria, or sudden increase in proteinuria or hypertension, new onset thrombocytopenia or increase in transaminase levels in a woman with chronic hypertension is defined as superimposed preeclampsia |
| Eclampsia | Eclampsia is the occurrence, in a woman with preeclampsia, of seizures that cannot be attributed to other causes |

(*Source*: National High Blood Pressure Education Program Working Group on High Blood Pressure in Pregnancy Report. *Am J Obstet Gynecol*. 2000; 183(1):S1–S22)

important to initiate early intervention to prevent maternal and fetal morbidity and mortality. The presence of hypertension and proteinuria is the most important clinical sign to diagnose preeclampsia. However, clinicians should remember that preeclampsia is a syndrome of endothelial dysfunction that can affect any organ system (RCOG 2006). Preeclampsia may also be associated with a variety of other signs and symptoms, such as edema, visual disturbances, headache and epigastric pain. Laboratory abnormalities may include hemolysis, elevated liver enzymes, and low platelet counts (HELLP syndrome). Proteinuria may or may not be present in patients with HELLP syndrome (ACOG 2002).

## Preeclampsia before 20 weeks

In certain clinical conditions, preeclampsia may develop before 20 weeks' gestation. This may occur with hydatidiform mole, multiple pregnancies, fetal or placental abnormalities, antiphospholipid syndrome or severe renal disease (Brown et al 2000).

Severe preeclampsia
- Blood pressure of 160 mm Hg systolic or higher or 110 mm Hg diastolic or higher on two occasions at least 6 hours apart while the patient is on bed rest
- Proteinuria of 5 g or higher in a 24-hour urine specimen or 3+ or greater on two random urine samples collected at least 4 hours apart
- Oliguria of less than 500 mL in 24 hours
- Cerebral or visual disturbances
- Pulmonary edema or cyanosis
- Epigastric or right upper-quadrant pain
- Impaired liver function
- Thrombocytopenia
- Fetal growth restriction

## Severe preeclampsia

Women should be considered as having severe preeclampsia if they have:

❖ blood pressure levels of 160 mmHg systolic or higher or 110 mmHg diastolic or higher on two occasions at least six hours apart while the patient is on bed rest,

❖ proteinuria of 5 g or higher in a 24-hour urine specimen or 3+ or greater on two random urine samples collected at least hour hours apart,

❖ oliguria of less than 500 ml in 24 hours,

- cerebral or visual disturbances,
- pulmonary edema or cyanosis,
- epigastric or upper right quadrant pain,
- elevated liver enzymes,
- thrombocytopenia, or
- fetal growth restriction (ACOG 2002).

## Eclampsia

The onset of convulsions in a woman with preeclampsia is termed eclampsia. These convulsions are generalised and though the majority of them occur before or during labour, less than 10 per cent will occur beyond 48 hours postpartum (Alexander et al 2006; Zwart et al 2008)

## Superimposed preeclampsia

The diagnostic criteria for superimposed preeclampsia include 'new-onset proteinuria' in a woman with hypertension before 20 weeks of gestation, a sudden increase in proteinuria if already present in early gestation, a sudden increase in hypertension or the development of HELLP syndrome (NHBPEP 2000). Women with chronic hypertension who develop headache, scotomata or epigastric pain also may have superimposed preeclampsia (ACOG 2002).

## Conditions that may mimic preeclampsia

It is important, from a clinical management perspective, to consider other conditions that may mimic preeclampsia or hypertension in pregnancy. These include renal disease, acute fatty liver and cholestasis of pregnancy, hemolytic uremic syndrome (HUS), thrombotic thrombocytopenic purpura (TTP), pheochromocytoma and cardiovascular diseases such as coarctation, subclavian stenosis, aortic dissection and vasculitis.

### Measuring blood pressure

Blood pressure should be measured with the patient seated in an upright position or lying at 45° with the arm at the level of the heart and after a rest period of at least 10 minutes' duration (Helewa 1997). A mercury sphygmomanometer is preferable over an electronic device. An appropriate-sized BP cuff is one with a length 1.5 times the upper arm circumference or a cuff with a bladder that encircles 80 per cent of the arm. The instrument should be placed on a steady and straight surface such that the subject is unable to view the reading panel. Diastolic pressure is measured using Korotkoff phase V. Multiple readings have to be taken, with the BP recorded to the nearest 2 mm (Duley 2006).

### Significant proteinuria

Proteinuria is a significant prognostic factor that suggests the presence of systemic involvement. The most commonly used test to identify proteinuria is a urine dipstick. A result of 1+ is considered equivalent to 0.3 g/l. Considering the poor predictive value of

> Conditions that may mimic preeclampsia:
> - Renal disease
> - Acute fatty liver and cholestasis of pregnancy
> - Hemolytic uremic syndrome
> - Thrombotic thrombocytopenic purpura (TTP)
> - Pheochromocytoma
> - Substance abuse
> - Cardiovascular diseases such as coarctation, subclavian stenosis, aortic dissection and vasculitis

> Correlation of dipstick to protein levels:
> - 1+ = 0.3 g/l
> - 2+ = 1 g/l
> - 3+ = 3 g/l

dipstick testing, a value of 2+ is considered significant for clinical management: 2+ is equivalent to 1 g/l and 3+ is equivalent to 3 g/l (Waugh 2004). The gold standard test to diagnose proteinuria is a 24-hours urine collection and protein estimation. Proteinuria of more than 5 g/24 hours (or ≥ 3+ on two random urine samples that are collected at least four hours apart) classifies a mother as having severe preeclampsia (Norwitz 2008). A spot protein–creatinine ratio of less than 0.03 g/mmol (equivalent to <0.3 g/24 hours) is also used primarily due to the convenience and reliability of the test (RCOG 2006).

## Diagnosis of severe preeclampsia

Preeclampsia is classified as 'mild' and 'severe' (there is no 'moderate' preeclampsia). A diagnosis of severe preeclampsia requires evidence of new-onset proteinuric hypertension along with at least one of a series of complications (Table 30.2). It should be emphasised that only one of the listed criteria is required for the diagnosis of severe disease. Mild preeclampsia refers to the disease that meets the criteria for the diagnosis of preeclampsia but is not severe. The distinction between mild and severe preeclampsia is important because it dictates management (Norwitz 2008; ACOG 2002).

In most women, progression through this spectrum of classification is slow, and the disorder may never proceed beyond mild preeclampsia.

> From a clinical perspective, over-estimating or over-diagnosing preeclampsia is preferable to under-estimating or under-diagnosing the condition, as the timing of delivery is among the most important components of the management protocol.

**Table 30.2** Criteria for categorising severe preeclampsia

- Blood pressure of 160 mmHg systolic or higher, or 110 mmHg diastolic or higher on two occasions at least 6 hours apart.
- Proteinuria of 5 gm or higher in a 24 hour urine specimen or 3+ or greater on two random urine samples collected at least 4 hours apart
- Oliguria of less than 500 ml in 24 hours
- Cerebral or visual disturbances
- Pulmonary edema or cyanosis
- Epigastric or right upper quadrant pain
- Impaired liver function
- Thrombocytopenia
- Fetal growth restriction

(*Adapted* from ACOG Practice Bulletin, Number 33, *Diagnosis and Management of Preeclampsia and Eclampsia*, 2002

Norwitz ER, Funai EF. 2008. Expectant management of severe pre eclampsia remote from term: hope for the best, but expect the worst. *Am J Obstet Gynecol*; 199 (3):209–12)

The disease may also progress rapidly, changing from mild to severe in days or weeks. Fulminant progression is possible, with mild preeclampsia evolving to severe preeclampsia or eclampsia within days or even hours. Multiple organs may be affected due to severe preeclampsia (Table 30.3).

## Risk factors

The most significant risk factors for preeclampsia are a history of preeclampsia and the presence of antiphospholipid antibodies. Pre-existing diabetes and a pre-pregnancy BMI ≥35 almost quadruple the risk. Nulliparity, family history of preeclampsia and twin pregnancy almost triple the risk. Maternal age ≥ 40, a booking BMI of ≥35 and a systolic pressure ≥ 130 at booking doubles the risk (Duckitt 2005). The other risk factors known to be associated

# Management of Severe Preeclampsia and Eclampsia

**Table 30.3** Maternal complications of severe preeclampsia

| Organ system | Manifestation |
| --- | --- |
| CNS | Eclampsia, hemorrhage, cortical blindness, retinal blindness, raised ICT |
| Renal System | Cortical necrosis, renal tubular necrosis |
| CVS | Left ventricular failure, aortic dissection |
| Respiratory system | Pulmonary edema |
| Liver | HELLP syndrome, Subcapsular hematoma |
| Coagulation system | DIC, hemorrhage |
| Multiple organs | MODS, death |

(*Adapted from* Duley L, Meher S, Abalos E. 2006. Management of preeclampsia. *BMJ*, 332; 463–468)

**Table 30.4** Risk factors for preeclampsia

First pregnancy
More than 10 years from first pregnancy
Advanced maternal age
BMI ≥ 35
Family history of preeclampsia
Diastolic BP of > 80 mmHg at booking
Proteinuria at booking
Underlying medical diseases – Chronic hypertension/ renal disease/diabetes mellitus
Antiphospholipid antibodies
Collagen vascular disease

(*Adapted from* Duckitt K, Harrington D. 2005. Risk factors for preeclampsia at antenatal booking: systematic review of controlled studies, *BMJ*; 330; 565)

with higher incidence of preeclampsia are given in Table 30.4.

## Monitoring preeclampsia

Antepartum monitoring of a woman who has developed preeclampsia has several goals:

1. To observe progression of the condition and to recognise imminent signs of eclampsia
2. To prevent maternal complications by assessing the optimum time of delivery
3. To monitor fetal well-being

## Evaluation of preeclampsia

Initial evaluation of preeclampsia involves

- Clinical assessment
- Laboratory investigations
- Ultrasound assessment
- Fundoscopy

### Clinical assessment

Hypertension and proteinuria in a mother warrant admission to the hospital to evaluate the severity of disease, to determine the trend of the disease and plan the most appropriate management. A detailed history, detailed clinical examination and laboratory assessment are required to detect multiorgan involvement.

Symptoms of imminent eclampsia such as headache, visual disturbances (scotomata or blurring), vomiting and epigastric pain should be specifically asked for and documented, even if negative. Epigastric pain

> Symptoms of imminent eclampsia
> - Headache
> - Visual disturbances
> - Vomiting
> - Epigastric pain

or upper right quadrant pain may be a sign of hepatocellular necrosis, ischemia and edema that stretches the Glisson capsule of the liver.

The general examination focuses on detecting other potential causes of hypertension, including cardiovascular and respiratory system examination, with palpation of all peripheral pulses. Deep tendon reflexes have not been found to be predictive of eclampsia, but the presence of clonus may be a predictor (RCOG 2006).

Abdominal examination is carried out to assess the fundal height, liquor volume and presence of epigastric tenderness.

## Laboratory evaluation

Laboratory tests include complete blood counts (including platelet count), liver function tests, renal function tests and complete urine examination. These are useful in assessing the severity of disease. Preeclampsia is usually associated with laboratory abnormalities that deviate significantly from those of normal pregnant women. The results of diagnostic tests can also be used to distinguish preeclampsia from either chronic or transient hypertension.

> Initial lab tests
> - Complete blood counts (including platelet count)
> - Liver function tests
> - Renal function tests
> - Complete urine examination

*Thrombocytopenia*: Thrombocytopenia is seen as a complication of severe preeclampsia. It is also a part of the HELLP syndrome, (*h*emolysis, *e*levated *l*iver enzymes, *l*ow *p*latelets), a term coined by Weinstein (1982). A platelet count of <100,000/μl indicates severe disease. Thrombocytopenia is an indication for performing coagulation studies besides suggesting terminating the pregnancy. This is due to the fact that as a rule, the lower the platelet count, the higher the rates of maternal and fetal morbidity and mortality (Leduc et al 1992). If the initial platelet count is normal, repeat counts are requested every four days as part of the expectant management protocol. But if the platelet counts are <100,000/μl, then it may need to be repeated every 6–12 hours, to monitor the coagulation system and plan for delivery. A rapidly falling platelet count indicates a worsening trend. Though the platelet count may decrease for the first 24 hours after delivery, it will start rising and reach normal levels within 3–5 days. It must be kept in mind that platelet counts may continue to drop significantly even after delivery in a woman with HELLP syndrome (Cunningham et al 2010).

> A rapidly falling platelet count indicates a worsening trend. It must be kept in mind that platelet counts may continue to drop significantly even after delivery in a woman with HELLP syndrome

*Hemolysis*: Hemolysis is a characteristic feature of severe preeclampsia and is suggested by abnormal fragmented red blood cells and elevated serum lactate dehydrogenase, spherocytosis and reticulocytosis (Cunningham and associates 1985).

*Renal function*: A serum creatinine of 0.9 mg/dl is considered the upper limit of normal in pregnancy. As a result of vasospasm, the normal expected increase in glomerular filtration rate and renal blood flow and the expected decrease in serum creatinine may not occur in women with preeclampsia, especially if the disease is severe (ACOG 2002). A value of more than 1.2 mg/dl signifies renal impairment. A 24-hour proteinuria collection and creatinine clearance also provide assessment of the renal status. Oliguria, commonly defined as less than 500 ml in 24 hours, may occur secondary to hemoconcentration and decreased renal blood flow. Rarely, persistent oliguria may reflect acute tubular necrosis, which may lead to acute renal failure (Cunningham et al 2010). Repeated testing of uric acid does not offer any additional information and is not used as a parameter for clinical decision making.

> Oliguria, defined as less than 500 ml in 24 hours, may occur in severe preeclampsia. Though rare, persistent oliguria may lead to renal failure due to acute tubular necrosis.

*Hepatic function*: Hepatic function may be significantly altered in women with severe preeclampsia. Involvement of the hepatic system by preeclampsia is diagnosed by elevation of alanine aminotransferase and aspartate aminotransferase. Serum bilirubin is rarely found to be elevated except in cases of severe hemolysis (Sibai 2004). Hepatic hemorrhage, which usually manifests as a subcapsular hematoma, also may occur, especially in women with preeclampsia and upper abdominal pain (Manas and colleagues 1985). Rarely, hepatic rupture, which is associated with a high mortality rate, may occur (Rinehart et al 1999).

**Fetal evaluation**

*Cardiotocography*: Though cardiotocography (CTG) is a common clinical tool to assess fetal well-being in a woman with severe preeclampsia, its value is questionable. In a systematic review, Grivell and colleagues (2010) found insufficient evidence to support the use of traditional cardiotocography (CTG) or computerised CTG in pregnancy for improving fetal outcomes. However, in a patient with severe preeclampsia and intrauterine growth restriction, cardiotocography may help rule out acute fetal compromise.

*Ultrasound evaluation and Doppler studies*: An ultrasound evaluation including growth assessment, amniotic fluid volume and Doppler flow studies provides information on fetal well-being. Fetal growth restriction (FGR) is seen in 30 per cent of all mothers with preeclampsia (Sibai and Barton 2007). When a pregnancy with severe preeclampsia is also complicated by fetal growth restriction, Doppler studies can be of great help in assessing fetal status and in the decision-making for delivery. An abnormal Doppler suggests that the pregnancy may be prolonged only for a few days, even if the mother is stable (Gonzalez 2007). In a systematic review of the Cochrane database, Alfirevic and colleagues (2010) suggest that the use of fetal (middle cerebral artery) and umbilical artery Doppler ultrasound in high-risk pregnancies reduces the risk of perinatal deaths and results in fewer obstetric interventions.

> The assessment of fetal middle cerebral artery and umbilical artery Doppler ultrasound in severe preeclampsia reduces the risk of perinatal deaths and results in fewer obstetric interventions.

*Amniotic fluid index*: Assessing the amniotic fluid index in a woman with severe preeclampsia may help in the decision-making for delivery. A rapid fall in amniotic fluid volume may occur with worsening disease as fetal renal perfusion drops. Schucker and co-workers (1996) found that for women with severe preeclampsia remote from term, an amniotic fluid index <= 5 cm was predictive of intrauterine growth restriction but lacked sensitivity. There was no association between the amniotic fluid index status and frequency of cesarean section for fetal distress or non-reassuring fetal testing.

After the initial assessment, subsequent management maybe continued either in a hospital, a day care facility or at home. It is preferable to hospitalise women who are assessed as likely to have difficulty with compliance, with signs of disease progression or who have severe disease.

> Indications for hospitalisation:
> - Difficulty with compliance
> - Signs of disease progression
> - Severe disease.

## Management of severe preeclampsia

Management of severe preeclampsia is based on the principle that *delivery is always appropriate therapy for the mother but may not be so for the fetus*. The pathological changes of preeclampsia are present long before the clinical diagnostic criteria are manifest. Irreversible changes affecting fetal well-being may be present before the clinical diagnosis. If there is a rationale for management other than delivery, it would be to palliate the maternal condition to allow fetal maturation and cervical ripening.

> When the gestational age is 34 weeks and above, the consensus is to expedite delivery. When severe preeclampsia occures remote from term (earlier than 34 weeks), expectant management may be attempted, as long as maternal well-being is not jeopardised.

The principles of management involve:

1. Control of hypertension
2. Prevention of seizures
3. Assessment of organ involvement
4. Determination of fetal well-being
5. Facilitation of fetal pulmonary maturity
6. Planning of the time and mode of delivery

### Control of severe hypertension

Severe hypertension is defined as a systolic BP ≥160 mmHg and/or a diastolic BP ≥110 mmHg. Severe hypertension is associated with an increased risk of intracerebral hemorrhage if left untreated (Lewis 2007). Reducing severe levels of hypertension decreases the risk of maternal death (Podymow and August 2008). A recent report on confidential enquiries into maternal deaths in the United Kingdom pointed out that controlling systolic blood pressure is as important as controlling diastolic pressure (Lewis 2007). Severe acute hypertension may also be associated with end organ complications, such as myocardial infarction, stroke, renal failure, uteroplacental insufficiency and placental abruption.

The Confidential Inquiry into Maternal Deaths Report, 2007, from the United Kingdom, had 18 deaths due to eclampsia or preeclampsia. Of these, ten were due to intracranial hemorrhage. The single major failing in clinical care was found to be inadequate treatment of systolic hypertension (CEMACH 2007). Similarly, Paily (2009) in a confidential review of maternal deaths in Kerala, India, found that inadequate control of hypertension played a role in the maternal mortality rate.

Most guidelines recommend lowering blood pressure to levels of 140–150 mmHg systolic and 90–100 mmHg diastolic in view of the risk of hemorrhagic stroke in the presence of systolic hypertension (Henry 2004; Martin et al 2005).

*Antihypertensive therapy*: A blood pressure of more than 160 mmHg systolic and 110 mmHg diastolic or a mean arterial pressure of >125 requires treatment with antihypertensives. *There is no evidence as yet for the best antihypertensive to use in pregnancy.* The aim is to bring about a smooth reduction in blood pressure to levels that are safe for the mother and the fetus, to lower the mean arterial pressure (2/3 diastolic + 1/3 systolic BP) by 25 per cent over minutes to hours, and subsequently to less than 160/100 mmHg.

The preferred antihypertensive agent should be based on the experience of the clinical unit and the familiarity of the clinician with each drug regimen. In treating severe hypertension, it is important to avoid hypotension, for it may lead to a decrease in uteroplacental blood flow and hence fetal distress. Labetalol, intravenous hydralazine and oral nifedipine are acceptable agents for this indication (Table 30.5). Hydralazine has been widely used as a short-acting IV preparation but recent studies have shown that labetalol and nifedipine are associated with milder maternal adverse effects. Esmolol (a cardioselective beta-1 receptor

> In correcting hypertension, care must be taken to avoid sudden hypotension which may compromise placental flow and hence fetal well-being.

**Table 30.5** Antihypertensives for treatment of severe hypertension

| Drug | Route of Administration | Recommended Dosage |
|---|---|---|
| Labetalol | IV | Bolus 20 mg, then 40, 40, 40 and 80 mg, every 15 minutes for a maximum of 220 mg |
| Hydralazine | IV | 5–10 mg bolus every 15–20 minutes for a maximum of 30 mg |
| Nifedipine | Oral | 10 mg every 30–45 minutes, maximum of 50 mg |

(*Adapted from* Podymov T, August P, 2008. Update on the use of Antihypertensive drugs in pregnancy, *Hypertension* 51:960–969)

blocker) and angiotensin-converting enzyme inhibitors/receptor blockers should be avoided in pregnancy. The latter are contraindicated in pregnancy because they have been associated with intrauterine fetal demise, renal dysgenesis, oligohydramnios and neonatal renal dysfunction (Podymow and August 2008; Duley 2006).

*Labetalol (Pregnancy Category C drug)*: Labetalol is a selective alpha-1 and non-selective beta adrenergic blocker, available both as an oral and an intravenous preparation. It decreases systemic vascular resistance and slows the heart rate, reducing myocardial oxygen consumption. It does not reduce peripheral, cerebral, renal, coronary and uteroplacental blood flow. The lack of reflex tachycardia, bradycardia, increased intracranial pressure and the rare occurrence of significant hypotension make labetalol a good choice for use in pregnancy. It can be given as a continuous infusion, but is most frequently used as IV bolus for rapid reduction of hypertension (Vidaeff 2005).

To avoid a precipitous fall in blood pressure, the initial dose should be an intravenous bolus of 20 mg. A progressive, incremental IV infusion regimen (infusing 20, 40, 80, and 160 mg/hour for 10 minutes at each dose level, or until the desired BP is achieved, to a maximum of 220 mg) has been used, and may result in more gradual BP reduction, minimising adverse effects, compared with repeated IV injections of the drug (NHBPEP 2000). The onset of action of intravenous labetalol is within five minutes, with a peak at 10–20 minutes and duration of action that may last up to six hours. Controlled comparisons of various IV administration methods are not available. The plasma half-life of labetalol following oral administration is about 6–8 hours.

In patients with decreased hepatic or renal function, the elimination half-life of labetalol is not altered; however, the relative bioavailability in hepatic impairment is increased due to decreased 'first-pass' metabolism. It is contraindicated in patients with pre-existing myocardial disease and decompensated cardiac failure. Because of its non-selective beta effect, it is contraindicated in patients with asthma.

Oral labetalol has been used to manage acute hypertension, but commonly for the long-term control of hypertension. It should be started at a dose of 200 mg twice daily with a maximum recommended dose of 1200 mg/day in 2–4 divided doses (Podymow and August 2008).

### Hydralazine (Pregnancy Category C drug):

Hydralazine selectively relaxes the arteriolar smooth muscle and is widely used for the acute management of severe hypertension. It is effective either orally or through the intramuscular and intravenous routes.

To rapidly lower dangerously elevated blood pressure, hydralazine is given at a dose of 5–10 mg intravenously every 15–20 minutes, reaching a maximum of 20 mg or until the desired response is achieved (Cunningham et al 2001). Magee et al (2003) pointed out that hydralazine was associated with worse maternal and perinatal outcomes than labetalol and nifedipine. Further, hydralazine was associated with more maternal side effects than labetalol and nifedipine. Intravenous hydralazine is not available in India.

The dose of oral hydralazine is 50–300 mg per day in two to four divided doses. Adverse effects are mostly due to excessive vasodilatation or sympathetic activation, and include headache, nausea, flushing and palpitations (Podymow and August 2008).

### Nifedipine (Pregnancy Category C drug):

Nifedipine is a calcium channel antagonist and is used as an oral preparation for the treatment of severe hypertension. Calcium channel blockers act on arteriolar smooth muscle and induce vasodilatation by blocking calcium entry into the cells. Nifedipine is

---

**Antihypertensive Treatment for Severe Preeclampsia**

**Labetalol:** 20 mg intravenous bolus dose followed by 40 mg if not effective within 10 minutes; then 80 mg every 10 minutes to a maximum total dose of 220 mg.

**Hydralazine:** 5–10 mg intravenously every 15–20 minutes until desired response is achieved.

Adapted from ACOG Practice Bulletin No. 33, 2002

given as an initial dose of 10 mg orally to be repeated in 30 minutes if necessary, up to a maximum of three doses (NHBPEP 2000; RCOG 2006). The side effects of calcium channel blockers include tachycardia, palpitations and headaches. Concomitant use of calcium channel blockers and magnesium sulphate is to be avoided. Nifedipine should not be given by the sublingual route as it can cause a precipitous fall in blood pressure.

Nifedipine is contraindicated in congestive cardiac failure and heart block. The possibility of synergistic action with magnesium sulphate, if nifedipine is used in labour, is a matter of concern (Podymow and August 2008).

Nifedipine is commonly used postpartum in patients with preeclampsia for blood pressure control. An oral maintenance dose of 30–120 mg per day is given as a slow release preparation (NHBPEP 2000).

## Treatment of mild–to-moderate hypertension

*The benefits of treating mild to moderately elevated BP in pregnancy (<160/110 mmHg) have not been demonstrated in clinical trials.* A Cochrane meta-analysis concluded that there is insufficient data to determine the benefits and risks of antihypertensive therapy for mild-to-moderate hypertension (Abalos et al 2007). Even though the outcomes were not different, the risk of developing severe hypertension was lower in the treated group. International guidelines vary with respect to thresholds for starting antihypertensives. Initiating antihypertensive therapy for mild-to-moderate hypertension has to take into consideration the gestational age at onset, presence of proteinuria, thrombocytopenia, renal disease and the woman's ability to monitor disease progression, especially if it is remote from term. The first-line agent for non- severe hypertension should be alpha methyldopa, with the second-line being labetalol and nifedipine.

*Methyldopa (Pregnancy Category B drug)*: Methyldopa has been used widely in the treatment of hypertension in pregnancy. It is a centrally acting $\alpha_2$ adrenergic agonist. The recommended dose is 500–2000 mg per day orally in 3–4 divided doses. Adverse effects are consequences of central $\alpha_2$ agonism or decreased peripheral sympathetic tone. These drugs act at the brainstem to decrease mental alertness and impair sleep, leading to a sense of fatigue and depression in a few patients (Podymow and August 2008).

## Prevention of seizures

Magnesium sulphate is recommended as prophylaxis for eclampsia in women with severe preeclampsia (ACOG 2002). Duley and Henderson-Smart in a systematic review of the Cochrane database (2003) showed that compared with placebo or no treatment, the use of magnesium sulphate more than halved the risk of eclampsia in women with severe preeclampsia. The number needed to treat (NNT) to prevent one seizure in this group of women was 50. Magnesium sulphate was also advantageous in reducing the intensity of the first seizure

---

**Antihypertensive Treatment for Severe Preeclampsia**

**Nifedipine:** Initial dose of 10 mg orally. Can be repeated after 30 minutes to a maximum of 3 doses.

Nifedipine should not be given by the sublingual route as it can cause a precipitous fall in blood pressure.

when compared with other agents. There is controversy regarding the use of magnesium sulphate in mild disease. The NNT to prevent one seizure was approximately 100 and side effects were more common in the magnesium sulphate group although none were life-threatening. Hence, magnesium sulphate prophylaxis is not recommended in mild preeclampsia.

## Management of eclampsia

Presence of seizures should be regarded as eclampsia in a setting of hypertension complicating pregnancy. *It is one of the obstetric emergencies where the A, B, C of resuscitation plays an important role, and requires regular drills to optimise management.* Oxygen with airway maintenance, protection from trauma, checking the pulse rate, respiratory rate and blood pressure and securing IV access are the initial steps of care in this emergency. A multidisciplinary team should be summoned early and should include an anesthetist and obstetric physician in addition to a consultant obstetrician. This helps in early decision making, and ensures the most optimal management plan.

### Control of seizures

Magnesium sulphate is the treatment of choice for eclampsia and reduces mortality. It most likely acts by exerting a specific anticonvulsant action on the cerebral cortex (Cunningham et al 2010). Magnesium sulphate is superior to diazepam, phenytoin and lytic cocktail (chlorpromazine, promethazine, pethidine) in significantly reducing the risk of seizure recurrence (Duley and Henderson-Smart 2003). Morbidity related to pneumonia, mechanical ventilation and admission to an intensive care unit is significantly reduced with the use of magnesium sulphate as compared with phenytoin.

Both the IV and the IM routes of administration have been used effectively. The regimen most commonly used is a 4 g loading dose of magnesium sulphate as a 20% solution given intravenously over 5–10 minutes, at a rate of not more than 1 g per minute (Cunningham et al 2010). This can be followed by an infusion of 1 g per hour in 100 ml of IV maintenance solution for 24 hours or until 24 hours post-delivery, whichever is earlier (RCOG 2006). The maintenance dose of magnesium sulphate can also be given intramuscularly. Immediately after the IV loading dose, 10 g of 50% magnesium sulphate solution is given deep IM, 5 g in each buttock. About 5 g of magnesium sulphate is then given deep IM in

---

**Steps in managing eclampsia**
- Airway maintenance with oxygen
- Monitoring oxygen saturation
- Monitoring pulse rate and respiratory rate, blood pressure
- Protection from trauma
- Securing IV access
- Control of seizures

---

**Administration of magnesium sulphate:**
1. 4 gm loading dose of magnesium sulphate as a 20% solution given intravenously over 5–10 minutes
2. Followed by an infusion of 1 g per hour in 100 ml of IV maintenance solution for 24 hours or until 24 hours post-delivery or
3. IM maintenance 10 g of 50% magnesium sulphate solution given deep IM, 5 g in each buttock. 5 g of magnesium sulphate is then given deep IM in the buttocks, every 4 hours

Adapted from ACOG Practice Bulletin No. 33, 2002

the buttocks, every four hours (Cunningham et al 2010). The addition of 1 ml of 2% lidocaine reduces the discomfort since IM magnesium sulphate can cause considerable pain.

### Monitoring for magnesium sulphate toxicity

Monitoring of magnesium sulphate should utilise clinical parameters of urinary output, respiratory rate, oxygen saturation and patellar reflexes. Serum magnesium levels should be measured if toxicity is suspected. Toxicity is most apparent with levels of >3.5 mmol/l. Features of toxicity include suppression or loss of patellar reflexes, respiratory depression, drowsiness and ultimately loss of consciousness. Toxicity is particularly likely in the presence of significant renal insufficiency. The antidote for magnesium sulphate toxicity is 10 ml of a 10% calcium gluconate solution (1 g) IV over 10 minutes.

> **Monitoring for magnesium sulphate toxicity**
> The next dose of magnesium sulphate should be administered only if
> 1. Patellar reflex is present
> 2. Respiratory rate is more than 16
> 3. Patient is alert
> 4. Urine output was >100 ml in the preceding 4 hours

If the seizures recur, an additional MgSO$_4$ dose of 2 g IV (20% solution) may be given (Collaborative Eclampsia Trial Group 1995). Thiopentone or diazepam derivative may be required if seizures persist. If the mother does not stabilise, intubation and ventilation may be required, with transfer to a tertiary care centre.

### Further management and decision for delivery

Once the mother stabilises, fetal assessment should be carried out along with preeclampsia evaluation for maternal end organ involvement. A decision for delivery should be taken after the initial assessment and stabilisation are completed. A delay of 24 hours may be possible to allow the use of corticosteroids for fetal lung maturity (for <34 weeks' gestation), if there is reassuring fetal status on cardiotocography. Expectant management in a mother with eclampsia is recommended only as part of experimental studies (Norwitz 2008) and does not form part of routine clinical management protocols.

## HELLP syndrome

The HELLP (*h*emolysis, *e*levated *l*iver enzymes, *l*ow platelet) syndrome is regarded as a variant or complication of severe preeclampsia. It is associated with severe maternal and fetal adverse events. There are two forms of HELLP: the complete form with all three components (H, EL and LP) and an incomplete form that consists of only one or two of the three elements (Audibert et al 1996). Partial or incomplete HELLP can progress to a complete HELLP syndrome.

HELLP occurs in 0.5–0.9 per cent of all pregnancies (Geary 1997), and in 20 per cent of cases with severe preeclampsia (Sibai et al 1993). The HELLP syndrome develops prior to delivery in about 70 per cent of pregnancies, often between the 27th and 37th week of pregnancy. The development of HELLP may be earlier than the 27th gestational week in about 10 per cent of pregnancies and later than the 37th week in 20 per cent of pregnancies (Sibai 1993; Geary 1997).

In a recent review of maternal deaths due to eclampsia and HELLP syndrome (Gracia 2009), in high-income countries, 3.9 per cent of deaths were due to eclampsia without HELLP syndrome, while in low-income countries, this figure was 42.5 per cent. The presence of the HELLP syndrome in the women who died of eclampsia was 90.6 per cent in high-income countries compared with 47.6 per cent in low-income countries. Concurrent eclampsia and HELLP syndrome was diagnosed in 5–6 out of 10 deaths associated with eclampsia or HELLP syndrome in this review.

Clinical signs of HELLP include upper right quadrant pain or epigastric fluctuating or colic-like pain, nausea and vomiting, headache, visual symptoms or even non-specific viral syndrome-like symptoms that are often exacerbated during the night with recovery during the day (Sibai 2004).

> Clinical signs of HELLP syndrome
> - Upper right quadrant pain
> - Epigastric pain
> - Nausea and vomiting
> - Headache
> - Visual symptoms

## Diagnostic criteria for HELLP syndrome

Sibai (2004) proposed strict criteria for 'true' or 'complete' HELLP syndrome (Tennessee Classification System):

1. Intravascular hemolysis diagnosed by abnormal peripheral blood smear
2. Increased serum bilirubin ≥20.5 μmol/l or ≥1.2 mg/100 ml
3. Elevated LDH levels (>600 units/l)
4. Platelet count of <100,000/microlitre
5. Serum AST (SGOT) levels >70 IU/l

The Mississippi Triple Class System further classifies the syndrome based on the platelet count: Class I <50 x 10$^6$/l, Class II – 50 x 10$^6$/l to 100 x 10$^6$/l and Class III –100 x 10$^6$/l to 150 x 10$^6$/l. Classes I and II are associated with hemolysis (LDH >600 U/l) and elevated AST (≥70 U/l) concentration, while Class III requires only LDH >600 U/l and AST ≥40 U/l in addition to the specific platelet count. Class III HELLP syndrome is indicative of a clinically significant transition stage or a phase of the HELLP syndrome that may progress (Martin et al 1999).

It is important to remember the differential diagnosis of the HELLP syndrome (Table 30.6) as the management strategy may differ for each condition.

The HELLP syndrome is associated with increased maternal and perinatal mortality as well as morbidity (Table 30.7). Maternal complications include severe ascites (4–11 per cent), eclampsia (4–9 per cent), pulmonary edema (3–10 per cent) and cerebral edema (4–9 per cent). Less common maternal liver complications include subcapsular

---

Table 30.6 Differential diagnosis for the HELLP syndrome

- Different types of thrombocytopenia
  - Benign thrombocytopenia of pregnancy
  - Immunologic thrombocytopenia (ITP)
  - Thrombocytopenia due to folate deficiency
  - Systemic lupus erythematosus (SLE)
  - Antiphospholipid syndrome (APS)
  - Thrombotic thrombocytopenic purpura (TTP)
  - Hemolytic uremic syndrome (HUS)
- Acute fatty liver of pregnancy
- Infectious and inflammatory diseases
  - Urinary tract infections
  - Acute pancreatitis
  - Gastritis and gastric ulcers
  - Cholecystitis or cholangitis
  - Hepatitis

(*Adapted from* Henry CS, Beidermann SA et al. 2004. Spectrum of hypertensive emergencies in pregnancy. *Crit Care Clin* 20;697–712.

Sibai BM, 2004. Imitators of eclampsia/severe preeclampsia. *Clin Perinatol* 31; 835–852)

# Management of Severe Preeclampsia and Eclampsia

**Table 30.7** Complications of HELLP Syndrome

| Maternal Complications | Frequency (%) |
|---|---|
| Disseminated Intravascular Coagulation (DIC) | 5–56 |
| Acute Renal Failure | 7–36 |
| Abruptio Placenta | 9–20 |
| Maternal Death | 1–25 |
| **Neonatal Complications** | |
| Preterm Delivery | 70 |
| Intra Uterine Growth Retardation | 38–61 |
| Neonatal thrombocytopenia | 15–50 |
| Respiratory distress syndrome | 5.7–40 |
| Perinatal death | 7.4–34 |

(*Adapted from* Sibai BM, Ramadan MK, Usta I, et al. 1993. Maternal morbidity and mortality in 442 pregnancies with hemolysis, elevated liver enzymes, and low platelets (HELLP syndrome). *Am J Obstet Gynecol* 169:1000.

Martin JN Jr, Rinehart B, May WL, Magann EF, Terrone DA, Blake PG. 1999. The spectrum of severe preeclampsia: comparative analysis by HELLP syndrome classification. *Am J Obstet Gynecol*; 180:1373–84.

Audibert F, Friedman SA, Frangieh AY, Sibai BM. 1996. Clinical utility of strict diagnostic criteria for the HELLP (hemolysis, elevated liver enzymes, and low platelets) syndrome. *Am J Obstet Gynecol* 175:460–4.

Abramovici D, Friedman SA, Mercer BM, Audibert F, Kao L, Sibai BM. 1999. Neonatal outcome in severe preeclampsia at 24 to 36 weeks' gestation: does the HELLP (hemolysis, elevated liver enzymes, and low platelet count) syndrome matter? *Am J Obstet Gynecol;* 180:221–5)

liver hematoma, liver rupture and hepatic infarction (Sibai et al 1993; Audibert et al 1996; Martin et al 1999).

### Management of HELLP syndrome

Management options (Sibai 2004; Martin et al 2006) for women with HELLP syndrome include:

1. Immediate delivery, which is the primary choice at 34 weeks' gestation or later.
2. Delivery within 48 hours after evaluation, stabilisation of the maternal clinical condition and corticosteroid treatment, especially between 27 and 34 weeks of gestation.
3. Termination of pregnancy may be considered if the diagnosis is made prior to 20 weeks of gestation.

The HELLP syndrome as a rule should have a planned immediate delivery except for a delay of 24–48 hours for a course of corticosteroids at 25–34 weeks' gestation. The role of high-dose steroids (dexamethasone) has been studied in a randomised controlled trial and the evidence does not suggest any improvement in outcomes with its use (Katz 2008). Expectant management has been studied in the HELLP syndrome at <34 weeks' gestation. Studies have shown the possibility of prolonging pregnancy, but not a significant improvement in perinatal outcomes, which is the aim of expectant management. Hence, this concept is still experimental and is to be carried out under research settings only. The mode of delivery depends on the urgency of delivery and the rapidity of worsening of the disease (Sibai and Barton 2007).

## Management of severe preeclampsia based on gestational age

*Delivery is the cure for preeclampsia, but expectant management is attempted with an effort to decrease the effects of prematurity or to optimally promote fetal maturation.* It is agreed that delivery should be planned if the mother reaches

34 weeks or develops the condition at >34 weeks, as severe preeclampsia is associated with severe maternal and fetal morbidity (RCOG 2006).

**Indications for expectant management**

Expectant management can be considered in pregnancies at less than 34 weeks of gestation if there is no evidence of:

1. Organ involvement
2. Thrombocytopenia
3. HELLP syndrome
4. Symptoms of cerebral irritation
5. Labour
6. Abruption
7. Immediate danger to the fetus if pregnancy is prolonged (no decelerations on CTG)

Sibai and Barton (2007) reviewed the expectant management of women with severe preeclampsia remote from term. In women who were treated conservatively, there was no increase in maternal complications, and there was a statistically significant prolongation of pregnancy (mean 15.4 vs 2.6 days), less time in the neonatal intensive care unit (20.2 vs 36.6 days) and a reduced incidence of respiratory distress syndrome (22.4 per cent vs 50.5 per cent). Although the average birth weight in this group was significantly higher (1622 g vs 1233 g), there was also a significantly higher incidence of small-for-gestational-age infants (SGA 30 per cent vs 11 per cent). Expectant management was found to be associated with increased perinatal complications if severe fetal growth restriction (less than the 5th centile) was present. Hence, severe fetal growth restriction and oligohydramnios are relative contraindications to expectant management (Sibai and Barton 2007).

Expectant management should be considered only in a select group of patients after maternal counselling about the benefits and risks of such treatment. *It has to be undertaken in a hospital with adequate monitoring facilities.* Anesthetic, neonatology, obstetric and operating room staff should be available round the clock. There should be defined surveillance guidelines for expectant management and delivery in these mothers (Norwitz 2008; Sibai 2007).

*Severe preeclampsia before 25 weeks*: Severe preeclampsia developing before 25 weeks has poor fetal prognosis and is associated with increased maternal morbidity and disastrous perinatal mortality. The incidence of perinatal death has been found to be 70–100 per cent, with very few babies surviving without complications (Sibai and colleagues 1985). Termination of pregnancy is sound clinical practice in this group. *Early onset severe preeclampsia should have an evaluation for secondary causes of hypertension, for it may be superimposed preeclampsia in a mother with chronic hypertension* (Jenkins 2002; Sibai 2007; Bombrys 2008).

*Severe preeclampsia between 26 and 34 weeks' gestation*: Expectant management plays a role in this group as it was found that pregnancy could be prolonged by about 15 days and perinatal morbidity and mortality decreased in selected populations (Sibai et al 1994). Corticosteroids are given for fetal lung maturity; the most commonly used regimen is two doses of betamethasone of 12 mg each, intramuscularly, at an interval of 24 hours. If the initial evaluation shows multiple organ involvement, it may be necessary to give the doses at 12-hour intervals, for both these regimens have been tried (Haas 2006). Expectant management should be carried out in a tertiary care hospital setting. Maternal monitoring should be done with BP monitoring every four hours, urine albumin every day, strict intake/output chart, with laboratory tests being repeated every 3–4 days. The tests ordered to evaluate the effects of the disease and progression of severity of organ involvement are platelet count, LDH, transaminases (SGOT, SGPT) and serum creatinine.

> **Monitoring of the mother during expectant management**
> - BP recorded every 4 hours
> - Twice-daily monitoring of urine albumin
> - Strict intake/output chart
> - Blood tests to evaluate platelet count, LDH, transaminases (SGOT, SGPT), creatinine

Monitoring of the fetus is done with subjective fetal kick count, daily assessment with cardiotocography, AFI and Doppler assessment twice a week (Sibai 1990). Estimated fetal weight by ultrasound is assessed every two weeks if the mother's condition remains stable.

> **Monitoring of the fetus during expectant management**
> - Subjective fetal kick count
> - Daily cardiotocography
> - Amniotic fluid index
> - Doppler assessment twice weekly

***Indications for delivery***: Indications for delivery have to be defined very clearly during expectant management of this high-risk group.

The maternal indications for immediate delivery are (Sibai and Barton 2007):

1. Uncontrolled severe hypertension despite treatment
2. Development of symptoms of cerebral irritation (headache, visual disturbances or eclampsia)
3. Persistent thrombocytopenia <100,000/σl.
4. Pulmonary edema (shortness of breath with basal lung crepitations, oxygen saturation <94% on room air).
5. HELLP syndrome (epigastric pain with transaminases twice the upper limit of normal)
6. Renal impairment (oliguria, <500 ml in 24 hours or serum creatinine >1.2 mg/dl)
7. Clinical signs of placental abruption

The fetal indications for delivery are (Sibai and Barton 2007):

1. Severe growth restriction (<5th per centile)
2. Decelerations on cardiotocography
3. Oligohydramnios (AFI <5)
4. Biophysical profile score of ≤ 4/10
5. Umbilical artery Doppler waveform showing reversed end diastolic flow
6. Fetal death

***Mode of delivery***: The mode of delivery is based on the urgency to deliver, cervical Bishop's score, gestational age, severity of fetal growth restriction and Doppler flow abnormality in the umbilical artery.

Induction of labour should be aggressive with an aim to deliver within 24 hours. Cesarean section is planned for those with severe fetal growth restriction or reversed end diastolic flow in the umbilical artery Doppler, or with any obstetric contraindication for vaginal delivery. Magnesium sulphate prophylaxis is started once the decision is made to deliver and continued till 24 hours post-delivery (Sibai 2007; RCOG 2006).

*Severe preeclampsia at more than 34 weeks' gestation*: Severe preeclampsia at 34 weeks or more of gestation requires delivery. Induction of labour with monitoring should be offered for all mothers eligible for vaginal delivery. Intensive maternal and fetal monitoring is continued, as the possibility of complications developing in the intrapartum period is high. Intrapartum and postpartum magnesium sulphate is given as prophylaxis.

## Planning delivery and intrapartum care

*The decision to deliver is the most important decision in the management of preeclampsia.* The timing, mode and place of delivery have to be the optimised. This may mean transfer to a tertiary unit if the facilities for care are not present in the primary institute.

A gestational age of >34 weeks mandates delivery, with the mode of delivery being guided by obstetric indications. A gestational age of <34 weeks has to be planned after corticosteroid therapy for fetal lung maturity. In most mothers, it is possible to delay delivery by at least 24 hours, to allow the steroids to have an effect on the fetus. The likelihood of success of induction has to be weighed against the need for urgent delivery. *If the mother's condition is unstable, it might be better for her to deliver in the primary institute rather than attempt transfer in an unstable state.*

Methyl ergometrine derivatives are avoided as these raise the blood pressure. All mothers should receive high dependency care and should be monitored using an obstetric early warning chart (CEMACH 2007). Continuous fetal monitoring must be used (RCOG 2006). Labour analgesia with an epidural gives good pain relief and has to be sited after thrombocytopenia/ coagulopathy is excluded. It may be judicious to cut short the second stage of labour with an instrumental delivery. The third stage of labour has to be managed with 5 units of oxytocin given intramuscularly. Methyl ergometrine derivatives are avoided as these cause elevation in blood pressure (RCOG 2006). As mothers with severe preeclampsia are at increased risk of venous thromboembolism, thromboprophylaxis is recommended (Walker 2009).

> Labour analgesia with an epidural gives good pain relief and should be used after thrombocytopenia/coagulopathy is excluded.

> Methyl ergometrine derivatives are avoided as these raise the blood pressure.

### Fluid management

Fluid management in preeclampsia is important since these mothers have vasoconstriction and reduced blood volume expansion when compared with normotensive mothers. The vasospasm in preeclampsia and subsequent hemoconcentration are associated with contraction of the intravascular space. Because of capillary leak and decreased colloid oncotic pressure often associated with this syndrome, attempts to expand the intravascular space in these women with vigorous fluid therapy may result in elevation of the pulmonary capillary wedge pressure and even pulmonary edema (ACOG 2002). Inappropriate use of fluids has been the cause of pulmonary edema and maternal death. Fluid expansion should not be used in severe preeclampsia/eclampsia and total fluid restriction to 80 ml/hour or 1 ml/kg/hour has been found to be beneficial (RCOG 2006).

> Women with severe preeclampsia have vasoconstriction and reduced blood volume expansion when compared with normotensive women. Attempts to expand the intravascular space in these women with vigorous fluid therapy may result in pulmonary edema.

## Postpartum care

The postpartum period can be a critical one for women with severe preeclampsia and eclampsia, for complications and maternal deaths may occur at this time. In recent years, there has been an increasing shift in the incidence of eclampsia in the postpartum period (Chames et al 2002). This is presumed to be because of improved access to antenatal care, earlier detection of preeclampsia and prophylactic use of magnesium sulphate. The same vigilance utilised in the antepartum period should be maintained for the first 24–72 hours postpartum. Discharge should be considered only after the fourth postpartum day after a review of the woman's condition as the risk of eclampsia is less after this.

### Antihypertensive therapy

Antihypertensive therapy has to be individualised in the postpartum period. Antihypertensive medications used in the antenatal period may be continued. Nifedipine, labetalol, thiazide diuretics and ACE inhibitors are safe for use in the postpartum period. Atenolol and other beta-blockers are not advocated since they are excreted in significant concentration in breast milk. The RCOG Guidelines for severe preeclampsia (2006) consider avoiding methyldopa as a good practice point in view of its adverse effect of depression. Antihypertensive therapy can be stopped if the blood pressure returns to normal, but is best continued for 2–3 weeks if the patient does not have the facility to monitor blood pressure at home. Pulmonary edema, oliguria and accelerated hypertension may occur and require a physician's review (Cunningham et al 1986).

> Nifedipine, labetalol, thiazide diuretics and ACE inhibitors are safe for use in the postpartum period. Atenolol and other beta-blockers are not advocated since they are excreted in significant concentration in breast milk.

## Follow up

All mothers with severe preeclampsia should have a review at the end of 6 weeks and 12 weeks. Up to 13 per cent of these women have renal disease or essential hypertension (Walker 2009). Those who have persistent proteinuria have to be evaluated further. Pre-pregnancy counselling should be offered before the next pregnancy. Risk factors and screening/prevention aspects of preeclampsia have to be discussed.

## Recurrence risk

The recurrence risk of severe preeclampsia is reported to vary from 5 per cent to 65 per cent depending on its severity and gestational age at onset (Sibai 1991; Lykke et al 2009a). Generally, the earlier the preeclampsia is diagnosed in the first pregnancy, the greater the chance of its recurrence. Preeclampsia between 18 and 27 weeks in a nulliparas has been found to have a recurrence risk of 40 per cent in subsequent pregnancies (Sibai 1991). In a recent study, the recurrence risk of severe preeclampsia was found to be relatively low (6.8 per cent), with advanced maternal age and pre-existing renal disease being the most important predictors (McDonald 2009). Women who developed the HELLP syndrome had a recurrence risk of 24 per cent and a 28 per cent risk of developing severe preeclampsia in a subsequent pregnancy (Habli 2009).

## Long-term prognosis of hypertension in pregnancy

Women with a history of hypertension in pregnancy have a significantly increased risk of chronic hypertension, myocardial infarction, ischemic heart disease, stroke and type II diabetes later in life (Lykke et al 2009b; Bellamy and colleagues 2007).

Mothers with preeclampsia are at four times the risk of developing end stage renal disease (Hannaford 1997; Leanne 2007; Thadhani 2008). Patients with a history of HELLP are found to be at a risk of long-term morbidities, such as depression and chronic hypertension (Habli 2009).

## Organisational issues

The importance of a multidisciplinary team approach to the management of preeclampsia has been highlighted in many recent publications. A common message is the importance of early referral and involvement of the anesthetist. This highlights the value of providing the anesthetist as much time as possible to stabilise the patient prior to delivery. The use of an obstetric early warning chart has been proposed as an important clinical tool, which may allow for more timely recognition of those women who are developing a critical illness (Lewis 2007). Institution of standardised evaluation and surveillance guidelines was associated with reduction in maternal morbidity (Menzies 2007).

## References

Abalos E, Duley L, Steyn DW, Henderson-Smart DJ. 2007. Antihypertensive drug therapy for mild to moderate hypertension during pregnancy. *Cochrane Database of Systematic Reviews*, Issue 1. Art. No.: CD002252. DOI: 10.1002/14651858. CD002252.pub2.

Alexander JM, McIntire DD, Leveno KJ, Cunningham FG. 2006. Selective magnesium sulfate prophylaxis for the prevention of eclampsia in women with gestational hypertension. *Obstet Gynecol* 108:826–32.

Alfirevic Z, Stampalija T, Gyte GML. 2010. Fetal and umbilical Doppler ultrasound in high-risk pregnancies. *Cochrane Database of Systematic Reviews* 2010, Issue 1. Art. No.: CD007529.

American College of Obstetricians and Gynaecologists. 2002. Diagnosis and Management of Pre eclampsia and Eclampsia. ACOG Practice Bulletin No.:33. *Obstet Gynecol* 99:159–67.

Audibert F, Friedman SA, Frangieh AY, Sibai BM. 1996. Clinical utility of strict diagnostic criteria for the HELLP (hemolysis, elevated liver enzymes, and low platelets) syndrome. *Am J Obstet Gynecol* 175:460–4.

Barton JR, Sibai BM. 2004. Diagnosis and management of hemolysis, elevated liver enzymes, and low platelets syndrome. *Clin Perinatol* 31;807–833.

Bellamy L, Casas JP, Hingorani AD et al. 2007. Pre-eclampsia and risk of cardiovascular disease and cancer in later life: Systematic review and meta-analysis. *BMJ* 335:974.

Bombrys AE, Barton JR, Nowacki EA et al. 2008. Expectant management of severe preeclampsia at less than 27 weeks' gestation: maternal and perinatal outcomes according to gestational age by weeks at onset of expectant management. *Am J Obstet Gynecol* 199:247.e1–247.e6.

Brown M, Hague WM, Higgins J, Lowe S, McCowan L, Oats J, Peek MJ, Rowan JA and Walters BN. 2000. The detection, investigation and management of hypertension in pregnancy: full consensus statement. *Aust N Z J Obstet Gynaecol*, vol. 40, 139–55.

Chames MC, Livingston JC, Ivester TS et al. 2002. Late postpartum eclampsia: a preventable disease? *Am J Obstet Gynecol* 186:1174.

Collaborative Eclampsia Trial. 1995. Which anticonvulsant for women with eclampsia? Evidence from the Collaborative Eclampsia Trial. *Lancet* 345 (8963):1455–63; erratum.

Cunningham FG, Gant NF, Leveno KJ, Gilstrap LC III, Hauth JC, Wenstrom KD. 2001. Hypertensive disorders in pregnancy. In: *Williams Obstetrics*, 21st ed, 567–618. McGraw-Hill: New York.

Cunningham FG, Leveno KJ, Bloom SL, Hauth JC, Rouse DJ, Spong CY. 2010. Pregnancy hypertension. In: *Williams Obstetrics*, 23rd ed, 706–756. McGraw-Hill: New York.

Cunningham FG, Lowe T, Guss S et al. 1985. Erythrocyte morphology in women with severe preeclampsia ans eclampsia. *Am J Obstet Gynecol* 153: 358.

Cunningham HG, Pritchard JA, Hankins GDV et al. 1986. Peripartum heart failure: Idiopathic cardiomyopathy or compounding cardiovascular events?. *Obstet Gynecol* 67:157.

Duckitt K, Harrington D. 2005. Risk factors for pre eclampsia at antenatal booking: systematic review of controlled studies. *BMJ* 330; 565.

Duley L, Henderson-Smart DJ, Meher S. 2006. Drugs for treatment of very high blood pressure during pregnancy. *Cochrane Database of Systematic Reviews*, Issue 3. Art. No.: CD001449. DOI : 10.1002/14651858.CD001449. pub2.

Duley L, Henderson-Smart DJ. 2003. Magnesium sulphate versus diazepam for eclampsia. *Cochrane Database of Systematic Reviews*, Issue 4. Art. No.: CD000127. DOI: 10.1002/14651858. CD000127.

Duley L, Henderson-Smart DJ. 2003. Magnesium sulphate versus phenytoin for eclampsia. *Cochrane Database of Systematic Reviews*, Issue 4. Art. No.: CD000128. DOI: 10.1002/14651858. CD000128.

Duley L, Meher S, Abalos E. 2006. Management of pre eclampsia. *BMJ* 332;463–468.

Geary M. 1997. The HELLP syndrome. *Br J Obstet Gynaecol* 104:887–891.

Gonzalez JM, David MS et al. 2007. Relationship between abnormal fetal testing and adverse perinatal outcomes in intrauterine growth restriction. *Am JOG* e48–e51.

Gracia, V P. 2009. Maternal deaths due to eclampsia and HELLP syndrome. *Int J Gynaecol Obstet* Feb; 104(2):90–4.

Grivell RM, Alfirevic Z, Gyte GML, Devane D. 2010. Antenatal cardiotocography for fetal assessment. *Cochrane Database of Systematic Reviews* 2010, Issue 1. Art. No.: CD007863s.

Haas DM et al. 2006. *Journal of Maternal-Fetal and Neonatal Medicine*, Vol. 19, No. 6, Pages 365–369, DOI 10.1080/14767050600715873.

Habli M, Eftekhari N, Wiebracht E et al. 2009. Long-term maternal and subsequent pregnancy outcomes 5 years after hemolysis, elevated liver enzymes, and low platelets (HELLP) syndrome. *Am J Obstet Gynecol* 201:385.e1–5.

Hannaford P, Ferry S, Hirsch S. 1997. Cardiovascular sequelae of toxemia of pregnancy. *Heart* 77:154–158.

Helewa ME, Burrows RF, Smith J et al. 1997. Report of the Canadian Hypertension Society Consensus Conference: 1. Definitions, evaluation and classification of hypertensive disorders in pregnancy. *Can Med Assoc J* 157:715.

Henry CS, Beidermann SA et al. 2004. Spectrum of hypertensive emergencies in Pregnancy. *Crit Care Clin* 20;697–712.

Jenkins SM. 2002. Severe preeclampsia at <25 weeks of gestation: maternal and neonatal outcomes. *Am J Obstet Gynecol* 186(4): 790–5.

Katz L, de Amorim JN et al. 2008. Postpartum dexamethasone for women with HELLP syndrome: a double blin,d placebo controlled, ramndomized clinical trial. *Am J Obstet Gynecol* 198:283.e1–283.e8.

Leanne B, Juan-Pablo C, Hingorani AD, Williams DJ. 2007. Pre eclampsia and risk of cardiovascular disease and cancer in later life: systematic review and meta-analysis, *BMJ* 335; 974.

Leduc L, Wheeler JM, Kirshon B et al. 1992. Coagulation profile in severe preeclampsia. *Obstet Gynecol* 79:14.

Lewis, G (ed). 2007. The Confidential Enquiry into Maternal and Child Health (CEMACH). Saving Mothers' Lives: Reviewing maternal deaths to make motherhood safer - 2003-2005. The Seventh Report on Confidential Enquiries into Maternal Deaths in the United Kingdom. CEMACH: London.

Lykke JA, Langhoff-Roos J, Sibai BM et al. 2009b. Hypertensive disorders and subsequent cardiovascular morbidity and Type II diabetes mellitus in the mother. *Hypertension*. 53:994.

Lykke JA, Paidas MJ, Langhoff-Roos J. 2009a. Recurring complications in second pregnancy. *Obstet Gynecol* 113:1217.

Magee LA, Cham C, Waterman EJ et al. 2003. Hydralazine for treatment of severe hypertension in pregnancy: meta-analysis. *BMJ*. Oct 25; 327(7421):955–60.

Manas KJ, Welsh JD, Rankin RA, Miller DD. 1985. Hepatic hemorrhage without rupture in preeclampsia. *N Engl J Med* 312:424–426.

Martin JN, Jr, Rose CH, Briery CM. 2006. Understanding and managing HELLP syndrome: the integral role of aggressive glucocorticoids for mother and child. *Am J Obstet Gynecol* 195:914–934.

Martin Jr JN, Rinehart B, May WL, Magann EF, Terrone DA, Blake PG. 1999. The spectrum of severe preeclampsia: comparative analysis by HELLP syndrome classification. *Am J Obstet Gynecol* 180:1373–84.

Martin Jr JN, Thigpen BD, Moore, Rose CH, Cushman J, and May W. 2005. Stroke and Severe Preeclampsia and Eclampsia: A Paradigm Shift Focusing on Systolic Blood Pressure. *Obstet Gynecol* 105:246–54.

McDonald S, Best C, Lam K. 2009. The recurrence risk of severe de novo pre-eclampsia in singleton pregnancies: a population-based cohort. *BJOG* 116:1578–1584.

Menzies J, Magee LA, Li J, MacNab YC, Yin R, Stuart H, Baraty B, Lam E, Hamilton T, Lee SK, and Dadelszen P. 2007. Pre eclampsia Integrated Estimate of Risk (PIERS) Study Group. Instituting Surveillance Guidelines and Adverse Outcomes in Pre eclampsia. *Obstet Gynecol* 110:121–7.

National High Blood Pressure Education Program Working Group on High Blood Pressure in Pregnancy Report. 2000. *Am J Obstet Gynecol* 183(1):S1–S22.

Norwitz ER, Funai EF. 2008. Expectant management of severe pre eclampsia remote from term: hope for the best, but expect the worst. *Am J Obstet Gynecol* 199(3):209–12.

Paily VP. 2009. *First Report of Confidential Review of Maternal Deaths*, Why Mothers Die, Kerala 2004–2005, ed Paily VP.

Podymov T, August P. 2008. Update on the use of Antihypertensive drugs in pregnancy, *Hypertension* 51:960–969.

RCOG. 2006. The management of severe pre eclampsia/eclampsia Guideline Number 10(A). *Royal College of Obstetricians and Gynaecologists Guidelines*.

Rinehart BK, Terrone DA, Magann EF, Martin RW, May WL, Martin JN Jr. 1999. Preeclampsia-associated hepatic hemorrhage and rupture: mode of management related to maternal and perinatal outcome. *Obstet Gynecol Surv* 54:196–202.

Saudan P, Brown MA, Buddle ML, Jones M. 1998. Does gestational hypertension become pre-eclampsia?. *BJOG: An International Journal of Obstetrics & Gynaecology* 105:1177–1184. doi: 10.1111/j.1471-0528.1998.tb09971.x

Schucker JL, Mercer BM, Audibert F, Lewis RL, Friedman SA, Sibai BM. 1996. Serial amniotic fluid index in severe preeclampsia: a poor predictor of adverse outcome. *Am J Obstet Gynecol* Oct;175(4 Pt 1):1018–23.

Sibai BM, Barton JR. 2007. Expectant management of severe pre eclampsia remote from term: patient selection, management and delivery indications. *Am J Obstet Gynecol* 196:514.e1–9.

Sibai BM, Mercer BM, Schiff E, Friedman SA. 1994. Aggressive versus expectant management of severe preeclampsia at 28 to 32 weeks' gestation: a randomized controlled trial. *Am J Obstet Gynecol* 171:818–22.

Sibai BM, Ramadan MK, Usta I, Salama M, Mercer BM, Friedman SA. 1993. Maternal morbidity and mortality in 442 pregnancies with hemolysis, elevated liver enzymes, and low platelets (HELLP syndrome). *Am J Obstet Gynecol* 169:1000–6.

Sibai BM, Spinnato JA, Watson DL et al. 1985. Eclampsia, 4. Neurological findings and future outcome. *Am J Obstet Gynecol* 152:184.

Sibai BM. 2004. Diagnosis, controversies, and management of the syndrome of hemolysis, elevated liver enzymes, and low platelet count. *Obstet Gynecol* 103:981–91.

Sibai BM. 2004. Imitators of eclampsia/severe pre eclampsia. *Clin Perinatol* 31;835–852.

Sibai BM. 2004. Diagnosis, controversies, and management of HELLP syndrome. *Obstet Gynecol* 103:981.

Thadhani R, Solomon CG. 2008. Pre eclampsia, a glimpse into the future? *NEJM* 359;8:858–860.

Vidaeff AC, Carroll MA, Ramin SM. 2005. Acute hypertensive emergencies in pregnancy. *Crit Care Med* Vol.33, No. 10 (Suppl.).

Walker JJ, arren R and Arulkumaran S. 2009. Management of Severe Preeclampsia / Eclampsia. In *Best Practice in Labour and Delivery*, 262–272. Cambridge University Press: Cambridge.

Waugh, Jason JS, Justin CT, Divakaran TG et al. 2004. *Obstetrics & Gynecology* 103(4):769–777.

Weinstein L. 1982. Syndrome of hemolysis, elevated liver enzymes and low platelet count: A severe consequence of hypertension in pregnancy. *Am J Obstet Gynecol* 142: 159.

World Health Report 2005. Make every mother and child count. WHO Press, World Health Organization.

Zwart JJ, Richters A, Ory F et al. 2008. Eclampsia in the Netherlands. *Obstet Gynecol* 112:820.

# CHAPTER 31

# NEONATAL RESUSCITATION AND THE MANAGEMENT OF IMMEDIATE NEONATAL PROBLEMS

*Ted Gasiorowski and Nigel Kennea*

## Introduction

Resuscitation of the newborn infant differs from that of any other age group. The newborn is small, wet and therefore prone to getting cold and has lungs that contain lung fluid. Therefore, the approach to resuscitation needs to be adapted to their needs.

While most infants will not require resuscitation at birth, approximately 3–5 per cent of newborns may need some support (Saugstad 1998). Most of the time, the potential need for resuscitation may be anticipated from maternal and obstetric history such as the presence of a congenital anomaly on the antenatal scans, preterm gestation, fetal distress (for example, as indicated by abnormal fetal heart rate pattern or abnormal fetal scalp blood sample), or by the presence of meconium-stained liquor. In these cases, trained members of the midwifery and/or neonatal team should be present prior to delivery. Very occasionally, a newborn infant may be unexpectedly delivered in poor condition and, while the neonatal team is being alerted, resuscitation will need to be started. It is therefore recommended that anyone who works in an environment where they may be required to resuscitate newborn babies should have training similar to the UK Newborn Life Support (NLS) course or the American Neonatal Advanced Life Support (NALS) Course.

> The need for neonatal resuscitation may be anticipated with:
> - the presence of a congenital anomaly on the antenatal scans
> - preterm gestation
> - fetal distress
> - the presence of meconium-stained liquor

## Physiology

The primary reason for resuscitation in the newborn differs from that in adults. While adults requiring resuscitation will most likely have had a primary cardiac event, the newborn infant's heart is healthy and it will usually initially be a hypoxic or ischemic event that will have compromised the newborn. Therefore, particular attention to the management of the **airway** and **breathing** is imperative.

In normal circumstances, during the first few minutes of life, the newborn baby will fill its lungs with air and establish resting lung volume. During this time, pneumocytes will change from actively secreting fluid to actively absorbing fluid under the influence of maternal hormones. Approximately 30 ml/kg of fluid (on average, approximately 100 ml for the average term infant) is absorbed through the alveoli, with a further 30 ml or so being present in the oropharynx and cleared more slowly. Routine suctioning could remove an insignificant amount of fluid from the oropharynx, but will not remove fluid from the alveoli. Routine suctioning of infants at birth may result in bradycardia and apnea, as a result of vagal stimulation, and is therefore not recommended (Richmond 2005).

> Routine suctioning of infants at birth may result in bradycardia and apnea, and is therefore not recommended

In order to initiate resuscitation at birth, it is vital to have an understanding of the pathophysiological consequences of hypoxia during birth. Such information has been derived from the work of physiologists in the 1960s such as Cross, Dawes and Godfrey that demonstrated the physiological responses of animals subjected to hypoxic stress at birth (Cross 1966; Dawes 1968; Godfrey 1968). The results of their experiments have been used to guide the teaching of a logical and effective approach to resuscitation now known as the ABC (D) of resuscitation.

These experiments demonstrated that when subjected to acute hypoxia by interrupting cord blood flow, the first response of the fetus is to breathe more deeply and rapidly. Within a few minutes of hypoxia, the activity of the respiratory centre switches off and the fetus stops breathing. This is known as primary apnea. The carbon dioxide levels in fetal blood ($pCO_2$) now slowly start to rise followed by a decrease in heart rate to about half the normal rate. The heart continues to beat slowly, rather than stop because of the presence of glycogen in the cardiac muscle, which provides an energy source via anaerobic metabolism. This anaerobic metabolism will subsequently contribute lactic acidosis and in turn leading to peripheral vasoconstriction, resulting in a clinically pale baby.

If the insult continues, the fetus begins to gasp as a result of primitive spinal reflexes. These gasps are shuddering, whole-body breathing movements that occur several times a minute. The effect of gasping may be enough for the infant to 'resuscitate itself' or, if given resuscitation in the form of airway management, to respond quickly. Cardiac output continues and blood pressure is maintained but if these gasps fail to aerate the lungs they fade away, hypoxia and acidosis become increasingly severe, all vital functions cease and terminal apnea supervenes. In the newborn human baby, this process probably takes about 20 minutes (Hey and Kelly 1968).

> With increasing hypoxia the baby goes through the following stages:
> - primary apnea
> - gasping
> - terminal apnea

A baby who is not breathing could be in primary apnea, about to gasp or in terminal apnea. Unfortunately, it is not possible to tell at the time, but it is reassuring to know that almost all babies respond rapidly once the lungs have been aerated.

## Equipment needed

The items mentioned are not an exhaustive list and when faced with the delivery of the newborn infant out of the hospital setting, making a note of the time, drying the infant and providing a warm environment with skin-to-skin contact between the infant and mother may be all that is needed. A tie should be used to clamp the umbilical cord, if possible while waiting for help to arrive.

In a planned delivery at home, midwives will take with them a bag-valve-mask device with suitable facemasks, oropharyngeal airways, a laryngoscope, a small oxygen cylinder and portable suction with large bore catheters. They should also have cord clamps, scissors and disposable gloves.

In the hospital setting, all of this equipment should be more easily available, including a resuscitaire to provide a flat surface, which is also able to provide warmth through radiant heat, a clock, pressure-limited delivery of air/oxygen and suction. In addition, a range of facemasks, oropharyngeal airways, laryngoscopes with blades and endotracheal tubes should be available. Equipment for placement of an umbilical venous catheter should also be made available if required and also emergency resuscitation drugs if needed.

Preparation for the early management of a newborn infant needs to include a review of the obstetric notes and discussion with colleagues regarding any foreseeable complications at delivery. It is also important to ensure good communication with the parents before birth and during resuscitation if at all possible.

## Priorities

### Warmth

Maintaining temperature is imperative, and indeed, hypothermia is associated with worsening morbidity and mortality (Bhatt et al 2007). Therefore, when present at the delivery of any newborn, irrespective of its need for resuscitation, drying the infant, disposing off the wet towels and wrapping the infant with a dry warm towel is necessary before further steps are taken. After drying and wrapping, the infant should be immediately assessed. This assessment comprises the respiratory effort, heart rate, tone and colour.

> Drying the infant, disposing off the wet towels and wrapping the infant with a dry warm towel is necessary before further resuscitation.

The heart rate is most accurately estimated using a stethoscope. Palpation of the apical cardiac impulse, umbilical or peripheral pulsation can be unreliable. Based on this assessment, the need for resuscitation will be determined. Should resuscitation be required, call for help early. Start the clock on the resuscitaire when the baby is born to guide resuscitation and also for documentation.

### Airway

Newborn infants have a large occiput, and when placed onto the resuscitaire or a hard surface, there is the tendency for their head to flex forward, thereby obstructing the airway. To overcome this, place the head in the neutral position by extending the neck very slightly (Fig. 31.1). This will result in the plane between the nose and mouth being parallel to the plane of the ceiling. This is different in adults where you tilt the head and apply a chin lift. Sometimes, this simple manoeuvre is all that is needed to assist the newborn's respiratory effort although there are further airway manoeuvres one can apply (see below).

If, having placed the head in the 'neutral position', the baby's respiratory effort

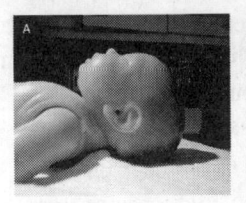

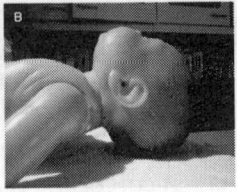

**Figure 31.1** Newborn infants have a large occiput, and when placed onto the resuscitaire or a hard surface, there is the tendency for the head to flex forward, thereby obstructing the airway (A). Placing the infant's head in the 'neutral position' opens the airway (B). Care must be taken not to over-extend the head.

remains poor or absent, with a heart rate that is slow (<100 beats per minute), the infant will need five inflation breaths. The idea of inflation breaths is to establish a residual volume and displace lung fluid. Therefore, these breaths are given with pressures set at 30 cm $H_2O$, each lasting 2–3 seconds, given using a bag and mask, or preferably a pressure-limited T piece, 'Tom Thumb' or other ventilation device. The reason for the five breaths is that the initial two or three breaths may only help in pushing lung liquid out of the alveoli and not expand the lungs with air.

Watch for chest wall movement as the inflation breaths are given to judge the effectiveness; the right-sized mask should be used which covers the nose and mouth but does not go over the end of the chin or encroach onto the eyes. Once these five inflation breaths are given, further assessment is necessary to see if this has aided the infant. While assessing the tone, colour and respiratory effort, the most important sign of effective inflation breaths is a rise in the heart rate. If there is no such rise and the chest was not seen to move, it is likely that the lungs have not been inflated. Other airway manoeuvres to open the airway and ensure that the infant receives the inflation breaths need to be considered.

> The right-sized mask should cover the nose and mouth but should not go over the end of the chin or encroach onto the eyes.

These airway manoeuvres include a single-handed jaw thrust: one places the third or fourth finger of the hand, used to keep the facemask on the infant, behind the angle of jaw and pushes it upward. This will aid in opening the airway by bringing the lower jaw in line with the upper jaw and will help to lift the tongue which may have dropped backwards obstructing the airway out of the way. Having performed this manoeuvre, five further inflation breaths should be given again. If this does not result in a rise in heart rate or chest wall movement, and if help is available, a two-person jaw thrust can be attempted to open the airway. In this manoeuvre, one person applies the jaw thrust behind both jaw angles and holds the face mask in place, while the other person gives the inflation breaths.

If this does not work or there is no help available, if competent, one should directly visualise the larynx and vocal cords using a laryngoscope placed in the left hand and perform suction if an obstruction such as a blood clot, vernix or meconium is seen. Alternatively, if there is no obstruction, an appropriately sized oropharyngeal airway should be placed using the laryngoscope or a tongue depressor. To size an oropharyngeal airway, hold it along the line of the lower jaw with the flange in the middle of the lips immediately below the tip of the nose and the end of the airway level with the angle of the jaw. The airway is inserted in the anatomical position you want it to be. That is, it is not rotated in the mouth due to the fragile palate.

Following these manoeuvres, five inflation breaths should again be given. One can only feel reassured if there is a rise in heart rate or chest wall movement is seen. If, using these manoeuvres, the chest wall moves with the inflation breaths but there is no rise in heart rate, one must undertake chest compressions. One may at any of these points intubate the baby using an appropriately sized endotracheal tube, if trained and skilled to do so. The advantage of being able to insert an endotracheal tube is that the airway is secured and, in an extended resuscitation, the hands can be freed to concentrate on circulatory resuscitation.

## Breathing

If the chest wall has moved with the inflation breaths with a rise in heart rate but the newborn continues not to breathe or has poor respiratory effort, ventilation breaths should be given. These breaths are to 'breathe for the baby' and therefore given with shorter inspiratory times, and given quicker, at a rate of 30 breaths per minute. Having overcome the initial stiffness of the lungs and dispersed some of the lung liquid, the inspiratory pressure given should also be reduced to a pressure sufficient to achieve adequate chest wall movement (normally around 20–25 cm $H_2O$).

If after 30 seconds of ventilation breaths the infant is still not breathing effectively, consider admission of the infant to the neonatal unit for continued ventilatory support and further management. Gasping suggests that the baby was in terminal apnea.

There is growing evidence from both animal and human studies that resuscitation of infants with room air is as effective as 100% oxygen. There is a theoretical risk that 100% oxygen can cause tissue damage via free radicals. Tan et al undertook a Cochrane review looking at air versus oxygen for resuscitation of infants at birth. They concluded that if one chooses to resuscitate using air, supplementary oxygen should be available as a back-up (Tan et al 2008).

> There is growing evidence that resuscitation of infants with room air is as effective as 100% oxygen.

Some devices are now available where one can set positive end expiratory pressure (PEEP) as well as a peak inspiratory pressure, such as the Neopuff®. There is a theoretical benefit to the infant when using PEEP, as this establishes and maintains functional residual capacity. While several papers have shown the benefit, particularly in preterm infants where there is an association between absence of functional residual capacity and subsequent respiratory distress syndrome in those requiring ventilation (Upton and Milner 1991), a Cochrane review undertaken in 2003 and recently updated in 2008 concluded that there was insufficient evidence to determine the efficacy and safety of PEEP in ventilation breaths given during resuscitation of the newborn infant and that further randomised clinical trials were needed (O'Donnell et al 2008).

## Circulation

The baby who does not respond to lung inflation at birth is very rare and the most likely reason for an inadequate rise in the heart rate is inadequate lung inflation. If despite good chest wall movement with inflation breaths, there is no rise in heart rate, chest compressions must be given. The aim of these chest compressions is to move oxygenated blood from the lungs to the coronary arteries. The best method of administering chest compressions is to encircle the whole of the infant's chest with both hands and place the tips of your thumbs just below an imaginary inter-nipple line (Fig. 31.2).

The chest compressions should ideally compress the chest by one-third to safely achieve maximum effectiveness (Meyer et al 2010) and are given at a ratio of one ventilation breath to three chest compressions. After approximately 15 cycles or 30 seconds, one needs to assess the infant's colour, tone, respiration and heart rate. If the heart rate has improved (>60/minite), then chest compressions can be stopped and, depending on the respiratory effort, ventilation breaths may or may not need to continue.

If, however, despite good airway management with chest movement and chest compressions the heart rate does not increase, drugs should be considered.

### Drugs

Emergency resuscitation drugs are very rarely required in the neonate. If you need to obtain vascular access and give drugs, the outcome for this newborn infant is likely to be poor. The drugs used in resuscitation are 4.2% sodium bicarbonate (1–2 mmol/kg), adrenaline (10 mcg/kg) and 10% dextrose (2.5 ml/kg). Occasionally, volume replacement (0.9% sodium chloride or O rhesus-negative blood) can be given, particularly if there is an obvious history of blood loss. As babies who require resuscitation often have poor peripheral circulation, the best method of administering drugs is via central access. This, in the newborn infant, will be by way of a catheter that has been inserted into the umbilical vein of the cord. Alternatively, an intraosseous needle may be used.

> In the newborn infant, drugs may be administered by way of a catheter that has been inserted into the umbilical vein of the cord.

If central venous access is difficult, the only drug that can be given via an endotracheal tube is adrenaline, but due to variable absorption, the efficacy of this route is questionable and therefore it is not recommended (Barber and Wyckoff 2006).

### Preterm infants

Infants that are born prematurely are even more vulnerable to heat loss and, therefore, attention to temperature control is important. Hypothermia not only increases the risk of death in very low birth weight babies (Stanley and Alberman 1978) but also significantly increases morbidity (Merritt and Farrell 1976). For those born at 30 weeks' gestation or less, immediately

> Hypothermia not only increases the risk of death in very low birth weight babies but also significantly increases morbidity.

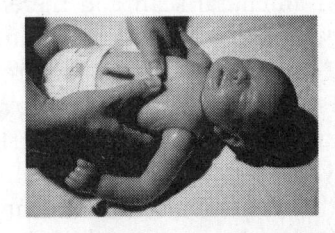

**Figure 31.2** Position of hands for cardiac compression in a newborn infant.

placing the body of the infant (without prior drying) into a plastic bag/wrap and subsequently under a radiant heater has been shown to improve maintenance of normothermia (Soll 2008). Preterm infants are more likely to require stabilisation rather than resuscitation. The approach to resuscitation is exactly the same as the approach to that of a term newborn.

Due to the fragility of their lungs, the pressures required to inflate their lungs and move the chest wall will be less, and if inflation breaths are required, starting with pressures of 20–25 cm $H_2O$ should be adequate. Having given inflation breaths, prematurity may cause their respiratory effort to be insufficient and hence intubation by a trained and skilled member of the team may need to be undertaken. One may also consider using a device that is able to provide PEEP when delivering ventilation breaths. If intubation is required, administration of surfactant at this time via the endotracheal tube should be considered. Having stabilised the infant, they should be transferred to the neonatal unit for ongoing assessment and management.

> If a premature infant requires intubation, administration of surfactant via the endotracheal tube should be considered.

## Meconium aspiration

Most babies that pass meconium *in utero* are either term or post-term. Its presence could be an indicator of fetal stress. The fetus must be gasping in order to aspirate meconium.

If a newborn cries at delivery despite the presence of meconium, it will imply that the infant has an open airway and therefore no action is required. If, however, the infant is born with no respiratory effort (apneic), there may have been a period of gasping *in utero* and this infant is at risk of meconium aspiration. Therefore, it is important, having firstly paid attention to keeping the infant warm, to directly visualise the larynx and vocal cords to suction any large plugs of meconium present using a large bore suction catheter. Having directly visualised the cords and either assessed that there is no obstruction or removed the obstruction, one can then continue with the normal approach to newborn resuscitation (NICE Guidance 2007). There is no evidence to suggest that upper airway suctioning during delivery reduces the number of babies with meconium aspiration syndrome.

> An infant which had gasping in utero due to hypoxia is at risk of meconium aspiration. This infant is likely to be born apneic.

## Known congenital problems

The majority of antenatal problems such as esophageal atresia with a tracheo-esophageal fistula or a congenital diaphragmatic hernia, that could alter the approach to resuscitation, will be picked up antenatally, and these babies should be delivered at an appropriate tertiary centre if indicated. However, potential congenital problems with the airway, such as Pierre-Robin sequence or Goldenhar syndrome, can be difficult to pick up on an antenatal scan and therefore the use of adjunct airways may be required if an infant needing resuscitation fails to inflate their chest with airway positioning and jaw thrust. Insertion of an appropriately sized oropharyngeal or nasopharyngeal airway can aid the maintenance of a patent airway by preventing the tongue, which is large in relation to the size of the oral cavity, flopping backwards and occluding the larynx.

# Neonatal Resuscitation and the Management of Immediate Neonatal Problems

## Stopping resuscitation

The Resuscitation Council (UK) has suggested that if there are no signs of life after 10 minutes of continuous and adequate resuscitation then discontinuation of resuscitation may be justified (Resuscitation Council UK 2008). This is supported with data published by Patel et al in 2004 which looked at the outcome of term newborn infants who had resuscitation beyond 10 minutes. Twenty-nine babies were included in their observation study; twenty babies died before leaving hospital. Of the nine that were discharged alive, eight had severe disability and one had moderate disability (Patel and Beeby 2004).

> If there are no signs of life after 10 minutes of continuous and adequate resuscitation then discontinuation of resuscitation may be justified.

## Summary

Newborn resuscitation follows a systematic stepwise approach with emphasis placed on temperature control, airway and breathing. Most newborns will not need resuscitation but should they do so, the vast majority will respond when airway and breathing are managed adequately. It is estimated that more aggressive resuscitation will be required in 1:2000 deliveries (Morley and Davis 2008). In the small minority who need further resuscitative measures, the outcome is likely to be poor and good documentation of the time from birth to resuscitation steps including intubation, cardiac compressions, administration of drugs and subsequent responses will help with further management and the counselling of parents. An approach to newborn resuscitation may be summarised as below by the algorithm provided by the Resuscitation Council (Resuscitation Council UK 2008). The importance of clear communication and documentation during and following resuscitation cannot be over-emphasised.

### An Approach to Newborn Resuscitation: Resuscitation Council Guideline

**Newborn Life Support**

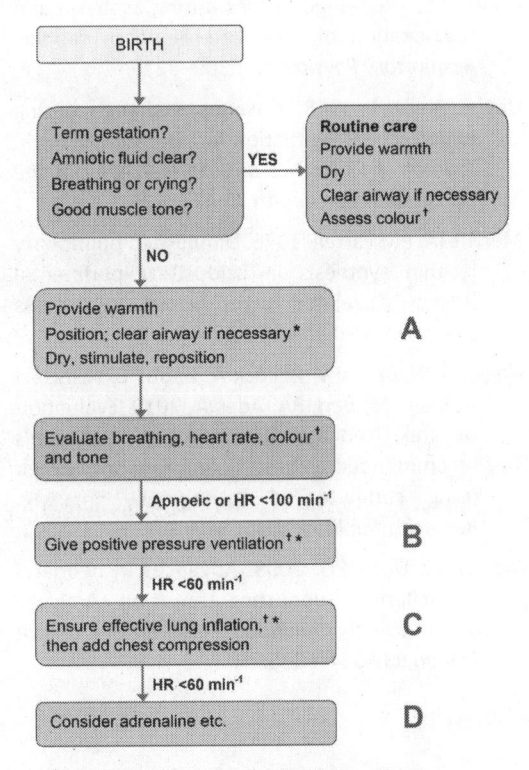

BIRTH
↓
Term gestation?
Amniotic fluid clear?
Breathing or crying?
Good muscle tone?
— YES → Routine care: Provide warmth, Dry, Clear airway if necessary, Assess colour[†]
↓ NO

**A** Provide warmth
Position; clear airway if necessary[*]
Dry, stimulate, reposition
↓
Evaluate breathing, heart rate, colour[†] and tone
↓ Apnoeic or HR <100 min$^{-1}$

**B** Give positive pressure ventilation[†][*]
↓ HR <60 min$^{-1}$

**C** Ensure effective lung inflation,[†][*] then add chest compression
↓ HR <60 min$^{-1}$

**D** Consider adrenaline etc.

[*] Tracheal intubation may be considered at several steps
[†] Consider supplemental oxygen at any stage if cyanosis persists

*Source*: The Resuscitation Council UK's website. Reproduced with permission.

## References

Barber CA, Wyckoff MH. 2006. Use and efficacy of endotracheal versus intravenous epinephrine during neonatal cardiopulmonary resuscitation in the delivery room. *Paediatrics* 118:1028–1034.

Bhatt DR, White R, Martin G, Van Marter L J, Finer N, Goldsmith J P, Ramos C, Kukreja S, Ramanathan R. 2007. Transitional hypothermia in preterm newborns. *Journal of Perinatology* 27:S45–S47.

Cross KW. 1966. Resuscitation of the asphyxiated infant. *British Medical Bulletin* 22:73–78.

Dawes G. 1968. *Fetal and neonatal physiology,* chapter 12:141–59. Year Book Publisher: Chicago.

Godfrey S. 1968. Blood gases during asphyxia and resuscitation of fetal and newborn rabbits. *Respiratory Physiology* 4:309–321.

Hey E, Kelly J. 1968. Gaseous exchange during endotracheal ventilation for asphyxia at birth. *Journal of Obstetrics and Gynaecology of the British Commonwealth* 75:414–423.

Merritt TA, PM Farrell. 1976. Diminished pulmonary lecithin synthesis in acidosis: experimental findings as related to the respiratory distress syndrome. *Pediatrics* 57:32–40.

Meyer A, Nadkarni V, Pollock A, Babbs C, Nishisaki A, Braga M, Berg RA, Ades A. 2010. Evaluation of the Neonatal Resuscitation Program's recommended chest compression depth using computerized tomography imaging. *Resuscitation* May; 81(5):544–8.

Morley CJ, Davis PG. 2008. Advances in neonatal resuscitation: supporting transition. *Archives of Disease in Childhood Fetal and Neonatal Edition* 93:F334–F336.

National Institute of Health and Clinical Excellence. 2007. Intrapartum care: management and delivery of care to women in labour. *Clinical Guidelines* (UK); p42

O'Donnell C, Davis P, Morley C. 2008. Positive end-expiratory pressure for resuscitation of newborn infants at birth. *The Cochrane Database of Systematic Reviews*; Volume 2.

Patel H, Beeby PJ. 2004. Resuscitation beyond 10 minutes of term babies born without signs of life. *Journal of Paediatrics and Child Health* 40:136–138.

Resuscitation Council (UK). 2008. (www.resus.org.uk)

Richmond S. 2007. ILCOR and neonatal resuscitation 2005. *Archives of Diseases in Childhood Fetal & Neonatal Edition* 92:F163–F165.

Saugstad OD. 1998. Practical aspects of resuscitating newborn infants. *European Journal of Pediatrics* 157:S11–S15.

Soll RF. *2008.* Heat loss prevention in neonates. *Journal of Perinatology* **28**:S57–S59.

Stanley FJ, ED Alberman. 1978. Infants of very low birth weight. 1. Factors affecting survival. *Developmental Medicine and Child Neurology* 20:300–12.

Tan A, Schulze A, O'Donnell CPF, Davis PG. 2008. Air versus oxygen for resuscitation of infants at birth. *The Cochrane Database of Systematic Reviews*; Volume 2.

Upton CJ, Milner AD. 1991. Endotracheal resuscitation of neonates using rebreathing bag. *Archives of Diseases in Childhood* 66:39–42.

# CHAPTER 32

# COMPLICATIONS OF THE PUERPERIUM

*Dhiraj Uchil*

The puerperium begins after delivery and lasts until six weeks postpartum. This is a period of extraordinary physiological and psychological changes. Postnatal care is, however, a sadly neglected field. The focus tends to be on the infant, with relatively little interest paid to the mother's health and needs. As a result, a significant proportion of maternal morbidity in the puerperium is undiagnosed and, therefore, untreated (Glazener and MacArthur 2001). While life-threatening complications are fortunately rare and well recognised, other 'minor' complications are often ignored with significant consequences to maternal well-being (Glazener 1997).

## Puerperal Genital Hematoma

These are relatively uncommon but can cause considerable maternal morbidity. Incidence ranges from 1 in 500 to 1 in 12,500 deliveries. Risk factors include nulliparity, prolonged

> Risk factors for hematomas:
> - nulliparity
> - prolonged second stage of labour
> - instrumental delivery
> - fetal weight > 4 kg
> - genital varicosities

second stage of labour, instrumental delivery, fetal weight > 4 kg and genital varicosities (Mawhinney and Holman 2007).

Anatomically, these hematomas can be vulvovaginal, paravaginal or supravaginal/subperitoneal in location. Vulval and vulvovaginal hematomas are visible on external inspection of the vulva. These occur as a result of injury to branches of the pudendal artery. Paravaginal hematomas, which result from damage to the descending branch of the uterine artery, are not obvious externally but can be diagnosed by vaginal examination, where they are felt as a bulging of the vaginal wall. These hematomas can extend into the ischiorectal fossa.

Supravaginal or subperitoneal hematomas result from damage to the uterine artery branches in the broad ligament. Due to the presence of loose areolar tissue in the broad ligament, these hematomas can reach considerable sizes and may present as an abdominal lump or postpartum collapse (Mawhinney and Holman 2007).

## Clinical features

Symptoms usually develop within a few hours after delivery. Most hematomas are associated with repaired perineal trauma. It is therefore essential to ensure meticulous hemostasis, as an unsecured vessel may continue to bleed, creating a hematoma. Excessive perineal pain is the characteristic symptom and its presence should prompt examination to exclude hematomas. It is necessary to perform a gentle vaginal examination to ascertain the extent of the hematoma. In large supravaginal hematoma, the uterus may be displaced to the opposite side by the enlarging broad ligament hematoma.

## Management

Resuscitative measures should be undertaken as blood loss is often under-estimated. In small vulvovaginal hematomas (< 5 cm) which are not expanding, conservative management may be appropriate. It is necessary to ensure adequate analgesia and insert a urinary catheter to prevent retention.

Large hematomas should be evacuated in the operating theatre, as conservative management is often not successful. Most hematomas can be evacuated using a vaginal approach, with the exception of a broad ligament hematoma, which would require an abdominal approach. Once the clots are evacuated, the visible bleeding points should be ligated and the dead space closed. Use of vaginal packs provides compression and minimises re-formation of the hematoma. The use of vaginal or vulval drains may be considered.

- Large hematomas should be evacuated in the theatre
- Most hematomas can be evacuated using a vaginal approach
- Broad ligament hematomas require an abdominal approach

In recurrent bleeding or a large hematoma in a stable patient, interventional radiology to embolise the bleeding vessels is an appropriate alternative (Mawhinney and Holman 2007).

# Secondary Postpartum Hemorrhage

Hemorrhage occurring more than 24 hours after birth is termed secondary postpartum hemorrhage. It complicates 0.5–1.5 per cent of all deliveries. The predisposing factors for this condition are retained placental fragments and uterine infection (Dewhurst 1966; King et al 1989).

## Clinical Features

Most of these cases occur during the second postpartum week and may be associated with the shedding of the placental 'eschar' that forms in the site of the placental bed.

When pyrexia is absent, the causes of bleeding are retained products causing subinvolution of the uterus or excessive bleeding after the eschar is shed. Rarer causes include coagulopathy and malignancies (Dewhurst 1966).

Examination may reveal a boggy uterus which is subinvoluted. Ultrasound may help identify the presence of retained tissue. However, an ultrasound examination of the postpartum uterus is often technically difficult due to the large number of artefacts.

## Management

The possibility of sepsis must be always entertained. Cervical and vaginal swabs should be taken followed by broadspectrum antibiotics. If there are general constitutional symptoms of fever and tachycardia or local uterine pain and tenderness, intravenous antibiotics are more appropriate. If delivery has been by cesarean section, the cavity would have been swabbed out during the procedure and, therefore, retained products are unlikely. In these cases, it is advisable to manage these patients conservatively with antibiotics. Uterotonics may be of value, but their use is controversial.

- Intravenous antibiotics should be used in the presence of sepsis
- Ampicillin (or clindamycin), metronidazole and gentamicin are recommended in combination

The recommended antibiotics are ampicillin (or clindamycin, if allergic to penicillin) and metronidazole. In the presence of obvious sepsis, gentamicin should be added to this regimen; it can be given as a single daily dose (5 mg/kg body weight) rather than in three divided doses. This combination of antibiotics does not preclude breastfeeding (RCOG 2009).

If there is a strong suspicion of retained products and ultrasound examination supports this diagnosis, then uterine evacuation must be performed. In addition, if there is persistent bleeding, surgical intervention should be considered irrespective of the ultrasound findings. A senior clinician should be involved in making this decision.

Curettage of the postpartum uterus is a procedure that is often fraught with complications and should not be undertaken lightly. Risks include perforation and Asherman's syndrome. It may be advisable to send the products for histopathology to exclude gestational trophoblastic disease (Park and Sachs 1999). Controversy also exists over whether to use a sharp or blunt curette because of the concern of uterine perforation.

Curettage of the postpartum uterus:
- Risk of perforation
- Risk of Asherman's syndrome
- Best performed with a sharp curette and gentle pressure

A sharp curette should be used with gentle pressure on the uterine wall. A blunt curette may need more pressure and may cause perforation. Curettage with vacuum aspiration may be more appropriate.

## Puerperal Pyrexia

Because most temperature elevations in the puerperium are caused by pelvic infection, this is often used as an index of their frequency. It is defined as the occurrence of a temperature elevation of 38°C (100.4°F) on any two days of the first ten days postpartum after the first 24 hours.

Although the pyrexia is usually due to uterine infection, it is important to remember that a wide variety of conditions can cause puerperal pyrexia. Differential diagnoses include deep vein thrombosis (DVT), abscesses, hematomas, infection of abdominal or perineal wounds, pulmonary complications like atelectasis, aspiration or bacterial pneumonia, urinary infection including pyelonephritis, breast conditions like engorgement, mastitis or abscess and rarer conditions like septic thrombophlebitis and ovarian vein thrombosis. Breast engorgement commonly causes brief temperature elevation. Almost 15 per cent of

- About 15 per cent of women develop breast engorgement
- The temperature rarely exceeds 39°C
- Usually does not last for >24 hours

women develop a temperature from breast engorgement, but this rarely exceeds 39°C or lasts more than 24 hours.

## Management

All women with puerperal pyrexia should be carefully assessed to ascertain the cause of the fever and appropriate management instituted. Although some of the conditions that cause this phenomenon are self-limiting, failure to diagnose sepsis or DVT can have disastrous consequences.

## Puerperal Sepsis

Alexander Gordon was the first to suggest that puerperal fever was contagious.

The work of Oliver Wendell Holmes and Ignas Semmelweis in this field is well recognised. Despite Semmelweis conclusively proving that puerperal fever could be minimised by the use of carbolic hand washes, he failed to convince the scientific community regarding its contagious nature and the efficacy of this simple intervention. Ironically, his death was due to sepsis that he acquired from a patient on whom he had operated (Steer 2001).

## Incidence

Puerperal sepsis continues to be a major cause of maternal death. As this is more commonly seen in developing countries, a misconception has taken root that this is a disease of the past. Reports of the Confidential Enquiry into Maternal Deaths (CEMD) have warned against such an assumption, pointing out that women continue to die from this illness even today (Thompson 2001). The incidence of uterine infection is 1–17 per cent, depending on antibiotic use (Glazener 1997).

## Predisposing factors

The route of delivery is the single most important risk factor for the development of postpartum uterine infection (endomyometritis). Compared with cesarean section, endomyometritis is uncommon following vaginal delivery (13 per cent versus 2.6 per cent) (Sweet and Ledger 1973). As cesarean section is the most commonly performed major operation, the burden of morbidity is quite significant.

> Risk factors for puerperal sepsis:
> - cesarean section
> - low socio-economic status,
> - prolonged rupture of membranes
> - chorioamnionitis
> - prolonged labour
> - operative delivery
> - bacterial vaginosis
> - urinary tract infection and asymptomatic bacteriuria

Other risk factors include low socio-economic status, prolonged rupture of membranes, chorioamnionitis, prolonged labour, operative delivery, bacterial vaginosis, urinary tract infection and asymptomatic bacteriuria.

## Microbiology

Endometritis is usually polymicrobial with a mixture of aerobic and anaerobic organisms.

> Endometritis is usually polymicrobial with a mixture of aerobic and anaerobic organisms.

In most women, the bacteria responsible for pelvic infection are those that are normally resident in the bowel and also colonise the lower genital tract. Of the aerobic organisms, Streptococcus groups A, B and Enterococcus predominate. Predominant anaerobic organisms include Gram-positive cocci like the Peptostreptococcus and Peptococcus species, Bacteroides and *Escherichia coli* (Park and Sachs 1999).

*Chlamydia trachomatis* can cause a late onset uterine infection in a third of women with antepartum cervical infection (Ismail et al 1985).

## Clinical features

Infection confined to the uterus may present with either local or systemic signs. Temperature commonly exceeds 38°–39°C. This is often associated with tachycardia that mirrors the temperature. Headache, malaise, nausea, rigors and abdominal pain are frequent.

The uterus is tender and larger than normal. However, because of incisional pain in patients with a cesarean, this is more helpful in the diagnosis of sepsis following vaginal delivery. The lochia may be profuse and malodourous. If the cervix is open, the cavity should be gently explored for the presence of retained products.

A particularly high fever within the first 24 hours may indicate a serious acute onset of infection. Gram-negative sepsis, group B streptococcus (GBS) disease, clostridial sepsis or toxic shock syndrome should be considered.

Septic shock is thankfully an infrequent presentation of puerperal sepsis. The patient presents with clinical features suggestive of infection with associated hypotension and oliguria. Fever after exclusion of other causes remains the most important criteria for the diagnosis of postpartum endomyometritis.

## Investigation and management

Urgent and repeated blood cultures should be taken in systemically ill women. Swabs should be taken from the genital tract to identify the offending organism. Ultrasound may help in identifying retained products, which may be the source of infection.

Treatment should be started promptly without awaiting the results of cultures (Steer 2001). In view of the polymicrobial nature of these infections, broadspectrum intravenous antibiotics should be commenced. The commonly used antibiotics are gentamycin with either ampicillin or clindamycin. Extended spectrum penicillins or cephalosporins may be used. The regimen with the highest efficacy is one using clindamycin with gentamycin. Prompt resolution of the infection is the rule. Improvement will follow in nearly 90 per cent of women within 48–72 hours.

If retained products are present, evacuation should be performed after antibiotics have been given for 24 hours. Earlier intervention in the presence of active sepsis may trigger septicemia and should be avoided.

Intravenous antibiotics are usually continued until the patient has been afebrile for 24 hours.

> Intravenous antibiotics are usually continued until the patient has been afebrile for 24 hours

The role of oral maintenance therapy after intravenous antibiotics is controversial, although they are often prescribed for a minimum of seven days.

If there is lack of improvement, causes of refractory pelvic infection should be looked for. These include intense parametrial cellulitis, abscesses, infected hematomas and septic thrombophlebitis.

Septic shock should be treated aggressively in an intensive care facility, as these patients will require accurate fluid replacement, respiratory and circulatory support and possible hemodialysis in addition to antibiotics.

## Prevention

In patients with spontaneous rupture of membranes, vaginal examinations should be avoided or kept to a minimum using appropriate aseptic precautions.

There is clear evidence that prophylactic antibiotics for cesarean section reduce the incidence of puerperal infection. This should form part of the protocol for patients undergoing emergency cesarean sections (Thompson 2001). Avoiding manual removal of placenta at cesarean section will also decrease the incidence of postpartum infection (Magann et al 1995).

## Deep Vein Thrombosis (DVT) and Thromboembolism

Pregnancy and the puerperium are one of the highest risks for otherwise healthy women to develop DVT and pulmonary embolism. The puerperium is the most hypercoagulable time of pregnancy. The puerperal conditions of trauma, stasis and hypercoagulability predispose to the development of DVT. Compared to non-pregnant women, pregnant women have a two and a half times increased risk of a thrombotic event. The risk increases 20-fold in the puerperium (Bonnar 2001).

Since 1985, pulmonary thromboembolism has been the one of the most important causes of direct maternal death in the United Kingdom (Drife 2001). The incidence of fatal pulmonary embolism is seven to eight times higher in the puerperium than in pregnancy. While pulmonary embolism can occur without warning, most women have clearly identifiable risk factors. As the puerperal period is the time of greatest risk of thrombosis, postpartum thromboprophylaxis for women deemed to be at significant risk can reduce the incidence of thrombosis and embolism.

## Incidence

The exact incidence of non-fatal thrombosis is not known. It is estimated to be between 0.05 per cent and 1.8 per cent. It is between 0.08 per cent and 1.2 per cent following vaginal delivery and 3.0 per cent following cesarean section (Greer 1996).

## Pathogenesis

Marked reduction in blood flow velocity had been documented in pregnancy and for six weeks following delivery. The reduction is more on the left side when compared to the right (Macklon and Greer 1997).

- Blood flow velocity decreases in pregnancy and the puerperium, more so on the left side
- 85 per cent of DVT in pregnancy occur in the left leg
- DVTs in pregnancy tend to involve the ileofemoral segment

This probably explains why 85 per cent of DVT in pregnancy occur in the left leg when compared to 55 per cent in the non-pregnant. In addition, the pressure of the pregnant uterus impedes venous return from the lower limbs with a greater effect on the left side due to the anatomical arrangements of the common iliac vessels.

In contrast with the non-pregnant, the majority of DVTs in pregnancy tend to involve the ileofemoral segment, which is more liable to embolise.

The hemostatic system undergoes major physiological changes in pregnancy. There is an increased concentration of coagulation factors I, VII, VIII, IX, X and XII and the von Willebrand factor (Greer 1997). Resistance to activated protein C and a marked reduction in protein S also contribute to the procoagulant features of pregnancy. Fibrinolytic activity in pregnancy is impaired due to the production of plasminogen activator inhibitor type 2 by the placenta. This rapidly returns to normal after delivery (Clark et al 1998).

## Predisposing Factors: Inherited and Acquired

Inherited factors include deficiencies of antithrombin, protein C and protein S and the presence of factor V Leiden, prothrombin gene variant, homozygosity for the thermolabile variant of methyl-tetrahydrofolate reductase (MTHFR) and the presence of lupus anticoagulant. Factor V Leiden is the most common inherited disorder and approximately five per cent of the Caucasian population carries this mutation.

Acquired risk factors which increase the risk of DVT include age above 35 years, obesity, parity greater than four, labour lasting more than 12 hours, gross varicose veins, current infection, preeclampsia, immobility prior to surgery, major current illness, emergency cesarean in labour and extensive abdominal or pelvic surgery (Drife 2001).

> Risk factors for DVT include:
> - age above 35 years
> - obesity
> - parity > four
> - labour lasting > 12 hours
> - gross varicose veins
> - preeclampsia
> - immobility prior to surgery
> - emergency cesarean in labour

## Clinical features

Clinical diagnosis of deep vein thrombosis is notoriously inaccurate. Less than half of all cases are identified clinically. However, when symptoms are present, these should be taken seriously and investigations done to confirm the diagnosis. Symptoms are usually unilateral and are more common on the left side. Physical signs like pyrexia, tenderness or induration of the calf muscles and edema help to identify patients who need urgent testing to confirm the diagnosis.

Any woman with signs and symptoms of DVT should have objective testing performed expeditiously to avoid the risks, inconvenience and costs of inappropriate anticoagulation. Real-time ultrasonography, using Duplex and colour Doppler ultrasound is currently the procedure of choice to confirm the diagnosis (RCOG 2007). This is non-invasive and has high sensitivity and specificity for the detection of proximal venous clots but is less accurate for the detection of calf vein thrombosis. Techniques like venography, MRI and CT scanning are not commonly used and are restricted to specific conditions where ultrasound findings are equivocal.

> Duplex and colour Doppler ultrasound is currently the procedure of choice to confirm the diagnosis f DVT

The clinical diagnosis of pulmonary thromboembolism (PTE) is similarly unreliable. About a third of cases are diagnosed clinically. Depending on the size of the embolus and the patient's condition, the symptoms vary considerably from silent emboli to sudden death. Common features include dyspnea, tachypnea, pleuritic chest pain, cough, hemoptysis, hypotension and tachycardia. In cases of massive embolism, air hunger, severe chest pain and sudden collapse may be encountered. Signs include the presence of cyanosis, rapid breathing, jugular vein distension and, in some cases, a friction rub.

> **Symptoms of pulmonary embolism include:**
> - dyspnea
> - tachypnea
> - pleuritic chest pain
> - cough
> - hemoptysis
> - hypotension
> - tachycardia

Assessment should include a chest radiograph, ECG and arterial blood gases. The chest x-ray may reveal the presence of consolidation, infiltration or an elevated hemidiaphragm on the affected side. The ECG changes include rhythm disturbances, ST and T wave changes. If there are changes on the x-ray suggestive of PE and Doppler ultrasound of the legs confirms a DVT, there is no need for further testing as treatment for DVT and PE is the same (anticoagulation). This would minimise the dose of radiation to the mother (RCOG 2007).

D-dimer estimation is a useful tool for detecting venous thromboembolism in non-pregnant populations. In pregnancy, the concentration of D-dimers is increased and this further increases in the puerperium, limiting the utility of this test and it is therefore not recommended (RCOG 2007)

In cases where the x-ray and ultrasound are inconclusive and there is a strong clinical suspicion of PE, further investigations should be undertaken. The ventilation/perfusion scan (V/Q scan) is usually the primary investigation in these cases. The scan may not, however, be able to give a conclusive result as other conditions like pneumonia also produce perfusion defects. Women who undergo V/Q scans should be advised not to breastfeed for 48 hours after the procedure as Technetium is excreted though breast milk.

Computed Tomography Pulmonary Angiography (CTPA) offers a definite method for diagnosis and is recommended in the non-pregnant state for massive PE. Radiation exposure to the fetus in CTPA is lower than that in a V/Q scan. However, CTPA involves more radiation exposure to the maternal breasts, increasing the long-term risk of breast cancer (RCOG 2007).

## Management

The mainstay of management in acute DVT and pulmonary embolism is full anticoagulation. This is either done with heparin or with low molecular weight heparin. Unlike the antenatal period, where warfarin is contraindicated, it can be safely used in the puerperium. Warfarin is usually commenced a few days after heparin and once the INR is in the therapeutic range, heparin can be discontinued. Warfarin is continued for three months in patients with DVT and for six months in patients with embolism.

> **Anticoagulation in DVT and PE:**
> - heparin or low molecular weight heparin
> - warfarin commenced a few days after heparin
> - heparin is discontinued once the INR is in the therapeutic range

In cases where the diagnosis is uncertain, it is safer to commence anticoagulation while awaiting confirmation by repeat testing. Therapeutic dose of heparin is loading dose of 5,000 IU intravenously followed by 15–25 units/kg/hour.

## Complications of the Puerperium

Low molecular weight heparins (LMWH) are now accepted as being more cost effective and efficacious than heparin and are the treatment of choice in the UK. When used for treatment, the drug is given twice daily by subcutaneous injection. The dose of LMWH is calculated depending on the woman's weight at booking or most recent weight (RCOG 2007).

In massive life-threatening PE, unfractionated heparin remains the treatment of choice in view of rapidity of action. These patients will require multidisciplinary specialist care in an intensive care setting.

> In massive life-threatening PE, unfractionated heparin is recommended due to rapidity of action

Neither heparin (unfractionated or LMWH) nor warfarin is a contraindication to breast feeding.

## Prevention

Women with antithrombin deficiency, previous venous thromboembolism (VTE) on anticoagulants, protein C deficiency, prothrombin mutation are homozygous for factor V Leiden and are at high risk of developing DVT in pregnancy and the puerperium. These women should be given prophylactic LMWH in the antenatal period with anticoagulation continuing into the puerperium.

> Women at high risk for DVT or PE should be given prophylactic LMWH in the antenatal period with anticoagulation continuing into the puerperium.

As most cases of DVT develop after cesarean section, careful consideration should be issued to the use of thromboprophylaxis after every case of cesarean section. A risk assessment of all women should be undertaken and appropriate prophylaxis instituted. These risk factors have been enumerated earlier. Women assessed to be at low risk (elective cesarean section with uncomplicated pregnancy) require only early mobilisation and hydration. Women at moderate risk should receive either mechanical methods of thromboprophylaxis or subcutaneous heparin. Women at high risk (three or more moderate risk factors or extensive abdominal/pelvic surgery) should receive LMWH prophylaxis, and in addition the use of leg stockings should be considered (Drife 2001).

The recommended prophylactic dose of heparin is 5,000–10,000 IU every 12 hours for seven days (with monitoring) or Enoxaparin 40 mg subcutaneously every 24 hours.

The widespread use of thromboprophylaxis has successfully reduced the number of fatal PE following cesarean section. In the last CEMD report, 71 per cent of postpartum deaths followed vaginal delivery (Drife 2001). This has led to recommendations concerning the use of thromboprophylaxis following vaginal delivery.

> Prophylactic dose:
> - Heparin 5,000–10,000 IU every 12 hours for 7 days
> - Enoxaparin 40 mg subcutaneously every 24 hours.

Regardless of their risk, immobilisation and dehydration of women in pregnancy, labour and delivery should be avoided. Women should be reassessed in labour for risk factors for thromboembolism. Age over 35 years and BMI >30 are important independent risk factors. In the presence of two or more risk factors, the clinician should consider the use of low molecular weight heparin (LMWH) for three to five days postpartum (RCOG 2009).

## Septic Pelvic Thrombophlebitis

### Incidence

The incidence is 1:3000 deliveries but is more common after cesarean section (Brown et al 1999).

### Pathogenesis

The bacterial infection that starts in the placental site or the uterine incision extends along the venous routes. The ovarian veins are commonly involved and, in a proportion of cases, the inferior vena cava.

### Clinical features

This usually presents about 4–8 days postpartum when the features of endometritis have resolved. These patients characteristically fail to respond to antibiotics and continue to have a swinging fever. They usually do not appear to be systemically ill. This has been termed as 'enigmatic fever' (Duff and Gibbs 1983). In patients with ovarian vein thrombophlebitis, pain is a significant feature. In some cases, a tender mass may be palpable just beyond the uterine cornu.

### Diagnosis and management

The diagnosis can be confirmed using CT scanning or MRI. Earlier, the 'heparin challenge test' was used to diagnose this condition. The administration of therapeutic doses of heparin was believed to lyse the clot and relieve the symptoms, thereby proving the diagnosis (Duff and Gibbs 1983).

Traditional management involves full anticoagulation until resolution of the symptoms. However, it has been suggested that the continued use of antibiotics may cure the condition without the need for anticoagulation (Brown et al 1999). A better approach may be the combined use of anticoagulation and antibiotics.

## Wound Infection

### Abdominal

The incidence of abdominal wound infection following cesarean section ranges from 3 to 15 per cent. When prophylactic antibiotics are used, the incidence is significantly reduced. Risk factors for wound infection include obesity, diabetes, corticosteroid therapy, immunosuppression, anemia, poor hemostasis and placement of open drains (Steer 2001).

Incisional abscesses usually cause fever after the fourth postoperative day. In many cases, this is preceded by uterine infection and there is persistent fever, despite antibiotic therapy. The wound is tender, erythematous and may be fluctuant. Treatment involves adequate drainage which may involve laying the incision open. Broadspectrum antibiotics should be used pending results of culture.

> Management of wound infection involves:
> - laying the incision open
> - broadspectrum antibiotics pending results of culture

### Perineal

Infection in the vagina and perineum are secondary to tears or episiotomy. They are associated with pain, discharge and swelling at the site of the infection. A common cause is delayed or improper suturing of a tear or episiotomy. The edges of the wound become indurated and red, the sutures often tearing through the tissues.

Treatment involves ensuring adequate drainage. This may entail removal of sutures to open the wound. Broadspectrum antibiotics are given to control infection. Secondary suturing of the perineum should only be attempted after infection has been controlled. Prior to suturing, the wound must be adequately debrided to remove the dead and necrotic tissue.

> Secondary suturing of the perineum should only be attempted after infection has been controlled.

## Disorders of the Breasts

### Breast Engorgement

This is a common occurrence and is a cause of postpartum pyrexia. This resolves spontaneously within a period of 24 hours. Treatment consists of wearing a supporting brassiere and analgesia.

### Mastitis and breast abscess

Approximately two per cent of patients will develop mastitis (Marshall et al 1975) and 5–10 per cent of these will develop an abscess.

*Etiology*: *Staphylococcus aureus* and *Staphylococcus epidermidis* are the most commonly isolated pathogens.

> Mastitis is caused by organisms from the nose and throat of the infant entering the breast through small fissures at the time of nursing.

The source of these organisms is usually the nose and throat of the infant. The organisms enter the breast through small fissures at the time of nursing. Milk stasis is also an important cause of mastitis.

*Clinical features and diagnosis*: Symptoms usually occur a few weeks into the puerperium. These are almost always unilateral and engorgement precedes the inflammation. The symptoms include fever, chills and rigors, pain and malaise. The affected breast becomes hard and erythematous. The presence of fluctuation or incomplete resolution with antibiotics warrants ultrasound examination to exclude abscess formation. The expressed milk should be cultured to identify the organism.

*Management*: Appropriate antibiotic therapy usually causes prompt resolution of mastitis. A penicillinase-resistant antibiotic like dicloxacillin or eythromycin (for patients who are sensitive to penicillin) should be used (Hindle 1994). Provided abscess formation has not occurred, rapid response is noted within 48 hours. It is very important to continue breastfeeding. If the infected breast is too tender to allow suckling, it should be emptied by manual expression or with a pump. It may be helpful to start nursing on the uninvolved breast to allow milk let-down to commence before nursing on the affected side.

> Dicloxacillin or erythromycin are antibiotics of choice for mastitis.

In cases where an abscess has formed, it should be drained under a general anesthetic. Any loculi should be broken. Ultrasound-guided placement of a

> Ultrasound-guided aspiration or placement of a suction system may help avoid open surgery

suction system may help avoid open surgery (Karstrup et al 1993). In cases of abscess formation, breastfeeding is usually stopped.

*Suppression of lactation*: If the mother decides to bottle-feed or stop breastfeeding, non-pharmacological methods of suppression should be used. This consists of using a well-supporting brassiere, ice packs and analgesia.

Bromocriptine, a dopamine agonist has been used successfully for the suppression of lactation. However, following reports of cerebrovascular accidents after its use in puerperal women, the manufacturers have withdrawn its use for this indication (Rayburn 1996). Cabergoline (1 mg orally) may be used if pharmacological prevention is required. In women who are lactating, suppression is achieved by a dose of 250 µg every 12 hours for two days.

> Suppression of lactation: Cabergoline 250 µg every 12 hours for two days.

## Urinary Complications

### Urinary retention

Postpartum urinary retention is a common complication. Postpartum voiding dysfunction, defined as failure to pass urine spontaneously within six hours of vaginal delivery or catheter removal occurs in 0.7–4.0 per cent of deliveries (Kearney and Cutner, 2008). The use of intravenous fluids in labour, coupled with decreased bladder sensation can predispose to retention. If this is not recognised and treated promptly, it can cause prolonged voiding dysfunction with recurrent UTI and incontinence.

Predisposing factors include first vaginal delivery, epidural anesthesia, cesarean section, operative vaginal delivery, prolonged labour, lacerations and hematomas (Glazener and MacArthur 2001).

*Management*: Prevention involves careful monitoring after delivery to ensure that the bladder does not overfill and that it empties completely after voiding. If the patient has not voided within 4–6 hours and has a palpable bladder, significant periurethral injury should be excluded. If the woman is unable to void within six hours, either the bladder should be emptied by catheterisation or the bladder volume assessed by ultrasound followed by catheterisation if necessary.

In cases of overdistention, the bladder should be rested by the use of an indwelling catheter. This should be left in place for at least 24 hours. Following removal of the catheter, the patient should be encouraged to void. The presence of large residual volumes (>200 ml) would require a further period of catheterisation. In such cases, the catheter may be left in situ for two weeks to allow return of bladder sensation. Infection should be excluded and a short course of antibiotics may be required. Adequate analgesia is essential as perineal pain increases the risk of retention (Kearney and Cutner 2008).

> Postpartum urinary retention can occur with:
> - first vaginal delivery
> - epidural anesthesia
> - cesarean section
> - operative vaginal delivery
> - prolonged labour
> - lacerations and hematomas

> An indwelling catheter can be left in place for at least 24 hours and up to 2 weeks if necessary.

## Urinary incontinence

The prevalence of postnatal urinary incontinence is 2–34 per cent according to various reports. Risk factors include obesity, high parity, vaginal delivery (especially instrumental), prolonged labour and large infant size. Cesarean section appears to reduce the risk of incontinence, although it is not completely eliminated. Postpartum incontinence is poorly reported by women due to a variety of factors, including embarrassment (Glazener and MacArthur 2001). Conservative therapies in the form of pelvic floor exercises are often effective.

## Bowel Complications

### Acute Colonic Pseudo-Obstruction (ACPO)

Acute colonic pseudo-obstruction or Ogilvie's syndrome is an acute surgical condition characterised by massive dilatation of the colon in the absence of mechanical obstruction. If untreated, it can cause perforation of the cecum and fecal peritonitis with subsequent high mortality.

ACPO is usually seen in the very ill postoperative patient and in the older age group. In young and healthy women, cesarean section is the operation most commonly associated with this syndrome, although cases have been reported after vaginal and instrumental deliveries (Karkarla et al 2006).

The exact pathophysiology is poorly understood but is believed to be due to an imbalance between the sympathetic and parasympathetic outflow to the colon. This leads to an adynamic colon causing a functional or 'pseudo' obstruction. The cecum is the area most likely to be involved, as, due to its large diameter, it dilates more rapidly than the rest of the colon. If untreated, the cecum ruptures causing fecal peritonitis. The overall mortality is around 15 per cent, but rises to 35–50 per cent when the bowel is perforated or is ischemic (Karkarla et al 2006).

### Clinical features

The syndrome typically presents 2–12 days after cesarean section, with signs and symptoms of mechanical large bowel obstruction. Most women have abdominal pain in the forms of cramps, nausea and cessation of bowel movements. Rapid abdominal distension then follows. Vomiting is a late sign as is fever which often denotes the presence of sepsis or perforation. There is often elevated heart rate and white cell count in the absence of obvious sepsis. Bowel sounds vary according to the duration of symptoms. The woman becomes acutely ill with dehydration and oliguria. Tenderness in the right iliac fossa is often a sign of impending cecal rupture.

The diagnosis is made using a plain x-ray of the abdomen. This will reveal the large bowel dilatation. Mechanical obstruction can be excluded by a contrast enema in which the contrast will be seen to flow freely to the cecum.

### Management

Conservative treatment is recommended for cecal dilatation less than 10 cm. The woman is kept nil by mouth, the stomach decompressed by a nasogastric tube and the fluid and electrolyte imbalance corrected by intravenous fluids. Drugs that hinder bowel mobility (like opioids) should be discontinued. Careful monitoring of urine output and prophylaxis for DVT should be undertaken. The reported success rate for conservative treatment ranges 20–92 per cent and this can be tried for 24–48 hours before attempting pharmacological treatment (Karkarle et al 2006).

Pharmacological treatment involves the use of intravenous neostigmine, in addition to conservative measures. Neostigmine acts by restoring the normal autonomic balance by inhibiting acetylcholinesterase activity. It is given in a dose of 2.5 mg IV over 3–5 minutes. Immediate clinical response is defined as a reduction in abdominal distension following the passage of flatus within 30 minutes of injection. X-rays should be taken at three hours to look for sustained response, indicated by reduction in cecal diameter. As neostigmine has significant muscarinic side effects, such treatment should only be carried out with careful cardiovascular monitoring and atropine available as an antidote.

In cases where there is no response to pharmacological intervention, colonoscopic decompression should be attempted to relieve the pressure in the bowel. This procedure has a success rate of 61–78 per cent, although it can be difficult due to the unprepared bowel. In suspected perforation and sepsis, the surgical approach involves a laparotomy. This often requires bowel resection with creation of a stoma.

The management of these patients requires multidisciplinary care ensuring that adequate support and counselling is available for the patient and her family.

## Fecal Incontinence

This is a debilitating problem that affects a significant proportion of women following childbirth. Its prevalence, including fecal urgency and soiling, has been estimated at 3–5 per cent (Fynes and O'Herlihy 2001). Ultrasound imaging of the anal sphincter has, however, revealed a large proportion of occult defects (35–44 per cent) (Glazener and MacArthur 2001).

> Fecal incontinence can be caused by:
> - obstetric trauma
> - maternal age >30 years
> - prolonged second stage
> - instrumental delivery
> - multiparity
> - fetal macrosomia
> - clinically apparent anal sphincter injury at delivery

There is substantial under-reporting of symptoms to health professionals, contributing to a previous lack of recognition of this condition as a major cause of postnatal morbidity.

Obstetric trauma is the most important causative factor. Increasing maternal age (>30 years), prolonged second stage, instrumental delivery, multiparity, fetal macrosomia and clinically apparent anal sphincter injury at delivery are the main risk factors. Fecal incontinence may occur due to disruption of the anal sphincter complex or by damage to the pudendal nerve.

Incontinence symptoms are often transient after the first vaginal delivery, but subsequent vaginal delivery may be associated with worsening of symptoms.

Prevention should be directed towards reducing the risk factors predisposing to anal sphincter injury, improving the recognition and management of acute anal sphincter tears and better postnatal surveillance.

Treatment consists of measures to improve fecal continence and advice concerning future deliveries. Biofeedback and pelvic floor exercises may be effective, with surgery reserved for the intractable cases. Elective cesarean section should be considered in women with persistent symptoms or large asymptomatic external anal sphincter defects (Fynes and O'Herlihy 2001).

## Sexual Difficulties

There is no definite time after delivery when coitus should be resumed. Reasons frequently cited for not resuming intercourse include concerns regarding perineal pain, bleeding, fatigue and depression (Glazener 1997). Unrealistic expectations regarding the time of resumption of intercourse may further aggravate the problem. After two weeks, coitus may be resumed at any time depending on the patient's desire and comfort.

A temporary decline in sexual interest is common in the postpartum period secondary to the physical and emotional changes. Dyspareunia following childbirth can be due to physical or psychological reasons, or a combination of both.

Physical causes include scar tissue formation or poor anatomical reconstruction following perineal trauma. Vaginal dryness is a very common cause for dyspareunia in the postpartum period, particularly in women who are breastfeeding. Increased prolactin levels decrease the maternal estrogen, progesterone and androgens levels, leading to a reduction in libido and lack of vaginal lubrication.

Psychological dyspareunia can occur secondary to a difficult birth and may be associated with anxiety and depression.

It is estimated that 17–23 per cent of women experience dyspareunia at three months following birth and 10–14 per cent at 12 months. The incidence of dyspareunia is associated with the type of delivery and extent of perineal trauma. While it may be expected that cesarean section may protect against such an outcome, there is no evidence to support this. In fact, the incidence of dyspareunia is higher after cesarean section compared to spontaneous delivery with an intact perineum (Kettle et al 2005).

Management should be directed towards treating the underlying cause. It is important to intervene early in order to prevent the development of complex sexual dysfunction. In cases of decreased libido, reassurance that this may be a normal phenomenon in the postpartum period may be all that is required. Vaginal dryness can be relieved by the use of water-based lubricants prior to intercourse. There is very little evidence regarding the use of topical estrogens in postnatal women (Kettle et al 2005).

Scar tissue at the introitus is a common cause of superficial dyspareunia. The scar tissue may be softened by massaging it with oil, prior to attempting surgical correction. Surgical correction is performed by a modified Fenton's operation.

## Psychiatric Disorders

Psychiatric illnesses contribute significantly to maternal morbidity and mortality. All sorts of psychiatric disorders can complicate the postpartum period, arising either de novo or as a relapse or a pre-existing condition. The first 90 days of the postpartum period are associated with an elevated risk of psychosis and severe depressive illness (Oates 2008a).

Psychiatric disorders are known to have caused or contributed to 12 per cent of maternal deaths in the period covered by the last Confidential Enquiry into Maternal Deaths in the United Kingdom. It is likely that mental illness is the leading cause of maternal mortality in the UK. Women who have had a past episode of severe mental illness following delivery have a one in two to one in three chance of recurrence (Oates 2001). It is therefore important that an adequate support structure to help these women is in place. Healthcare professionals should actively attempt to identify women at high risk of the development of these problems during the antenatal period.

All women with illness of varying severities and those that are not ill but experiencing the common episodes of distress and adjustment need good psychological support. This has to be based on an understanding of the normal emotional and cognitive changes that happen in pregnancy and the puerperium (Oates 2008b).

## Postnatal Blues

The postpartum period is a time of psychological vulnerability. A majority (50–80 per cent) of women will experience 'postnatal blues'. This occurs in the first postpartum week, around the fifth day. Core symptoms include insomnia, weepiness, depression, anxiety, poor concentration and fatigue. In some cases, there is a period of unnaturally elevated mood, accompanied by irritability, known as 'the highs'. This affective lability is a characteristic feature of this condition. Symptoms are mild and transient, lasting around 48 hours. This may, however, recur over the next 6–8 weeks,

> 'Postnatal blues' may be associated with:
> - insomnia
> - weepiness
> - depression
> - anxiety
> - poor concentration
> - fatigue

particularly when the mother is very tired (Oates 2008a).

Treatment consists of reassurance and emotional support (Liddle and Oates 2002). Those caring for women who have recently delivered must be able to distinguish between the common symptoms seen in new mothers and those that suggest a more severe illness (Oates 2008a).

## Postpartum Depression

This occurs in 13 per cent of women, making it one of the most common complications of childbirth (Wisner et al 2002). Depression usually develops within two to three months of delivery. Depression following childbirth has the same range of severity and subtypes as non-postnatal depression (Oates 2008a).

### Predisposing factors

It is likely to result from interactions between genetic, neuroendocrine and psychological factors. A previous history of depressive illness or family history of severe unipolar depression predisposes to this condition (Oates 2008a).

Risk factors for the development of postnatal depression can usually be identified during prenatal care. These include previous history of depression, ambivalence about the pregnancy, unemployment, poor social or partner support and stressful life events. There is also evidence to suggest that emergency delivery may precipitate this condition. In the months following childbirth, the mother experiences not only the physically exhausting demands of caring for a young baby, but is also vulnerable to negative self-evaluation. This may occur due to the discrepancy between the expectations of motherhood and the realities of coping with a newborn (Liddle and Oates 2002).

It was previously thought that postnatal depression was related to progesterone deficiency, and progesterone was frequently used to prevent or treat the condition. There is, however, no evidence that the levels of progesterone are lower in women with postnatal depression, and progesterone is not efficacious in treating the condition. In fact, progesterone may actually aggravate the condition and it should therefore not be used (Oates 2008a).

## Clinical features

Onset tends to be gradual and usually does not manifest itself until 4–6 weeks after birth. These include depressed or anxious moods, irritability, anhedonia, guilty or pessimistic preoccupations, poor appetite, disturbed sleep, psychomotor agitation and fatigue. Features specific to postpartum depression include preoccupation with inadequacy as a mother, undue anxiety about the infant and, in severe cases, hopelessness about the future of the infant. In extreme cases, this may lead to suicide or infanticide.

> Features specific to postpartum depression include:
> - preoccupation with inadequacy as a mother
> - undue anxiety about the infant and,
> - in severe cases, hopelessness about the future of the infant.

## Prognosis

The illness usually persists for several months and often for more than a year, especially if untreated. There is evidence for adverse effects on the baby and on the relationship with the partner. Mothers show evidence of less social interaction with the children and the child may show delayed development (Stein et al 1991). These patients have a significant risk of recurrence in a subsequent pregnancy (50–70 per cent).

## Management

The condition needs to be quickly identified and treated by a specialist perinatal mental health team. The value of early contact with professionals who can recognise and validate the symptoms and distress and offer hope for the future cannot be underestimated (Oates 2008a). The optimum balance between social, psychological and pharmacological management depends on individual patients. Hospitalisation may be required for observation and treatment. These patients should be cared for in special 'mother and baby' units. This allows the mother to gain confidence in her ability to care for her child and provides valuable support (Liddle and Oates 2002).

There have been no adequate trials to determine the best drug for the treatment of this condition. Treatment with tricyclic antidepressants produces substantial improvement in 70 per cent of cases. These drugs are excreted in breast milk and should be used at the lowest effective dose (Wisner et al 2002).

> Treatment with tricyclic antidepressants produces substantial improvement in 70 per cent of cases.

The role of estrogen and progesterone in the management of postpartum depression is controversial. Due to the supposed hormonal etiology behind this condition, there has been considerable interest in the use of these drugs. Progesterone does not seem to be effective but estrogens may be more effective. However, presently their use remains experimental.

## Puerperal psychosis

This has an incidence of 1 in 500 deliveries (Kendall et al 1987).

### Predisposing factors

Women with pre-existing psychotic illness are at highest risk, with bipolar and schizophrenia being strongly associated (Kumar et al 1993).

Approximately, a quarter of women who have had puerperal psychosis will have a recurrence in a subsequent pregnancy.

### Clinical features

Fifty per cent develop within the first week after birth, 75 per cent in the first 6 weeks and 90 per cent within 90 days (Oates 2008a).

In most cases, the first few days are characterised by an acute undifferentiated psychosis with confusion and disturbance. Thereafter, the clinical features are of manic-depressive illness. There is a marked disturbance of mood ranging from profound depression to elation or irritability. This is often associated with delusions and hallucinations. These may include delusions that the baby is dead or defective and suspicions regarding the motives of family and professionals. Attention is seriously impaired. Sleep is disturbed and the patient often paces about in an agitated manner. Risk of suicide or infanticide, although low, should be considered (Liddle and Oates 2002).

Puerperal psychosis typically undergoes rapid deterioration. The woman does not sleep, eat or drink and neglects her self-care. The illness gradually becomes more recognisable as a variant of bipolar illness (Oates 2008a).

### Management

These patients should be admitted to a specialist mother and baby unit. Close supervision and support is essential as the patient's ability to care for herself and her baby is severely limited. Treatment with chlorpromazine or haloperidol forms the mainstay of treatment. Electroconvulsive therapy (ECT) is likely to provide the most certain and safe resolution of symptoms and should be considered in refractory cases.

### Prognosis

About 95 per cent will improve within two to three months of treatment.

However, the risk of recurrence may be as high as 50 per cent in a subsequent pregnancy.

About 50 per cent of women who have an episode of puerperal psychosis have a further episode of serious mental illness at some point. The older the woman is when she had her first postpartum episode, the less likely she is to have another non-postpartum illness (Oates 2008a).

## CEMD recommendations for the management of mental illness

Protocols for the management of women at risk should be in place in each hospital providing maternity care. Systematic and sensitive enquiries regarding psychiatric history should be done routinely during the antenatal period. Women with a significant history should be assessed by a psychiatrist during the antenatal period to formulate a plan of care and counselled regarding the risk of recurrence during pregnancy and following childbirth.

A specialist team should be available to care for these women. Women who require admission following childbirth for psychiatric illness, should be admitted to a special mother and baby unit along with their infant. If necessary, they should be transferred to such a unit, if facilities are not available locally (Oates 2001).

## References

Bonnar J. 2001. Venous thrombosis and pulmonary embolism. In *Turnbull's Obstetrics*, ed G Chamberlain, PJ Steer, 671–80. Churchill Livingstone: London.

Brown CE, RW Stettler, D Twickler, FG Cunningham. 1999. Puerperal septic pelvic thrombophlebitis: Incidence and response to Heparin therapy. *Am J Obstet Gynecol* 181(1):143–48.

Clark P, J Brennand, JA Conkie et al. 1998. Activated protein C sensitivity, protein C, protein S and coagulation in normal pregnancy. *Thromb Haemost* 79:1166–70.

Dewhurst CJ. 1966. Secondary postpartum hemorrhage. *J Obstet Gynaecol Br C'wlth* 73:53–58.

Drife J. 2001. Thrombosis and thromboembolism. In Why Mothers Die 1997–1999. *Confidential Enquiries into Maternal Death in the United Kingdom*, 49–75. RCOG Press: London.

Duff P, RS Gibbs. 1983. Pelvic vein thrombophlebitis: diagnostic dilemma and therapeutic challenge. *Obstet Gynaecol Surv* 38:365–73.

Fynes M, C O'Herlihy. 2001. The influence of mode of delivery on anal sphincter injury and faecal continence. *Obstet Gynaecol* 3:120–25.

Glazener CMA, C MacArthur. 2001. Postnatal morbidity. *Obstet Gynaecol* 3(4):179–88.

Glazener CMA. 1997. Sexual function after childbirth: Women's experiences, persistent morbidity and lack of professional recognition. *Br J Obstet Gynaecol* 104:330–35.

Greer IA. 1996. Special case of venous thromboembolism in pregnancy. In *A textbook of vascular medicine*, ed JE Tooke, GDO Lowe, 538–61. Edward Arnold: London.

Greer IA. 1997. Epidemiology, risk factors and prophylaxis of venous thromboembolism in Obstetrics and Gynaecology. *Balliere's Clin Obstet Gynaecol* 11:403–30.

Hindle WH. 1994. Other benign breast problems. *Clin Obstet Gynecol* 37(4):916–24.

Ismail MA, AE Chandler, MO Beem, AH Moawad. 1985. Chlamydial colonisation of the cervix in pregnant adolescents. *J Reprod Med* 30(7):549–53.

Karkarla A, Posnett H, Jan A, George M, Ash A. 2006. Acute colonic pseudo-obstruction after caesarean section. *The Obstetrician and Gynaecologist* 8:207–13.

Karstrup S, J Solvig, CP Nolsoe, P Nilsson, S Khattar, 1993. Acute puerperal breast abscesses: US guided drainage. *Radiology* 188:807–09.

Kearney R, Cutner A. 2008. Postpartum voiding dysfunction. *The Obstetrician and Gynaecologist* 10:71–74.

Kendall RE, JC Chalmers, C Platz. 1987. Epidemiology of puerperal psychosis. *Br J Psychiatry* 150:662–73.

Kettle C, Ismail K, O'Mahony. 2005. Dyspareunia following childbirth. *The Obstetrician and Gynaecologist* 7:245-49.

King PA, SJ Duthie, ZG Dong, HK Ma. 1989. Secondary postpartum hemorrhage. *Aust NZ J Obstet Gynaecol* 29:394–98.

Kumar R, M Marks, A Wieck, D Hirst, I Campbell, S Ceckley. 1993. Neuroendocrine and psychosocial mechanisms in postpartum psychosis. *Prog Neuropsychopharmacol Biol Psychiatry* 17(4):571–79.

Liddle PF, MR Oates. 2002. Psychiatry in pregnancy. In *Medical disorders in obstetric practice*, ed M de Sweit, 578–91. Blackwell Science: London.

Macklon NS, IA Greer. 1997. The deep venous system in the puerperium: An ultrasound study. *Br J Obstet Gynaecol* 104:198–200.

Magann EF, JF Washburne, RL Harris, JD Bass, WP Duff, JC Morison. 1995. Infectious morbidity, operative blood loss and length of operative procedure after Caesarean section by method of placental removal and site of uterine repair. *J Am Coll Surg* 181:517–20.

Marshall BK, JK Hepper, CC Zirbel. 1975. Sporadic puerperal mastitis: An infection that need not disrupt lactation. *J Am Med Assoc* 233:1377–79.

Mawhinney S, Holman R. 2007. Puerperal genital haematoma: a commonly missed diagnosis. *The Obstetrician and Gynaecologist* 9:195–200.

Oates M. 2001. Deaths from Psychiatric causes. In *Why Mothers Die 1997–1999. Confidential Enquiries into Maternal Death in the United Kingdom*, 165–87. RCOG Press: London.

Oates M. 2008a. Postnatal affective disorders. Part 1: an introduction. *The Obstetrician and Gynaecologist* 10:145–50

Oates M. 2008b. Postnatal affective disorders. Part 2: prevention and management. *The Obstetrician and Gynaecologist* 10:231–35

Park EH, BP Sachs. 1999. Puerperal problems. In *High risk pregnancy management options*, ed DK James, PJ Steer, CP Weiner, B Gonik, 1269–80. WB Saunders: London.

Rayburn WF. 1996. Clinical commentary: the bromocriptine (Parlodel) controversy and recommendations for lactation suppression. *Am J Perinatol* 13:69–71.

Royal College of Obstetricians and Gynaecologists. 2007. Thromboembolic disease in pregnancy and the puerperium: Acute management. *Guideline No 28*. RCOG Press: London.

Royal College of Obstetricians and Gynaecologists. 2009. Thromboprophylaxis during pregnancy, labour and after vaginal delivery. *Guideline No 37*. RCOG Press: London.

Royal College of Obstetricians and Gynaecologists. 2009. Prevention and management of postpartum haemorrhage. *Guideline No 52*. RCOG Press: London.

Steer PJ. 2001. Puerperal sepsis. In *Turnbull's Obstetrics*, ed G Chamberlain, PJ Steer (eds), 663–70. Churchill Livingstone: London.

Sweet RL, WJ Ledger. 1973. Puerperal infectious morbidity: A two year review. *Am J Obstet Gynaecol* 117:1093–1100.

Stein A, DH Gath, J Bucher, A Bond, A Day, PJ Cooper. 1991. The relationship between postnatal depression and mother–child interaction. *Br J Psychiatry* 158:46–52.

Thompson W. 2001. Genital tract sepsis. In *Why mothers die 1997–1999. Confidential Enquiries into Maternal Death in the United Kingdom*. RCOG Press: London.

Wisner KL, BL Parry, CM Piontek. 2002. Postpartum depression. *N Engl J Med* 347:194–99.

# INDEX

Abnormal labour patterns 431
Abdominal examination 34, 221
Abdominal palpation 34, 115, 158
Actin 4, 113
Acute colonic pseudo-infection (ACPO) 507–508
Adenosine triphosphate (ATP) 4
Adnexal masses 261
Adrenergic stimulation 11
Air embolism 326
Amnioinfusion 131
Amniotic fluid embolism 326
Amniotic fluid estimation 426
Amniotic fluid index 469
Amniotic fluid leakage 398
Amniotomy 376, 434
Analgesia 37
    inhalational 37
    local 37
    systemic 37
Anaphylactoid reactions 331
Anaphylaxis 331
Anencephaly 215
Anesthesia 37
    epidural 38
    lumbar epidural 38
Aneurysm 324
Antenatal corticosteroid therapy 393

Antepartum cardiotocography (CTG) 426
Antepartum hemorrhage (APH) 277
Antihypertensive therapy 471
Aortic dissection 333
Apgar score 420, 426
Arachidonic acid 14
Arrest disorders 434–435
Arteriovenous malformations 324
Artificial rupture of membranes (ARM) 46
Atonic PPH 305
Atosiban 413
Augmentation of labour 41
    duration of 48
    in the active phase 45
    in the latent phase 45
    in special circumstances 49
        breech 50
        malposition 51
        multiparas 49
        previous cesarean section 49
Autonomic nervous system 11

Bacterial vaginosis 405
Bandl's ring 438
Barnum maneouvre 199

Beta sympathomimetic drugs 412
Betamethasone 414
Birth asphyxia 218
Birth defects 406
Birth injuries 218
Bishop's score 359, 382
Bleeding, indeterminate origin 286
B-Lynch suture 311
Breast abscess 505, 506
Breast engorgement 505
Breech presentation 215–217
    diagnosis 221
    delivery of shoulders 220
    complications 218
    delivery 220
    delivery by forceps 232
    delivery of head 220
    incidence 215
    maternal complications 217
    perinatal morbidity and mortality 217
    risk factors 215
        fetal factors 215
        maternal factors 215
Burn's Marshall technique 232

Calcium channel blockers 412–413

Calder's modified Bishop's score 382
Carboprost 294, 306
Cardiac disease 334
Cardiomyopathy 333
Cardio-pulmonary resuscitation 337
Cardiotocograph (CTG) 85
    accelerations 91
    baseline heart rate 90
    baseline variability 90
    decelerations 91
    definitions 90
    interpretation 90, 94
Cardiotocography 469
Caudal block 37
Central venous pressure (CVP) 148
Cerebral venous thrombosis 337
Cervical cerclage 397
Cervical dilatation 31
Cervical incompetence 404
Cervical length, assessment of 408
Cervical ripening 14
Cervical scoring 382
Cervix 2
Cesarean delivery 248–262
    types of incision 253
        Cherney incision 254
        Joel-Cohen incision 253
        Maylard incision 253
        Pfannensteil incision 253
    opening the abdomen 252
    abdominal irrigation 259
    closure of peritoneum 259
    delivering deeply impacted head 257
    delivering the fetus 256
    delivering the placenta 257
    incidental surgery 261
    inspection of adnexae 259
    opening the peritoneum 254
    prophylactic antibiotics 260
    postoperative care 261
    procedure and technique 248

raising the bladder flap 254
rectus muscles 259
skin incision 252
subcutaneous tissue closure 260
technique 252
    pre-operative care 252
uterine incision 254
    transverse incision 255
    vertical incision 256
uterine wound closure 258
    double layer 259
    single layer 258
wound dressing 260
Cesarean section on demand 250
Cesarean section rate 237
    information collection 237
    emergency or intrapartum 251
    10-group classification 238
    classification 238
    indications for 250
    reducing the rate of 245
    rising rates of 248
    instrumental delivery at 256
Cho's square suture 312
Cholinergic system 12
Chromosomal abnormalities 215
Clavicular fracture 194
Clamping the cord 294
Combined Rubin's and Wood's maneouvre 198
Complete breech 216
Congenital anomalies 215
Connexins 3
Consent 77–84
    informed consent 78
    theoretical models 79
        functionalist model 80
        postmodern theories 80
Consenting women in labour 78
Continuous electronic fetal monitoring 87
Continuous suturing 212

Controlled cord traction 295
Cord accidents 218
Cord prolapse 129
Corticotrophin-releasing hormones (CRH) 10
Corticosteroids 1, 10, 393, 394, 396, 397, 398
Court-enforced cesarean sections 82
Cyclic adenosine monophosphate (cAMP) 3
Cytokines 20
Curve of Carus 176

Deep vein thrombosis (DVT) 500–504
Delivery of the fetus 134
Dexamethasone 414
Diabetes 144
    initial treatment 145
Diabetic ketoacidosis (DKA) 145
Diagnosis of labour 32
Dinoprostone 360
Drug overdose 337
Drug toxicity 332
Duhrssens' cervical incision 441
Dye test 390
Dyspnea 65, 335, 502
Dystocia 39, 251

Eclampsia 331, 465 (See also Preeclapsia)
    management 474–475
Elective cesarean delivery 192, 250
Elective induction 192
    advantages 370
    disadvantages 370
Electronic fetal monitoring (EFM) 85
Entrapment of the head 218
Epidural analgesia 160
Epidural, drugs used for 67
Episiotomy 161, 196, 205
    clinical approach 207

definition 205
epidemiology 205
etiology 206
mediolateral 208
methods of repair 209
midline 207
pathology 205
performing an 207
post-repair management 213
prognosis 206
repairing an 208
the role of 176
Ergometrine 291
Ergot alkaloids 291
Estrogen 1
External cephalic version 223
    contraindications 224
    procedure 224
    risks of 223
External vacuum generator 177
Extra-amniotic saline infusion (EASI) 376

Factor V Leiden 501
Factor VII A therapy 315
Failed induction 381
Failed instrumental delivery 181
Fecal incontinence 508–509
Ferguson's reflex 17
Fern test 389
Fetal asphyxia 126, 194
Fetal acidosis 88, 100, 153
Fetal blood sampling 98
Fetal distress 126, 251, 423
    causes 128
        cord compression 128
        labour dystocia 129
        maternal position 128
        sudden dramatic events 129
        uterine contractions 128
    management 127
        fetal reserve 127
    medicolegal implications 134
Fetal Doppler 426–427

Fetal ECG waveform analysis 101
    ST segment analysis 101
Fetal fibronectin 407
Fetal gender 191
Fetal heart rate (FHR) 31
Fetal heart rate (FHR) monitoring 85
Fetal hyperinsulinemia 190
Fetal macrosomia 349
Fetal membrane structure 387
    amnion 387
    chorion 387
    intermediate layer 387
Fetal monitoring 161
Fetal morbidity 182
    cephalhematoma 182
    forceps marks 182
    intracranial hemorrhage 183
    nerve injury 182
    ocular trauma 183
    subgaleal/subaponeurotic hemorrhage 183
Fetal movement counting 425–426
Fetal pulse oximetry (FPO) 103
Fetal weight 423
Fetus, legal standing of 81
Fibroids 261
First stage of labour 289–301
    acceleration phase 431
    active phase 431
    deceleration phase 431
Fluid management in labour 138
    hydration 139
    maternal ketonuria 140
    physiological considerations 138
Fluid–electrolyte balance 36, 138
Forceps delivery 175
Forceps 171
    non-rotational 171
        Naegle 171
        Neville-Barnes 171

        Piper's 171
        Wriggley's 171
    rotational 171
        Kielland's 171
        Tucker-McLane 171
Frank breech 216
Friedman's curve of labour 156, 158
Full cervical dilatation 154
Functional synctitium 1
Fundal height 34
Fundal pressure 165

Gap junctions 2
Gaskin's maneouvre 200
Genital tract, injuries to 314
Genital tract sepsis 328
Glycosaminoglycan 14, 15, 16
Goldenhar syndrome 492
Grand multigravida 437
Group B streptococcus 405
Gynecoid pelvis 152, 193

HELLP syndrome 315, 467, 468, 475–477
Hematoma 277, 304, 314, 315
    hepatic subcapsular 324
Hemolysis 468
Hemorrhagic shock 322
Hemorrhagic stroke 336
Herpes genetalis 398
HIV 398
Huntington's technique 326
Hyaluronidase 23
Hydralazine 472
Hydrocephalus 215
Hypertension 463–464
    chronic 464, 465
    gestational 464, 465
Hypertensive disorders 146
Hyperventilation 320
Hypoglycemia 335
Hypothermia 488, 491
Hysterectomy 313, 459

Iatrogenic prematurity 381
Incomplete (footling) breech 217
Inducing agent 369
Induction of labour 422
  contraindications 375
  indications 370
    medical 371
    non-medical 371
      post-term/prolonged labour 370
  non-pharmacological interventions 380
    sexual intercourse and breast stimulation 380
    uterine hyperstimulation 380
  pharmacological interventions 377
    mifepristone 379
    misoprostol 379
    oxytocin 378
    prostaglandins 377
Inflammatory mediators 22
Instrument types 170
Interleukins 22
Intermittent auscultation (IA) 85
Intermittent EFM 87
  admission cardiotocograph 87
Interpartum umbilical artery Doppler waveforms 105
Interrupted suturing 209
Intrapartum fetal distress 96, 126–135
  diagnosis 127
  management of 126
Intrapartum fetal scalp stimulation tests 98
Intrauterine fetal death 374
Intrauterine growth restriction 372
Intrauterine pressure catheters (IUPC) 116
Intravenous fluids 131
Ischemic stroke 336

Isolated oligohydramnios 373

Korotoff sounds 465

Labour progress, assessment 431–432
Labour, first stage 30
  active phase 31
  consent in 77
  diagnosis of 32
  false or spurious 32
  induction of 368
  latent phase 31
  management of first stage 34
    abdominal examination 34
    general examination 34
    investigations 35
    vaginal examination 35
  poor progress 38
    passages 40
    passenger 40
    poor practice 40
    powers 40
  spontaneous 30
  the third stage of 289
    active management 290
    expectant management 290
    physiological mechanisms 289
  induced and augmented 120
Large for gestation (LGA) 425
Lovset's maneouvre 230

Macrosomia 189, 373
Magnesium sulphate toxicity 475
Magnesium toxicity 331
Major postpartum hemorrhage 308
Mariceau-Smelli-Veit technique 232
Marfan syndrome 333
Mastitis 505
Maternal diabetes 190

Maternal hyponatremia 381
Maternal morbidity 183, 319
  lacerations 183
  perineal and cervical tears 183
  psychological trauma 183
  urinary and fecal incontinence 183
Maternal mortality 319
Maternal obesity 190
Maternal oxygen administration 132
Maternal position 130
Maternal position in labour 158
  clinical implications 159
  hands and knees 160
  hemodynamic implications 158
  lying on the side 159
  squatting 160
McGill pain rating index 57
McRoberts' manoeuvre 197
Meconium 38
Meconium aspiration 492
Mediolateral episiotomy 350
Membrane sweeping 375, 421–422
Mendelson's syndrome 36
Messenger RNA (mRNA) 3
Minor postpartum hemorrhage 308
Misoprostol 362
Mobility in labour 36
Modified Early Obstetric Warning Scoring (MEOWS) system 342
Monroe-Kerr incision 255
Moulding 42
Mueller–Hillis syndrome 433
Multiple gestation 273
Multiple pregnancy 406
Musculoskeletal morbidity 392
Myocardial infarction 335
Myomectomy 261
Myometrium 2
Mytonic dystrophy 215

Naloxone 65
Narcotics 64
Natural childbirth 45
Near infra-red spectroscopy (NIRS) 105
Neonatal hyperbilirubinemia 382
Neonatal indications 393
Neonatal resuscitation 486–493
　airway 488
　breathing 490
　circulation 490
　drugs 491
　equipment 487–488
　warmth 488
Neurological damage 392
Nifedipine 472, 473
Nitrazine text 389
Nomogram 31
　action line 32
　alert line 31
Non hemorrhagic shock 322
Normal labour 30
Normal labour curve 431
Nulliparity 349

O'Leary technique 311
Obstetric hemorrhage 444
Obstetric perineal trauma 349–353
　clinical approach 350
　definition 348
　epidemiology 348
　etiology 349
　first degree tears 348
　fourth degree tears
　management of 348
　pathology 349
　postoperative management 352
　prognosis 350
　repair 351
　　end-to-end repair technique 352
　　overlapping technique 352
　second degree tears 348
　third degree tears 348
Obstructed labour 436–441
　causes 437
　　cephalopelvic disproportion 437
　　fetal malformations 437
　　malpresentations 437
　　reproductive tract abnormalities 437
　consequences 439
　management 439–441
　　cesarean 440
　　destructive operations 440
　　instrumental vaginal delivery 440
　　symphysiotomy 440
　risks 437
Oliguria 148
Operational vaginal surgery 170
　classification 171
Operative vaginal delivery 191
Oral carbohydrate drinks 141
　carbohydrate solutions 141
　isotonic sports drinks 141
Oxytocics 5, 20, 291, 292
Oxytocin augmentation 433–434
Pain pathways 58
Pain relief in labour 56, 59
　first stage 58
　inhalational methods 65
　　entonox 65
　nonpharmocological methods 60
　　acupuncture 61
　　continuous labour support 60
　　hypnosis 61
　　touch and massage 60
　　transcutaneous nerve stimulation (TENS) 61
　　vertical maternal positioning 60
　parenteral agents 62
　　butorphanol 64
　　fentanyl 63
　　morphine 63
　　opioid anatagonists 65
　　pethidine 62
　　remiphentanil 64
　　systemic opioids 62
　　tramadol 64
　second stage 58
Pain scores 57
Partogram 39, 272, 431, 432, 439
　active line 431
　alert line 431
Patwardhan technique 257
Pelvic brim 35
Pelvic floor 164
Pelvimetry 51
Peptide hormones 5
Perinatal mortality 249
Perineal infiltration 37
Perineal tears 163
Perineum, care of 163
Peripartum hysterectomy 445–451
　complications 449
　definition 445
　indications 445, 446
　technique 447–449
Pierre-Robin sequence 492
Piracetam 133
Placenta accrete 285, 299
Placenta and membranes, examination of 296
Placenta previa 280
　classification 280
　clinical presentation and diagnosis 282
　etiology and associated factors 282
　management 283
Placental abruption 129, 277, 391
　clinical presentation 278
　incidence 277

management 279
mild (Grade 1) 279
moderate (Grade 2) 279
pathology and etiology 277
severe (Grade 3) 279
Placentation, abnormalities of 304
Planned elective repeat cesarean section (ERCS) 267
Poisoning 337
Positive end respiratory pressure (PEEP) 490
Post-maturity 420
Postpartum care 480
Postpartum collapse 319
    causes 320
    clinical presentation 320
    hemorrhagic causes 323
        PPH 323
        uterine rupture 323
    management 337
        antenatal care 343
        risk factor assessment 343
    non-hemorrhagic causes 325
        uterine inversion 325
Postpartum collapse, training issues 343
Post-term pregnancy, incidence 420
Post-term pregnancy, risks 421
Posture in labour 36
Potter syndrome 215
Postpartum hemorrhage (PPH), 30, 148, 381
    arresting the bleeding 309
        mechanical methods 309
        pharmacological measure 309
        tamponade test 309
    causes 304
    complications of third stage 298
    defects in coagulation 315
    definition 303

genital tract injuries 314
initial evaluation 305
management 303, 306
placenta accrete 313
prevention 306
resuscitation 307
retained placenta 313
risk factors 305
uterine inversion 314
Preterm prelabour rupture of membranes (PPROM) 374, 387–399
    antibiotic prophylaxis 395
    timing of delivery 395
    use of tocolytics 394
PR interval 102
Prague manoeuvre 234
Preeclampsia 146 (see also Eclampsia; Hypertension in pregnancy; Pregnancy induced hypertension)
    evaluation 467–470
        fetal 469
    fluid management 148, 480
    monitoring 467
    risk factors 466
Pregnancy after surgical repair of rupture 460
Preinduction cervical ripening 375
    membrane sweeping 375
Prelabour 32
Prelabour rupture of membranes (PROM) 387, 374
    clinical risk factors 388
    incidence 387
    terminology 387
Prematurity 215
Preterm birth rates 403
Preterm breech 219
    mode of delivery 225
Preterm infants 491–492
Preterm labour 273, 402–416
    definition 402–403
    delivery 414–416
    diagnosis 409

    management 411–414
        tocolytics 412–413
    mode of delivery 415–416
    prevention 409–411
        antibiotics 410
        cervical cerclage 409–411
        progesterone 410–411
    risk factors 403–406
        cervical insufficiency 404–405
        ethnic origin 404
        iatrogenic 403
        infection 405–406
        previous obstetric history 404
        social factors 404
Previous cesarean section 373
Previous scar 359
Primary apnea 487
Primary postpartum hemorrhage 304, 444
    thrombin 304
    tissue 304
    tone 304
    trauma 304
Progesterone block theory 17
Progesterones 1
Prolactin 9
Prolongation disorder, prolonged latent phase 432–433
Prolonged labour 429–436
    classification 432–436
    consequences 436
    etiology 429–430
        passage 429, 430
        passenger 429, 430
        power 429, 430
    incidence 429
    second stage abnormalities 435
Prolonged pregnancy 420–427
    pathophysiology 421
        amniotic fluid volume reduction 421

# Index

continued growth of baby 421
placental ageing 421
Prolonged second stage 191
Prostaglandins 12, 19, 293, 355
  distribution in normal tissues 357
  E series 355
  F series 355
  metabolism 356
  PPH and 363
  properties 357
  role in labour 357
    cervical ripening 358
    induction 359
    third stage 358
  structure and classification 356
Proteinuria 467, 469, 473
Protraction disorders 433–434
Psychiatric disorders 509–513
  postnatal blues 510
  postpartum depression 510–511
  puerperal psychosis 512
Pudendal block 37
Puerperal genital hematoma 495–496
Puerperal pyrexia 497–498
Puerperal sepsis 498–500
Puerperium, complications 495–513
Pulmonary embolism 330
Pulmonary hypoplasia 392
Pushing 154
  duration 155
  techniques 155
Pyridoxine 133

Regional analgesia 66
  complications and side effects 72
    accidental dural puncture 72
    backache 72
    bladder dysfunction 73

hypotension 72
labour in 66
neuraxial techniques 66
  combined spinal-epidural analgesia (CSEA) 66, 67
  continuous spinal analgesia 67
  epidural analgesia 66
  lumbar sympathetic block 66

Regional anesthesia 142
Relaxin 8
Renal function 468
Respiratory distress syndrome (RDS) 413
Restitution 195
Restrictive episiotomy 350
Resuscitation, neonatal 486–493
  stopping resuscitation 493
  structured approach 337
Retained placenta 298
Risk scoring 407
Rotational instrumental delivery 181
Rubin's maneouvre 198
Rupture uterus 453–460

Salivary estriol 407
Scarred uterus 455
Screening tests 407–408
Second stage of labour
  diagnosis 154
  management of 152
  mechanism 152
  phases 153
    active phase 153
    passive phase 153
Second stage partogram 164
Second stage, delayed descent 157
  maternal position 158
  oxytocin augmentation 158

Secondary postpartum hemorrhage 315, 444, 496–497
Seizures 474
Septic pelvic thrombophlebitis 504
Septic shock 329
Severe hypertension, control of 470
Severe preeclampsia 464–465
  diagnosis 466, 477
  management 470–473
Shoulder dystocia 182, 188
  complications 194
  definition 188
  diagnosis and management 195
  fetal complications 194
  incidence 189
  maternal complications 195
  mechanism in 193
  previous history of 190
  risk factors 189
Sinusoidal trace 94
Small for gestation (SGA) 423, 424–425
Splenic rupture 324
Spontaneous hepatic rupture 324
Spontaneous labour, mechanism of shoulder delivery 193
Stillbirth 422, 423
Sub-arachnoid hemorrhage 336
Subtotal hysterectomy 449
Suicide 337
Superimposed preeclampsia 465
Suprapubic pressure 199
Suture material 213
Syntometrine 293

Term Breech Trial 226
Term breech 226
  cesarean section for 227
  indications for 228
Terminal apnea 487

Third stage of labour 289–301
The PEOPLE (Pushing late or pushing early with epidural) Trial 154
Thrombocytopenia 468
Thromboembolism 501
Tocolysis 130
Trial of labour after previous cesarean delivery (TOLAC) 266
　analgesia 272
　continuous fetal monitoring 272
　contraindications 269
　intrapartum management 271
　maternal risks 267
　　failed TOLAC 267
　　uterine rupture 267
　risks to fetus/neonate 268
　selecting women for 269
Tom Thumb 489
Total hysterectomy 449
Training issues 184
Transcervical catheters 376
Turtle sign 195

Ultrasound 192
Ultrasound imaging 390
Umbilical cord prolapsed 381
Urinary incontinence 507
Urinary retention 506
Urokinase plasminogen activator receptor (UPAR) 23
Uterine activity 42, 47–49, 113, 114–122
　excessive uterine activity 119
　in the presence of cesarean section scar 121
　incoordinate 119
　medico-legal implications 121
　monitoring 121
　normal labour in 118

　quantification 114
Uterine anomalies 406
Uterine artery embolisation 312
Uterine atony 182
　surgical techniques 310
　　internal iliac artery ligation 310
　　uterine artery ligation 310
Uterine compression sutures 311
Uterine contractility 4
Uterine contractions 112
　measurement of 48
　methods of measurement 115
　　external tocography 116
　　importance 115
　　internal tocography 116
　　manual palpation 115
　　maternal perception 115
　parameters 113
　physiology 112
Uterine electromyography (EMG) 117
Uterine hemorrhage, prevention of 258
Uterine invasion 300
Uterine rupture 129, 373, 381
　complete uterine rupture 453
　diagnosis 457–458
　incomplete rupture 453
　management 457
　maternal and perinatal complications 459
　prevention 460–461
　risk factors 454
　　induction of labour in a scarred uterus 455
　　Mullerian anomalies 457
　　myomectomy 455
　　obstructed labour 456
　　previous cesarean section 454

　　previous repair 456
　　spontaneous rupture in pregnancy 457
　　trauma 456, 457
Uterine scar dehiscence 453
Uterine scar rupture 272
Uterotonics 291

Vacuum extraction 165, 174, 181, 191
Vaginal birth after cesarean section (VBAC) 49, 266
　advantages of 269
　antenatal counselling 271
　delivery 273
　factors influencing success 269
Vaginal breech delivery 228
　assisted breech delivery 229
　breech extraction 228
　spontaneous breech delivery 228
Vaginal drain 213
Valid consent 77
　adequate information provision 78
　capacity 77
　voluntariness 78
Vasa previa 129, 286
Vasoactive intestinal polypeptides (VIP) 9
Vasopressin 8
Vasovagal syncope 320
Ventouse delivery 174
Ventouse/vacuum extractor 170
von Willebrand's disease 316

Wood's corkscrew maneouvre 198
Wound infection 504–505

Zavanelli maneouvre 200